Core Textbook of
PEDIATRICS

Core Textbook of
PEDIATRICS

Robert Kaye, M.D.

Professor and Chairman
Department of Pediatrics
Hahnemann Medical College and Hospital
Philadelphia, Pennsylvania

Frank A. Oski, M.D.

Professor and Chairman
Department of Pediatrics
State University of New York
Upstate Medical Center
Syracuse, New York

Lewis A. Barness, M.D.

Professor and Chairman
Department of Pediatrics
University of South Florida
Tampa, Florida

With 23 Contributors

J. B. Lippincott Company
Philadelphia • Toronto

ISBN 0 397 52084 0

Library of Congress Catalog Card Number 78-18683

Printed in the United States of America

1   3   5   6   4   2

Library of Congress Cataloging in Publication Data

Main entry under title:

Core textbook of pediatrics.

  Bibliography: p.
  Includes index.
  1. Pediatrics. I. Kaye, Robert. II. Oski, Frank A. III. Barness, Lewis A.
RJ45.C78   618.9'2   78-18683
ISBN 0-397-52084-0

To:

Edwards A. Park, Joseph Stokes, Jr., Paul Gyorgy, Louis K. Diamond, and Charles A. Janeway, all Howland Awardees of the American Pediatric Society who have been our most significant teachers and sources of inspiration, and to the medical students who will become the pediatricians of the future.

ROBERT KAYE, M.D.
FRANK A. OSKI, M.D.
LEWIS A. BARNESS, M.D.

Contributors

David Baker, M.D.
Associate Professor of
  Pediatrics
Hahnemann Medical College
  and Hospital
Philadelphia, Pennsylvania

Lester Baker, M.D.
Professor of Pediatrics
University of Pennsylvania
  School of Medicine
Acting Director, Division of
  Endocrinology/Diabetes
Director, Clinical Research
  Center
Senior Physician,
The Children's Hospital of
  Philadelphia
Philadelphia, Pennsylvania

Lewis A. Barness, M.D.
Professor and Chairman
Department of Pediatrics
University of South Florida
Tampa, Florida

Herman S. Belmont, M.D.
Professor and Deputy
  Chairman for Child and
  Adolescent Mental Health
  Sciences
Hahnemann Medical College
  and Hospital
Philadelphia, Pennsylvania

Peter H. Berman, M.D.
Associate Professor of
  Neurology and Pediatrics
University of Pennsylvania
  School of Medicine
Director, Division of
  Neurology
The Children's Hospital of
  Philadelphia
Philadelphia, Pennsylvania

John S. Curran, M.D.
Associate Professor of
  Pediatrics
University of South Florida
Tampa, Florida

Eliot H. Dunsky, M.D.
Assistant Professor of
  Pediatrics
Director, Section of Allergy
  and Immunology
Hahnemann Medical College
  and Hospital
Philadelphia, Pennsylvania

Sidney Friedman, M.D.
Professor of Pediatrics
University of Pennsylvania
  School of Medicine
Chief Cardiologist
The Children's Hospital of
  Philadelphia
Philadelphia, Pennsylvania

Ian S. E. Gibbons, M.D.
Associate Professor of
   Pediatrics and Medicine
Chief, Division of Pediatric
   and Adolescent
   Gastroenterology
Hahnemann Medical College
   and Hospital
Philadelphia, Pennsylvania

James A. Hallock, M.D.
Associate Professor of
   Pediatrics
University of South Florida
Tampa, Florida

Douglas S. Holsclaw, M.D.
Associate Professor of
   Pediatrics
Director, Cystic Fibrosis and
   Pediatric Pulmonary
   Centers
Hahnemann Medical College
   and Hospital
Philadelphia, Pennsylvania

J. Martin Kaplan, M.D.
Associate Professor of
   Pediatrics
Hahnemann Medical College
   and Hospital
Philadelphia, Pennsylvania

Robert Kaye, M.D.
Professor and Chairman
Department of Pediatrics
Hahnemann Medical College
   and Hospital
Philadelphia, Pennsylvania

John I. Malone, M.D.
Associate Professor of
   Pediatrics
University of South Florida
Tampa, Florida

William J. Mellman, M.D.
Professor and Chairman
Department of Human
   Genetics
University of Pennsylvania
   School of Medicine
Chief, Division of Genetics
The Children's Hospital of
   Philadelphia
Philadelphia, Pennsylvania

Michael A. Mitchell, M.D.
Assistant Professor of
   Pediatrics and Neurology
Hahnemann Medical College
   and Hospital
Philadelphia, Pennsylvania

Hugh L. Moffet, M.D.
Professor of Pediatrics
University of Wisconsin -
   Madison
Madison, Wisconsin

Frank A. Oski, M.D.
Professor and Chairman
Department of Pediatrics
State University of New York
Upstate Medical Center
Syracuse, New York

Edward O. Reiter, M.D.
Associate Professor of
   Pediatrics
University of South Florida
Tampa, Florida;
Assistant Director of
   University Service
All Children's Hospital
St. Petersburg, Florida

Allen W. Root, M.D.
Professor of Pediatrics
University of South Florida
Tampa, Florida;
Director of University
   Service
All Children's Hospital
St. Petersburg, Florida

Thomas F. McNair Scott, M.D.
Professor of Pediatrics
Director, Pediatric
   Ambulatory Clinic
Hahnemann Medical College
   and Hospital
Philadelphia, Pennsylvania

Charles A. Stanley, M.D.
Associate Professor of
   Pediatrics,
University of Pennsylvania
   School of Medicine
Staff Physician
The Children's Hospital of
   Philadelphia
Philadelphia, Pennsylvania

Peter W. Vanace, M.D.
Associate Professor of
  Pediatrics
Director, Division of
  Pediatric Rehabilitation
Hahnemann Medical College
  and Hospital
Philadelphia, Pennsylvania

Mary L. Voorhess, M.D.
Professor of Pediatrics
State University of New York
  at Buffalo
School of Medicine;
Co-Director, Division of
  Endocrinology
Buffalo Children's Hospital
Buffalo, New York

Margaret L. Williams, M.D.
Professor of Pediatrics
State University of New York
Upstate Medical Center
Chief, Division of
  Neonatology
Director of Nurseries
Crouse-Irving Memorial
  Hospital
Syracuse, New York

Elaine H. Zackai, M.D.
Assistant Professor of
  Pediatrics and Human
  Genetics
University of Pennsylvania
  School of Medicine
Associate Physician
The Children's Hospital of
  Philadelphia
Philadelphia, Pennsylvania

Acknowledgments

We would like to express our gratitude to Lewis Reines and Karen Okie, both of the Lippincott Company: Lewis, Editor-in-Chief, for having conceived of this book in the first place, and for having nourished it through its years of development; Karen, Assistant Medical Editor, who edited the text with skill and professionalism, and who was unfailingly both pleasant and helpful.

We would also like to thank Mary Cecero, who diligently with resourcefulness assisted Dr. Kaye; Marjorie Gillette, who with patience and capability aided Dr. Oski; and Nancy Watson, who enabled Dr. Barness to keep up with his co-authors.

Special thanks are given to those friends and colleagues who contributed separate chapters to this book. If our objectives are realized, it will be due to their very splendid efforts.

ROBERT KAYE, M.D.
FRANK A. OSKI, M.D.
LEWIS A. BARNESS, M.D.

Preface

Each of the editors of this book has had the responsibility of organizing and presenting the introductory course in pediatrics to medical students. We undertook the preparation of this volume in the belief that there was an unmet need for a book that would help students to acquire a beginning familiarity with the major topics in the health needs of children, and we intended that the book be of a size that could be read during the limited time alloted to the pediatrics rotation.

A problem-oriented presentation was used whenever appropriate, since parents usually seek medical care for their children because of the appearance of a worrisome symptom or sign rather than for treatment of a specific disease. We hope that this approach assists the students in developing competence and satisfaction in the decision-making process, leading from the identification of the patient's problems to diagnosis.

This book is not intended to supplant the major textbooks in pediatrics . . . those books should serve as sources of supplemental information to the reader. We hope that this book will help students enjoy their first professional contacts with children, while sparing them dismay at the multitude and variation of illnesses with which the complete pediatrician is faced.

ROBERT KAYE, M.D.
FRANK A. OSKI, M.D.
LEWIS A. BARNESS, M.D.

Contents

Core Textbook of
PEDIATRICS

1

History and Physical Examination

Lewis A. Barness, M.D.

HISTORY

Taking an adequate history is essential to making a diagnosis of pediatric diseases. Since most infants and children are unable to give good histories, the anomalous situation is overcome by formulating an order of taking a history, interpreting the remarks of an observer, and synthesizing these into a relatively accurate data base.

Until the novitiate learns the significance of signs and symptoms, it is reasonable to ask all questions in an orderly fashion. As the student learns the different diseases, lines of questions may be pursued to make or eliminate specific diagnoses. Even then, it is important not to miss negative historical information which may be significant to a future date or future illness.

Interest in the well-being of the child as well as your interest in the illness should be conveyed to the parent. The informant should be allowed to talk freely at first about the child's problem; further information is then obtained by direct questioning. A service will be performed for your patient if this information can be transcribed into a meaningful medical record, which aids and complements the medical care to be delivered.

The medical record is the basis for medical care, and every effort should be made to organize the record and include all pertinent information. The following guidelines aid in organizing the history and physical data.

ELEMENTS OF A COMPLETE HISTORY

General Information

This should include the name, the age and birth date, the sex, the race, the admission date, the referral source, for example, a clinic or physician, and relation of informant to the child, including a statement of the reliability of the informant.

Chief Complaint (C.C.)

This is a brief statement, in the informant's or patient's own words, of the reason the child was brought to the hospital or clinic. The duration of the problem should also be noted.

History of the Present Illness (H.P.I.)

This portion of the history tells, in chronological sequence, the problem or problems for which the child is being seen. It should begin with a statement of the child's general status and onset of illness, such as "This is the first admission of this 5-year-old white boy who was well until 3 days prior to admission . . ." Each problem defined in the history should include the following information:

1. Date of onset
2. Chronological development of symptoms and duration of symptoms
3. Treatment and response to treatment
4. Change or changes in condition (course of the illness)

If the past medical history is significant to the development of the current illness, a brief summary may be included. Old charts may be used for this information and they may be included in this section or they may be included during the review of the past medical history. However, this information need not be recorded in both places. Pertinent negative findings should be included in this section.

Past Medical History

Prenatal History. The informant should supply information as to which pregnancy this was for the mother and what the health of the mother was during pregnancy; these data include any infections, illnesses, vaginal bleeding or toxemia. If radiographs were taken or medications given, this information should also be included. The results of serology tests as well as the blood types of the mother and the baby should be recorded. Details of the baby's movement in the uterus should be also recorded.

Birth History. The examiner should ascertain the duration of pregnancy, the ease or difficulty of labor, and the duration of labor. Whether the delivery was spontaneous, forceps-assisted, or by Caesarean section should be recorded, as should the type of anesthesia used during delivery. The place and date of birth and the birth weight are also pertinent.

Neonatal History. Inquire as to the condition of the baby after birth, recording such information as difficulty in starting to breathe, and the presence of cyanosis or convulsions. If the baby was jaundiced during the neonatal period, ascertain the date of onset, duration, and need for treatment. The baby's length of stay in the nursery and need for special care, such as an incubator, transfusions, medications, should be included.

Feeding History. It should be noted whether the baby was breast or bottle fed and how well the baby took the first feeding. If the infant is bottle fed, the type of formula, amounts of components used, and total amount of formula taken in 24 hours must be recorded. Details of the introduction of solid food and the use of vitamins and fluorides are pertinent. Problems with food intolerance or vomiting should be included in this section.

For an older child the diet history may be ascertained by asking the informant to supply sample breakfast, lunch and supper menus.

In any child with feeding difficulties or a nutritional problem, the following information should be detailed: the onset of the problem, methods of feeding, types of formula used, reasons for changes, interval between feedings, amount taken per feeding, vomiting, crying, and weight change.

Developmental History. The progression of weight gain is important in a developmental assessment. Therefore, birth weight, the weight at 6 months, the weight at 1 year, and the weight at 2 years should be ascertained. Any sudden gain or loss of weight should be listed first. The informant should compare the child's general growth with that of his siblings. In all instances, and in older children with a developmental problem, the dates of the following developmental milestones should be included in the history: followed person with eyes, held head erect, transferred objects, walked with support, spoke first words and sentences, sat alone, smiled responsively, reached for objects, and walked alone. For children 2 years of age and older, pertinent developmental landmarks should be recorded. For a school age child, his grade and marks received in school should be ascertained and compared with those of his siblings.

Behavior History. The informant should supply information as to whether the child is a happy one or is difficult to manage. The child's response to other children, to new situations, to strangers, and to school are clues to behavior problems. If the child manifests successive demands for attention such as showing off, nagging, temper tantrums, and crying, these should be recorded. Problems with bowel or bladder training and habits such as thumb-sucking, nail-biting, and masturbation are important. The examiner should discover if the child has nightmares and whether he suffers from pica, particularly from paint or plaster.

Immunization History. The types of immunization, the number and dates given and the child's reactions, if any, should be recorded.

History of Past Illnesses. A statement should be made here as to the health of the patient before this illness. Specific inquiry should be made as to the child's having had: roseola, rubeola, rubella, pertussis, mumps, varicella, scarlet fever, tuberculosis, anemia, recurrent tonsillitis, otitis media, pneumonia, meningitis, encephalitis or other nervous system disease, gastrointestinal tract disease, and any other disease. The history of each past illness should include the date of onset, symptoms, course, termination, and whether there were complications or sequelae. If the child was hospitalized or had surgery in the past, the diagnoses for these events should be stated. The results of surgery should be ascertained. Details of allergy include: the occurrence and type of drug reactions, and the presence of food allergies, hay fever, and asthma. All accidents, injuries, and poisonings should be included.

Review of Systems (R.O.S.)

This should supplement the history of present illness, and information included there need not be repeated, but merely referred to as "See P.I."

Head. Injuries, headache.

Eyes. Visual changes, crossed or tendency to cross, discharge, redness, puffiness, any injuries, glasses.

Ears. Difficulty in hearing, pain, discharge, past history of ear infections.

Nose. Discharge (watery or purulent), difficulty in breathing through nose, epistaxis.

Mouth and Throat. Sore throat or tongue, difficulty in swallowing, dental trouble.

Lungs. Difficulty in breathing, cough (time and character), hoarseness, wheezing, hemoptysis, pain in chest.

Heart. Cyanosis, edema, history of heart murmurs or "heart trouble," ability to keep up with other children in active play, shortness of breath, chest pains.

Gastrointestinal. Appetite, nausea, vomiting (relation to feeding, amount, character), bowel movements (number and character), abdominal pain, distention, jaundice.

Genitourinary. Frequency, dysuria, hematuria, character of urinary stream, bedwetting, urethral or vaginal discharge, menstrual history.

Extremities. Weaknesses, deformities, difficulty in moving extremities or in walking, joint pains or swelling.

Neurologic. Headaches, dizziness, incoordination, convulsions.

Skin. Rashes, hives.

Family History (F.H.)

A genetic chart may be used here. (Fig. 1-1) and should include parents, siblings, and grandparents, with their ages, health, or cause of death.

When problems with genetic implications exist, inquiry should be made about other relatives. If a genetic chart is used, the pregnancies should be listed in a series, and include the health of the siblings, e.g.:

1. 1954—stillbirth at. . .month of gestation

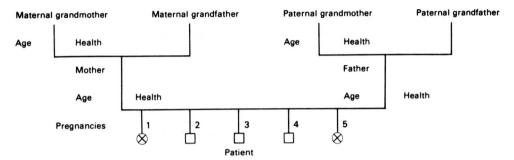

Maternal grandmother Maternal grandfather Paternal grandmother Paternal grandfather

Age Health Age Health

Mother Father

Age Health Age Health

Pregnancies 1 2 3 4 5

Patient

Fig. 1-1. Genetic chart.

2. 1956—boy with hay fever
3. 1958—boy (the patient)
4. 1960—a boy who is well
5. 1966—girl who died at age 2 days with hyaline membrane disease

Inquiries should be made about a family history of allergy, blood disease, heart disease, lung disease, kidney disease, tuberculosis, diabetes, rheumatic fever, convulsions or mental disorders, skin or gastrointestinal disorders, cancer, venereal disease or behavioral disorders, or any other diseases in the family.

Social History

Record details of the family unit in this section. Include information on the presence of grandparents and the marital status of the parents (living together, separated, divorced). Data on home living conditions should include such details as whether the family lives in a house or an apartment, whether the mother works and if so who looks after the patient when she is working, and the father's employment. If pertinent to the child's problem, detailed inquiry should be made about the family's attitudes toward each other and towards the child. A typical day in the child's life may be outlined.

PHYSICAL EXAMINATION

The physical examination of a child cannot be approached in the same manner as that of an adult, i.e. starting with the head and ending with the feet. The child is in a new situation and may be apprehensive. An attempt should be made to befriend the child before examining him, and the order of the examination should fit the child and the circumstances. In general, it is wise to make no sudden movements, and to first complete those parts of the examination for which the child's cooperation is needed. All painful or disagreeable procedures should be deferred until the end of the examination, and the child should be warned before the start of these procedures. Thoroughness is essential. The child should be completely undressed, but not necessarily all at once. In recording findings of physical examination, descriptions should be exact as to size, color, and so forth.

Although the physical examination may not necessarily be conducted in this order, the recorded information should follow the outline below.

Measurements. These should include height, weight, head circumference (all given with percentile for age), temperature (oral or rectal), pulse, respiration, blood pressure (site used and position in which taken, e.g. left arm supine position).

General Appearance. A statement should be included of the child's general development and nutrition, any unusual positions he assumes, his mental status, activity and evidence of how the child apparently feels. The apparent degree and acuteness of illness and the presence of any distress should be noted.

Skin. Include color, the presence of cyanosis, jaundice, eruptions, edema, skin turgor, amount of subcutaneous tissue, and evidence of recent weight loss.

Lymph Nodes. Their location, size, and presence of tenderness should be recorded.

Head. The head should be examined for shape, symmetry, sutures, bone defects, and size and tension of fontanels (posterior fontanel usually closed by 2 months, anterior fontanel usually closed by 12 to 18 months, but occasionally as early as 9 months). The hair and scalp should also be examined, with pertinent findings recorded.

Eyes. Make a gross test of vision. Visual field should be tested in all children old enough to cooperate. The eyes should be evaluated for strabismus by position of the light reflex in both eyes, and the cover test. The range of eye movements should be evaluated. The presence of nystagmus should be noted. Other structures to be examined around the eyes include the conjunctivae, and sclerae, the cornea for haziness and opacities, the pupils for size and shape, and the iris and lens. The reaction to light (direct and consensual) and accommodation should be noted. A funduscopic examination should be performed, noting the presence of the red reflex, the condition of the veins and arteries (they should be of almost equal caliber, or veins slightly larger than arteries), the presence of hemorrhages or pigmented or depigmented areas. Visualization of the disc should detect sharp or blurred borders. The macula is examined to detect possible degenerative changes. Testing of the corneal reflex may also be part of the examination.

Ears. Evaluate hearing and the condition of the external ear (deformity or unusual shape, pain with movement of the ear), the canal wall, the drum, and the mastoid.

Nose. The nasal examination is performed to detect deformities, condition of the airway, color and state of the mucosa and turbinates, discharge (amount and character), sinus tenderness or swelling. At birth, the maxillary antrum, the anterior and posterior ethmoid cells and sphenoid sinus are present. However, the latter does not assume clinical significance until approximately 5 years of age. At 2 to 4 years of age, pneumatization of the frontal sinus occurs, but it is rarely a site of infection until after ages 6 to 10.

Mouth and Throat. This examination should detect the number and condition of the teeth, the condition of the gums, the buccal mucosa, the tongue, palate, tonsils, and posterior pharynx. Listening to the voice reveals the presence of hoarseness, the quality of the cry, and the presence of stridor.

Neck. Examination of the neck may reveal rigidity or swelling, abnormalities in the lymph nodes, salivary glands, thyroid, and position of the trachea.

Chest. The general shape and the presence of any deformities should be noted. In infancy the chest is almost round. As the child grows, the chest normally expands in the transverse diameter. Abnormal signs to look for are beading, asymmetry of expansion, and suprasternal, intercostal, and subcostal retractions.

Lungs. The type of breathing (regular, Cheyne-Stokes) and rate of respiration should be recorded.

Auscultation. Breath sounds are usually bronchovesicular in children. To be noted are whether they are increased or decreased. Rales, rhonchi, friction rub, and inspiratory or expiratory wheezes are abnormal findings. Also listen for vocal resonance.

Palpation. Chest palpation detects tactile fremitus and masses on the chest wall.

Percussion. This is done to detect areas of dullness or hyperresonance. Normally the top of the liver is percussed anteriorly at about the level of the sixth rib from the mid-axillary line to the sternum. The lower edge of the lung or the top of the diaphragm is usually percussed to the level of the 8th to 10th ribs posteriorly on both sides.

Heart and Cardiovascular System. A thorough examination should include the following:

Inspection. The presence of cyanosis, edema, clubbing of fingers, and respiratory distress suggest a cardiac etiology.

Palpation. Part of the cardiac examination is locating the apex beat. The apex beat is normally felt in the fourth interspace just to the left of the mid-clavicular line in children under 7 years of age. After 7 years, it is felt in the fifth intercostal space in the mid-clavicular line. Thrills at the apex are best felt with the child lying on the left side, basal thrills are felt with the child sitting up.

Percussion. An attempt should be made to percuss the heart borders. Learn scratch percussion which is accurate in crying children and children with thick pectoralis muscles or heavy breasts.

Auscultation. Detects the heart rate and rhythm, and is performed over the entire chest, anteriorly and posteriorly, with particular attention at the listening posts of the four valve areas. The quality of the heart sounds is normally sharp and clear; splitting of the first or second heart sounds may be heard.

Murmurs. The presence of heart murmurs must be documented by noting location, intensity (I to VI), quality, duration, and transmission. Also note the effect of change of position and exercise.

Radial and Femoral Pulses. These are palpated and the blood pressure taken. The blood pressure should be taken in both arms and one leg if the child has a cardiac problem, hypertension, or if only weak femoral pulses are palpated.

Abdomen. In the abdominal examination, look for: shape (distended or flat), tenderness (include costovertebral), rigidity, palpable organs or masses, hernia, visible peristalsis, ascites, and bowel sounds.

Back. By employing both observation and palpation, the spinal shape and posture (lordosis, kyphosis, scoliosis), masses, tenderness, limitation of motion, spina bifida, and pilonidal dimples or cysts may be detected.

Genitalia. In the male, descent of the testes, presence of hydrocele, state of the foreskin, adequacy of urethral meatal orifice, and malformations such as hypospadius should be recorded. In the female, abnormalities such as fused labia minora or imperforate hymen, urethral or vaginal inflammation or discharge, pubic and axillary hair are recorded. A vaginal examination is not done routinely.

Anus. This should be examined for patency, the presence of fissures, fistulae, or hemorrhoids, and for the state of the sphincter. Rectal examination is performed whenever the child has an abdominal problem.

Extremities. All extremities are observed for asymmetry, anomalies, unusual length, pain and tenderness, temperature, swelling, deformities, and shape (genu varum, genu valgum, tibial torsion, metatarsus varus). The presence of a limp should be recorded. Abnormal findings of the joints include heat, tenderness, swelling, effusion, redness, and limitation or pain on motion. In infants, the examiner must always test for congenital dislocation of the hips.

Muscles. Muscle development and tone are noted, as is the presence of tenderness, spasm, paresis (weakness) or paralysis, flaccidity, spasticity, rigidity, and muscle atrophy.

Neurologic Examination. The mental status and orientation are recorded, stating how this was determined.

Abnormal Movements. These include tremors, twitchings, choreiform movements, and athetosis.

Coordination. The gait is observed and the Romberg and finger-to-nose tests are performed.

Cranial Nerves. All of the cranial nerves are tested: I (olfactory), II (optic), III (oculomotor), IV (trochlear), V (trigeminal), VI (abducens), VII (facial), VIII (auditory and vestibular divisions), IX (glossopharyngeal), X (vagus), XI (accessory), XII (hypoglossal).

Reflexes.   The biceps, triceps, radial, finger flexion, patellar, Achilles tendon, plantar, abdominal, and cremasteric reflexes are recorded after evaluation on both the right and left side. Other reflexes in a young infant include sucking, rooting and Moro reflex. In cases of suspected meningeal irritation, the Brudzinski and Kernig signs must also be checked.

Sensory examination includes evaluation of touch, pain, vibration, and position.

Muscle strength may be evaluated here if not done under the examination of the extremities.

SUMMARY

A thorough history and physical examination aid in making a differential diagnosis and in delineating problems. A problem list is then drawn up, based on the history and physical examination. The problems are numbered and subjective findings (see symptoms), objective signs (physical) and laboratory results, assessment and plan are included. Progress notes should be kept for each problem until it is resolved.

BIBLIOGRAPHY

Barness, L.A.: Manual of Pediatric Physical Diagnosis, 4th ed. Chicago, Year Book Medical Publishers, 1972.

This is a manual detailing how to perform and record a complete physical examination with suggestions for approaching the patient at various ages. Differential diagnosis of significant signs is given.

Weed, L.L.: Medical Records, Medical Education and Patient Care. Chicago, Year Book Medical Publishers, 1971.

This short book delineates the method and value of obtaining a problem-oriented history and the usefulness of a problem-oriented record in following the course of a patient in health or disease.

2

Genetic Disorders

Elaine H. Zackai, M.D., and William J. Mellman, M.D.

Recent studies indicate that 25–30 per cent of hospitalized children have genetic conditions. Genetics is particularly important in pediatric practice when an infant or child is malformed with or without serious developmental problems. The parents of such patients want to learn not only about cause and treatment, but risks to other children in their present and future family. Genetic screening is an expanding form of preventive medicine, a traditional concern of the pediatrician. In order to decide who should be screened, the physician needs to understand the genetic risks of specific population groups. We now realize that many people with relatively high risk of bearing children with specific genetic diseases may not have an affected relative.

Counseling the families of children affected with heritable diseases should involve the pediatrician or family physician primarily responsible for the care of such patients. Their intimate knowledge of and continuing relationship with these families are unique assets of this type of health care.

Categories of Clinical Genetic Problems

Mendelian—Autosomal or X-linked
Chromosomal—Sex (X or Y) chromosome or autosome
Polygenic
Non-genetic

GENETIC COUNSELING OF PATIENTS WITH BIRTH DEFECTS

Genetic counseling is an attempt to help the family understand a disease problem or malformation present in their family and the risk of recurrence of that particular disorder. To do this effectively requires an accurate and specific diagnosis, as well as the ability to place this condition into one of the categories of clinical genetic problems listed below. Some problems may be easy to categorize, e.g. when a chromosomal syndrome (Down's syndrome or mongolism) is recognized and the chromosome analysis (trisomy 21) is confirmatory, or when a mendelian trait is diagnosed both clinically and by the appropriate biochemical analysis (Lesch-Nyhan Syndrome with hypoxanthine-guanine phosphoribosyltransferase [HGPRT] deficiency in the patient's red cells), or the pedigree and pathology support a mendelian mechanism (aqueduct stenosis in X-linked hydrocephalus). More often than not the problem is rare and may not be immediately obvious; if this is the case, all the tools listed below need to be utilized in making the diagnosis.

CLINICAL EVALUATION

(The geneticist refers to the patient as "index case," "proband," or "propositus.") A thorough physical examination should include a dissection of the dysmorphic features of the patient—head shape, evidence of hypo- or hypertelorism, shape and position of ears (see Feingold, 1974, for normative values of these physical parameters), dermatoglyphics of hands and feet. Physical features should be carefully compared with first degree relatives (both parents and sibs), since many anomalies are dominant traits (e.g., syndactyly, polydactyly, ear lobe anomalies, missing teeth, etc.) and can be diagnostic "red herrings." Appropriate radiological and pathological analyses are often required.

Tools Available for Diagnosis of Genetic Conditions

1. Clinical evaluation	3. Literature search
2. Pedigree analysis	4. Special laboratory procedures

Family Analysis

Family history should include a complete pedigree with a record of abortions (and the length of gestation of abortions), both normal and abnormal persons in the generations of the index case, the parents and grandparents. Evidence of consanguinity should be specifically asked for as well as the ethnic origin of parents. Rare genetic disorders are more common in certain population groups (e.g., Ellis von Creveld syndrome in the Amish). Rare autosomal traits are more likely to be homozygous if there is a common ancestor.

Literature Search

Armed with information obtained by physical examination and family analysis, the literature must be screened for evidence that similar malformations have been observed in other index cases. A number of compendia of malformation syndromes is now available in both book and computerized forms. The latter method produces a differential diagnosis for a particular constellation of physical findings with references to pertinent literature for the various diagnostic entities.

Laboratory Studies

Although specific entities may be suggested by the above analysis of the problem with their appropriate laboratory analyses (e.g., a specific enzyme analysis), more often the laboratory must be used as a screening activity. Chromosomal analysis, biochemical screening (urine and blood amino acid, organic acid, urine mucopolysaccharides, etc.) may produce evidence of a diagnosis that was not specifically suggested by the clinical presentation. However, the type of laboratory study most likely to be informative can be predicted from the history and physical examination, (e.g., three or more physical malformations suggest a chromosomal abnormality), while a family history of consanguinity suggests an inborn error of metabolism (an autosomal recessive gene disorder).

GENETIC PRINCIPLES APPLIED TO CLINICAL PROBLEMS

The following discussion illustrates how genetics is applied to clinical problems included under the various categories listed previously.

Mendelian Traits

See McKusick's *Mendelian Inheritance in Man* for a compendium of the more than 2,000 identified human traits believed to be determined by single genes.

Autosomal. An autosomal trait may be manifested when only one dose of a mutant gene (in the *heterozygous* state) is present. This is referred to as a "dominant" trait. If a disease occurs only when the patient has two doses of the mutant gene (*homozygous* state), it is considered a recessive disorder. Both heterozygous and homozygous states may be expressed, but the clinical picture may be different. The homozygote may have a more severe disease than the heterozygote. An example is familial hypercholesterolemia that is associated with lipid-containing skin tumors (xanthomas) and is caused by a defect in a gene that affects the control of cholesterol biosynthesis. The following outline contrasts the manifestations of those who are heterozygous for the defective gene and those who are homozygous for the same mutant gene.

Familial Hypercholesterolemia

Disease in Heterozygotes
  Hypercholesterolemia
    300—600 mg./dl. in adults
    230—500 mg./dl. <20 yrs.
  Tendon xanthomas
    lipid-containing skin tumors
  Coronary heart disease
    3rd—6th decade

Disease in Homozygotes
  Profound hypercholesterolemia
    >500 mg./dl.
  Cutaneous planar xanthomas
    appear before age 10—palms, buttocks,
    knees and tendon xanthomas
  Progressive coronary heart disease
    death often by 20 years

In contrast to familial hypercholesterolemia, most inborn errors of metabolism in man are caused by autosomal recessive genes. For example, phenylketonuria (PKU) is a defect in the conversion of phenylalanine to tyrosine (phenylalanine hydroxylase). Children with PKU are usually mentally retarded unless phenylalanine is sharply restricted from early infancy. They are homozygous (have a double dose of the mutant gene). Heterozygotes, or carriers for this trait, are not diseased, although some heterozygotes are found to be phenylalanine intolerant, e.g. when a load of phenylalanine is administered it disappears at a slower rate from the blood than it does in persons who do not carry this gene.

Dominant traits are frequently puzzling in terms of pedigree analysis because of their variation in clinical expression. *Penetrance* refers to the situation where the gene is not expressed at all in the person, but is certainly present by virtue of the transmission of the disease to offspring who manifest (express) the disorder. Single dominant traits often have several forms of expression, referred to as *pleiotrophy*. The Waardenburg syndrome illustrates these principles. Families with this dominant trait usually come to clinical attention because of congenital deafness in several members of the family. Figure 2-1 is the pedigree of a family with

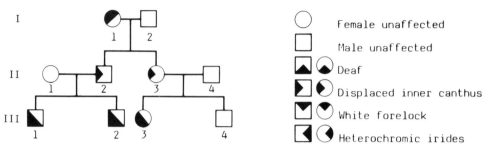

Fig. 2-1. Waardenburg syndrome.

this gene disorder; deafness is not expressed in many members of this family who are carrying the gene. But it is clear that they are carrying the gene because they have children who are deaf. The gene might be considered "non-penetrant" in those persons who are not deaf, if deafness were the only expression of the gene. However, the gene results in a syndrome whose expressions are listed in Table 2-1. The various expressions are the *pleiotrophic traits* of this gene and nearly all persons carrying the gene have at least one expression—broad nasal bridge, lateral displacement of the inner canthus, etc.

Diagnosis of this particular syndrome demands clinical skill; it does little good to look at a child and comment on his "odd" or "funny-looking" or "dysmorphic" appearance. But a description of a widened nasal root and lateral displacement of the inner canthus, along with a test of hearing can prove diagnostic *if* the parents and siblings are also carefully examined. The father may well have the same facies, e.g. anomalies of the midface, but normal hearing (II-2, Fig. 2-1), or he may have other expressions of Waardenburg syndrome such as heterochromia of the irides. With this information about the syndrome, it is clear how to counsel this family in terms of explaining the mechanism of inheritance and

Table 2-1. Waardenburg Syndrome: Frequency of Clinical Features

Clinical Features	Percentage
Lateral displacement of inner canthi	99
Broad and high nasal bridge	78
Medial hyperplasia eyebrows	45
White forelock	17
Partial or complete loss of pigment in the iris	25
Congenital deafness	20

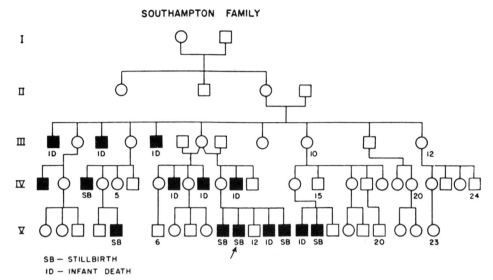

Fig. 2-2. X-linked hydrocephalus. (Darkened boxes denote hydrocephalus, ID denotes infant death and SB denotes stillbirth.) (From Edwards, J. H., Norman, R. M., and Roberts, J. M.: Sex linked hydrocephalus. Report of a family with 15 affected members. Arch. Dis. Child., 36:481, 1961.)

the risk of recurrence. The pediatrician with an epidemiologic orientation would advise the parents as to how other children such as first cousins might also be affected by the disorder. (A first cousin, III-3, of the index case in Fig. 2-1 was labelled mentally retarded until the diagnosis in the index case led to the realization that deafness was responsible for that child's "retardation.")

X-linked traits are transmitted from an unaffected carrier mother to her son when the trait is recessive. A number of pathologically important genes has been localized to the X-chromosome (e.g., those for coagulation factors, deficiencies of which lead to hemophilia A and B respectively; HGPRT [hypoxanthine-guanine phosphoribosyl transferase] deficiency that leads to the Lesch-Nyhan Syndrome [ataxia, self-mutilation and overproduction of uric acid], and ornithine carbamyl synthetase deficiency, a fatal liver dysfunction with hyperammonemia.) With the exception of the last example, where the female heterozygous for the mutant gene is affected (although she may not have a fatal disease), the other conditions are only expressed in the hemizygous male whose one X-chromosome carries the mutant gene. The heterozygous female is clinically unaffected, even though specific biochemical analysis often can detect a partial defect.

An example of an X-linked recessive trait that is expressed as a congenital malformation is a particular form of hydrocephalus. Most hydrocephalus is unexplained, while non-communicating hydrocephalus due

Table 2-2. Newborn Surveys

Sex Chromosome Abnormality		Number	Frequency (%)
Females:	XO	2	
	XXX	13	
	Other	5	
Total		20	.13
Males:	XYY	26	
	XXY	30	
	Other	17	
Total		73	.26

Autosomal Abnormality			
Structural rearrangements			
Euploid		81	.19
Aneuploid		21	.05
Total		102	
Trisomies			
13		3	
18		4	
21		45	
Other		2	
Total		54	.12
Total		249	.57

Total: 43,558 (28,582 males, 14,976 females)

to stenosis of the aqueduct of Sylvius occurs in families with the pattern of an X-linked recessive trait (Fig. 2-2). Infants with this disorder often develop such massive head enlargement before birth that vaginal delivery is not possible.

Chromosomal Disorders

Chromosomal *aneuploidy* usually refers to the state when the chromosome number is greater or less than the *euploid* number of 46. The chromosome involved may be one of the 22 pairs of autosomes or the sex chromosome pair (XX in the female and XY in the male). Structural rearrangements also occur that may alter the amount of genetic information without changing the chromosome number.

The chromosomes of a large number of newborn infants have been examined in recent years. Studies performed in several centers throughout the world have obtained similar results, which are summarized in Table 2-2. Approximately 1/200 newborns have chromosomal abnormalities and about half involve sex chromosomes. A newborn with physical anomalies has about a 4 per cent chance of having a chromosome aberration.

The autosomal trisomies that are found regularly among liveborn infants are trisomy 13, 18, and 21. Syndromes ascribed to the various autosomal trisomies are reasonably specific. Table 2-3 lists their features.

Table 2-3. Features of Autosomal Trisomies 13, 18, and 21

Disorder	Clinical Manifestations

Trisomy 13	Developmental retardation
	Facies
	    Microcephaly—sloping forehead (holoprosencephaly type
	      brain defect)
	    Microphthalmia
	    Cleft lip and palate
	    Low-set malformed ears
	Extremities
	    Polydactyly of hands and feet
	    Rocker bottom feet
	    Position anomaly of fingers—flexed
	      with overlapping index over third
	Cardiac
	    Abnormality in 80%
	Renal
	    Polycystic kidneys in 31%
	      (and other malformations—hydronephrosis,
	      horseshoe kidney, duplicated ureters)

Trisomy 18	Developmental retardation—difficulty feeding, poor suck, low
	    birth weight
	Facies
	    Prominent occiput
	    Low-set malformed ears
	    Small mouth
	    Micrognathia
	Extremities
	    Rocker-bottom feet
	    Position anomaly of fingers—flexed
	      with overlapping index over third
	Dermatoglyphics
	    Simple arches on 6 or more digits >80%
	Cardiac
	    VSD, PDA >95%
	Renal
	    Renal malformation—horseshoe kidney,
	      hydronephrosis, hydroureter

Trisomy 21	Developmental retardation, hypotonia
	Facies
	    Flattened facies
	    Flat occiput
	    Oblique palpebral fissures
	    Epicanthal folds
	    Brushfield spots
	    Protruding tongue
	    Excess skin nape of neck (infants)
	    Three fontanels (infants)
	    Ears—small, box-like configuration
	Extremities
	    Short broad fingers ⎫
	    Clinodactyly ⎬ Hands
	    Transverse palmar crease ⎭
	    Increased space 1st & 2nd toes
	Dermatoglyphics
	    Distal axial triradii—palm
	    Ulnar loops—digits
	    Open field—hallucal area
	Heart
	    Cardiac abnormality in 35% of cases (most common—
	      endocardial cushion defect)

The clinical diagnosis of these trisomies requires that the physician be able to recognize a typical facies, associated anomalies of the extremities, and specific dermatoglyphic features (particularly with trisomies 18 and 21).

Trisomy 21 is the most prevalent autosomal disorder in clinical medicine. It is responsible for the syndrome currently called Down's syndrome, known for over a century as mongolism. Down's syndrome is usually a sporadic error in gametogenesis that causes trisomy 21 in a single affected fetus of the involved couple. Occasionally the extra chromosome is present as part of a compound or "translocated chromosome" (3.5% of all patients), most commonly translocated with another small acrocentric (G group) chromosome (56% of translocations) or a large acrocentric (D group) chromosome (44% of translocations). Such "translocation mongols" have 46 chromosomes, yet have the extra chromosomal material to account for the trisomy 21 syndrome. Some trans-

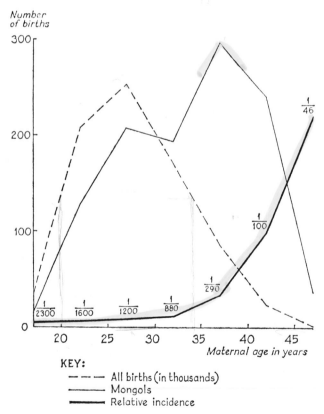

Fig. 2-3. Incidence at birth. (From Colman, R. D., and Staller, A.: Am. J. Public Health, *52*:813, 1962.)

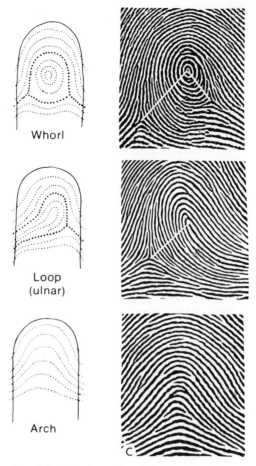

Fig. 2-4. The three dermal ridge patterns—whorl, loop and arch. (From Holt, S.: The Genetics of Dermal Ridges. Br. Med. Bull., 17:247, 1961.

location trisomies are the consequence of the carrier state in one of the parents (for D/G translocations, 49% are inherited, for G/G—5.6%). In such cases there is a significant recurrence risk to that particular couple and their relatives who might also be carriers of the translocation. (D/G mother = 10.9% risk of affected offspring; D/G father = 2.4% risk of affected offspring.)

Trisomy 21 (as well as other trisomies, XXY and XXX) occurs more frequently in the offspring of women of advanced childbearing age. Figure 2-3 indicates the relative risk at varying maternal ages for trisomy 21. Even though the relative risks are significantly greater for women over

35, the absolute number of pregnancies are distributed by maternal age in such a way that more than half the infants with trisomy 21 are born to women under 35. Translocation trisomies are less common among the offspring of women over 35 years. *Mosaicism* refers to the situation where there are two (or more) populations of cells with different chromosome compositions. *Mosaic mongolism* usually refers to patients whose cells have a proportion with trisomy 21 and another with the normal number of chromosomes.

The clinical expression of trisomy 21 is highly variable in terms of physical and mental development. Adults with trisomy 21 have a wide range of IQs; although the range is considerably below that of a normal population. The distribution of IQs of mosaic mongols tends to be closer to that of the general population, even though it is rare for individuals in this group to have a "normal IQ."

Dermatoglyphics. The dermal ridge patterns that are formed in early embryonic life vary considerably due to differences that are inherited, disturbances in the normal differentiation of the peripheral limb buds (such as the influences of intrauterine infections like rubella) and chromosome abnormalities. The *distal phalanges* have a variety of dermal ridge patterns that can be classified into three major patterns—arches, whorls and loops (Fig. 2-4). The occurrence of *arches* on eight or more digits would be a rare event, yet in trisomy 18 this is the usual finding. The *palmar* patterns usually are absent or small in the hypothenar area, the ulnar portion of the proximal palm. When the pattern is large, a junction pattern (triradius or delta) formed by the hypothenar, thenar and distal palmar patterns occurs in the middle one-third of the palm along an axis that passes through the fourth digit and the middle of the wrist. This *distal palmar axial triradius* (Fig. 2-5) is found in 75 per cent of patients with trisomy 21 and in less than 3.5 per cent of control subjects. In the foot there is a pattern in the dermal pad at the base of the great toe. In 50 per cent of patients with trisomy 21 there is a simple arch pattern in the hallucal region (Fig. 2-6) that is found in less than 1 per cent of control subjects. This unusual dermal pattern in the foot of patients with trisomy 21 is associated with hypoplasia of the hallucal pad and a wide space between the great and second toes.

Sex chromosome aneuploidy is less appreciated as a clinical problem than trisomy 21 even though it occurs more frequently. XXY and XYY occur in male newborns at a combined incidence of about 1/400; XXX and XO occur in female newborns at a combined incidence of 1/800. The clinical significance of XYY and XXX is still poorly defined, but appears to be associated with learning and perhaps behavioral disorders.

Klinefelter's (XXY) and Turner's (XO) syndromes are summarized in Table 2-4. Both syndromes should be recognized so that appropriate hormonal therapy can be instituted. For the former there is still controversy as to when and how androgen therapy should be administered, and its

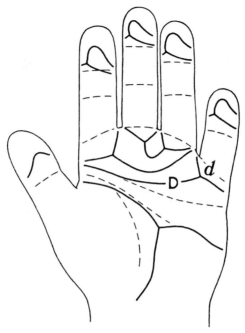

Fig. 2-5. Distal palmar axial triradius. (From Holt, S.: The Genetics of Dermal Ridges. Springfield, Ill., Charles C Thomas, 1968.)

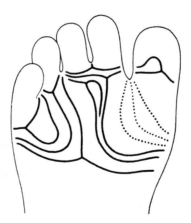

Fig. 2-6. Hallucal area—simple arch pattern (open fields). (From Holt, S.: The Genetics of Dermal Ridges. Springfield, Illinois, Charles C Thomas, 1968.)

Table 2-4. Differentiating Features of Klinefelter's and Turner's Syndromes

Syndrome	Clinical Features

XXY (Klinefelter)	Buccal smear chromatin positive
	Phenotype
	  External and internal male ductal system
	Hypogonadism ($<$ 2 cm diameter postpubertal testes)
	  Firm to palpation
	  Biopsy—hyalination and hypoplasia of seminiferous tubules
	Azospermia (90%)
	Gynecomastia (25–40%)
	  2° sexual development—variable (completely normal to infantile)
	Height
	  Taller than average
	  Decreased U/L segment ratio
	Intelligence
	  Variable (normal to moderate retardation)
	Behavioral abnormalities
	  Lack of goal orientation
	  Social ineptness
	  Poor school performance
	  Speech difficulty

XO (Turner)	Buccal smear chromatin negative
	Phenotype
	  Female
	    Absence of definitive gonad ("streak ovaries")
	    Infantile uterus in presence of female external genitalia
	Lack of 2° sex characteristics
	1° amenorrhea
	Height
	  Short stature (mean adult height 55")
	  Birth length below 18.5"
	Normal intelligence
	Variable findings
	  Shield chest
	  Congenital lymphedema
	  Low posterior hairline
	  High arched palate
	  Hyperconvex nails
	  Cubitus valgus
	  Webbed neck
	  Pigmented nevi
	  Small mandible
	  Short 4th metacarpal
	  Renal anomaly
	  Cardiac anomaly (coarctation of aorta most frequent)

influence on the general psychological and social maladjustments commonly found with XXY. Turner's syndrome patients need estrogen therapy to artificially stimulate sexual maturation and menarche. Because of the slow linear growth of these patients from infancy, early diagnosis is important to avoid unnecessary anxiety and diagnostic activity. Infertility is a manifestation of both syndromes.

Polygenic Inheritance

This is perhaps the most difficult category of inherited disorders to explain mechanistically. Since a significant proportion of inherited congenital malformations is included in this class of disorders, it cannot be neglected. The genetic principles involved are based solidly on scientific evidence in both man and experimentally bred animals. There are several genetic factors that determine an individual fetus' susceptibility to a number of specific malformations (e.g., cleft lip, neural tube defects, congenital hip dislocation, hypertrophic pyloric stenosis). This susceptibility has a continuous distribution in the general population and the factors involved determine this susceptibility. Persons with certain hereditary endowments may exceed the "threshold" of susceptibility, but this threshold may also be exceeded by environmental influences that shift an individual's position in the susceptibility distribution. Relatives of affected persons also have a range of susceptibility similar to the general population but the mean susceptibility is greater than that of the general population. The more distantly related a person is to an affected subject, the more his risk approaches that of the general population (see Fig. 2-7). This same theory of polygenic inheritance also applies to height and IQ (e.g., the relatives of tall or very intelligent persons have a greater "risk" of being tall or very smart than the general population; the converse is

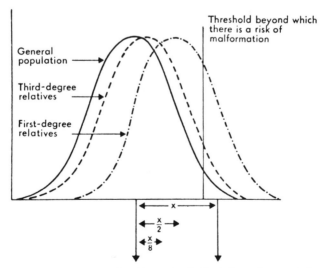

x: deviation of mean of malformed individuals from the population mean

Fig. 2-7. Model for polygenic inheritance of cleft lip, with, or without, cleft palate. (From Carter, C. O.: Genetics of common disorders. Br. Med. Bull., 25:52, 1969.)

true for shortness and stupidity). This "threshold theory" can account for the observed risks to relatives of different degrees—grandparents, aunts, and uncles—and to malformations believed to be polygenically inherited. (See Table 2-5 for empiric risk of cleft lip and cleft palate to various degrees of relatives.)

Although most occurrences of cleft lip are based on a polygenically inherited mechanism with a 3–5 per cent risk of recurrence to parents of an affected child, cleft lip can be one of the findings in a child with multiple malformations. Careful classification of these multiple malformations may lead to a previously described syndrome. A syndrome is a grouping of congenital malformations that show a "tendency to run together" and have a uniform etiology. Once a syndrome has been identified it should be examined in terms of the principles outlined in the list on page 10 (Mendelian trait, chromosomal disorders, polygenic disorder, non-genetic). The family can then be properly counseled with information based on previously reported cases and, when available, etiologic factors.

Non-Genetic Causes of Congenital Anomalies

These causes are almost certainly manifold even though the identified ones are few; included are congenital infections (rubella, cytomegalo-inclusion disease, syphilis, toxoplasmosis) and teratogenic drugs (aminopterin, thalidomide). Other drugs inspire less confidence. Anticonvulsant drugs are currently highly suspected (diphenylhydantoin, trimethadione). There are problems in incriminating drugs as teratogens: two are the relatively high incidence of malformations in random pregnancies (Table 2-6) and the near certainty that teratogenic drugs only cause problems in a proportion of fetuses. These differences in susceptibility to potential teratogens may well be genetic, either at the maternal or fetal

Table 2-5. Risk of Cleft Lip and Cleft Palate

Risk in:	Cleft lip with or without cleft palate
General Population	0.001
Monozygotic twins	×400
First-degree relatives (siblings, parents, offspring)	× 40
Second-degree relatives (aunts, uncles, nieces, nephews, grandchildren)	× 7
Third-degree relatives (first cousins)	× 3

Table 2-6. Malformations in Random Pregnancies

Genetic problem	% of newborns afflicted
Congenital malformations (polygenic disorders)	2–2.5
Chromosomal abnormalities	.5
Single gene disorders	< .1
	2.5–3

level of response to the drug. As pharmacogeneticists develop more data about individual responses to drugs and other environmental agents, there may well be an improved understanding of why one fetus is damaged by certain drugs taken by the mother, while another is unaffected by the same agents. With such insights the category of "non-genetic" may well be changed to "environmental with genetic predisposition."

RECURRENCE RISKS

· Once a patient's condition has been diagnosed and classified accurately, parents can be provided with specific risk rates for certain disorders, e.g., 25 per cent for autosomal recessive disorders, 50 per cent for males when the mother carries an X-linked recessive trait, 50 per cent for autosomal dominant disorders with an affected parent, 3–5 per cent for cleft lip and palate, anencephaly, meningomyelocele and other polygenic disorders when sib is affected, 10 per cent for offspring of women with a D/G translocation, 2.5 per cent for offspring of men with the same translocation. Often specific risk cannot be ascribed. In other situations there may be no specific risks to the family seeking counsel (e.g. "sporadic" translocation mongolism with chromosomally normal parents; achondroplasia when the parents are normal, therefore the index case is the result of a fresh dominant mutation). Risks may be those of the general population (1/100 for a woman of 39 who is concerned that her infant may be born with trisomy 21 and who bore a child with this condition at age 35).

Prenatal diagnosis can now be used to identify some disorders of an affected or unaffected fetus by removing amniotic fluid after the fourteenth week of gestation. Conditions that can be diagnosed from amniotic fluid study are listed below (biochemical assay, chromosome analysis, α-feto protein determination).

Amniotic Fluid Study for Prenatal Diagnosis

Chromosome disorders
  Indications
    Familial translocation
    Advanced maternal age
    Previous trisomy
Metabolic disorders
  Specific biochemical diagnosis is possible for over 60 inborn errors
    of metabolism
Neural tube defects (anencephaly, meningomyelocele)
X-linked disorders
Determination of sex of the fetus by chromosome analysis. The male
  has a 50 per cent chance of being affected. Not a diagnostic test
  for a specific X-linked disorder, in most cases.

SCREENING THE FAMILIES OF PATIENTS WITH GENETIC DISORDERS

Thus far we have been dealing with the propositus (affected patient) and the risk of recurrence in his future siblings. The scope of the pediatrician should extend beyond the nuclear family to include other relatives who may have a greater risk of bearing affected offspring than the general population.

Chromosome Translocations

Many people with mental retardation and dysmorphic features have been identified as having unbalanced translocations, i.e., having extra or missing portions of the chromosomes involved in the translocation. With the advent of specialized chromosome banding techniques (giemsa and fluorescent banding) the specificity of these anomalies has improved dramatically, and, therefore, many new "partial trisomy" syndromes are being described. In most instances, one parent of a patient is then detected as the balanced carrier. The transmission of translocations in the balanced form may resemble that of a dominant trait. Siblings and cousins of a translocation-bearing parent may be carriers also and susceptible to the production of a chromosomally abnormal fetus. Once these "at risk" carrier individuals have been identified, prenatal diagnosis of the chromosomally unbalanced fetus can be offered. For example, a severely retarded dysmorphic proband was identified as trisomic for the distal part of long arm of chromosome 10 (46, XY, −17, +t) (17p:10q); (see Fig. 2-8A). His mother is a balanced carrier for the translocation which involved the short arm of 17 and long arm of chromosome 10 (17p+ 10q−); (Fig. 2-8 B and C). This balanced translocation was traced through three gen-

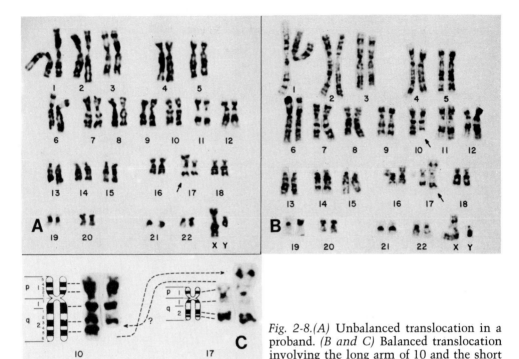

Fig. 2-8.(A) Unbalanced translocation in a proband. *(B and C)* Balanced translocation involving the long arm of 10 and the short arm of 17.

erations of this family (Fig. 2-9). The proband's fourth cousin, also severely retarded with a strikingly similar dysmorphia, had the same unbalanced translocation.

Family Risks for Autosomal Recessive Disorders

The special risk for families in which the proband has a rare autosomal recessive disease should be considered when caring for a diseased patient. The gene frequency of a rare trait in the population is surprisingly common. It can be calculated by estimating the frequency of the disease (individuals homozygous for the gene) and determining its square root. Carrier frequency is twice the gene frequency since, for autosomal genes, two loci are involved. Table 2-7 compares the frequency of some diseases with their gene and carrier frequencies in the population. The parents are almost certainly carriers of rare diseases. Their siblings have a 50 per cent, uncles and aunts a 25 per cent, and first cousins a 12½ per cent risk of also being carriers. Spouses of these relatives, unless related by blood (consanguinous), have the same probability of being carriers as the general population. Based on these probabilities, the risk of close relatives producing offspring diseased with rare recessive conditions is usually

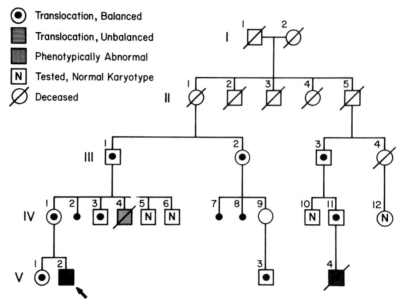

Translocation, Balanced
Translocation, Unbalanced
Phenotypically Abnormal
N Tested, Normal Karyotype
Ø Deceased

Fig. 2-9. Familial translocation 10q:17p. Note unbalanced 4th cousins V2 & V4.

small but often more likely than in the general population. (See Table 2-8). This information demonstrates why physicians with an epidemiological orientation to health care should be able to estimate the risk and be alert to the diagnosis in relatives other than the siblings of an affected individual (e.g. first cousins of patients with phenylketonuria, Tay-Sach's disease, sickle-cell anemia are much more likely to be affected with these diseases than random individuals in the population).

Table 2-7. Frequency of Disease with Gene and Carrier Frequency

Disease and Ethnic Group	Estimated Incidence of Homozygotes Among Newborns	Population Gene Frequency	Population Carrier Frequency
Cystic fibrosis (Northern Europeans)	1:2500	1 in 50	1 in 25
Sickle-cell anemia (Blacks)	1:600	1 in 25	1 in 12
Tay-Sachs (Ashkenazic Jews)	1:3600	1 in 60	1 in 30
β thalassemia (Greeks, Italians)	1:3600	1 in 60	1 in 30
Phenylketonuria	1:11,500	1 in 100	1 in 50
Maple syrup urine disease	1:200,000	1 in 450	1 in 225
Homocystinuria	1:230,000	1 in 480	1 in 240
Galactosemia	1:187,171	1 in 435	1 in 218

Table 2-8. Risk to Offspring for Phenylketonuria

Population at Risk	Risk Ratio
General population $\frac{1}{50} \times \frac{1}{50} \times \frac{1}{2} \times \frac{1}{2}$	~ 1:10,000
Parents of affected $\frac{1}{2} \times \frac{1}{2}$	1:4
Siblings of carriers $\frac{1}{50} \times \frac{1}{2} \times \frac{1}{2} \times \frac{1}{2}$	1:400
Uncles and aunts of carrier $\frac{1}{100} \times \frac{1}{2} \times \frac{1}{2} \times \frac{1}{2}$	1:800
First cousins of carrier $\frac{1}{200} \times \frac{1}{2} \times \frac{1}{2} \times \frac{1}{2}$	1:1600

SPECIAL POPULATIONS AT RISK OTHER THAN RELATIVES OF AFFECTED PATIENTS

In addition to being "proband-oriented," the pediatrician must realize that he may be dealing with many people who do not have an affected relative yet are at a relatively high risk of bearing children with specific genetic diseases. Genetic screening or pre-proband identification of the at-risk person or family is an expanding form of preventive medicine. This involves the identification and screening of high-risk subpopulations. One such subpopulation discussed earlier is women over the age of 35 who are at a substantially greater risk relative to younger women of bearing children with non-disjunctional chromosomal aberrations (especially Down's syndrome). (Fig. 2-3) The counseling of this population as to risk and availability of prenatal diagnosis is a key in the prevention of such disease.

Various subpopulations have high carrier frequencies of specific recessive traits that are rare in the general population (see Table 2-7 for ethnic group) and high frequencies of specific gene abnormalities. The identification of carriers within these high-risk subpopulations, identification of at-risk couples, genetic counseling, and in some instances prenatal diagnosis (Tay-Sachs disease) is another aspect of preventive medicine within the scope of the genetically oriented physician.

BIBLIOGRAPHY

Bergsma, D.: Birth Defects: Atlas and compendium. Baltimore, Williams and Wilkins Co., 1972.

Carter, C.O.: Multifactorial genetic disease. In: Medical Genetics, V.A. McKusick, and R. Claiborne, ed. New York, Hospital Practice, 1973, p. 199.

Feingold, M., and Bassert, W.: Normal values for selected physical parameters. An aid to syndrome delineation. In Birth Defects—Original Article Series Vol. X, No. 13, 1974.

Holt, S.: The Genetics of Dermal Ridges. Springfield, Illinois, Charles C Thomas, 1968.

Lewandowski, R.C., and Yunis, J.: New chromosomal syndromes. Am. J. Dis. Child. *129*:515, 1975.

McKusick, V.A.: Mendelian Inheritance in Man. 4th ed. Baltimore, Johns Hopkins Press, 1974.

> A useful catalogue from which one is able to learn the pattern of inheritance of all known genetic disorders. In addition, it gives a summary of the disease entity with pertinent references.

Milunsky, A., and Atkins, L.: Prenatal diagnosis of genetic disorders. In: The Prevention of Genetic Disease and Mental Retardation, A. Milunsky, ed. Philadelphia, W.B. Saunders, 1975, p. 221.

Rimoin, D.L., and Schimke, R.N.: Genetic forms of hypogonadism in phenotypic males. Genetic disorders of the endocrine glands. St. Louis, C.V. Mosby, 1971.

Smith, D.W.: Recognizable Patterns of Human Malformation; Genetic Embryologic and Clinical Aspects. Philadelphia, W.B. Saunders, 1970–1976.

> Comprehensive picture and clinical summary including features, prognosis, pattern of inheritance, and recurrence risk of all dysmorphology syndromes.

Stanbury, Wyngaarden and Fredrickson (eds.) Metabolic Basis of Inherited Disease. 3rd ed. New York, McGraw Hill, 1972.

> Excellent coverage of all inborn errors of metabolism from a biochemical and genetic viewpoint.

Thompson, J.S., and Thompson, M.W.: Genetics in Medicine. 2nd ed. Philadelphia, W.B. Saunders, 1973.

> Written for the student in medicine with a brief discussion of genetics and emphasis on clinical problems.

Warkany, J.: Congenital Malformations. Chicago, Year Book Medical Publishers, 1971.

> Complete discussion of all birth defects from historical, embryologic, and etiologic viewpoints. Good discussions of familial patterns and risk of recurrence.

———: Syndromes. Am. J. Dis. Child. *121*:365, 1971.

3

Motor and Intellectual Development

David Baker, M.D., and Peter Vanace, M.D.

PRINCIPLES OF CHILD DEVELOPMENT

Development is an interacting dynamic process that begins with fertilization and is molded by genetic and environmental influences. Although genetic factors may be viewed as setting upper limits to development, bio-environmental factors figure powerfully in the expression of genetic influences and also may cause injury to the central nervous system and to somatic systems as well. In addition to these biological factors, socio-environmental and emotional factors play a major role in determining the outcome of development.

Development follows a dynamic sequential pattern with the time table varying not only in normal vs. abnormal individuals, but also reflecting individual differences between children. The newborn, equipped with innate instinctive reflex responses, develops in a pattern of cephalocaudal and proximodistal progression of function. The massive diffuse responses of the newborn become more differentiated with progressive myelination and inhibition from higher centers. Intersensory and sensorimotor integration emerge while synaptic connections are elaborated in the association cortex.

Genetic Factors

Genetic factors that influence development operate through a wide continuum including, on one extreme, conditions in which environmental factors are minimally involved and, on the other extreme, those in which environmental conditions are necessary to produce clinically evident alterations. Furthermore, because of variable penetrance and expressiveness, a wide spectrum of clinical manifestations may be seen.

31

For example, in a child with neurofibromatosis, severe mental retardation, convulsions, and sensorimotor signs may be seen as one extreme, while other members of the family may have cutaneous lesions only.

Genetic disorders can be of four types: (1) single gene defects transmitted by recessive or dominant inheritance (recessive disorders are related to inborn errors of metabolism, [enzyme defects], and may be autosomal or sex-linked, dominant genetic conditions are related to structural malformations); (2) polygenic defects resulting in familial retardation; (3) chromosome defects transmitted on autosomal or sex chromosomes; and (4) congenital malformations in which there is an empirical high risk of recurrence. These include meningomyelocele (neural tube defects) and some cases of hydrocephalus. Some genetic disorders only become clinically evident after birth (such as PKU), when the maternal metabolism is no longer available to metabolize the neurotoxic substance.

A careful family history, noting consanguinity especially, is of extreme importance. Laboratory tests necessary to ascertain genetic disorders are: (1) metabolic screening tests, (2) buccal smear and karyotypes, (3) enzyme studies, (4) dermatoglyphics, and (5) amniocentesis and examination of amniotic fluid for specific risk situations.

Environmental Factors

The environment exerts an influence that extends from preconception through pregnancy (intra-uterine environment) and continues postnatally. The infant who has an intact central nervous system and who is exposed to a nurturing, stimulating environment should grow and develop normally. Defects in development, then, may be related to impairment of the primary neural apparatus, to maturational lag or to an unfavorable environment. The normal infant will reach out to explore his environment and thus develop a sense of reality and mastery of tasks. Motility plays a vital part in development of the learning process.

Environmental stimulation as well as parental goals and expectations play a powerful role in shaping linguistic, intellectual, emotional and social functions in preparing the child for school experience (learning readiness). On the other hand, sensory and emotional deprivation (deprivation not only in terms of quantitative reduction of stimuli, but also in the qualitative sense of disordered, chaotic stimulation) may induce varying degrees of retardation which, if sustained early and for a prolonged period, may be irreversible. The child with a *pre-existing* visual, auditory or neurological handicap may suffer compounding increments of retardation with still further loss of developmental potential. Hence, such a child needs to be detected early and stimulated at the earliest possible age.

THE DEVELOPMENTAL EVALUATION

Clinical Assessment

The history follows a traditional format, but focuses on specific issues related to development. It begins with the reason for referral or the presenting complaints (perhaps the parents or the staff of the school noticed that the child was not developing normally). Obviously, the plan of workup depends upon the age of the child.

The prenatal and perinatal history should stress high-risk factors associated with developmental disabilities. This includes inquiry into the social environment (age and marital status of parents, living conditions), the prenatal environment (circumstances of this pregnancy, nature of prenatal care, the mother's health). The perinatal history should include complications and progress of labor and delivery. The neonatal history includes a thorough account of neonatal and maternal complications such as separation from a sick baby or postpartum depression.

A postnatal history is taken to elicit evidence of impaired development, such as poor feeding, hyper- or hypo-activity, and convulsions. The child with delayed developmental milestones is at high risk for developmental impairment, especially if the child does not sit alone before 9 months, does not walk or speak before 18 months, and does not form sentences before 3 years. A history of trauma, poisoning, or meningitis, encephalitis, or other severe infections should be noted. Some behavior patterns seen in retarded, deprived or disturbed children are rocking, head-banging, pica, breath-holding, temper tantrums, and unusual approaches to the environment, such as touching, tasting, or smelling objects (use of proximal sensory receptors rather than distal). These should be noted if they extend beyond the normal age.

Family history includes not only the age and health of all family members, and genetic aspects, but also the environmental background. Environmental stresses and the observed impact on the child should be noted.

Social history should include peer interaction and the ages of playmates (often younger or older than the patient).

The Physical Examination

After taking the history, a complete physical examination is performed, noting special points that may be related to the development of the child. Attempts should be made to examine the child before using instruments that might frighten him. The developmental examination may be done best prior to the general physical examination. The head, eyes, ears, nose and throat should be examined last.

The special points to be observed are: (1) general growth failure, and (2) morphologic stigmata of congenital defects and mental retardation.

The Neurological Examination

Accurate examination of the nervous system in infants and children is dependent upon the degree of relaxation and cooperation of the child. Thus, the first task of the examiner is to avoid frightening the child. It is best to make general observations and to observe how the child reacts to the parents, siblings and other children.

The general habitus and posture of the child can be observed. Weakness and hypotonia may also be evident during the child's spontaneous behavior. The examiner should note the activity of the child and his ability to shift and adjust to a change in stimulation (habituation and perseveration). Is the child alert, does he have an ability to focus, concentrate, and maintain attention span, or is he overly distractible? How does the child react to people? Does he withdraw, is he shy, does he have appropriate affect, does he maintain eye contact? Does he show an interest in his surroundings; does he show curiosity? On the other hand, does he appear to be unresponsive and indifferent to external stimuli? Many retarded, neurologically impaired or severely emotionally disturbed children have ritualistic, repetitive mannerisms. Occasionally there will be evidence of seizure activity, and it should be noted whether the child is responsive to external stimuli during seizure activity. In the child suspected of petit mal seizures, a 3- to 5-minute period of hyperventilation may evoke an absence spell.

The child's speech and communication skills, including non-verbal communication, should be observed. Is the child's thinking concrete; can he abstract and conceptualize?

Visual and hearing acuity should be assessed carefully. In the assessment of the cranial nerves, the visual fields should be checked by confrontation. Eye tracking movements should be noted. The immature response is for the head and eyes to move synchronously, but later, as the child matures, he initially moves his eyes with the head following after a brief interval.

Examination of the motor system includes assessment of muscle tone, bulk and strength. Changes in muscle tone may be elicited by changes in position. Subtle spasticity in the adductors of the hips and gastrocnemei become more evident when the child is held upright in vertical suspension. The muscles should be palpated for abnormal consistency, a condition seen in myopathies. Fasciculations and fibrillations should be noted, especially in the tongue. The examiner should also check for easy fatigability, myotonic phenomena and percussion myotonia.

Observe gross motor behavior, including the gait with normal walking, walking on tip-toes and walking on heels. Children with spastic diplegia myopathies and autistic children may prefer toe-walking. Heel-walking is difficult for the child with a spastic paresis or any condition that produces contractures of the ankles in plantar flexion. Ataxia should be noted. Associated arm-swinging movements should be observed, as they may give a clue to a subtle hemiparesis. In addition to walking on heels, many children with extrapyramidal involvement may show abnormal posturing. The child should be observed while standing.

Gross movements such as running, hopping on either foot and skipping should be observed. For the older boy who finds it embarrassing to skip, the examiner has noted that jumping jacks, with which school-age children are familiar, afford an opportunity to observe synchronized movements of the upper and lower extremities.

Fine motor activities can be observed while watching the child dress and undress. Buttoning and tying shoelaces may be extremely difficult for the child with subtle impairment of fine motor function.

Cerebellar signs such as rebound phenomenon, pendular reflexes, intention tremors, dysmetria and tandem walking should be observed.

The child should be observed while standing with feet together, arms outstretched in front of him, to the side, and upward to observe for jerking choreiform movements, abnormal posturing, motor impersistence and dystonia.

Visual motor coordination can be observed while the child copies geometric figures, writes, and performs manual construction skills.

Sensory examination includes not only assessment of primary sensory modalities, but also tests of higher sensory integration such as stereognosis, graphesthesia and finger agnosia. One should note the preferred eye, hand and foot. This may give a clue to a subtle hemiparesis or amblyopia. In addition, the child's sense of direction should be tested by having him point to his left ear with his right hand; with an older child, have him identify the right hand of the examiner when the examiner is facing the child.

"Soft" neurological signs are those that are truly indicators of development in that they are normal at a certain age, but disappear with maturation. They are not to be confused with "hard" neurological signs such as hemiparesis, cranial nerve palsy, sensory deficits, and asymmetric and pathological reflexes which are abnormal at any age. The soft neurological signs include the synkinesias (associated movements) and overflow movements, including choreiform-like movements of the upper extremities. The presence of these phenomena at an age when they should have disappeared suggests developmental immaturity of the nervous system and may be seen in children with so-called minimal brain dysfunction and children with learning disabilities.

Neurological Assessment of the Newborn and Young Infant

The infantile reflexes and automatisms are grouped into (1) inherent primitive responses, which wane during the first 3 to 4 months, and (2) secondary responses, which emerge later.

The primitive responses include general reactions (the Moro response and the asymmetric tonic neck reflex) and local responses (the righting response of the head, the primitive grasp of the fingers, and the forward movement of the arms when the baby is placed in the prone position). In the lower limbs, the local responses are the primitive grasp reflex of the toes, placing response of the lower limbs, and supporting and primary stepping responses. Asymmetry in the grasp reflex, in the placing and stepping reactions and in the Moro response may be of value in detecting or localizing an early hemiparesis.

The Moro reflex traditionally is elicited by lifting the infant's head 30 to 45° and allowing it to fall gently, but also may be elicited by lifting the baby slightly by the hands and releasing or by sudden jarring movements of the examining table and sudden auditory stimuli. The Moro reflex consists of two phases, the first of which is sudden symmetrical abduction and extension of all extremities. The second phase consists of a more gradual flexion and adduction movement of the extremities, with slight shaking movements. In addition to hemiparesis, injuries of the brachial plexus and various orthopedic disorders may cause an asymmetrical Moro response.

The asymmetric tonic reflex is elicited by rotating the head to one side. The ipsilateral (chin) arm will extend and the contralateral (occipital) arm will flex. An obligatory response, in which the infant is unable to change posture during elicitation of the reflex, is abnormal.

By 6 to 12 weeks, it should be possible to elicit all deep reflexes. A few beats of ankle clonus is permissible if present bilaterally, but unilateral sustained responses are abnormal. The plantar reflex is one of withdrawal simulating the Babinski reflex; there is extension of the great toe and there may be extension and fanning of the other toes as well. This response is normal up to age 2 years, but if present unilaterally in association with marked ankle clonus, spasticity or asymmetrical reflexes may be indicative of brain damage.

Other reflexes which reflect the immature development of the pyramidal pathways are the palmar and plantar grasp reflexes, the adductor spread of the knee reflex, and the crossed extension and automatic walking reflexes. These are basically spinal automatisms, or the so-called spinal defense reflexes.

The avoidance response is prepotent in early infancy and childhood. In the course of normal maturation, the avoidance response becomes integrated with the grasping automatisms to permit control of voluntary prehension. It may persist in the child with brain damage and produce abnormal postures and movements.

Another group of special reflexes of the newborn and young infant are the so-called postural and righting reflexes. One group of reflexes of posture and movement are independent of gravity. This includes the Moro reflex, the compensatory ("doll's eye") movements of the eyes when the head is shifted in position, postural reflexes including the tonic neck reflex, spinal or trunk incurvation reflex, and righting reflexes of the neck on the body and of the body on the head.

The postural reflexes dependent upon gravity include the labyrinthine reflexes of the head which orient the head with respect to the gravitational field and ultimately allow the infant to assume an upright position (bipedal) so that his arms are free to explore his surroundings. His head is held upright by 4 to 6 months and, subsequently, chain reflexes are involved in sitting and standing. Gravity-stimulated reflexes of station and gait are seen in the readiness to stand at 4 to 6 months; the infant extends his legs when the soles touch the horizontal surface and after 6 months has true supporting reactions of the legs.

The secondary responses, which appear at 4 to 7 months of age and persist to some degree, include the rolling, balancing and protective reactions.

The rolling response permits the infant to roll from supine to prone position. After the fourth month, the supine infant whose head is turned will exhibit the body-on-head and head-on-body righting response requisite for rolling over. The balancing (righting) reactions serve to right the head with respect to gravity and can be elicited by tilting the infant to one side.

Protective reactions include the propping and/or parachute reactions; these are reactions to acceleration forces. When the prone infant is thrust toward the examining table he extends both arms and fingers toward the table. The lateral propping reaction is elicited by suddenly tilting the baby (in a sitting position) to one side. The arm on that side will extend. It is necessary for the child to develop balancing and protective reactions in order to be able to walk.

The Landau reflex, which is seen from about 8 to 24 months, is based on the otolith and tonic neck reflexes. When the infant is held in a prone position parallel to the floor, he will dorsiflex his head and extend his spine so that the curve of the spine is convexly downward. If the head is ventriflexed, the vertebral column and extremities will flex, producing an upward convexity of the spine.

Associated or synkinetic movements are those which involve automatic movements of one part of the body in response to voluntary movements of other parts. They can be ipsilateral or symmetrical. These associated movements may be seen physiologically in infants in whom movements of one limb are accompanied by similar ("mirror") involuntary movements of the opposite limb. These gradually disappear with maturity (about age 9). They appear when learning new patterns of movements or during excessive physical or mental effort.

Although the simple reflex phenomena of the newborn are closely related to gestational age and are independent of birth weight, differences in motor behavior relating to phenomena which are more dependent on spinal integration and supraspinal control of motor neurons have been reported in babies small for gestational age.

Assessment of the newborn should include observations of the baby's cry, measurement of the head circumference and any abnormal cranial features, transillumination of the head, the character of spontaneous and provoked movements, the waking and sleeping pattern, estimations of alertness and abnormal muscle tone, and especially asymmetry in muscle tone.

Estimation of visual function in the newborn can be obtained by rotating the baby; this should produce deviation of the eyes in the direction of movement followed by nystagmus in the opposite direction when the movement ceases. Photic stimulation evokes eye-blink and pupillary reflexes. Opticokinetic nystagmus can be elicited by moving a striped cloth or a revolving drum. The baby can fix, follow, and be alert to the stimulus of a bright red ball 2 inches in diameter suspended 6 to 10 inches from his face.

The Infant and the Preschool Child

Assessment of developmental progress should be incorporated into the usual timetable of child care, but special notes should be made at certain

Table 3-1. Infantile Reflexes and Automatisms

Response	New-born	1	2	3	4	5	6	9	12
Primitive Responses									
Moro	+	+	+	70%	+	±	0	0	0
Rooting and sucking	+	+	+	+	+	+	+	0	0
Palmar grasp	+	+	+	+	+	0	0	0	0
Asymmetric tonic neck	+	+	+	50%	±	±	±	0	0
Plantar grasp	+	+	+	+	+	+	+	0	0
Placing	+	+	+	+	+	+	+	decreased but persists to 24 months	
Stepping	+	+	+	+	+	0	0	0	0
Supporting reaction	±	50%	+	+	+	+	66%	100% true supporting	
Secondary Responses									
Neck righting reactions									
Head	0	0	+	+	+	+	+	+	+
Body	0	0	0	+	+	+	+	+	+
Body derotative	0	0	0	0	+	+	+	+	+
Body rotative	0	0	0	0	0	0	0	+	+
Parachute reaction									
Downwards	0	0	0	0	+	+	+	+	+
Sideways (propping)	0	0	0	0	0	0	+	+	+
Forwards	0	0	0	0	0	0	0 (at 7 months)	+	+
Backwards	0	0	0	0	0	0	0	+	+
Landau	0	0	0	0	0	0	42%	+ to 24 months	+

key ages: 4, 16, 28, 40, and 52 weeks and 18, 24, 36, 48, and 60 months (Tables 3-1, 3-2, 3-3).

In the first year of life, motor achievements concur with the disappearance of primitive infantile reflexes and automatisms and the evolution of secondary responses. The persistence of primitive reflexes reflects CNS pathology, which will prevent normal maturation in motor areas.

Manual Dexterity. The development of manual dexterity illustrates the ontogeny of development. At 4 weeks of age, the hands are fisted, clench on contact (grasp reflex), but a rattle is not retained. At 8 weeks a rattle is retained briefly. The hands open by 12 weeks and by 16 weeks the arms activate when an object is regarded, and the infant reaches in a poorly coordinated fashion. The grasp then becomes palmar (24 weeks) to radial palmar (28 weeks) to radial digital (36 weeks) to scissors to inferior pincer (36 weeks) and pincer (40 to 48 weeks). The approach is at first two-handed (20 weeks), later one-handed (28 weeks). Transfer across the midline is a significant advance (28 weeks). The ability to handle multiple objects improves: one cube (20 weeks), two cubes (32 weeks) and three cubes (36 weeks). Voluntary releasing function appears at about 28 weeks—at the same time as transfer—and matures progressively (voluntary release at 40 weeks).

Increasing development of fine motor, visual motor coordination and perception can be tested in the preschool child by cube play (tower, bridge building), manipulation of pellet and bottle and the use of a crayon.

The School Age Child

Developmental assessment of school age children involves assessment of cognitive abilities, and testing is usually performed by psychologists. Developmental abnormalities are often related to problems of minimal brain dysfunction and learning disabilities, the typical presenting complaint being poor school performance despite intelligence within the normal range.

It should be noted that in childhood many central nervous system abnormalities are diffuse or global and do not produce focal abnormalities but rather signs of immature development in various spheres. Associated movements normally present in 3- to 4-year old children decrease with age and should disappear by 9 years. Mirror movements may be present until age 10 years. After age 3 years, the width of the gait should not exceed 11 to 20 cm. In children up to age 4 to 5 years, the plantar response may reveal inconsistent dorsiflexion and also fanning or spreading of the small toes.

Tests Used in Developmental Assessment

The Denver Developmental Screening Test (DDST) is the one most widely used by pediatricians. It is made up of 105 test items culled from 12 developmental and preschool intelligence tests. It is not an

Table 3-2. Events in Postural and Motor Development

Response	Newborn	1	2	Age in Months 3	4	5
Gross Motor						
Ventral suspension						
Head	hangs down		in plane of body	above body plane		
Extremities	flexor tone		extensor tone			
Prone position						
Head	to one side	lifts chin	midline to 45°	chin and shoulder up	head up 90°; chest up	rolls over prone to supine
Extremities	knees under abdomen			pelvis flat	extension	up on forearms
Sitting; traction from supine	head lag complete			slight head lag		no head lag
Standing and walking	automatic walk; legs flexed	diminished	absent		legs extend	legs straight
Fine Motor						
Manipulation of hands	grasp reflex; hands closed	grasp reflex	grasp reflex; hands open	diminished grasp reflex;	diminished grasp reflex; reaching	voluntary grasp; puts objects in mouth; bidextrous approach

"intelligence" test, however, and it does not establish a diagnosis. Its purpose is to screen children for the detection of deviation from normal development and to provide a baseline for further investigation of the problem.

Strict adherence to the instructions and interpretation of the DDST is necessary. Its use further requires that the child be retested in 1 month if the initial findings were abnormal and that suitable referral consistent with the overall clinical picture be followed.

Other commonly used developmental tests are the Stanford-Binet, the Wechsler, and the draw-a-man test.

LEARNING DISABILITY

A child may have a normal capacity or potential to perform but may be learning at reduced efficiency and, hence, underachieving. This may be due to factors involving general health, specific sensory disorders or reactive disorders related to the situation at home or in school. The child

Table 3-2. Events in Postural and Motor Development (continued)

		Age in Months			
6	9	12	15	18	24
pushes up on hands	crawls backward	bear walk	walking; kneeling		
lifts head from supine; sits propped; rolls over supine to prone at 7 months	sits without support	pivots	seats self in chair		
initial weight bearing	bears full weight; pulls to stand	walks with support at 11 months	walks without support at 13 months	up and down stairs; jumping	backwards; runs; kicks ball
palmar grasp radial at 8 months; transfer objects to opposite hand at 7 months	finger to thumb (pincer) grasp releases ± 10 months; unidextrous approach	throws	tower 2-3 cubes	tower 3-4 cubes; removes pellet from bottle; draw a stroke	tower 6-7 cubes; imitates circular stroke

may have a central nervous system problem that can result in global mental retardation, or he may have specific deficits interfering with learning, as in the case of the child with minimal brain dysfunction or the child with a learning disability. The examination may disclose hints of a seizure disorder or a neuromotor disorder.

Differential Diagnosis of Learning Disability

Many factors come into play when determining whether or not a child has a learning disability. Low overall intelligence or psychiatric disorders could be responsible. On the other hand, a child of normal intelligence might be suffering due to unreasonable demands and expectations on the part of parents or teachers. Culturally different children may appear to have a learning disability when confronted with a new school or learning situation.

A learning disability can be the result of a physical disability, either systemic, neurological, or sensory. Epilepsy, defects of special senses or rare neurological disorders can also manifest as a learning disability.

Table 3-3. Developmental Milestones: 2 to 5 Years

Age	24 months	36 mo.	48 mo.	60 mo.
Gross Motor	Runs, walks backwards Kicks large ball	Steps: Up: Alternates feet Balances one foot 2–5 sec.	Alternates feet up and down 4–8 Hops 2–8 times	Skips both feet, alternating 8–10 9–12 Skips alternating feet
		Throws ball one hand Rides tricycle	Overhand throw Catches ball	
Fine Motor	Cubes: tower of 6-7	9-10 Imitates bridge	Copies bridge Imitates gate	Serial finger to thumb sequencing movements; holds pencil in mature fashion
Adaptive	Inserts square block in performance board Imitates vertical stroke	Repeats 3 digits Matches 3 colors Copies circle	Counts 3 objects Copies a cross	Counts to 10 Copies square Knows morning, afternoon
Language: Vocabulary	200-300 words	900	1500 words	2000
Sentence Length	2 words	3 words	4 words	5 words
Articulation	Repetitions	90% intelligible		100% intelligible
Comprehension & syntax	Obeys one directional preposition* and 2 commands Identifies familiar objects	Uses we, us, you, I; 3 prepositions; names objects	Size labels. Numbers 1,2,3 and all; obeys 3 commands	4 prepositions Describes a picture
Personal-Social	Improved feeding; pulls on simple garment; mimics domestic tasks. Parallel play	Knows own name & sex; feeds self; unbuttons. Associative play	Washes and dries face; brushes teeth, laces shoes Cooperative play	Dressing self-sufficient Tells fanciful tales; plays games
Vision	Convergence-accommodation weak; may develop esotropia	V.A. 20/40. Test with Sjogren Hand Card, Illiterate E chart, STYCAR or Allen picture card test; Denver eye screening test	20/30	True stereopsis & color perception Tests with + lens for hyperopia
Developmental Neurological Signs				After 5, spooning of outstretched fingers is abnormal; can identify bilateral simultaneous visual stimuli.

*"On" or "under"

Language Disability

The language pathways begin at the peripheral receptive organ, and receptive language disorders occur when there is pathology of the peripheral auditory apparatus, including the middle ear (conductive hearing loss) or the inner ear and cochlear nerve (sensorineural loss) or its central connections. This may be very difficult to assess in the newborn or very young infant. A history of maternal exposure to rubella or a family history of hearing disorder mandates consultation with an experienced audiologist. The cortical-evoked response to sound stimuli and assessment of auditory reflexes may be useful in equivocal cases.

There are children who seem to have more difficulty with expressive than with receptive language; this group includes those with articulation difficulties and those who are immature in their syntactic construction of sentences. Such children respond better to speech therapy than do children who appear to have a central auditory imperception. Any child not using a few intelligible phrases or sentences by 30 months should be of concern to his physician.

In the differential diagnosis of the child who is not talking appropriately, the following must be considered:

1. Hearing loss, which may be due to conduction defects or sensorineural involvement and which may vary from mild to profound. The child who has a high frequency hearing loss may omit consonants.

2. Mental Retardation. Although it is true that delayed speech and language development is seen uniformly in children who prove to be mentally retarded, there are children with delayed speech and language development who may develop normal intellect.

3. Specific impairments of speech and language, either developmental or acquired.

4. Situational disorders, including multi-lingualism in the home, cultural differences, "private language of twins" and social and environmental deprivation.

5. Children who are severely emotionally disturbed, including autistic children.

6. Children with the inborn error, histidinemia.

In summary, the child who fails to respond to sound (and by 6 months of age this should be clearly ascertained; congenitally deaf children will make cooing and babbling sounds initially but then will cease to make progress) should be referred for audiological evaluation.

It is extremely important to have a proper hearing and speech evaluation of any child who is not developing properly. Often children may be misdiagnosed as having mental retardation or autism who, in reality, have an underlying hearing or language disturbance.

As there is no satisfactory technique for a routine hearing screening of all newborns, certain infants at risk for hearing impairment should be tested within 2 months after discharge from the nursery and at regular intervals thereafter. These infants include those with a genetic history of hearing impairment, rubella or other nonbacterial intrauterine fetal infections, congenital defects of the ears, nose and throat, birthweight less than 1500 g, and a bilirubin concentration that is potentially toxic.

Assuming that the integrity of the auditory pathway is intact, one should look into the environment of the child to see whether he is getting adequate stimulation and nurture; include here an assessment of the maternal-infant interaction. The development of speech and language needs to be related to other aspects of development to give clues as to whether one is dealing with a specific deficit in this area alone or whether it is part of a global retardation. Early intervention, including infant stimulation programs and speech therapy, should be considered. It would be better to over-refer such children to competent centers than the reverse.

Mechanical speech problems are not truly included in the group of language disorders but deserve early recognition and appropriate therapy. Disorders of articulation and phonation and anatomical disturbances such as cleft palate and severe malocclusions are commonly seen.

Functional speech problems such as stuttering, stammering and cluttered speech (other than the repetitions seen normally in the 2½- to 3-year-old) are characterized as dysfluency or disturbance in rhythm. Aberrations in intonation and regional variations (accent) are readily recognized.

Developmental Language Disabilities. The prognosis in the group with delayed speech but adequate comprehension may be favorable for the later development of speech, but these children may have language learning disabilities involving higher order processing of concepts. On the other hand, the child with language retardation who has *difficulty understanding language* and, therefore, cannot develop expressive speech has a poor prognosis. Such children may have structural abnormalities of the central auditory pathways and do not have the neurological substrate for decoding language symbols.

Acquired language disturbance is a concept implying that the child who was developing normally in the language area sustained an insult to the central nervous system, as a result of which he suffered a loss of these skills.

A word about the so-called plasticity of the nervous system may be appropriate. The left hemisphere is dominant for speech and language in almost all right-handed and in the majority of left-handed individuals. The cerebral hemispheres are equipotential for language development in the infant. If damage is sustained early in life to the dominant hemisphere there is the possibility of recovery with the nondominant hemisphere subserving language function. This may occur up to age 3 and even perhaps to age 8 or more years.

If the child sustains damage with retrograde amnesia, he will also suffer a loss of memory of previously learned material. Bilateral focal lesions involving the limbic system may cause this type of memory loss.

BIBLIOGRAPHY

General

Knobloch, H., and Pasamanick, B. (eds): Gessell and Amatruda's Developmental Diagnosis. 3d. ed. Hagerstown, Md., Harper & Row, 1975.

> This up-to-date revision of a classic work is an essential reference for the student who wishes to pursue the subject in depth. Background information is clearly presented with respect to normal development, major clinical disorders and detailed instructions for clinical evaluation.

Illingworth, R. S.: The Development of the Infant and Young Children, Normal and Abnormal. Baltimore, Williams & Wilkins, 1972.

> The author, a colleague and student of Gesell, discusses theoretical and practical issues in detail. Enjoyable and indispensable reading for anyone concerned with the care of children.

Meir, J.: Developmental and Learning Disabilities: Evaluation, Management and Prevention in Children. Baltimore, University Park Press, 1976.

> A remarkable compendium of basic developmental psychology and a concise overview of the subject with a complete bibliography.

Neurological Examination

Paine, R. S., and Oppe, T. E.: Neurological examination of children. *In* Clinics in Developmental Medicine, (Double Volume 20/21). London, Spastics Society and Wm. Heinemann, Ltd., 1966.

Prechtl, H., and Beintema, D.: The Neurological Examination of the Full-Term Infant. London, William Heinemann, Ltd., 1964.

Thomas, A., Chesni, Y., and Dargassies, S.: The Neurologic Examination of the Infant. London, National Spastics Society, 1960.

Tollwen, C. L., and Prechtl, F. R.: The neurological examination of the child with minor nervous dysfunction. *In* Clinics in Developmental Medicine, No. 38. London, Spastics International Publications and London, Wm. Heinemann, Ltd., 1970.

> These publications are unique in setting up criteria for systematic and standardized neurological examinations.

Developmental Screening

Brazelton, T. B.: Neonatal Behavioral Assessment Scale. London, William Heinemann, Ltd., 1973.

> A systematic approach for studying individual characteristics of the newborn, useful for counselling parents to anticipate and meet the needs of their infant.

Frankenberg, W. K.: Pediatric Screening Tests. Springfield, Ill, Charles C Thomas, 1976.

Frankenberg, W. K. *et al.*: The revised Denver Developmental Screening Test. J. Pediatr., 79:988, 1971.

> Authoritative discussion of the rationale and practical applications of screening tests by the mentor of the Denver Screening Test.

Schwartz, A. H., and Murphy, M. W.: Cues for screening language disorders in pre-school children. Pediatrics 55:712-722, 1975.

A useful summary and check-list for early detection of language disorders.

Minimal Brain Dysfunction

Clements, S. D., and Peters, J. E.: Minimal brain dysfunction in the school age child. Arch. Gen. Psy. 6:185-197, 1962.

This paper represents a milestone in formulating and popularizing the concept of MBD.

De La Cruz, F. F., Fox, B. H., and Robert, R. H.: Minimal brain dysfunction. Ann. NY Acad. Sci., *205*:1-396, 1973.

An excellent compilation of background papers with an exhaustive bibliography.

Learning Disorders

Denhoff, E., and Tarnapol, L.: Medical responsibilities in learning disorders. *In* Tarnapol, L. (ed.): Learning Disorders in Children. Boston, Little, Brown, 1971; pp. 65-118.

The author spells out procedures for evaluation and management of the child with a learning disorder.

Goldberg, H. K., and Schiffman, G. B.: Dyslexia. New York, Grune & Stratton, 1971.

Illuminates a very confusing field with factual material and clear thinking. A joint collaboration by an ophthalmologist and an educator.

Kinsbourne, M.: School problems. Pediatrics, *52*:697-710, 1973.

Provocative and exciting in terms of the keen insights the author conveys. Highly recommended for those who are skeptical about the role of the physician in this area.

Shain, R. J.: Neurology of Childhood Learning Disorders. Baltimore, Williams & Wilkins, 1972.

A "hard" neurological look at a "soft" subject and a monograph well worth reading.

4

Principles of Immunization

Hugh L. Moffet, M.D.

Immunization can be defined as an effort to prevent or modify natural infection by administration of antibody or antigen. Passive immunization is defined as the administration of antibody, either by intramuscular injection or by intravenous infusion. This temporary protection lasts as long as the antibody survives (half-life about 3 to 4 weeks).

Active immunization is defined as the administration of antigen as a killed microorganism, a component of a microorganism, or as a live, attenuated microorganism. Active immunization should provide permanent immunity by stimulation of the host to produce its own antibody, and other components of immunity.

ANTIBODY PREPARATIONS

Human Convalescent Plasma

This is plasma obtained from individuals recovering from a naturally occurring illness. For example, plasma obtained from an adult recovering from chickenpox may be useful in modifying or preventing chickenpox in a child with leukemia, if given shortly after the child is exposed.

Animal Hyperimmune Serum

This is serum obtained after active immunization of animals. For example, diphtheria antitoxin is produced by immunization of a horse with diphtheria toxoid. Animal hyperimmune sera, such as for rabies, have a high risk of serum sickness and anaphylactoid reactions; human hyper-immune serum is always preferable if it is available.

Immune Serum Globulin

This is the gamma globulin fraction obtained from unselected blood donors. It also has been called "gamma" globulin or "immune human" globulin. The type and quantity of antibodies present are variable, and depend on the past infections or immunizations of the donors. In past years, it could be assumed that ordinary gamma globulin contained antibodies protective against poliovirus, measles, and infectious hepatitis. In recent years, the preparations available usually have been titered to standardize the antibody content against measles.

Human Hyperimmune Globulin

This gamma globulin fraction is obtained from humans who have a very high titer of antibody. The source of these preparations can be individuals who have recovered from the natural illness (zoster immune globulin), or who have been immunized with a live virus (vaccinia immune globulin), a killed bacteria or virus (pertussis immune globulin or rabies immune globulin), or a toxoid (tetanus immune globulin).

Passive Immunity from Transplacental Antibodies

The very young infant is often protected by maternal antibodies which pass transplacentally from the pregnant woman to the fetus before birth. Only the smaller antibodies (IgG) pass the placental barrier. The duration of protection by transplacentally acquired antibodies depends on the initial concentration (titer) of antibodies of the mother. The antibody titer of transplacentally acquired antibodies then decreases gradually during the first year of the infant's life. Measles, tetanus, and polio are examples of diseases from which the infant is often protected for a variable period in the first year of life, usually about 6 months. Maternal antibodies can also prevent immunization of the infant by live vaccines, such as attentuated measles vaccine, until as late as 13 months of age.

ACTIVE IMMUNIZATION

The decision to use a vaccine should depend on a balance between the need for the vaccine and the risk of the vaccine (Fig. 4-1). These general principles are particularly important in the evaluation of the indications for use of new vaccines. The balance between need and risk may be shifted by changes in these factors, so that routine use of a vaccine may be discontinued, as in the case of smallpox vaccine. The balance between

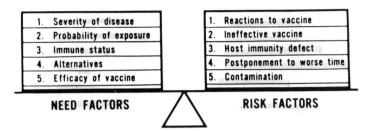

1. Severity of disease	1. Reactions to vaccine
2. Probability of exposure	2. Ineffective vaccine
3. Immune status	3. Host immunity defect
4. Alternatives	4. Postponement to worse time
5. Efficacy of vaccine	5. Contamination
NEED FACTORS	**RISK FACTORS**

Fig. 4-1. Need and risk factors in immunization. (From Moffet, H. L.: Pediatric Infectious Diseases, p. 409. Philadelphia, J. B. Lippincott, 1975.)

need and risk factors is a useful concept when explaining immunization of children to the parents.

NEED FACTORS

Severity of the Natural Disease

The severity is best defined in terms of the mortality rate or the damage done by the naturally occurring disease. Rabies is the most severe disease for which immunization is used, since it is virtually always fatal. In children, mumps and rubella are the least severe diseases for which live virus vaccines are available. However, the possible complications of orchitis in adult males and congenital rubella syndrome in the infant born to a pregnant woman with rubella make immunization desirable at some time before adulthood is reached.

Probability of Exposure

This depends on the degree to which the agent is contagious and the age, occupation, and geographic exposures of the patient. For example, there is a relatively high risk of exposure to measles in the United States, especially in areas where many children have not received adequate immunization.

Immune Status of the Individual

Although determination of a person's immune status is usually not convenient, it may be useful in several situations. For example, rubella antibodies should be measured before giving rubella vaccine to a woman of childbearing age because the vaccine is not necessary if antibodies indicate past natural infection. In addition, natural infection requires no boosters, and rubella vaccine possibly may require boosters if long-term studies indicate the need.

Alternatives to Immunization

Immunization is not the only method available to prevent infections, although few of the alternatives are superior.

Avoid Exposure. Some infections can be prevented by education of people to avoid unnecessary exposures. Measles is an example of the importance of the exposure factor. Measles may occur in infants between 6 months and 1 year of age, at a time when they have lost some or most of their transplacentally acquired maternal antibodies. If exposure to measles can be avoided, measles vaccine is usually postponed until 15 months of age when all maternal antibodies are gone; these antibodies may prevent infection and immunization by the vaccine.

Chemoprophylaxis. Antibiotics or other drugs can be given to persons in advance of any exposure and can effectively prevent infections, if directed at a specific pathogen. Chemoprophylaxis with erythromycin to prevent pertussis in an exposed susceptible sibling is an example.

Deliberate Exposure to Natural Disease. Controlled exposure is a possible method of protecting the person from a more severe form of infection. Examples include the past practice of deliberate exposure of susceptible individuals to rubella or mumps during childhood to avoid complications which may occur if these diseases are acquired as an adult. Deliberate exposure is not used now for these diseases, since the vaccine is less likely to produce complications in children than is the natural disease.

Effectiveness of the Available Vaccine

Sometimes a vaccine has limited effectiveness and may be used only for special needs. Typoid vaccine is an example of a vaccine with a limited need because of limited effectiveness.

RISK FACTORS

Contamination

Bacterial contamination is extremely unlikely in modern commercial vaccines, but viral contamination can occur. Administration of yellow fever vaccine stabilized with human serum contaminated with hepatitis virus resulted in an outbreak of viral hepatitis. There were about 28,000 cases and 62 fatalities in 1942, during World War II.

In 1973, 17 of 71 tested lots of live virus vaccines for polio, measles, mumps, and rubella contained bacteriophage. These viruses that infect bacteria usually come from the fetal calf serum used to support the growth of the cell cultures in which the vaccine viruses are grown. There has been no evidence that these bacteriophages have a harmful effect on humans. Endotoxin also has been detected in small quantities in some viral vaccines.

Virulent Vaccine

In 1969, an attenuated live measles virus vaccine used in Great Britain was withdrawn due to some cases of measles encephalitis which occurred immediately following administration of the vaccine.

Worsened Natural Disease

Early field trials of a killed respiratory syncytial virus vaccine indicated that more severe bronchiolitis occurred in immunized infants than in unimmunized. This was attributed to an antigen-antibody reaction between natural wild virus and serum antibodies.

Lack of Protection

This can be an unexpected risk. Use of live measles vaccine in the first year of life may not result in infection by the attenuated virus because of residual transplacentally acquired maternal antibodies. This may leave the infant unprotected against measles, and when the infant is exposed, unmodified measles may occur.

Postponement of Natural Disease to a Worse Time

This risk is largely theoretical. It has been suggested that mumps or rubella immunization in early childhood may postpone the natural disease until adulthood, at which time the complications of orchitis (mumps) or fetal infection (rubella) may occur. However, postponement of natural disease has not yet been observed.

Host Defects and Pregnancy

Existing disease in the host may result in complications from immunization. For example, eczema is a contraindication to smallpox vaccination because the affected skin may become extensively infected by the vaccinia virus. In addition, smallpox vaccination may produce progressive, and even fatal, disease in individuals with a defect of cellular immunity.

No live vaccine should be given during pregnancy. Immunosuppressive drugs or diseases are also important contraindications to immunization. Known or suspected hypersensitivity to a vaccine or one of its components is also a contraindication to the use of the vaccine.

Vaccine Reactions, Complications, or Side Effects

All vaccines contain small to moderate amounts of antigens other than the agent being immunized against. Most killed vaccines or toxoids are given in multiple doses; this can result in the development of hypersensitivity, with subsequent local or anaphylactoid reactions.

Some complications of attenuated virus vaccines are similar to effects of the wild virus but occur much less frequently than after the natural disease. These include the extremely rare complication of flaccid paralysis after poliovaccine, which may sometimes be related to an immunologic problem of the host. Rubella vaccine may produce arthritis, but with current vaccines this occurs less frequently than the arthritis after the natural disease.

Contagion

Some vaccines have a risk because the vaccine virus can be contagious. Vaccinia virus can be transmitted by direct contact with the inoculation site, so a child with eczema must be protected from exposure to another person with a recent smallpox vaccination.

EFFICACY

Efficacy of a vaccine can be quantitated by comparing the frequency of the illness in immunized and unimmunized individuals during an outbreak.

Indirect Efficacy (Herd Immunity)

Herd immunity refers to protection of a patient indirectly by reduction or prevention of exposure by immunization of the patient's contacts. If a very high percentage of a "herd" is immune, some diseases may not be transmitted to the susceptible individuals. This concept was used to predict that there should be significant protection of pregnant women; they are protected from exposure to rubella by immunization of children. However, recent observations have indicated that rubella spreads rapidly through exposed susceptibles even if 85 per cent of the group is immune. Furthermore, the concept of protection by herd immunity assumes random contacts, and does not apply to the non-random interaction that occurs between the many small groups in most societies.

Vaccine Failure

This can be defined as the occurrence of unmodified natural disease in vaccinated individuals. It can be a result of failure to include all important antigens in the vaccine, as has been observed in pertussis and influenza. It can be caused by inadequate preservation of the vaccine by deficient refrigeration or freezing, as has been observed for measles and smallpox vaccines. It can be caused by failure of the vaccine virus to infect the subject because of the presence of antibodies in the person being immunized, as has been observed after measles immunization in the first year of life.

Overattenuation

Some investigational vaccines have not been released because they have been overattenuated by too many passages in tissue culture and fail to produce an adequate frequency of infection in subjects. In the case of rubella vaccine, the vaccine has been attenuated enough to be noncontagious, but is not so overattenuated that it fails to infect the subject. It is possible that this desired degree of attenuation found in the final vaccines available may be appropriate for most hosts, but it may represent overattenuation for a few.

PRACTICAL PROBLEMS

Availability of Vaccine

The first vaccine available usually gets the most early use. Killed virus vaccines usually have been available before live vaccines, as in measles, poliovirus, and mumps vaccines. The first vaccine tends to get a safety record established and continues to be used more often until the newest vaccine has been proved better in some way.

Cooperation of Susceptible Groups

Social factors are extremely important in immunization. Some socioeconomic or ethnic groups are notoriously underimmunized, either because the vaccine is not available, or the individual will not accept immunization, even when offered without charge. The physician should always be alert for the opportunity to immunize susceptible children; this often can be done when the child is seen during convalescence from another illness. Minor respiratory symptoms should not be used as a reason to defer immunizations in infancy if the physician knows that the child is usually not seen for supervisory health care. Unfortunately, any immunization given during a prodrome of a serious illness is likely to be blamed for the illness. Viral interference between vaccines is not a practical problem.

The major emphasis of immunization programs in the United States should now be the identification and immunization of susceptible subgroups. An immunization program directed at susceptible people is more important than mass programs which may give repeated immunization to cooperative people who may already have had the vaccines. Recent antibody surveys indicate that many young children in lower socioeconomic groups have no protective antibodies against polio or measles; increased efforts are necessary to reach these children.

Immunization Schedules

Often used by physicians, particularly for infants (Tables 4-1 and 4-2), these schedules need to be revised every few years because of the introduction of new vaccines or modified vaccines, or newly recognized side effects of vaccines. Unfortunately, the complexity of such schedules tends to make the physician overlook the general principles involved. It

Table 4-1. Recommended Schedule for Active Immunization of Normal Infants and Children

2 mo	DTP[1]	TOPV[2a]
4 mo	DTP	TOPV
6 mo	DTP	[2b]
1 yr		Tuberculin Test[3]
15 mo	Measles,[4] Rubella[4]	Mumps[4]
1½ yr	DTP	TOPV
4–6 yr	DTP	TOPV
14–16 yr	Td[5]—repeat every 10 years	

[1] DTP—diphtheria and tetanus toxoids combined with pertussis vaccine.
[2a] TOPV—trivalent oral poliovirus vaccine. This recommendation is suitable for breast-fed as well as bottle-fed infants.
[2b] A third dose of TOPV is optional but may be given in areas of high endemicity of poliomyelitis.
[3] Frequency of repeated tuberculin tests depends on risk of exposure of the child and on the prevalence of tuberculosis in the population group. For the pediatrician's office or outpatient clinic, an annual or biennial tuberculin test, unless local circumstances clearly indicate otherwise, is appropriate. The initial test should be at the time of, or preceding, the measles immunization.
[4] May be given at 15 months as measles-rubella or measles-mumps-rubella combined vaccines (see Rubella, section 9, and Mumps, section 9, for further discussion of age of administration).
[5] Td—combined tetanus and diphtheria toxoids (adult type) for those more than 6 years of age, in contrast to diphtheria and tetanus (DT) toxoids which contain a larger amount of diphtheria antigen. *Tetanus toxoid at time of injury:* For clean, minor wounds no booster dose is needed by a fully immunized child unless more then 10 years have elapsed since the last dose. For contaminated wounds, a booster dose should be given if more than 5 years have elapsed since the last dose.

Concentration and Storage of Vaccines
  Because the concentration of antigen varies in different products, the manufacturer's package insert should be consulted regarding the volume of individual doses of immunizing agents.
  Because biologics are of varying stability, the manufacturer's recommendations for optimal storage conditions (e.g., temperature, light) should be carefully followed. Failure to observe these precautions may significantly reduce the potency and effectiveness of the vaccines.
  (Report of the Committee on Infectious Diseases, American Academy of Pediatrics, 1977.)

is important to be aware of the principles of immunization and avoid the rigidity of schedules if they become outdated.

The most important single principle in the immunization of any person is to adapt the schedule to the person's particular needs and risks.

Immunization Records

Records kept by the patient or parent are extremely important and in the past have been greatly neglected by many physicians and patients. Such records are useful in reminding the patient of the need for immunizations, and in preventing unnecessary treatment; they can be used as a record of allergies, chronic illnesses, or medications.

Excessive Immunization

The risks of excessive immunization are primarily related to allergic reactions, although any *unnecessary* immunization producing an untoward reaction can be regarded as excessive. Several vaccines and situations are often unnecessary. Paratyphoid vaccine is not indicated in the United States. Typhoid vaccine has no indications in the United States,

Table 4-2. Primary Immunization for Children not Immunized in Early Infancy

Under 6 Years of Age	
First visit	DTP, TOPV, Tuberculin Test
Interval after first visit	
1 mo	Measles,† Mumps, Rubella
2 mo	DTP, TOPV
4 mo	DTP, TOPV‡
10 to 16 mo or preschool	DTP, TOPV
Age, 14–16 yr	Td–repeat every 10 yr
6 Years of Age and Over	
First visit	Td, TOPV, Tuberculin Test
Interval after first visit	
1 mo	Measles, Mumps, Rubella
2 mo	Td, TOPV
8 to 14 mo	Td, TOPV
Age, 14–16 yr	Td–repeat every 10 years

*Physicians may choose to alter the sequence of these schedules if specific infections are prevalent at the time. For example, measles vaccine might be given on the first visit if an epidemic is underway in the community.

†Measles vaccine is not routinely given before 15 months of age (see Table 1).

‡Optional.

(Report of the Committee on Infectious Diseases, American Academy of Pediatrics, 1977)

except in a household exposure to known typhoid fever, or in travel to an area where there is an outbreak of typhoid fever. It is unnecessary for people in flooded areas or for those taking camping trips.

Tetanus toxoid boosters should not be given routinely each year for the convenience of summer camps. Rabies vaccine is seldom if ever indicated for rodent bites. Skunks (which are not rodents), however, have a high risk of transmitting rabies. Combinations of live virus vaccines, such as rubella and measles, should not be given if the patient needs only one of the vaccines.

VACCINES COMMONLY USED

DPT

This vaccine contains diphtheria and tetanus toxoids and killed pertussis bacteria. Pertussis is the most likely component to produce hypersensitivity reactions such as fever, local pain and swelling. Encephalopathy is a very rare complication of pertussis immunization. Pertussis vaccine is not recommended for use after 6 years of age, because then the risks of hypersensitivity reactions are thought to exceed the need for protection against pertussis (which can produce serious disease or even death in infants and young children).

Routine tetanus toxoid boosters are given every 10 years after the initial series of five injections with DPT. Whether or not an "emergency" tetanus toxoid booster is recommended after injury depends on the severity and contamination of the wound, and the number and timing of past doses of tetanus toxoid. In equivocal situations, a dose of 0.1 ml. of toxoid is as effective as the usual 0.5 ml. and is less likely to produce a local reaction. Human tetanus immune globulin should be given if the patient has had no previous toxoid, and has a deep puncture or other significant wound.

Poliovaccine

Poliovaccine provides excellent protection against one of the dread diseases of the past. The live attenuated vaccine virus is excreted in the feces of immunized children and can infect exposed susceptible contacts. Paralytic disease is very rarely caused by the vaccine virus and sometimes an immunologic defect can be detected in the individuals who develop paralysis. Whether or not this risk of paralysis is greater than the need for the vaccine depends on the risk of exposure to wild poliovirus. Very likely the severity of the natural disease would be much worse than paralysis from the vaccine, if the susceptible person were exposed to the wild virus.

Measles

This is a very important vaccine, because the risk of naturally occurring measles virus infection is significant and often results in brain damage or death. Because the disease is very contagious, exposed children will contract measles if they are not immunized by past infection or immunization. Very rarely will a child who has received measles vaccine develop a progressive fatal encephalitis 2 to 10 years later. This subacute sclerosing panencephalitis is a rare late complication of naturally occurring measles. It is possible that children who develop this complication after vaccine do so because of naturally occurring measles in the first year of life that was made milder by maternal antibodies and was not recognized as measles.

Rubella

This vaccine is used to prevent fetal damage by direct administration to susceptible but non-pregnant females. It also is given to male children so they will not be a source of wild rubella exposure to susceptible pregnant woman (who should have been immunized but have not been). Immunization of male children also protects them against complications of rubella infection, such as arthritis and the rare complication of encephalitis.

Mumps

This vaccine appears to produce minimal discomfort and no serious complications. Although the need to protect children from naturally occurring mumps virus infection is limited to prevention of aseptic meningitis and perhaps a few rare complications, this need appears to exceed the very low risk of the vaccine. The skin test is not useful as a guide to susceptibility of adults.

Rabies

The availability of duck embryo vaccine and human rabies immune globulin has made rabies immunization much less of a risk than when horse serum and nervous system (Semple) vaccine were used. The decision to use rabies vaccine or globulin is quite complicated; current guidelines should be consulted for most situations.

Vaccines for Foreign Travel

The Center for Disease Control guidelines should be consulted for most recent recommendations for specific countries.

BIBLIOGRAPHY

Center for Disease Control: Health information for international travel. Morbidity Mortality Weekly Report 26 (Suppl.):1-97, 1977.

Very useful guide for travellers. It is revised each year.

Levine, M. M., Edsall, G., and Bruce-Chwatt, L. J.: Live-virus vaccines in pregnancy. Risks and recommendations. Lancet, 2:34-38, 1974.

A review of data on vaccines in pregnancy.

Moffet, H. L.: Pediatric Infectious Diseases: A Problem-Oriented Approach. Chapter on Immunization. Philadelphia, J. B. Lippincott, 1975.

A detailed discussion of general principles and specific need and risk factors for each vaccine.

Report of the Committee on Infectious Diseases. Evanston, Illinois, American Academy of Pediatrics, 1974, 1977.

The "Redbook." Authoritative recommendations, revised about every 3 years.

Wilson, G. S.: The Hazards of Immunization. University of London, Athlone Press, 1967.

A broad and historical approach to complications of immunization.

5

Feeding

Lewis A. Barness, M.D.

A limited number of guidelines is necessary for the feeding of low birth weight infants, term infants and older children. A few principles of infant nutrition help to determine how these have been formulated.

The natural food of term infants is human milk. While certain formulas have been developed that can lead to more rapid growth in infants than those breast fed, no formula has ever been shown to be superior to human milk for the human infant. Most of the newer formulas have been developed to simulate human milk.

Certain aspects of breast feeding have not yet been approached by artificial feeds. Among these are the low incidence of allergy, the presence of antibodies to common viruses, the high biological value of the protein, the low electrolyte content, the favorable calcium:phosphorus ratio to produce high calcium absorption, and probably other factors not yet delineated. Nursing in the postpartum period helps the mother contract the uterus.

Aspects of artificial feeding that have been developed to approach human milk include lowering of the saturated fat in artificial milks, increasing the unsaturated fat, lowering of the protein and salt content to

Table 5-1. Composition of Human Milk, Simulated Human Milk, and Cow's Milk Formulas

Nutrient (per dl.)	Human Milk	Simulated	Cow's Milk
Calories	67	67	65
Protein	0.8–1.1	1.5	3.5
Carbohydrate (Lactose)	7	7	4.5
Fat	3.5	3.5	3.5
Minerals	0.2	0.3–0.7	0.7–0.9

approach human milk, providing the carbohydrate almost entirely as lactose, and in some, adjusting the calcium:phosphorus ratio.

Most term infants gain satisfactorily for the first half-year if they consume 90–120 cal./kg. and 150–200 ml./kg./day. Thus, the caloric and water requirements are both met with 150–200 ml./kg./day of breast milk or formula.

Wide variation in the requirements of infants may be due not only to the variability of infants and their families but also to metabolic factors that are not well defined.

BREAST FEEDING

Breast feeding can be successfully accomplished by most mothers if support is given during the first weeks. Mothers are encouraged to feed from both breasts during the first week, 10 minutes on each side, and then to alternate breasts. The baby should be fed if crying or hungry; intervals should be 3 to 5 hours with six feedings a day for the first month. Generally, during the second month, the 2 a.m. feeding can be stopped, and by the fifth month, the 10 p.m. feeding can cease so that the baby is fed four times a day. The back should be patted every 10 minutes to burp the baby, helping him to get rid of swallowed air.

Vitamins should be added at about the fifth day; a multivitamin preparation which delivers 30 mg. of vitamin C and 400 IU. of vitamin D is satisfactory. In areas where the water supply is not fluoridated, the same preparation should contain approximately 0.25 mg. of fluoride.

Solid feedings may be begun at 10 weeks to 4 months of age. Because they may have increased caloric density, the likelihood of early obesity is increased. The baby's extrusion reflex, the reflex which causes the baby to push out any material on the anterior third of the tongue, normally disappears at about 6 weeks to 3 months of age.

No more than one new food should be introduced a week. If reaction occurs, the food should not be offered again for 3 months. Foods with the least allergenicity should be offered first. Although the infant is born with apparently normal intestinal trypsin and lipase and deficient amylase, customarily cereal is introduced early.

A typical feeding schedule is:

6:00 a.m.	breast
10:00 a.m.	breast
2:00 p.m.	breast
6:00 p.m.	breast
10:00 p.m.	breast
2:00 a.m.	breast

Offer water twice daily and add vitamins at five days.

At 1 month omit the 2 a.m. feeding. At 10 weeks to 4 months add rice cereal, 2 tablespoons in diluted form at 10 a.m. and 6 p.m. Add fruits, ⅓–½ jar or equivalent at 2 p.m. (apples, pears, peaches) when the baby is 4 months old. At 5 months add meats, ⅓–½ jar or equivalent at 2 p.m. (beef, lamb, liver). Vegetables can be added at 6 months: ⅓–½ jar or equivalent at 6 p.m. (peas, beans, carrots). Omit the 10 p.m. feeding. Add an egg yolk at the 10 a.m. feeding when the baby is 7 months old. At 8 months "chewy" foods (e.g., Zweibach, cottage cheese) can be added. Change to junior foods and wean to a cup at 9 months. An egg white can be added at 12 months.

BOTTLE FEEDINGS

At present, available evidence indicates that breast feeding remains the superior feeding for human infants. While evaporated milk formulas are somewhat cheaper than the simulated formulas, the next most desirable form of infant feeding, according to current information, is a simulated human milk formula. The more nearly it approaches the composition of human milk, the better. Life and growth are, at present, measurements of a baby's well-being; in developed countries there does not seem to be a difference among those fed human milk, cow's milk, or simulated human milk formulas. However, as measurement techniques improve other more subtle differences, such as those below, indicate that one or another feeding is more desirable. These include: decreased infections, repair of injury, avoiding special disease states, imprinting for high sodium diets, allergies, mental status, learning ability, hyperkinesis, onset of degenerative diseases.

Simulated human milks are diluted to contain 67 cal./100 ml. and are fed as human milk to provide 150–200 ml./kg./day in divided feedings. These formulas contain sufficient vitamins so that no vitamin supplements are given. If fluoridated water is not used for diluting the formula, give the baby fluoride drops daily.

Satisfactory evaporated milk formulas can be made with one ounce of evaporated milk per lb./day. Sugar is added to make a 5 per cent addition, e.g.:

10 lbs. (5 kg.)		cal.	13 lbs. (6.5 kg.)		cal.
E.M.	10 oz.	400	E.M.	13 oz.	520
Sugar	1½ oz.	180	Sugar	1 oz.	120
Water	20 oz.	0	Water	17 oz.	0
		580			640

Formulas should be sterilized and kept in the refrigerator.

OLDER INFANTS AND CHILDREN

Calories

The daily caloric requirement decreases to 80–120 cal. at 1 year. A simple estimate for the caloric requirement past 1 year is:

1000 cal + age in years x 100 cal

This is only an estimate and most children adjust caloric requirements to need. The doctor should check that weight gain is satisfactory but not excessive.

Much has been written about the type of diet a child should eat. Presently, factual dietary advice goes no further than providing a balanced diet which includes:

4 daily servings of colored vegetables, fruits

2 or more daily servings of meat, eggs, fish, liver

4 or more daily servings of cereal, bread

not more than 1 pt. daily from the milk group

These diets should provide sufficient calories, and will contain sufficient known vitamins if the foods are not overcooked. Excess milk may decrease intake of necessary foods, decrease iron absorption, and provide a high saturated fatty acid diet.

Vitamins and Minerals

The Recommended Daily Dietary Allowances of the NAS-NRC (1974) are found in Table 5-1. Vitamins are necessary for a number of biochemical and biological effects. (See Table 5-2.)

Minerals are also required; these minerals, with their major function and manifestations are listed in Table 5-3.

DEFICIENCY AND EXCESS STATES

Calories

Caloric deficiency, a form of starvation, is probably the leading cause of failure to thrive in young children. In severe states it is known as marasmus. Causes include emotional problems and educational defects in the family.

In addition, calorie requirements may be elevated or calories may be lost. If these increased requirements are not met, signs of deficiency become obvious: failure to gain, weight loss, failure to grow, failure of chest circumference to increase, wasting of buttocks, cheeks, and fat pads, failure of head circumference to increase.

Increased caloric requirements are seen in hypermetabolic states: fever, emotional distress, infection, hyperthyroidism, renal disease, heart dis-

Table 5-2. United States Recommended Daily Allowances of Vitamins and Minerals

	Unit	Infants (0–12 mo.)	Children under 4 yrs.	Adults & children 4 or more years	Pregnant or lactating women
Vitamin A	IU	1500	2500	5000	8000
Vitamin D	IU	400	400	400	400
Vitamin E	IU	5	10	30	30
Vitamin C	mg	35	40	60	60
Folic acid	mg	0.1	0.2	0.4	0.8
Thiamine (B$_1$)	mg	0.5	0.7	1.5	1.7
Riboflavin (B$_2$)	mg	0.6	0.8	1.7	2.0
Niacin	mg	8	9	20	20
Vitamin B$_6$	mg	0.4	0.7	2	2.5
Vitamin B$_{12}$	mcg	2	3	6	8
Biotin	mg	0.05	0.15	0.3	0.3
Pantothenic acid	mg	3	5	10	10
Calcium	g	0.6	0.8	1.0	1.3
Phosphorus	g	0.5	0.8	1.0	1.3
Iodine	mcg	45	70	150	150
Iron	mg	15	10	18	18
Magnesium	mg	70	200	400	450
Copper	mg	0.6	1.0	2.0	2.0
Zinc	mg	5	8	15	15

ease, hypothalamic lesions, ectodermal dysplasia, hemolytic anemia, other anemia states, drug ingestion.

Wasting of calories occurs with: celiac disease, cystic fibrosis, renal disease, antibiotic administration, ulcerative colitis, regional enteritis, diarrheal states, iron deficiency, diabetes.

Calorie excess occurs when caloric intake is greater than calorie utilization and waste. Excessive calorie intake can result in vomiting, diarrhea or obesity.

Causes of excessive calorie intake and obesity are not well understood. Some causes include: familial patterns, habit, ? genetics, hypothalamic lesions, rapid growth *in utero*, rapid growth in first few months, familial emotional problems, patient emotional problems, infections (resulting in bed rest), social factors, hypothyroidism, sedation.

Protein Deficiency

When caloric requirement is almost sufficient but protein intake is low, weight loss may not be too prominent. In severe form, kwashiorkor occurs. Symptoms and signs include: lethargy, hyperactivity, distended abdomen, skin rash, decreased hair coloration, low serum proteins, anemia, edema, diarrhea, frequent infections.

In children consuming a high carbohydrate, low protein diet, multiple deficiencies occur. Excessive protein intake is described below.

Table 5-3. Summary of Vitamins in Nutrition

Vitamin	Manifestation	Function	Source	Test
A		Rhodopsin formation Epithelialization Lysomal instability	Fish liver oil Carotene containing vegetables	
Deficiency	Failure to gain, vaginitis, bronchitis, etc. Bitot's spots, xerophthalmia, Night blindness, Keratinization			Blood level Flicker fusion
Excess	Carotenemia, hepatospleno-megaly, anemia, coarse hair, periosteal swelling, pseudo-tumor cerebri, hypercalcemia			
B_1 (Thiamine) deficiency	Beriberi, neuritis, edema, cardiomegaly	Cocarboxylase	Cereals, meats, legumes	Lactate-pyruvate ratio, urine excretion
B_2 (Riboflavin) deficiency	Conjunctivitis, glossitis, cheilosis, dermatitis, keratitis	Coenzymes, flavin enzymes	Eggs, milk, yeast	Excretion
Niacin deficiency Toxicity-vascular dilatation	Pellegra, diarrhea, dermatitis, dementia	Coenzymes: NAD, NADP	Liver, meat, eggs	Therapeutic
Pantothenic acid	?	Coenzyme A	Liver	
Pyridoxine (B_6) deficiency	Anemia, polyneuritis, seizures, dermatitis	Coenzyme Transaminases	Yeast, meat, cereal	Therapeutic, blood
Biotin deficiency	? Dermatitis, ? neuritis	CO_2 fixation	Liver	Blood propionate
Inositol	? Fatty liver	Phospholipid formation	Grain	
Folic acid	Macrocytic anemia	Purine precursor	Yeast, vegetables	Blood, forminibo-glutamin acid excretion
B_{12} deficiency	Pernicious anemia, B_{12} neuropathy	Methylation	Liver, animal protein	Methylmalonic acid excretion
Choline deficiency	Fatty liver	Methylation	Yeast	
C deficiency	Scurvy, hemorrhage, irritability, pseudopara-lysis, spongy gums, rosary	Collagen formation	Fruit juice	Blood level, radiograph Tourniquet
D deficiency	Rickets, craniotabes, rosary, large fontanelle, tetany	Mineralization, calcium absorption	Fish liver oil, sunlight	Radiograph, blood phosphorus, phosphatase
Excess	Calcification of soft tissues, kidneys, pallor weakness, anorexia			Calcinuria, albuminuria
E	Hemolysis in premature	? Respiratory enzyme	Vegetables	
K deficiency	Hemorrhagic disease	Prothrombin formation	Fish meal	Prothrombin time

Table 5-4. Minerals and Their Functions

Mineral	Major function	Deficiency	Excess
			Clinical Manifestations
Sodium	Osmotic regulation	Weakness Hypotension Convulsions	Edema Hypertension Intracranial bleed
Potassium	Intracellular enzyme activity	Weakness Heart failure Alkalosis	Paralysis Heart block Alkalosis
Chloride	Osmotic regulation	Similar to sodium	
Calcium	Bone metabolism Nerve conduction	Tetany Seizures	Renal failure Aberrant ossification
Phosphorus	Bone metabolism Energy transfer enzymes	Weakness Bone pain	Hyperparathyroidism Hypocalcemia
Magnesium	Electric potential Intracellular enzymes	Seizures Neuritis	Catharsis Paralysis
Iron	Hemoglobin formation	Anemia	Hemosiderosis
Copper	Enzymes, collagen formation	Anemia Skeletal defects	
Iodine	Thyroid function	Hypothyroidism	Hyperthyroidism? Skin lesions
Fluorine		Caries	Hypoglycemia Bone lesions
Zinc	Major metabolic enzymes	Hypogonadism Failure of wound Healing	
Chromium	Glucose metabolism	Diabetes?	
Cobalt	Vitamin B_{12}	Anemia	
Manganese	Enzymes	Bone defects	
Molybdenum	Xanthine oxidase		

Essential Fatty Acids

Small amounts of long-chain polyunsaturated fats cannot be formed in humans. Deficiency results in seborrhea-like skin rash and failure to grow (probably due to inefficient utilization of calories).

Fat and Carbohydrate

Since these are the main sources of utilizable calories, deficiency signs may be restricted to those of calorie deficiency or, if calories are supplied as protein, of protein intoxication. These include: lethargy, hyperammonemia, abnormal liver function tests, asterixis, failure to gain, diarrhea. Signs of excess are those of calorie excess.

Water

While man may be able to live 40 days without food, he cannot live more than 2 to 3 days without water. Dehydration in infants is always a critical problem, requiring immediate attention.

Excessive water ingestion results in water intoxication. Signs include: weight gain, edema, decreased serum electrolytes, seizures, anuria-oliguria, heart failure, signs of increased intracranial pressure.

Causes of increased water intake may be: iatrogenic—excessive or improper parenteral fluids, psychogenic, or caused by heat.

PROBLEMS RELATED TO FEEDING

Colic

The symptoms of colic are paroxysmal crying and drawing up of the legs—symptoms apparently associated with pain. The cause is unknown, but factors which produce this complex include: overfeeding, underfeeding, tension or other psychological factors, food allergy or intolerance, peritonitis, incarcerated umbilical or inguinal hernia, eyelash in the eye.

Holding the infant or placing warmth over the abdomen may relieve symptoms. Medications or formula changes do not help. The condition usually disappears by three months.

Constipation

Constipation refers to hard stools. Stools can be softened by increasing dietary carbohydrates. However, rectal examination may reveal tight anal sphincter or megacolon. Tests for hypothyroidism and observation for dehydration or underfeeding may be indicated.

BIBLIOGRAPHY

Fomon, S.: Infant Nutrition. 2nd ed. Philadelphia, W. B. Saunders, 1974.

One of the few available books on infant nutrition which gives some of the bases of current feeding practices.

6

Fever

J. Martin Kaplan, M.D., and T. F. McNair Scott, M.D.

THE CLINICAL PROBLEM

A child is often brought to the physician because the parent believes "he has a fever." Under these circumstances, the physician should ascertain what is considered fever. There are several possibilities.

A parent's understanding of "normal" for the three common methods of determining the temperature must be determined. For children over the age of 5, the oral route is usually preferred. The thermometer is placed under the tongue for 4 minutes while the lips are closed; "normal" is 37° ±0.3 C (98.6°F). Rectal temperatures are utilized for younger children. The lubricated thermometer is placed in the rectum for 4 minutes; "normal" equals 37.6° ±0.3 C (99.6°F). Axillary temperatures are taken only when the rectal route is impractical (e.g., imperforate anus, diarrhea). Parents will sometimes use it when they are hesitant to try the rectal method. The thermometer is placed under the arm which is held close to the trunk; in this case, "normal" is 36.5° ±0.3 C (97.6°F). Deviations from the normal occur for various reasons and require an understanding of the physiology of temperature control. These deviations will be discussed later in the chapter.

TEMPERATURE CONTROL

The naked body is able to maintain its temperature at or about 37° ±0.6 C in environmental temperatures ranging from 16°–55°C. This stability is maintained by a continuous balance between heat loss, mainly through the skin and lungs, and heat production by the muscles and liver. The entire system is under the control of a "thermostat" in the hypothalamus.

Heat Loss

Twenty-five per cent of heat generated is normally dissipated by evaporation of water from the body surface and lungs; the remainder is lost by radiation (60 per cent), convection (12 per cent) and conduction (3 per cent). Any rise in temperature above 37°C (98.6°F) sets the mechanism of heat loss in motion. Centrally, in the hypothalamus, there is a simultaneous inhibition of vasoconstriction and activation of the sympathetic innervation to the sweat glands. This leads to dilatation of the peripheral vessels and increased moisture from sweat. With the increment in vapor pressure from heat generated by peripheral vasodilatation, there is a rise in insensible losses (1°C elevation in temperature increases insensible losses by 10 per cent); a further dissipation of body heat takes place by evaporation of sweat.

Heat Conservation and Generation

Heat conservation or generation start after a drop of temperature below 37°C (98.6°F). The body responds either by decreasing heat loss or by activating heat production.

A decrease in heat loss is accomplished in two ways: (1) Allowing peripheral vasoconstriction to occur under the influence of the sympathetic areas in the hypothalamus by turning off the previously mentioned active inhibition of this mechanism; or by (2) concurrently diminishing cholinergic stimulation of sweat glands, thus decreasing water evaporation from the skin. Heat production is activated by shivering or chemical thermogenesis. Shivering can increase heat production by 500 per cent. It results when the inhibition of the primary motor center in the dorsomedial area of the posterior hypothalamus is shut off, leaving the motor center to be driven by signals from cold sensors in the skin and spinal cord. Chemical thermogenesis accounts for a 50 per cent increase in heat production, and is the result of increased cell metabolism in the muscles and the liver which is initiated by the action of centrally released norepinephrine. There is also a small contribution from the thyroid, secondary to an increase of thyroid releasing factor. These control mechanisms can be modified by age, transitory physiologic factors and disease.

Age. Neonates exposed to a cold environment will drop their core temperature more rapidly than a 2- or 3-month-old infant. A chilled newborn becomes restless but cannot shiver; heat production is not regulated by increased metabolism of muscles and liver but by the breakdown of "brown fat." This tissue begins to form at about 26 to 30 weeks of gestation and reaches its peak 3 to 5 weeks postpartum. Though a major collection is found between the scapulae, there are deposits along the major blood vessels and the perinephric region. The thermolability of the neonate is enhanced by the facility for heat loss provided by the large surface area/weight (SA/wt) ratio and the small amount of subcutaneous (yellow) fat. For the premature, these factors are exaggerated, because of less "brown fat," less subcutaneous fat and greater SA/wt ratio.

In the older infant and child, the importance of brown fat and SA/wt ratio decreases with the increase of subcutaneous fat, and control of temperature gradually approaches that of the adult as normal growth proceeds.

Transient Physiologic Factors. *Diurnal variation.* Depending on age, there is a normal temperature fluctuation between a low at 4:00 A.M. and a peak at 6:00 P.M. This variation is very slight under the age of 2 but may reach a maximum of 1.2°C (2°F) by 6 years. It remains at this level through adolescence, decreasing to 0.8°C (1.4°F) in adulthood. The "normal" temperature range is between 35.5° and 38.4°C (96.0–101.1°F).

Activity. It is well known that in athletes, after strenuous exercise, there is a rise in temperature of several degrees. An active child probably outdoes the athlete, so that an increase in temperature can be expected after normal activity.

Emotion. A sudden rise of temperature by several degrees is not an uncommon accompaniment of acute anxiety. This disappears rapidly as the anxiety is dissipated. The mechanism may be that vasoconstriction, resulting from the sudden catecholamine production caused by the emotional outburst, activates the cold sensors to initiate heat production.

Disease. Most disease states cause a rise in temperature (hyperthermia); a fall (hypothermia) is unusual except in the neonate in whom a hypothermic response is common because of the factors discussed above. Hyperthermia is the result of the reaction of the hypothalamus to "pyrogens."

These fever-inducing substances are of two types: (1) exogenous, in the form of endotoxins derived directly from certain bacteria; or (2) endogenous, released from the patient's leucocytes following combination of the white cells with such agents as viruses, bacteria, or antigen-antibody complexes.

Endogenous, rather than exogenous, pyrogen (EP), is the more common contributor to the production of a temperature rise. It is postulated that EP causes the release of the prostaglandins of the E group which in turn raises the set point of the hypothalmic thermostat. The body responds by conserving heat through peripheral vasoconstriction. Symptomatically, this is felt as a "chill"; shivering is also experienced from the body's response for more heat through increased muscle contraction. As the new level of temperature demand is reached, any excess heat will be given off by vasodilatation and sweating, and the patient feels "feverish."

APPROACH TO THE PROBLEM

Parents' Interpretation

Many parents consider any deviation of temperature from the commonly accepted normal of 37°C (98.6°F) means that the child has a "fever" and is sick. This anxiety can often be dissipated by a discussion of how the temperature was taken and the possibility of physiologic variation as explained above.

Evidence of Toxicity

This is one of the most important judgments that the clinician must make. Overestimate can result in unnecessary investigation or admission to the hospital while failure to recognize toxicity may seriously jeopardize the child's life or health. An assessment of the child's functional capacity is therefore essential, regardless of the height of the fever. The lack of correlation of the height of the temperature and its depressant effect on functioning depends on the individual child's temperature-regulating mechanism as well as his response to fever.

Infants less than 1 month of age with systemic infection frequently do not have a febrile response. On the other hand, children up to 4 weeks old with elevated temperatures more often have serious disease than an older child with the same temperature. Therefore, in the first month of life fever is usually an indication for admission and further investigation.

In most children, variations in the height of fever lie within a fairly narrow range but some children tolerate higher elevations without serious consequences. On questioning, the parents may state the child "always runs a high temperature" with an apparently trivial infection. Indeed some children can have documented temperatures of 39.5°C (103°F) and above without appearing sick, while others manifest symptoms of marked toxicity at these levels. Even in these temperature-prone children, extreme elevations should be an indication for therapy, as temperatures of approximately 41.3°C (106°F) and above may cause neurone damage from denaturation of cellular proteins.

In the absence of dehydration, lethargy, irritability, or toxicity, which would warrant admission, the clinician is faced with the considerations discussed below in treating the child as an outpatient.

Diagnosis and Therapy

Because these are so interrelated they can be discussed together. The first problem is an approach to diagnosis. If the history suggests exposure to a sibling with an infection, the patient should be carefully examined for physical signs pointing to a specific infection (e.g., measles, streptococcal pharyngitis, or a non-specific viral infection). If no specific physical signs are detected, then it follows that therapy is nonspecific. If there is only mild irritability or lethargy, the child is taking fluids well and appears alert and vigorous during the examination, the mother can be reassured and symptomatic treatment initiated. This consists of appropriate doses of an antipyretic, acetylsalicylic acid (aspirin) or acetaminophen (tylenol, tempra etc). The dose of each is 10 mg./kg. up to 650 mg/dose; this may be repeated in 4 to 6 hours, not to exceed 60 mg./kg./24 hours. Both medications are equally effective as antipyretics. Parents should be discouraged from using antipyretics for temperatures under 39.5°C (103°F) and from repeating the dose every 4 hours without sufficient indication; these indications are continued high fever or irritability, symptoms which call for further contact with the physician.

Other supportive measures in addition to the antipyretic must be considered in light of clinical objectives. Temperatures of 40°C (104°F) probably call for rapid reduction without regard to the patient's comfort. It has been shown that sponging with ice water is an efficient method regardless of the shivering it causes; however, most children exhibit symptoms of discomfort. If urgent reduction is not called for, sponging with tepid water reduces the fever more slowly, but causes little distress. Weinstein has recommended brisk rubbing with Turkish towels and tepid water to produce general erythema.

Ice water enemas should be avoided because of the risk of water intoxication. Rubbing with alcohol, which causes toxicity through inhaling fumes, should also be avoided. Free access to fluids should be encouraged. Do not advise pushing or forcing fluids because they may lead to a negative reaction, especially in the toddler age group.

The parent should be asked to record the temperatures at specified intervals and call the physician if the temperature rises past a given point despite antipyretic measures.

If the etiology is still unclear, a urinalysis should be done, particularly in a female where urinary tract infections are common and the symptomatology may be nonspecific. A blood count may also be performed and is definitely indicated if the urinalysis is negative and symptoms continue for another 48 hours without definite physical signs appearing. A leucocytosis with a shift to the left might suggest an occult bacterial infection, while a leukopenia with a high lymphocyte count could indicate a continuing viral infection. Such viral infections may cause fever for 7 to 10 days with few specific physical signs. Infectious mononucleosis or leukemia might be indicated by finding the characteristic cells on the smear.

If a specific diagnosis is arrived at by means of these procedures, appropriate therapy can be administered. If an etiology cannot be established, and there are no suggestive physical findings after repeated examinations, radiographs of the chest, sinuses or teeth may reveal a hidden pathology which can be appropriately treated.

If no diagnosis can be established, the situation should be re-evaluated with the recognition that parental anxiety grows with uncertainty. First the extent of the child's toxicity should be reviewed with the parent. Frequently, the child is not looking or acting "sick," in spite of the fever. Under these circumstances, the temperature record should be examined critically and the parent-child interaction assessed. Two observations may then clarify the problem: (1) the parent's concentration on temperature taking, however justifiable at the onset, may now be resulting in misinterpretation of physiologic variations as indications of disease, and (2) the child may perceive secondary gains from the constant attention and support the parental interpretation of illness.

An explanation may alleviate anxiety sufficiently so that the parents can follow a suggestion to put aside the thermometer and thereby minimize the child's complaints. If the parents do not comply, a more serious problem of parent-child interaction is indicated and may require evaluation.

If after 10 days a review of the situation indicates either increasing toxicity, or, despite apparent absence of toxicity, a continuing fever for which the above explanations are inadequate, the child should be admitted with the diagnosis of "fever of unknown origin" (FUO). Admission provides an opportunity for continuous monitoring and more elaborate diagnostic investigation.

After admission, the steps taken must reflect the clinical appearance of the patient. A toxic child requires the expeditious initiation of appropriate diagnostic procedures. The preferred treatment of the nontoxic individual is to delay the initiation of extensive laboratory evaluation. This allows observation of the fever during hospitalization, and may suggest the following two important causes of fever:

1. *Emotional Fever*: A child who at home has been running a documented fever as high as 38.3–40° C (103–104°F) will, in the neutral atmosphere of the hospital, have recorded temperatures within the normal range. Such an occurrence requires a search for a source of stress in the home environment. As Apley points out, "recurrent pyrexia" is one of several recurrent symptoms associated with emotional stress, such as "recurrent abdominal pain" and "recurrent limb pain."

2. *Factitious Fever*: In 10 per cent of 200 patients admitted for FUO of greater than 1 year's duration, the fever was factitious (self-induced). An older child can achieve this by various means. Sometimes self-inflicted infections are utilized to produce a true fever, but more often manipulation of the thermometer is the mechanism employed. Such "factitious fever" can be confusing unless its possibility is considered early in hospitalization.

Diagnosis rests on the recognition that the temperature elevations are the rule only when the nurse leaves the room during the temperature determinations. No child with an FUO should be left alone while his temperature is being taken. It is usually wise to take both oral and rectal temperatures every 4 hours (or at other prescribed intervals) for a day or two after admission. Even the presence of an observer, which obviates the use of the radiator or the hot water bag, can not prevent oral temperatures being manipulated by a prior mouthful of hot water or rapid rubbing of the end of the thermometer by the tongue. A diagnosis of "factitious fever" should be considered a "cry for help" and appropriate steps taken to understand what is troubling the patient.

DISEASE STATES OFTEN PRESENTING AS AN FUO

If the child shows evidence of toxicity, or if the above causes of fever are eliminated, the clinician is faced with an extensive differential diagnosis. The most frequent etiologies may be considered under three general headings: connective tissue disease, malignancy, or infection.

Connective Tissue Disease

Juvenile Rheumatoid Arthritis (JRA). In one series, 75 per cent of children seen because of unexplained fever suffered from JRA. Eventually, these children develop joint signs and symptoms, but the only evidence of disease for weeks or months may be intermittent fever, especially in young children with the systemic type of disease. Suggestive clinical evidences of the disease are the following:

Type of fever. Intermittent, occurring late in the afternoon.

Rash. This is present in 20 to 70 per cent of patients. It is salmon colored, macular or maculopapular, may be discrete or form patches 5 to 6 cm. in diameter. It is not pruritic and is evanscent, tending to accompany temperature elevations and disappearing as the fever falls. It is distributed mainly on the upper back, but may be present on the extremities.

Generalized lymphadenopathy and splenomegaly may be associated with fever in patients with JRA but this finding is nonspecific. Supporting laboratory findings are: (1) an elevated sedimentation rate, which is always found in such patients; and (2) a rheumatoid factor, which is usually absent in younger patients.

Systemic Lupus Erythematosis. This is uncommon before puberty and, as in adults, is more frequent among females. The presence of fever was reported in 90 per cent of patients in one series. Suggestive diagnostic clues are: malar butterfly rash, joint pains, and nonspecific psychiatric/neurologic symptoms. The diagnosis is confirmed by the presence of antinuclear antibodies in the serum.

Granulomatous Bowel Disease or Ulcerative Colitis. Early in the disease, distinction between these is difficult. It is more common for granulomatous disease to present as an FUO. Suggestive clues are a history of diarrhea or abdominal pain which may be intermittent and not sufficiently symptomatic to be mentioned in the initial history. FUO with abdominal pain may be the only presenting symptom early in the disease. Repeated examinations may be required before more supportive evidence is obtained. These examinations would include: a characteristic radiologic picture on the upper gastrointestinal tract or barium enema studies and pathological changes seen on sigmoidoscopy. Weight loss, arthritis and perianal fissures may occur.

Malignancy

Fever may occur in any type of malignancy because of infection superimposed on impaired immunity, or secondary to tissue breakdown as the tumor outruns its vascular supply. Specifically, fever may be the presenting sign in the following:

Leukemia. This possibility must always be entertained in any child with prolonged fever. It will occur to the parents, probably before it does to the clinician, as a result of the publicity it receives. Diagnostic clues are: increasing pallor, petechiae or ecchymosis, and bone pain.

Laboratory confirmation may come from: (1) the blood count which might reveal thrombocytopenia with changes in leucocyte count, a low hemoglobin and abnormal cells on the smear. These changes may not have been evident in a blood count taken early in the investigation while the child was an outpatient. (2) Bone marrow aspiration. In the unusual form of leukemia, abnormal cells may not be found in the peripheral smear but will be found in the bone marrow. (3) Radiographs of the long bones where characteristic metaphyseal changes will be found.

Lymphoma. Fever may be the presenting sign. This has no particular pattern although historically the Pel Ebstein fever (a fever recurring at regular intervals) was considered characteristic of Hodgkin's disease. Diagnostic clues include: (1) the presence of generalized lymphadenopathy; (2) a paraspinal mass on deep abdominal palpation; (3) persistent enlargement of one tonsil; (4) evidence of recent nasopharyngeal obstruction; (5) evidence of intestinal obstruction; (6) the rapid appearance of ascites; (7) onset of wheezing. ("All that wheezes is not asthma"). Suggestive laboratory data include: radiographic examinations, especially the finding of a mass in the chest or lateral neck; a distorted intravenous pyelogram that may indicate a retroperitoneal mass. However, a biopsy of an accessible mass is essential for the diagnosis. Repeated biopsies may be necessary.

Neuroblastoma. This is the most common solid tumor in childhood. It can arise wherever sympathetic nervous tissue is present but most commonly is derived from the adrenal gland. FUO may be its presenting sign. Diagnostic clues are: an abdominal mass, malabsorption syndrome, hypertension, or upper airway obstruction. Laboratory confirmation is sought from an x-ray examination that may show mediastinal, retroperitoneal, or adrenal masses, and a bone scan that may demonstrate osseous metastases. Increased vanillylmandelic acid concentration in the urine, after the patient has been on an appropriate diet, is highly suggestive.

Wilms' tumor is the second most common solid tumor of infants and children, and usually presents as an abdominal tumor on routine examination; however, an FUO is occasionally the first sign. Diagnosis is based on a characteristic intravenous pyelogram.

Infection

Most fevers are caused by infection. In many, the febrile illness is limited to a few days. Viral infections usually respond without specific therapy but may continue for 7 to 10 days. Bacterial infections generally respond rapidly to antibiotic therapy. Without such therapy many of the short-lived illnesses will proceed to a chronic phase with prolonged fever. Among those which may cause a diagnostic puzzle are the following:

Urinary Tract Infection. Many children with this problem will have a normal urinalysis. Children with FUO deserve at least two appropriately collected urine cultures.

Respiratory Tract Infection. These include: occult pneumonia, tracheobronchitis, chronic streptococcal disease and sinusitis. Appropriate radiographs and cultures along with antibody determinations against Group A streptococcal antigens will establish the diagnosis.

Viral Infection. Occasionally a viral infection such as that caused by many of the Coxsackie A organisms will cause fever for 2 weeks or even longer. Cultures of the throat and stool and rising antibody titers may reveal the etiologic agent in retrospect. In one series of childhood FUOs, this was the most common etiology.

Salmonellosis. *Typhoid Fever (S. typhi).* This may present as an intermittent fever, usually without diarrhea. Constipation, in fact, is more common. Diagnostic clues are: epidemiologic evidence of exposure, e.g., travel in an endemic area; tender splenomegaly; rose spots; and a relative bradycardia. Diagnosis is based on positive cultures from blood, urine, bone marrow, and stool; a rise in antibody titer against salmonella O and H antigens is suggestive evidence.

Systemic salmonellosis due to other salmonellae, (e.g., *S. typhimurium*. Supportive findings include the presence of sickle cell anemia since such patients are peculiarly prone to this systemic infection, and a swollen painful joint or bone pain. Laboratory confirmation is obtained from: (1) blood, urine, bone marrow and stool cultures; or (2) evidence of osteomyelitis or septic arthritis from a radiograph.

Brucellosis. Diagnostic clues come from epidemiologic considerations (e.g., drinking unpasteurized milk). Confirmation rests on a positive blood culture using a special medium and evidence of serum agglutinins against the organism at a greater than 1:160 dilution.

Tuberculosis. While cases are rarely found in the United States, it is still a common disease world wide. The asymptomatic child will be detected by routine tuberculin testing. FUO may be the presenting sign in a young child with miliary tuberculosis or bronchial node infection; in an older patient, renal involvement may be the cause of the fever. Diagnostic clues are: (1) an epidemiologic history of exposure; (2) positive tuberculin test; (3) enlarged liver and spleen; (4) a pertussis-like cough; (5) painless hematuria. Laboratory confirmation is obtained by: (1) radiographs of the chest showing a characteristic picture of miliary tuberculosis; (2) cultures of sputum (if available), or gastric juice in young children who swallow their sputum; (3) lymphnode, liver or bone marrow biopsy for culture, presence of giant cells and acid-fast bacilli.

Fungal Infections. Of these Histoplasmosis in the eastern United States and Coccidiomycosis in the West are the prominent causes. Diagnostic clues depend on an epidemiologic history of living in an endemic area. Confirmation depends on an appropriate serologic examination.

Intra-Abdominal Infection. *Ruptured Retroceal Appendix With a Localized or Subphrenic Abscess.* Diagnostic clues are: (1) history of a recent attack of abdominal pain, with or without diarrhea, which subsided before fever started (the diagnosis of a retrocecal appendicitis can be missed by the most careful clinician); (2) a tender mass in the right side of the pelvis on rectal examination; (3) dullness on percussion and impaired movement of the base of one lung. Laboratory investigation includes: (1) a complete blood count which would reveal a marked polymorphonuclear leucocytosis with a shift to the left; (2) flat plate of the abdomen revealing diaphragmatic elevation or subdiaphragmatic air, or a fecalith in a soft tissue mass; (3) an intravenous pyelogram that could yield evidence of the kidney's displacement by a retroperitoneal mass; (4) retroperitoneal aspiration of purulent material; (5) a laparotomy.

Pelvic Inflammatory Disease (PID). This must be considered in the pubertal female. Diagnostic clues are: a history of sexual activity, vaginal discharge, and a tender mass on pelvic examination. Laboratory investigations include: (1) Culture of vagina, rectum and throat for gonococcus; (2) Blood count for evidence of polymorphonuclear pleocytosis with a shift to the left.

Cholecystitis. Although rare in children, this should be suspected in a patient with hemolytic anemia of any sort because of the common presence of stones. Diagnostic clues are the presence of marked tenderness in the right upper quadrant with or without palpable mass. Laboratory investigations include: (1) complete blood count for polymorphonuclear leucocytosis; (2) elevated serum bilirubin; (3) cholecystogram; (4) a laparotomy, which may be required for a definitive diagnosis.

Chronic Active Hepatitis. FUO may be the presenting sign. Diagnostic support includes: jaundice; a tender palpable liver, especially the left lobe; loss of weight and appetite. Laboratory confirmation is obtained from: (1) rise of serum bilirubin, SGOT, SGPT, and alkaline phosphatase as well as the presence of bilirubin in the urine. (2) liver biopsy showing characteristic morphologic changes or Hepatitis B antigens on immunofluorescent examination.

Other Infections. *Subacute bacterial endocarditis* should be suspected in any child with FUO who has a known congenital heart lesion. Diagnostic clues are: (1) evidence of emboli, (e.g., splinter hemorrhages in the nails) and hematuria, although these are rarely found in prepubertal children; and (2) changing heart murmurs. Laboratory confirmation depends on obtaining a positive blood culture. This often necessitates repeated attempts and observation of cultures for 10 to 14 days since it may take this long for the presence of a few organisms in the blood to manifest themselves.

Osteomyelitis must be suspected in any child developing an FUO particularly after trauma. Limitation of spontaneous movement in a limb should direct investigation to this end. Diagnostic clues are tenderness in the neighborhood of one or more joints and limitation of passive motion. Laboratory investigation includes: (1) complete blood count to detect polymorphonuclear leucocytosis; (2) sedimentation rate, which should be elevated; (3) bone scan; (4) radiographs of the suspected site, for periosteal elevation or bone erosion (if taken early they are often negative and must be repeated in 10–14 days); (5) aspiration to detect subperiosteal pus when there is a mass adjacent to a bone.

"PERIODIC FEVER"

Periodic recurrences of fever may occur as part of the clinical picture in the conditions considered above. In rare and otherwise healthy persons, bouts of fever may recur at regular intervals for which no etiology can be found. The condition can begin at any age, continue for decades, have long periods of remission and cease spontaneously. There seems to be an hereditary factor.

PROGRAM OF INVESTIGATION

With these possibilities in mind, the following diagnostic procedures may be introduced, either sequentially or simultaneously, depending on the severity of the child's illness and the clinical clues that have developed:

1. Complete blood count. Look for changes since previous ones.
2. Urinalysis and culture. Look for changes since previous ones.
3. Sedimentation rate. The uncorrected figure is a more useful guide except in patients with severe anemia. It will be elevated in connective

tissue disease, infection and in most but not all malignancies. It will not be elevated in emotional or factitious fever, or in some viral diseases. A normal sedimentation rate suggests that organic disease is not present.

4. Tuberculin test. An intermediate strength PPD should be introduced intradermally. An area of induration of 10 mm. or greater should direct investigation to finding the site of tuberculous infection.

5. Tests for fungi. Serologic and intradermal tests are available for histoplasmosis, coccidiomycosis and blastomycosis and may provide a diagnostic clue.

6. Radiographs (A) of the chest to look for changes since previous ones; (B) skeletal survey for evidence of malignancies or infection; (C) intravenous pyelogram for evidence of chronic renal infection, tumor, retroperitoneal or adrenal masses; (D) gastrointestinal series or barium enema preceded by flat plate; and (E) radiographs of teeth and sinuses.

7. Blood culture. At least two carefully taken cultures should be obtained using media that will support the growth of aerobic and anaerobic organisms. A positive culture of a significant organism can provide an important diagnostic lead for further clinical evaluation.

8. Bone marrow. Culture, aspiration and biopsy for detection of the abnormal cellular picture and for culture, including that for anaerobes, mycobacteria and fungi.

9. Bone scan where indicated.

10. Antinuclear antibody. The presence or absence rules in or out the great majority of patients with lupus erythematosis. It can be positive in a certain number of the other recognized connective tissue diseases.

11. Rheumatoid factor. This may be useful in pinpointing a diagnosis of JRA in older children. However, it is usually negative in young children with this disease and may be positive in patients with other connective tissue diseases.

12. Lumbar puncture. This should be almost routine in newborn infants up to 1 month of age and strongly considered in children up to 18 months even in the absence of obvious meningeal signs. For older children the presence of meningeal signs should be the indication. The fluid is examined for protein, glucose and cells as well as bacteria, mycobacterial organisms, fungi and viruses.

13. Sigmoidoscopy or colonoscopy. For visualization of intestinal mucosa with or without biopsy.

14. Operative procedures: (a) biopsy of a mass, an enlarged lymphnode (which may have to be repeated several times) or an enlarged or too small liver; (b) as a last resort, laparotomy, for the possibility of an intra-abdominal abscess or tumor.

With the indicated procedures, it is usually possible to make a specific diagnosis. However, in some children, despite appropriate diagnostic evaluation, a specific etiology cannot be established. The passage of time and careful repeated examinations may be required before arriving at a diagnosis.

BIBLIOGRAPHY

Apley, J., and MacKeith, R.: The child and his symptoms. ed. 2. Philadelphia, F. A. Davis Company, 1968.

Atkins, E., and Bodel, P.: Fever. N. Engl. J. Med., 286:27, 1972.

A review of the pathophysiology of fever.

Pizzo, P. A., *et al.*: Prolonged fever in children. Review of 100 cases. Pediatrics, 55:408, 1975.

A clinical article reviewing the final diagnosis of pediatric patients with FUO. The authors point out those laboratory procedures that were particularly helpful.

Steele, R. W., *et al.*: Evaluation of sponging and of oral antipyretic therapy to reduce fever. J. Pediatr., 77:824, 1970.

Vane, J. R.: The mode of action of aspirin and similar compounds. J. Allergy Clin. Immunol., 58:691, 1976.

This article discusses the recent work on the pyrogenic action of prostaglandins and the mechanism of the antipyretic effect of aspirin and like drugs.

7

Pallor

Frank A. Oski, M.D.

Pallor does not necessarily indicate that an infant or child is anemic. A child may appear pale due to lack of sufficient exposure to sunlight, chronic illness, the presence of edema, or asphyxia. Observation of the color of the mucous membranes of the mouth, the conjunctiva, or the creases in the hyperextended palm of the hand, are all far better indicators of anemia than the color of the skin. Even these maneuvers may fail to detect the presence of anemia when the hemoglobin value is above 8 g./dl.

Because physical examination alone will fail to detect the presence of mild anemia, a laboratory test such as the hemoglobin or hematocrit should be performed on all infants at some time during their nursery stay and again at 6 months, 12 months, and 2 years of age.

The normal hemoglobin value and the definition of anemia change with the age of the patient. Failure to appreciate this developmental fact generally results in the underdiagnosis of anemia in the newborn period and the overdiagnosis of anemia during the period from 3 months to 2 years of age. Normal values for hemoglobin as a function of age are listed in Table 7-1.

Once it has been established that the infant or child is anemic, an orderly approach to the diagnosis of the disease should begin with an examination of the peripheral blood smear, a reticulocyte count, and a measurement of the red cell indices. The interpretation of these results is facilitated by an understanding of the more probable causes of anemia at the varying stages of infancy and childhood.

This knowledge coupled with the information obtained from the history and physical examination will generally enable the physician to make a correct presumptive diagnosis that can be confirmed by a minimum of additional laboratory tests.

In the physical examination, attention should be paid to the color of

Table 7-1. Average Normal Blood Values at Different Age Levels
(for Term Infants)

Value	At birth	2 days	14 days	3 months	6 months	1 year	2 years	4 years	8–12 years
Red cells/mm.³ (in millions)	5.1	5.3	5.0	4.3	4.6	4.7	4.8	4.8	5.1
Hemoglobin (g./dl.)	17.6	18.0	17.0	11.4	11.5	12.2	12.9	13.1	14.1
Percentage of reticulocytes in total red cells	4.2±1.6	3.2±1.4	0.5±0.3	0.5±0.3	0.8±0.3	1 ±0.3	1 ±0.3	1 ±0.3	1 ±0.3
Anemia if hemoglobin less than	14.0	14.0	12.0	10.0	10.0	10.5	10.5	11.0	12.0

the mucous membranes, the presence of lymphadenopathy, the size of the liver and spleen, the presence of bruises or petechiae, and the detection of jaundice.

The history should include information regarding the patient's racial background, information concerning the presence of anemia, jaundice, or gallstones in other family members, a detailed dietary history, inquiries regarding the frequency and color of the child's stools, the presence of pica, drug ingestion, previous episodes of jaundice, and the frequency of infections.

ANEMIA IN EARLY INFANCY

The diagnosis of anemia in early infancy is a far more complicated process than it is at any other time of life. During the first 3 months of extrauterine existence, continuous changes produced by growth and development result in week-to-week variations in what may be regarded as the normal hemoglobin value. In addition, unique pathologic processes are operative at this age that also contribute to diagnostic confusion. These unique processes are a consequence of maternal-fetal interactions, the rapidity of growth with its attendant nutritional requirements, and the proclivity of newborns to acquire a variety of infections.

After the 34th to 35th week of gestation, the mean cord blood hemoglobin value is approximately 17.0 g./dl. Values of less than 14.5 g./dl. at birth may be regarded as abnormal. During the first hours of life, the hemoglobin value may rise by as much as 20 per cent in those infants whose umbilical cords were not clamped immediately at birth. During the first week of life in both the term and premature infant, there is very

Table 7-2. Serial Hemoglobin Values (g %) in Low Birth Weight Infants

Birth weight (g)	Age (in weeks)				
	2	4	6	8	10
800—1000	16.0 ± 0.6	10.0 ± 3.2	8.7 ± 1.5	8.0 ± 0.9	8.0 ± 1.1
1001—1200	16.4 ± 2.3	12.8 ± 2.5	10.5 ± 1.8	9.1 ± 1.3	8.5 ± 1.5
1201—1400	16.2 ± 1.3	13.4 ± 2.8	10.9 ± 1.2	9.9 ± 1.9	—
1401—1500	15.6 ± 2.2	11.7 ± 1.0	10.5 ± 0.7	9.8 ± 1.4	—

little change in the hemoglobin concentration, and values at 7 days of age are very similar to those values present at birth.

Beyond the first week of life, the hemoglobin values begin to decline rapidly. In the term infant, the hemoglobin value reaches its lowest level at 8-9 weeks of age (Table 7-1). At this time, hemoglobin values as low as 9.5 g./dl. can be viewed as normal. Hemoglobin values tend to fall more rapidly and reach lower levels in apparently healthy premature infants (Table 7-2). Between 6 to 8 weeks of age, the hemoglobin value of infants weighing 1200 g. or less at birth averages about 8.0 g./dl. and values of 7.0 g./dl. are frequently observed in the absence of any recognizable pathologic process.

Regulation of Erythropoiesis

This fall in hemoglobin levels appears to be a normal physiologic process that is influenced by both the oxygen requirements of the infant and the mechanisms governing oxygen release to the tissues. Although it seems clear that the regulation of erythropoiesis in the adult is under the influence of erythropoietin, the modulation of fetal and newborn erythropoiesis has been more difficult to understand because of the many complex factors affecting red cell formation during this stage of development. These factors include the influence of maternal erythropoiesis, variations in placental function, multiple sites of red cell production in the fetus, changes in arterial oxygenation at birth, the gradual replacement of fetal hemoglobin by adult hemoglobin, and alterations in the concentration and effects of red cell 2,3-diphosphoglycerate.

Red cell formation *in utero* begins at approximately day 14 of gestation and occurs successively in the yolk sac, liver and bone marrow. Erythropoietin is produced by the fetus and appears to be responsive to the usual factors stimulating its production. Both term and preterm infants have normal or elevated erythropoietin levels when compared with normal adults. Infants with erythroblastosis fetalis increase erythropoietin production in the presence of anemia. Infants with polycythemia at birth also demonstrate elevations in erythropoietin levels. This is seen in infants who are small for gestational age or who are post-mature, and is associated with placental insufficiency and presumed intrauterine hypoxia.

The erythropoietin present in the plasma of the newborn appears to be produced endogenously and under fetal control. Although maternal plasma erythropoietin levels are slightly elevated during pregnancy, the cord blood samples from anemic infants with erythroblastosis show even greater erythropoietin activity.

The normal or elevated plasma erythropoietin level present at birth declines to undetectable levels within several days of birth and rises again between 60 and 90 days of life. During this period the hemoglobin level falls progressively, accompanied by a decreased rate of erythropoiesis. The bone marrow at this time is capable of increased erythropoiesis mediated via erythropoietin if appropriate stimulation is present such as is observed with anemia or the hypoxemia of cyanotic heart disease. Thus it would appear that the fall in hemoglobin level that is observed during the first 2 to 3 months of life occurs as a result of increased oxygen delivery to the tissues with removal of the stimulation to erythropoietin production. At birth, arterial oxygen saturation promptly rises from the intrauterine value of 45 per cent to 95 per cent. During the next several months of life, the position of the oxygen-hemoglobin dissociation curve gradually shifts to the right as the hemoglobin falls. This gradual shift in the curve facilitates oxygen release to the tissues. As a result, the term infant at 3 months is capable of releasing as much oxygen to his tissues, at a mixed venous oxygen tension of 40 mm. Hg, as the normal newborn infant despite a pronounced fall in the oxygen-carrying capacity of the blood. This shift in the position of the curve to the right is mediated by the replacement of fetal by adult hemoglobin and its interaction with red cell 2,3-diphosphoglycerate.

The causes of true anemia both at birth and during the first several months of life can be considered against this background of normal developmental changes.

Anemia at Birth

Anemia at birth or appearing during the first week of life is generally the result of hemolysis or hemorrhage. Hemolytic anemias occurring during this early period of life are of multiple etiologies and generally are associated with serum bilirubin levels in excess of 6 to 8 mg./dl. Hemolytic disease in the newborn can be broadly classified into three large categories: isoimmunization, inherited defects of the red cell, and acquired defects of the red cell. In most parts of the world, isoimmunization as a result of maternal-fetal incompatibilities in either the Rh or ABO blood group systems is the leading cause of hemolytic disease. Of the inherited defects of the red cell, red cell glucose-6-phosphate dehydrogenase deficiency appears to be the abnormality most commonly associated with both anemia and hyperbilirubinemia. Virtually all of the red cell enzyme deficiencies described to date have been associated with anemia and hyperbilirubinemia during the early days of life. The red cell membrane disorders, which include hereditary spherocytosis, elliptocytosis, and stomatocytosis, may also be associated with anemia in early life. Approximately 50 per cent of patients with hereditary spherocytosis experience hyperbilirubinemia during the first week of life.

Anemia and jaundice frequently accompany profound acidosis and hypoxemia in the young infant. In many instances, this hemolytic anemia may be a consequence of the associated pathologic process of disseminated intravascular coagulation. Infections, most notably those produced by congenital cytomegalovirus, toxoplasmosis, rubella, syphilis, and gram negative bacteria, are other causes of anemia during this period. Red cell hypoplasia (the Blackfan-Diamond syndrome) may also manifest itself at the time of birth as anemia and reticulocytopenia.

Other inherited abnormalities that may result in anemia during the first several days of life include defects in alpha chain synthesis (alpha-thalassemia trait) or gamma chain synthesis (gamma-thalassemia).

Hemorrhage leading to anemia at birth or in the first few days of life may be broadly grouped into three major etiologic categories. These include hemorrhage associated with obstetric accidents or malformations of the placenta and cord, occult hemorrhage from the fetus into the maternal circulation or from twin to twin, and internal hemorrhages (Table 7-3). In these situations, pallor and signs of circulatory collapse are prominent clinical features and jaundice is generally absent.

Anemia at 1 to 3 Months of Life

Anemia that is first detected at 1 to 3 months of life may represent the sequel of previously undiagnosed events in the immediate newborn period. Most commonly, these include mild isoimmunization, fetal to maternal hemorrhage, or chronic congenital infections.

By this period of life, hemoglobinopathies involving defects of the beta chain become clinically apparent. Both thalassemia major and sickle-cell anemia produce anemia by 3 months of age.

In the rapidly growing premature infant, both folic acid deficiency and vitamin E deficiency also may produce true anemia by 8 to 10 weeks of life. Folic acid deficiency is most commonly observed in those infants whose clinical course has been complicated by diarrhea and infections. Vitamin E deficiency occurs almost exclusively in infants with birth weights less than 1500 g. The anemia is primarily the result of excessive hemolysis and is accompanied by reticulocytosis, poikilocytosis, red cell fragmentation, mild spherocytosis, thrombocytosis, and in the more severely deficient infants, edema may be observed.

Vitamin E deficiency results from a combination of factors which include: low vitamin E stores at birth, inadequate dietary intake, and poor absorption of this fat-soluble vitamin. The administration of iron during

Table 7-3. Common Causes of Anemia in Early Infancy

Age	Diagnosis	Supporting data
At birth	Hemorrhage Obstetric accidents (placenta previa, abruptio placenta, incision of placenta, rupture of cord, rupture of anomalous placental vessel)	History and visual inspection of placenta and cord
	Occult hemorrhage Fetomaternal Twin-to-twin	Demonstration of fetal cells in maternal circulation Demonstration of significant difference in hemoglobin values of identical twins
	Internal hemorrhage (intracranial, retroperitoneal, intrahepatic, intrasplenic, cephalohematoma)	Physical examination
	Isoimmunization	Blood groups of mother and infant evidence of antibody on infant's red cells
	Inherited defect of red cell (induces G-6-PD deficiency, pyruvate kinase deficiency, hereditary spherocytosis, elliptocytosis, stomatocytosis, etc.)	Red cell morphology, family history, and appropriate screening tests
	Acquired defect (generally in association with hypoxemia, acidosis, or infection)	Physical findings, red cell morphology, coagulation disturbance, blood and urine cultures, and serologic studies and Gamma M determination
	Red cell hypoplasia (Blackfan-Diamond syndrome, congenital leukemia, osteopetrosis)	Rare disorders. Bone marrow aspirate

the first weeks of life, either in the form of a medicinal supplement or incorporated into the formula, tends to aggravate the anemia in these vitamin E-deficient premature infants.

In Table 7-3, the more common cause of anemia during the first 3 months of life are listed. Because of the plethora of diagnostic possibilities, the physician must approach this challenging problem with a clear understanding of what "true" anemia is, diligently collect relevant information concerning family history, obstetric history, the early neonatal course of events, and dietary history before instituting a myriad of unnecessary and ill-suited diagnostic procedures.

ANEMIA AFTER 3 MONTHS OF AGE

The rational approach to diagnosis at this age again begins with an attempt to classify the anemia based on its morphologic characteristics.

Table 7-3. Common Causes of Anemia in Early Infancy (*Continued*)

Age	Diagnosis	Supporting data
2–3 months	Iron deficiency as a consequence of previous hemorrhage	Obstetric history when available
	Late manifestation of previous isoimmunization	Blood types of mother and infant; maternal and antibody titers
	Hereditary defects of the red cell	Persistence of hemolytic anemia. Red cell morphology and laboratory tests
	Thalassemia major	Red cell morphology, splenomegaly, persistence of fetal hemoglobin elevation, family studies
	Sickle-cell anemia	Red cell morphology, hemoglobin electrophoresis
	Vitamin E deficiency	Infant of low birth weight. Red cell morphology, low serum E level, positive hydrogen peroxide hemolysis test
	Folic acid deficiency	Premature infant, history of infections or diarrhea, red cell and marrow morphology, response to folic acid
	Persistent infection	Elevated titers to rubella, cytomegalovirus, toxoplasmosis
	Renal tubular acidosis	Acidosis, hypochloremia, mild azotemia, urine pH of 6.0 or greater in presence of acidosis

A simple flow diagram for this purpose is depicted in Figure 7-1. The anemias are subdivided into those in which the red cells are small in size (microcytic), normal in size (normocytic), or large in size (macrocytic). In addition, the anemias that are generally normocytic are further subdivided into those anemias that are primarily a result of accelerated red cell destruction as contrasted with those that are primarily a result of impaired red cell production.

Between 3 months and 2 years of age, and particularly between 9 months and 2 years of age, iron deficiency, is the leading cause of anemia. During this period of life, an infant will outgrow his iron endowment. Normal newborns are born with an iron endowment of approximately 75 mg./kg. Almost two-thirds of this iron endowment is present in the infant's red cell hemoglobin. Very little iron is normally lost from the body so that the infant can increase his birth weight approximately 2½-fold before his iron stores are depleted and iron deficiency begins to limit the

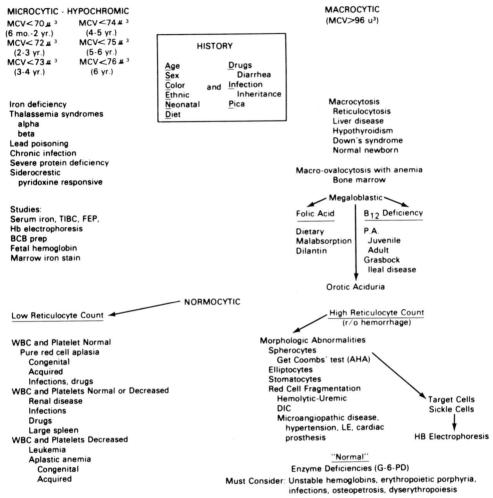

MICROCYTIC - HYPOCHROMIC

MCV<70μ³   MCV<74μ³
(6 mo.-2 yr.)   (4-5 yr.)
MCV<72μ³   MCV<75μ³
(2-3 yr.)   (5-6 yr.)
MCV<73μ³   MCV<76μ³
(3-4 yr.)   (6 yr.)

Iron deficiency
Thalassemia syndromes
  alpha
  beta
Lead poisoning
Chronic infection
Severe protein deficiency
Siderocrestic
  pyridoxine responsive

Studies:
Serum iron, TIBC, FEP,
Hb electrophoresis
BCB prep
Fetal hemoglobin
Marrow iron stain

HISTORY

Age   Drugs
Sex   Diarrhea
Color and   Infection
Ethnic   Inheritance
Neonatal   Pica
Diet

MACROCYTIC
(MCV>96 u³)

Macrocytosis
Reticulocytosis
Liver disease
Hypothyroidism
Down's syndrome
Normal newborn

Macro-ovalocytosis with anemia
Bone marrow

Megaloblastic

Folic Acid | B₁₂ Deficiency

Dietary | P.A.
Malabsorption | Juvenile
Dilantin | Adult
              | Grasbock
              | Ileal disease

Orotic Aciduria

NORMOCYTIC

Low Reticulocyte Count

WBC and Platelet Normal
  Pure red cell aplasia
    Congenital
    Acquired
    Infections, drugs
WBC and Platelets Normal or Decreased
  Renal disease
  Infections
  Drugs
  Large spleen
WBC and Platelets Decreased
  Leukemia
  Aplastic anemia
    Congenital
    Acquired

High Reticulocyte Count
(r/o hemorrhage)

Morphologic Abnormalities
  Spherocytes
    Get Coombs' test (AHA)
  Elliptocytes
  Stomatocytes
  Red Cell Fragmentation
    Hemolytic-Uremic
    DIC
  Microangiopathic disease,
    hypertension, LE, cardiac
    prosthesis

Target Cells
Sickle Cells

HB Electrophoresis

"Normal"
Enzyme Deficiencies (G-6-PD)
Must Consider: Unstable hemoglobins, erythropoietic porphyria,
infections, osteopetrosis, dyserythropoiesis

Fig. 7-1. A diagnostic approach to anemia. (Must get red cell indices, retiocolocyte count and smear.)

rate of hemoglobin synthesis. For this reason, nutritional iron deficiency is rarely observed during the first 6 months of life. Only in infants who are growing rapidly (e.g., infants born of low birth weights who may quadruple their birth weights within the first 6 months of life) will nutritional causes of iron deficiency occur early in life.

Other causes of microcytic anemias that may be confused with iron deficiency are listed in Figure 7-1.

Another major subdivision of anemia is the macrocytic and megaloblastic anemias. Macrocytes in and of themselves are not diagnostic of a megaloblastic anemia. Macrocytes are large erythrocytes and may be seen in anyone with reticulocytosis. As young cells are larger cells, they may be seen in patients with hemolytic diseases. They may also be seen in patients with hypothyroidism, liver disease, and in the normal new-born. The hallmark of a macrocytic-megaloblastic anemia is the presence of macro-ovalocytes in the peripheral blood smear. In addition, changes in white cell morphology are extremely important in substantiating the diagnosis of megaloblastic anemia. The normal individual has a mean neutrophil lobe count of approximately 3.2. In general, a normal individual may have as many as three, five-lobed polymorphonuclear leukocytes in a peripheral smear when 100 cells are counted. The presence of more than this number of five-lobed polys or the presence of polys with six or more lobes should alert the physician to the possibility that the patient may have a megaloblastic anemia.

Dietary folic acid deficiency can occur in young infants, particularly those raised on goat's milk, which is very low in this vitamin. It is more commonly seen in patients with malabsorptive states. Folic acid is absorbed primarily in the jejunum and vitamin B_{12} is absorbed primarily in the ileum. Diseases in these portions of the gastrointestinal tract can result in the appearance of a deficiency of these vitamins. In patients with macro-ovalocytes or white cell changes suggestive of a megaloblastic anemia, bone marrow studies should be performed to confirm the fact that megaloblastic erythropoiesis is present. Once this is established, attention should be directed to the cause of the deficiency.

The normocytic anemias are a heterogenous group of disorders. Although every anemic patient should have a reticulocyte count performed, it is particularly important in facilitating a diagnosis in patients in this category. When anemia is associated with a low reticulocyte count, one must seriously suspect some form of bone marrow dysfunction. Attention should be paid to the white cell and platelet count in an effort to determine if all the formed elements are involved in the bone marrow failure. Both congenital and acquired diseases may produce disturbances in erythropoiesis. Many of these diagnostic possibilities are listed in Figure 7-1. Confirmation requires bone marrow examination coupled with other appropriate laboratory studies.

Another large group of patients with normocytic anemias is associated with reticulocytosis and a shortened red cell lifespan. Here the morphology of the red cells provides an important clue as to etiology. Based on the appearance of the red cells, the physician may decide to request additional confirmatory studies such as hemoglobin electrophoresis, enzyme assays, and study of other possibly affected family members.

It must be realized that anemia is never a diagnosis. It is only evidence of the presence of a disease whose cause must be ascertained. Through a series of generally simple and logical steps a diagnosis can be established in most patients. Treatment can then be directed in an appropriate fashion.

BIBLIOGRAPHY

Oski, F. A.: Anemia in children. Hosp. Prac., *11*:63, 1976.

    A review of the causes and diagnosis of anemia in infants and children.

Oski, F. A., and Lubin, B.: Hemolytic anemias in infants and children. Mod. Treat., *8*:436, 1971.

    A review of the causes of hemolysis in pediatrics.

Oski, F. A., and Stockman, J. A.: Congenital hemolytic anemias and red cell enzyme deficiencies. Cur. Prob. Pediatr., *4*:(2), 1973.

    A monograph detailing the recognition and metabolic basis of hereditary abnormalities of the red cell.

8

Bruising and Bleeding

Frank A. Oski, M.D.

Parents of young toddlers often remark that their child bruises easily. Children with recurrent epistaxis are referred frequently for evaluation of a possible bleeding disorder. An accurate and detailed history often discloses justification for suspecting an underlying inherited or acquired bleeding disturbance. A history coupled with a careful physical examination generally eliminates the need for further laboratory investigation.

The parents and the family should be specifically questioned about all past injuries including needle punctures, minor cuts in the mouth and the skin, and all instances of surgery including dental extractions, tonsillectomy, and circumcision. The absence of excessive bleeding after dental extractions, tonsillectomy, surgical incisions, or major trauma eliminates the possibility of a long-standing or inherited defect in coagulation.

Excessive bruising and bleeding can be the result of: (1) a deficiency of one of the coagulation factors, (2) a quantitative deficiency of platelets, (3) a qualitative abnormality of platelets, or (4) an abnormality of the vessels—either excessive capillary fragility or the presence of vasculitis.

Some features of the history and physical examination allow you to separate the suspected bleeding disturbance into one of the two groups— a defect of the fluid phase of coagulation or an abnormality of platelets or vessel wall. The distinguishing characteristics are described in Table 8-1. The steps in the coagulation pathway are illustrated in Figure 8-1.

When one suspects a bleeding disorder, initial laboratory studies should include a partial thromboplastin time, a prothrombin time, a platelet count, a smear to examine platelet morphology, and a standardized Ivy Bleeding Time. This battery of tests allows a presumptive diagnosis of a bleeding disturbance. The only defect not detected by one of these procedures is an inherited deficiency of Factor XIII (fibrin stabilizing factor). The use of such tests in arriving at a presumptive diagnosis

Table 8-1. Clinical Features That Serve to Distinguish Bleeding as a Result of a Defect in the Fluid Phase of Coagulation from a Platelet or Capillary Defect

Clinical features	Coagulation defects	Platelet and Capillary defects
Bleeding from superficial cuts and abrasions.	Usually not excessive.	Often profuse and prolonged.
Spontaneous bruises and hematomas.	Often deep and spreading hematoma. Only a few at any one time.	Usually small, superficial, and multiple.
Hemarthroses	Common in severe cases.	Very rare.
Bleeding from deep cuts and tooth extractions.	Onset often delayed for minutes or hours. Not permanently controlled by local pressure.	Onset usually immediate. Frequently permanently arrested by local pressure.
Most common bleeding manifestations.	Deep tissue hemorrhages, often involves joints and muscle. Prolonged bleeding after injury.	Epistaxis, menorrhagia, and gastrointestinal bleeding.
Petechiae	Rare	Common

is illustrated in Table 8-2. Once a provisional diagnosis has been made, it can be confirmed by assay of specific clotting factors. The mode of transmission of the inherited defects of coagulation is listed below.

Mode of Transmission of the Hereditary Coagulation Disorders

Sex-linked recessive (disorders primarily of males)
    Factor VIII (AHF) deficiency
    Factor IX (PTC) deficiency

Autosomal dominant (disorders of both sexes; one parent affected)
    Factor XI (PTA) deficiency
    Von Willebrand's disease

Autosomal recessive (disorders of both sexes; parents appear normal)
    Prothrombin deficiency
    Factor V (proaccelerin) deficiency
    Factor VII (proconvertin) deficiency
    Factor X (Stuart-Prower) deficiency
    Factor XII (Hageman) deficiency—no bleeding associated with this disorder
    Factor XIII (fibrin stabilizing factor) deficiency
    Afibrinogenemia, congenital

Table 8-2. A Diagnostic Approach to the Bleeding Patient

Platelets decreased PT prolonged PTT prolonged	Platelets normal PT prolonged PTT prolonged	Platelets normal PT normal PTT prolonged	Platelets normal PT prolonged PTT normal	Platelets normal PT normal PTT normal	Platelets decreased PT and PTT normal
Consider: disseminated intravascular coagulation, particularly in patients with sepsis or hypoxia. ↓ ↓ ↓ ↓ ↓ ↓	*Consider:* Vitamin K deficiency. ↓ ↓ ↓ ↓ ↓ ↓ ↓ ↓	*Consider:* Congenital Factor VIII deficiency. Congenital Factor IX deficiency. Congenital Factor XI deficiency. Congenital Factor XII deficiency. Von Willebrand's disease. Heparin treatment. ↓	*Consider:* Congenital Factor II deficiency. Congenital Factor VII deficiency. ↓ ↓ ↓ ↓ ↓ ↓	*Consider:* Factor XIII deficiency. Platelet dysfunction. Von Willebrand's disease. ↓ ↓ ↓	Determine cause of thrombocytopenia.
Tests to confirm: Thrombin time. Fibrin split products. Factor V assay Red cell fragmentation.	If vitamin K has not been given, administer vitamin K₁, 2.0 mg. I.V. Repeat PT and PTT in 4 hours.	*Tests to confirm:* Factor VIII, IX, XI, XII assay. Bleeding time (prolonged in Von Willebrand's desease).	*Tests to confirm:* Factor II assay. Factor VII assay.	*Tests to confirm:* Factor XII assay. Bleeding time. Platelet adhesiveness. Maternal and infant drug history.	

Bleeding stops.
PT normal.
PTT normal.
↓
Diagnosis:
Vitamin K deficiency.

→ Bleeding continues.
PT abnormal.
PTT abnormal.
↓
Consider:
Congenital Factor V deficiency.
Congenital Factor X deficiency.
Congenital fibrinogen deficiency.
Severe liver disease.
↓
Tests to confirm:
Factor V assay.
Factor X assay.
Fibrinogen assay.

If the patient is found to be thrombocytopenic, a decision must be made as to whether the low platelet count is the result of inadequate platelet production or accelerated platelet destruction. Simple studies that assist the physician in this determination include a bone marrow examination to determine the adequacy of megakaryocyte number, and an examination of the peripheral smear. Young platelets tend to be large (greater than 2.5 μm in diameter). In patients with destructive thrombocytopenias, young platelets are usually evident on the blood film. If the results of the bone marrow examination and peripheral smear are indecisive, the patient can be administered platelets and their survival determined.

Causes of thrombocytopenia are listed below. In addition to these more common causes of bleeding, a large variety of rare disorders of platelet function have now been described.

Causes of Thrombocytopenia

Decreased rate of production
  Leukemia
  Aplastic anemia (inherited and acquired)
  Drug-induced
  Prolonged steroid therapy

Increased rate of destruction
  Idiopathic thrombocytopenic purpura
  Disseminated intravascular coagulation
  Hypersplenism
  Systemic lupus erythematosus
  Wiskott-Aldrich syndrome
  Inherited platelet defects
  Evan's syndrome (thrombocytopenia in association with autoimmune
    hemolytic anemia)

Bleeding in the newborn infant presents some unique problems of interpretation and management.

It has been estimated that approximately 1 per cent of all nursery admissions are complicated by problems of hemorrhage or thrombosis. With the prolongation of life in small and desperately ill premature infants, the incidence of clinical coagulation problems appears to be even greater.

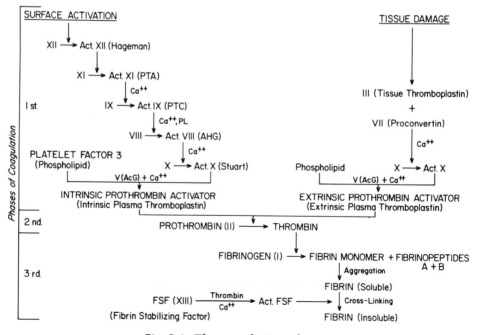

Fig. 8-1. The coagulation scheme.

Table 8-3. Coagulation Factors and Test Values in Term and Premature Infants

Factor	Normal	Term infant (cord blood)	Premature infant (cord blood)
Fibrinogen (mg/dl.)	200–400	200–250	200–250
Factor II (%)	50–150	40	25
Factor V (%)	75–125	90	60–75
Factor VII (%)	75–125	50	35
Factor VIII (%)	50–150	100	80–100
Factor IX (%)	50–150	25–40	25–40
Factor X (%)	50–150	50–60	25–40
Factor XI (%)	75–125	30–40	—
Factor XII (%)	75–125	50–100	50–100
Factor XIII (titer)	1:16	1:8	1:8
Partial thromboplastin time (sec)	30–50	70	80–90
Prothrombin time (sec)	10–12	12–18	14–20
Thrombin time (sec)	10–12	12–16	13–20

The bleeding problems of the newborn can be conveniently divided into the following broad categories: (1) inherited defects of the coagulation mechanism, (2) accentuation of the normally occurring transitory deficiencies of the coagulation mechanism characteristic of this period of life, (3) transitory disturbances secondary to an associated disease process, (4) quantitative or qualitative abnormalities of the platelets.

Many of the coagulation factors are not present in normal concentrations in the blood of the newborn infant. These deviations from normal adult values are particularly marked in the premature infant. Several recent publications have described these developmental changes. The usual values encountered in the term and preterm infant are summarized in Table 8-3. It should be noted that the vitamin K dependent factors (Factors II, VII, IX, and X) and Factors XI, XII, and XIII are generally decreased while the levels of fibrinogen (Factors V and VIII) and platelets are in, or near, the normal adult range.

Despite deficiencies of many of these factors, the whole blood of the newborn infant appears hypercoagulable. This hypercoagulability appears related most closely to a deficiency of antithrombin-III being observed in infants who developed the respiratory distress syndrome.

INHERITED DEFECTS OF THE COAGULATION MECHANISM

Although the majority of infants with congenital deficiencies of the coagulation factors do not bleed during the first weeks of life, all of the congenital defects can manifest themselves with hemorrhage in the newborn period.

It is not clear why hemorrhage does not occur more frequently. None of the coagulation factors crosses the placenta, so infants with hemophilia can be diagnosed at birth and are presumably at risk from hemorrhage.

From studies of patients with Factor VIII deficiency (classical hemophilia), it would appear that only the most severely affected persons bled during the newborn period. When bleeding occurs in the newborn, it is most commonly a result of a circumcision. More serious bleeding may take the form of giant cephalohematoma, intracranial hemorrhages, hemarthroses, and intramuscular hematomas. Petechiae and flat ecchymotic areas are uncommon isolated manifestions of hemophilia.

VITAMIN K DEFICIENCY

Vitamin K deficiency, or true "hemorrhagic disease of the newborn," is caused by an accentuation of the normally occurring transient deficiencies of the coagulation mechanism that characterize this period of life. Bleeding due to vitamin K deficiency is completely preventable if the recommendations of the American Academy of Pediatrics are followed. The administration of 1 mg. of the naturally occurring vitamin K_1 (phytonadione) corrects the deficiency and has not been reported to produce undesirable side effects.

Bleeding due to vitamin K deficiency can occur on the first day of life but is more commonly observed on the second or third day of life. Bleeding from the gastrointestinal tract, umbilical cord, circumcision site, nose, and into the scalp, as well as generalized ecchymosis, are the most frequent external manifestations of the disease. Internal hemorrhages can also occur. Prolonged oozing from capillary punctures may be the first clue to its presence.

The laboratory features of the disease are summarized in Table 8-4 and contrasted with those observed in neonates with disseminated intravascular coagulation. Vitamin K deficiency is characterized by a marked prolongation in the prothrombin time and partial thromboplastin time. Slight prolongations of either of these tests should not be used as an explanation for serious hemorrhages.

Treatment of bleeding due to vitamin K deficiency consists of the in-

Table 8-4. Differential Features of Hemorrhagic Disease of the Newborn

Features	Vitamin K deficiency	Disseminated intravascular coagulation
Uniformity of clotting defect	Constant	Variable
Capillary fragility	Normal	Usually abnormal
Bleeding time	Normal	Often prolonged
Clotting time	Prolonged	Variable
One-stage prothrombin	Very prolonged (5% or less)	Moderately prolonged
Partial thromboplastin time	Prolonged	Prolonged
Thrombin time	Normal for age	Usually prolonged
Fibrin degradation products	Not present	Present
Factor V	Normal	Decreased
Fibrinogen	Normal	Often decreased
Platelets	Normal	Often decreased
Red cell fragmentation	Not present	Usually present
Response to vitamin K	Spectacular	Diminished or absent
Associated disease	Usually trivial (trauma may be precipitating factor)	Severe. May include sepsis, hypoxia, acidosis, or obstetric accident
Previous history	No vitamin K given or mother receiving barbiturates or anticonvulsants	Above illnesses Vitamin K given

travenous administration of 1 mg. of vitamin K_1. If this deficiency is responsible for the abnormal test results, dramatic correction may be observed in a period as short as 2 hours. Maximal correction may be observed in 24 hours. It is important to remember that neither the prothrombin time, the partial thromboplastin time, nor the level of Factor II may reach the expected adult normal values for a period of several weeks to months. The response to vitamin K is less marked in the premature infant, but even in these infants, if otherwise well, a therapeutic response can be anticipated.

DISSEMINATED INTRAVASCULAR COAGULATION

Disseminated intravascular coagulation (DIC) is an acquired patho-physiologic process characterized by the intravascular consumption of platelets and plasma clotting factors, most notably Factors II, V, VIII, XIII, and fibrinogen. This widespread coagulation within the circulation results in the deposition of fibrin thrombi in small vessels and the production of a hemorrhagic state when the level of platelets and clotting factors drop to values that are insufficient to maintain hemostasis. The accumulation of fibrin in the microcirculation also produces mechanical injury to the red cells, leading to erythrocyte fragmentation and a hemolytic anemia.

Disseminated intravascular coagulation is recognized with increasing frequency as an associated event in a variety of disorders and has been the subject of several excellent reviews. Clinical conditions in the newborn period that may be accompanied by DIC are summarized in Table 8-5. Gram-negative septicemia, acidosis, hypoxia, and hypotension appear to be the most common initiating events during the first several days of life. Coagulation disturbances characteristic of disseminated intravascular coagulation are seen in many of the sickest infants with the respiratory distress syndrome. Most evidence to date indicates that the disturbance in coagulation reflects the severity of the disease process and in no way is responsible for the idiopathic respiratory distress syndrome. Hemorrhage, however, may be a terminal event in many of these sick infants.

The clinical manifestations are variable, and in part are determined by the associated disease process, in part by the severity of the coagulation disturbance. In a typical case, oozing at puncture sites is noted in a sick infant. Closer examination usually reveals the presence of petechiae and scattered purpura. Clinical manifestations may include pulmonary, cerebral, and intraventricular hemorrhages. Also observed are bleeding from the umbilical stump and body orifices, and thrombosis of peripheral or central vessels with tissue necrosis and gangrene.

Laboratory abnormalities include the presence of a hemolytic anemia with red cell fragmentation visible on the peripheral smear, variable degrees of thrombocytopenia, and a prolongation of the prothrombin, partial thromboplastin and thrombin time. The level of Factor V and fibrinogen are most commonly decreased in the sickest infants. This decrease may reflect impaired hepatic synthesis in a very sick, immature infant and does not establish the presence of disseminated intravascular coagulation. The presence of elevated levels of fibrin-split products occurs invariably in older infants, children, and adults with disseminated intravascular coagulation, but may not always be present in the neonate. This can be a result of a relative deficiency of plasminogen and plasminogen

Table 8-5. Conditions Associated with Disseminated Intravascular Coagulation in the Newborn

Obstetric complications	Neonatal Infections	Miscellaneous conditions
Abruptio placentae	Bacterial, both gram-negative and gram-positive	Respiratory distress syndrome
Preeclampsia and eclampsia	Disseminated herpes simplex	Severe erythroblastosis fetalis
Dead twin fetus	Cytomegalovirus infections	Giant hemangioma
Fetal distress during delivery	Rubella	Renal vein thrombosis
Amniotic fluid embolism	Toxoplasmosis	Severe acidosis and hypoxemia
Breech delivery	Syphilis	Indwelling catheters

activators during this period of life. The laboratory features characteristic of disseminated intravascular coagulation are described in Table 8-4.

Treatment must be directed at both the underlying disease process and the coagulation abnormality. Success, in general, depends on the ability to correct the condition that initiated the process of disseminated intravascular coagulation rather than merely on the management of the hematologic abnormalities. Management of the patient thus may include the administration of appropriate antibiotics, correction of abnormalities of pH and electrolytes, and maintenance of adequate oxygenation and blood pressure. The decision to treat the abnormalities of coagulation must be based on the clinical findings as well as on the laboratory results. If the infant is bleeding or has evidence of thrombotic complications, and laboratory studies support the diagnosis of disseminated intravascular coagulation, then treatment appears indicated. Exchange transfusion with blood that is less than 48 hours old is the simplest and most effective means of treating DIC.

PLATELET DISTURBANCES

A platelet count of less than 100,000/mm.^{3} is abnormal in either the term or premature infant. The level of platelets in the blood reflects a balance between their production and their destruction. Thrombocytopenia, therefore, may result from a decreased production of platelets, increased destruction of platelets, or a combination of the two. Platelet production is evaluated chiefly by inspection of the number and appearance of megakaryocytes in a carefully collected sample of bone marrow. This is not always easy to accomplish in a small infant. Platelet destruction may be evaluated by determination of the platelet survival, using platelets labeled with isotopes such as chromium-51 or by merely monitoring the disappearance rate of platelets following a transfusion of unlabeled platelets. An additional clue to the mechanism of thrombocytopenia may be obtained from an evaluation of platelet size. Young platelets are larger than old platelets. The predominance of large platelets in a peripheral smear of blood collected in EDTA, to prevent platelet aggregation, suggests that the thrombocytopenia is a result of peripheral platelet destruction with a compensatory increase in young platelets from the bone marrow.

There are many causes of thrombocytopenia in the newborn. The most common of these disorders are outlined below and have been reviewed in detail elsewhere.

Etiologic Classification of Neonatal Thrombocytopenia

Immune disorders
Passive (acquired from mother)—ITP, drug-induced thrombocytopenia, systemic lupus erythematosus.
Active
Isoimmune—platelet group incompatibility.
Associated with erythroblastosis fetalis—due to the disease or to exchange transfusion.

Infections (? mediated in part by intravascular coagulation)
Bacterial—generalized sepsis, congenital syphilis.
Viral—cytomegalic inclusion disease, disseminated herpes simplex, rubella syndrome.
Protozoal—congenital toxoplasmosis.

Drugs (administered to mother)—nonimmune mechanism (e.g., thiazide diuretics, tolbutamide)

Congenital megakaryocytic hypoplasia
Isolated—congenital hypoplastic thrombocytopenia.
Associated with: absent radii, microcephaly; rubella syndrome; pancytopenia and congenital anomalies (Fanconi's anemia).
Associated with pancytopenia but no congenital anomalies.
Associated with trisomy syndromes—D_1 (13, E 18).

Bone marrow disease
Congenital leukemia.

Disseminated intravascular coagulation (DIC)
  Sepsis.
  Obstetrical complications—abruptio placentae, eclampsia, amniotic fluid
    embolism, dead twin fetus.
  Anoxia.
  Stasis—giant hemangioma (including placental chorangioma), renal vein
    thrombosis, polycythemia.

Inherited (chronic) thrombocytopenia
  Sex-linked:
    Pure.
    Aldrich's syndrome.
  Autosomal:
    Pure—dominant or recessive.
    May-Hegglin anomaly—dominant.

Miscellaneous
  Thrombotic thrombocytopenic purpura.
  Inherited metabolic disorders—glycinemia, methylmalonic acidemia,
    isovaleric acidemia.
  Congenital thyrotoxicosis.

Immune Thrombocytopenia

A variety of conditions are associated with the passage of antibody from the mother across the placenta to the infant that result in immunologic destruction of the infant's platelets. The antibody may be formed against an antigen on the mother's platelets (autoimmune) or those of the infant (isoimmune).

The maternal disorders in which thrombocytopenia may occur in both the mother and infant include idiopathic thrombocytopenic purpura, drug-induced thrombocytopenia, and systemic lupus erythematosus.

In isoimmune thrombocytopenia, the thrombocytopenia is confined to the infant. In this condition, the infant possesses a platelet antigen lacking in the mother and the infant's platelets cross the placenta into the maternal circulation, resulting in the formation of antibodies by the mother against the foreign platelet antigen. This immunologic mechanism is analogous to that of red cell sensitization that occurs in erythroblastosis fetalis.

Infants born with immune thrombocytopenia show wide variation in their clinical manifestations, although bleeding manifestations appear to be more severe in the isoimmune form of the disease. Infants tend to show maximal signs of bruising and bleeding shortly after birth as a consequence of the mechanical trauma of the birth process. The most common type of bleeding consists of generalized petechiae and purpuric spots. Bleeding from other sites may be observed (e.g., oozing from the cord, epistaxis, hematuria, melena, and bleeding from needle punctures). Intracranial hemorrhages may also occur.

Jaundice may develop as a consequence of the increased breakdown of red cells within entrapped hemorrhages. Hepatosplenomegaly is absent in these conditions. Bone marrow examination usually reveals the presence of normal to increased numbers of megakaryocytes.

It has been estimated that approximately 10 per cent of infants born to mothers with autoimmune thrombocytopenia die in the neonatal period as a consequence of hemorrhage, while 15 per cent of infants with isoimmune thrombocytopenia succumb. These figures appear excessive. The thrombocytopenia of passively acquired thrombocytopenia may persist for 1 to 4 months, while the course of isoimmune thrombocytopenia is generally only 1 to 6 weeks' duration.

Treatment is generally reserved for the infant with bleeding. In infants with passive forms of thrombocytopenia, exchange transfusion, followed by platelet transfusion, appears to be most effective in management. In infants with isoimmune thrombocytopenia, transfusions of platelets obtained from the mother will normalize the platelet count and produce a cessation of bleeding. Neither steroids nor splenectomy has been demonstrated to be of benefit, and splenectomy should never be considered in management of the newborn.

In pregnancies complicated by isoimmune thrombocytopenia, it would appear advantageous to reduce the hazards of bleeding in subsequent children by delivering the infant by Caesarean section.

Other Forms of Thrombocytopenia

As indicated above, a variety of other disorders may produce a reduction in platelet count. Infections are a leading cause of thrombocytopenia. Inherited defects in platelet production or platelet function may also manifest themselves at this period of life. An approach to the multiple diagnostic possibilities is outlined in Figure 8-2.

In this scheme, it is as important to study the mother as it is to study the infant. Points requiring specific inquiry include: (1) a history of previous bleeding in the form of purpura, bruising, or nosebleeds that might suggest a diagnosis of maternal ITP at some time in the past; (2) ingestion of drugs that might cause thrombocytopenia in the mother and infant (for example, quinidine and quinine) or in the infant alone (thiazide diuretics, tolbutamide); (3) previous infants affected with purpura, suggesting either one of the immune or inherited thrombocytopenias; (4) skin rash or exposure to rubella in the first 8 weeks of pregnancy. The results of the routine test for syphilis should be sought and recorded rather than left buried among the other routine laboratory results performed earlier in pregnancy. Finally, an accurate platelet count should be performed on the mother as soon as possible after delivery to separate immune neonatal thrombocytopenia due to maternal ITP from that due

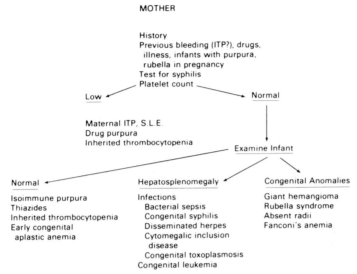

MOTHER

History
Previous bleeding (ITP?), drugs,
  illness, infants with purpura,
  rubella in pregnancy
Test for syphilis
Platelet count

Low ← → Normal

Maternal ITP, S.L.E.
Drug purpura
Inherited thrombocytopenia

Examine Infant

Normal ← Hepatosplenomegaly ← Congenital Anomalies

Normal	Hepatosplenomegaly	Congenital Anomalies
Isoimmune purpura	Infections	Giant hemangioma
Thiazides	Bacterial sepsis	Rubella syndrome
Inherited thrombocytopenia	Congenital syphilis	Absent radii
Early congenital	Disseminated herpes	Fanconi's anemia
aplastic anemia	Cytomegalic inclusion	
	disease	
	Congenital toxoplasmosis	
	Congenital leukemia	

Fig. 8-2. Approach to the diagnosis of the thrombocytopenic newborn.

to platelet isoimmunization (in which case the mother's platelet count is normal).

Physical findings of importance in differential diagnosis in the affected newborn include the presence or absence of hepatosplenomegaly and congenital anomalies. Hepatosplenomegaly is often accompanied by jaundice and suggests an infectious process as the most likely cause of thrombocytopenia. In some cases, congenital leukemia may also have to be considered. Among the congenital anomalies associated with neonatal thrombocytopenia, the most common group recognizable at birth is that occurring in the rubella syndrome (congenital heart defects, cataracts, and microcephaly). Deformity and shortening of the forearms should suggest bilateral absence of the radii with associated megakaryocytic thrombocytopenia. A single large hemangioma or multiple smaller hemangiomas point to these tumors as the problem site of platelet trapping leading to thrombocytopenia.

Complete blood count on the infant should include hemoglobin, white cell count, platelet count, and smear. Associated anemia may be due to blood loss, concurrent hemolysis (as might occur in one of the infectious processes), or marrow infiltration due to congenital leukemia. Leukocytosis of a mild degree may accompany infection or blood loss, but when this exceeds 40,000 to 50,000/mm³. it should point either to congenital leukemia or to the absent radii syndrome. Bone marrow examination is essential not only for assessment of megakaryocytes, but also to exclude underlying infiltrative disorders such as leukemia. Increased numbers of megakaryocytes suggest either consumption coagulopathy or one of the immune thrombocytopenias, although megakaryocytes may be diminished in number in some infants with these disorders. A decrease in the number of megakaryocytes generally suggests one of the types of congenital megakaryocytic hypoplasia. It is important, however, to exclude the immune disorders, if possible, by serologic tests before arriving at this diagnosis because of its ominous prognosis. When in doubt, it is wise to defer such a diagnosis until follow-up observations clarify the situation. Repeat bone marrow examination may be necessary.

Serologic tests for platelet antibodies are at present difficult, time-consuming, and available only in a small number of laboratories. Should isoimmune thrombocytopenia be suspected by the finding of an otherwise normal thrombocytopenic newborn of a healthy mother with a normal platelet count, blood should be drawn from the mother soon after delivery and serum frozen and saved until antibody testing can be carried out. Because results of such studies are usually not available for some time, their chief value lies in the management of subsequent pregnancies, much in the manner of maternal Rh antibody tests in predicting the occurrence of erythroblastosis fetalis.

The response to platelet transfusions may be of both therapeutic and diagnostic aid. Platelet counts following transfusion have been shown to correlate with the known pathogenetic mechanisms in several infants with either increased platelet destruction or impaired platelet production.

BIBLIOGRAPHY

Gross, S. J., and Stuart, M. J.: Hemostasis in the premature infant. Clin. Perinatol., 4:259, 1977.

> An in-depth review of the developmental physiology of coagulation and the disorders encountered in the newborn infant.

Stuart, M. J.: Inherited defects of platelet function. Sem. Hematol., 12:233, 1975.

> A review of the common and uncommon disorders of platelet function.

Tullis, J. L: Clot. Springfield, Ill. Charles C Thomas, 1976.

> A lucid account of the physiology, clinical diagnosis, and management of the disorders of blood coagulation.

9

Lymphadenopathy

Frank A. Oski, M.D.

The presence of lymphadenopathy, either localized or generalized, is generally greeted with fear and apprehension on both the part of the parent as well as the physician. This is due to the mistaken impression that lymph node enlargement generally signifies the presence of a malignant process.

It must be appreciated that the lymphatic tissue forms a larger percentage of the total body weight during infancy and childhood than in adult life and as a result lymphoid tissue is easily palpable in many areas of the body. The relative abundance of lymphoid tissue is reflected by the size of the pharyngeal tonsillar tissue. The tonsils generally reach their maximal size about the age of 7 years and gradually atrophy. Cervical, axillary, and inguinal nodes are palpable in almost all infants and children. Occipital nodes may be palpable in about 5 per cent of children less than 12 years of age. Enlargement of postauricular, supraclavicular, epitrochlear, popliteal, mediastinal, and abdominal nodes is uncommon and suggests the presence of an associated pathologic process.

Lymph node enlargement results from one of two basic processes. These processes are *proliferation* of cells intrinsic to the lymph node or *infiltration* by extrinsic cells. Cells intrinsic to the lymph node that may undergo proliferation include lymphocytes, plasma cells, and histiocytes. This form of proliferation occurs in response to antigenic stimulation. All types of antigens may provoke such a response. Infiltration of a lymph node involves invasion by malignant cells or by polymorphonuclear leukocytes in response to a local infection.

In attempting to determine the significance of lymphadenopathy, a number of simple facts should be ascertained which will facilitate a decision as to what should be done next in terms of reaching a diagnosis and instituting appropriate therapy.

The following questions should be answered:

1. Is the lymphadenopathy generalized (enlargement of more than two non-contiguous lymph node regions) or is it localized? Generalized lymphadenopathy is caused by generalized disease.

2. If the lymphadenopathy is localized, is it accompanied by signs of infection in the involved node? Is the node tender, is the skin over the node warm or red?

3. If the lymphadenopathy is localized, is there evidence of infection in the drainage area of the lymph node or a history of recent antigenic introduction in the drainage area?

4. Which lymph nodes are involved in the process?

5. If the lymphadenopathy is generalized, what are the associated symptoms and signs? Of importance in the physical examination are the presence of hepatic and splenic enlargement, size of the thyroid gland, and the presence of disease involving the heart, lungs, or joints. Is there evidence of pallor and easy bruising?

GENERALIZED LYMPHADENOPATHY

Generalized lymphadenopathy does not usually present the same diagnostic dilemma to the physician as the presence of local lymphadenopathy. Generalized lymphadenopathy is usually associated with other abnormalities in the history, physical examination, or initial laboratory tests and thus enables the physician to reach a probable diagnosis.

The more common causes of generalized lymphadenopathy are listed below.

Infections must always be seriously considered in patients with generalized lymphadenopathy. Viral infections are probably the most common group of infections responsible for such a response. Viral infections associated with an exanthem such as rubella and rubeola should produce no diagnostic confusion. Infants and children with acquired cytomegalovirus infections or infectious mononucleosis may have nonspecific eruptions. The presence of more than 10 per cent atypical lymphocytes in the peripheral blood smear should alert you to this diagnostic possibility.

With acute overwhelming infections, the presence of fever, leukocytosis, signs of toxicity, and perhaps evidence of a focal lesion responsible for the dissemination process will generally alert the physician to the nature of the underlying disease.

Chronic infections with tuberculosis or syphilis may be causes of generalized lymphadenopathy. This is a very unusual manifestation of these disorders in children.

In patients with rheumatoid arthritis or lupus erythematosus, the history is characterized by the presence of chronic, intermittent fever, eva-

---

Causes of Generalized Lymphadenopathy

Infections
  Pyogenic infections
  Tuberculosis
  Syphilis
  Toxoplasmosis
  Brucellosis
  Histoplasmosis
  Malaria
  Typhoid fever
  Cytomegalovirus infection
  Infectious mononucleosis
  Exanthems (scarlet fever, rubella, rubeola)
  Infectious hepatitis

Collagen vascular diseases
  Lupus erythematosus
  Rheumatoid arthritis

Immunologic reactions
  Serum sickness
  Drug reactions
  Granulomatous diseases (sarcoid)

Drug-induced
  Dilantin

Storage diseases
  Gaucher's disease
  Niemann-Pick's disease

Malignancies
  Leukemia
  Neuroblastoma, metastatic
  Lymphomas
  Histiocytosis

---

nescent rashes, and arthralgia and arthritis. Physical examination and laboratory tests may indicate the presence of disease involving the joints, kidney, lungs, liver, myocardium, and pericardium.

In patients with storage disorders that are associated with lymphadenopathy, the spleen and liver will also be enlarged. In young infants and children with these generalized disorders, evidence of cerebral involvement may dominate the clinical picture.

Although it is estimated that as many as 70 per cent of pediatric patients with acute lymphoblastic leukemia will have generalized lymphadenopathy, this finding is rarely the initial manifestation of the disease. The clinical picture in these patients is dominated by a history of unexplained fever, general malaise, pallor, and easy bruising. With generalized lymphadenopathy, splenomegaly is invariably present.

The patient with histiocytosis frequently has associated skin involvement, a history of chronic otitis media, and evidence of disease involving the lungs, liver, and spleen.

In view of these considerations, it is unusual for patients with generalized lymphadenopathy to require a lymph node biopsy to establish a diagnosis.

REGIONAL LYMPHADENOPATHY

Regional lymphadenopathy, and most particularly lymphadenopathy in the cervical area, produce the greatest diagnostic dilemma to the physician. The physician in this circumstance must decide if the lump is malignant or not and how long he can observe the patient before resorting to a biopsy or lymph node excision.

Again, the area of involvement and the associated findings will facilitate a logical decision. For example, isolated supraclavicular lymph node involvement should always suggest the presence of malignancy. This will usually be accompanied by signs of mediastinal disease and generally is a result of Hodgkin's disease or non-Hodgkin's lymphoma.

Cervical Lymph Node Enlargement

Isolated enlargement of the cervical nodes is generally the result of localized infection. The most common agents producing adenitis in this region are the staphlococcus and streptococcus. Often a history of a recent upper respiratory infection will be elicited. The major causes of cervical adenopathy and their distinguishing characteristics are described in Table 9-1.

A systematic approach to patients with cervical adenitis is extremely important and a time-table that may ultimately lead to biopsy should be established.

When the cervical nodes are warm and tender and evidence of overlying infection is present in the overlying skin, then diagnosis is relatively simple. These nodes should be aspirated for purposes of bacterial culture and smear for bacteriologic identification. In addition, a search should be made for a primary focus of infection in the scalp, mouth, pharynx, and sinuses. The sub-mandibular nodes are most frequently enlarged in patients with infections in the ethmoid and maxillary sinuses. A history of cat scratch should also be elicited.

When the cervical node enlargement is non-tender and not associated with signs of infection, other diagnostic procedures should accompany the initial evaluation. The following should be included: a complete

Table 9-1. Causes of Cervical Adenitis

Cause	Comment
Viral upper respiratory infections	Most common cause. Nodes soft, minimally tender, and not associated with evidence of redness and warmth of overlying skin.
Bacterial infection	Streptococcus and staphylococcus most common etiologic agents. Usually secondary to previous or associated infection in drainage area of node. More frequently unilateral. Signs of infection—tenderness, warmth and redness—generally present.
Tuberculosis	Mycobacteria tuberculosis infections generally bilateral, involve multiple nodes. Associated with evidence of chest disease and systemic signs. Atypical mycobacteria infections more commonly unilateral initially. Not associated, in general, with other foci of disease. With either agent, evidence of local warmth and redness uncommon.
Infectious mononucleosis	Fever, malaise, preceding upper respiratory infection often noted. Splenomegaly common. Atypical lymphocytes present. Epstein-Barr virus titers required for diagnosis in younger children.
Cytomegalovirus Toxoplasmosis	Clinically indistinguishable from Epstein-Barr virus infections. Requires serologic studies to make the diagnosis.
Cat scratch disease	History of contact with young cat. May be preceded by history of fever and malaise. Adenopathy restricted to area drained by initial cat scratch.
Sarcoidosis	Disease bilateral. Chest film almost always abnormal. May have keratitis, iritis and evidence of bone disease.
Hodgkin's disease	Common presenting symptom. Frequently unilateral at time of initial manifestation. Node is rubbery, non-tender, and not associated with signs of inflammation. Make certain that supraclavicular involvement is not present. When present, strongly suspect lymphoma.
Non-Hodgkin's lymphoma	Bilateral at time of initial presentation in approximately 40% of patients. Cervical and submaxillary nodes commonly involved together.

blood count and smear looking for evidence of atypical lymphocytes, a heterophile test or a titer for the presence of Epstein-Barr virus antibodies, skin tests for both mycobacteria tuberculosis and atypical mycobacteria, and a chest film.

If the cervical enlargement is accompanied by supraclavicular enlargement, or if splenomegaly is present in the absence of evidence of a viral illness, recent immunization, or signs of drug allergy, then an early lymph node biopsy should be obtained.

Table 9-2. Localized Non-Cervical Lymphadenopathy

Supraclavicular	Always consider mediastinal disease (tuberculosis, histoplasmosis, coccidiomycosis, sarcoidosis). Always consider lymphoma. In absence of evidence of pulmonary infection, early node biopsy indicated.
Axillary	Secondary to infections in the hand, arm, lateral chest wall or lateral portion of the breast. May be result of recently administered immunizations in the arm. Very common with BCG innoculations.
Epitrochlear	Secondary to infections on ulnar side of hand and forearm. Observed in tularemia when bite occurs on finger. Also observed in secondary syphilis.
Inguinal	Look for evidence of infection in the lower extremity, scrotum and penis in the male, vulva and vagina in the female, the skin of the lower abdomen, perineum, gluteal region, or anal canal.
	May be manifestation of lymphogranuloma venereum.
	May represent metastatic disease from testicular tumors or bony tumors of the leg.

If all diagnostic studies reveal nothing, the patient can be treated safely for several weeks on the presumption that an undiagnosed, deep-seated bacterial infection is present in the node. Treatment should be with penicillin or a penicillin derivative in large doses. Careful measurements of the node should be performed. If at the end of 2 to 4 weeks of observation the node has not changed in size or character or has grown painlessly larger, then node biopsy or excision should be performed.

It must be remembered that not all masses in the neck are of lymphoid origin. Palpable lumps in the neck may represent a cervical rib, thyroglossal cysts, branchial cleft cysts, cystic hygromas, goiters, and thyroid carcinomas.

LYMPHADENOPATHY ELSEWHERE IN THE BODY

The presence of localized lymphadenopathy in non-cervical regions does not generally produce the same diagnostic dilemma. Generally this reflects infection or the introduction of an antigen into the area drained by the nodes. The principal causes of localized non-cervical lymphadenopathy are described in Table 9-2. Management of this form of lymphadenopathy is dictated by the associated findings.

BIBLIOGRAPHY

Barton, L. L., and Feigin, R. D.: Childhood cervical lymphadenitis: A reappraisal. J. Pediatr., *84*:846, 1974.

> A study of the infectious agents that produce lymphadenopathy in children and a guide to their diagnosis and management.

Jones, P. G.: Swellings in the neck in children. Med. J. Aust., *1*:212, 1963.
Snapper, I.: The bedside diagnosis of cervical lymphadenopathies. Med. Clin. North Am., *51*:627, 1962.

> A review of the most common form of adenopathy in children—cervical adenopathy.

Zeulzer, W. W., and Kaplan, J.: The child with lymphadenopathy. Semin. Hematol., *12*:323, 1975.

> A comprehensive discussion of the causes of lymphadenopathy in infants and children with suggestions regarding diagnosis and management.

10

Splenomegaly

Frank A. Oski, M.D.

The spleen is one of the major components of the reticuloendothelial system. The spleen is comprised of two distinct but closely related elements: the white pulp and the red pulp. The white pulp represents histiocytic macrophages, lymphocytes, and plasma cells, while the red pulp is composed of the Billroth cords and splenic sinuses. As a consequence of its dual anatomic construction, it serves dual functions. The two primary functions of the spleen are the filtration of particulate matter and formed elements from the blood and the production of humoral factors required for the opsonization of infectious organisms. Splenic enlargement can be observed in disease states in which either the clearing function of the spleen is excessive or in circumstances in which antigenic stimulation is either massive or prolonged. During fetal life and early infancy, the spleen is also the site of erythropoiesis. In response to needs for augmented red cell production, the spleen may continue to serve as a site for erythrocyte production and this also is reflected by the presence of splenomegaly.

The spleen is normally palpable as a soft organ in most infants born prior to 40 weeks gestation. In this circumstance, the spleen can be felt 1 to 2 cm. below the left costal margin in the mid-clavicular line. The spleen can be palpated in approximately 30 per cent of normal term infants and in 10 per cent of healthy infants at 1 year of age. By the age of 12 years, about 1 per cent of normal children still have a spleen that is palpable approximately 1 cm. below the left costal margin. In healthy infants and children, the spleen, when palpable, is soft and non-tender and feels much like a normal lymph node.

There are many diseases in which the spleen may be palpable. It is useless to try to memorize lengthy lists of this sort in a attempt to reach a diagnosis of splenomegaly. It is far more helpful to visualize the different processes that result in splenomegaly by using the letters in the word SPLEEN.

SEQUESTRATION

The spleen sequesters effete red cells at the end of their normal 120-day lifespan. Abnormal red cells are also retained within the red pulp of this organ. Two main mechanisms are operative under conditions that result in splenic sequestration of erythrocytes. The first is an alteration in the surface properties of the red cell. The presence of immunoglobulins or complement on the surface of the red cell results in their recognition, detention, and ultimate phagocytosis by the monocytes and macrophages within the endothelial lining of the spleen. Diseases accompanied by antibody coating of red cells are generally associated with some degree of splenomegaly. Examples of such diseases include Rh and ABO isoimmunization during the newborn period and "autoimmune" hemolytic anemias later in life.

Splenic sequestration causes a loss of the normal deformability of the erythrocyte. Red cells may lose their normal deformability as a result of alterations in membrane proteins, intracellular deposition of precipitated or aggregated hemoglobin, or as a result of alterations in cell water, cations, or metabolic intermediates such as adenosine triphosphate.

Hereditary hemolytic anemias that are accompanied by alterations in red cell deformability include sickle-cell anemia, hemoglobin C disease, thalassemia major, many of the unstable hemoglobins, some of the enzyme deficiencies such as pyruvate kinase deficiency, hereditary spherocytosis, hereditary elliptocytosis, and hereditary stomatocytosis.

The enlargement of the spleen should not be accompanied by generalized lymphadenopathy in patients in whom splenomegaly is produced by sequestration of red cells. A history of anemia or jaundice may be present in the patient or in other family members. Examination of the well-prepared peripheral blood smear and a determination of the patient's hemoglobin, red cell indices, and reticulocyte count should enable the physician to make a preliminary decision that the patient's splenomegaly is primarily a result of an alteration of the red cell.

PROLIFERATION

Many viral and bacterial infections result in a proliferation of the white pulp of the spleen. Chronic immunologic stimulation from any cause can also result in splenomegaly.

Examples of viral infections that most commonly result in splenic enlargement in pediatric patients include infectious mononucleosis (Epstein-Barr virus) and cytomegalovirus infections. Splenic enlargement in these situations is usually accompanied by lymphadenopathy, a history of fever and sore throat, a nonspecific rash in some instances, laboratory evidence of hepatic dysfunction, and the presence of atypical lympho-cytes in the peripheral blood smear.

Bacterial infections frequently accompanied by splenic enlargement include severe pneumonias, typhoid fever, bacterial endocarditis, and in-dolent septicemias. The other manifestations of the disease usually dom-inate the clinical picture and isolated splenomegaly is rarely present as a diagnostic enigma.

LIPID

This designation refers to the large and heterogenous group of disorders in which "foam cells" or lipid-laden macrophages accumulate within the spleen and bone marrow resulting in splenomegaly. Lipids appear to ac-cumulate in the spleen in these disorders because of defects in catabolism of sphingolipids or other related metabolic intermediates. Many of these disturbances have sufficiently distinct clinical manifestations which may lead to a presumptive diagnosis. Tables 10-1 to 10-5 attempt to summarize their salient features.

ENGORGEMENT

Engorgement of the spleen may produce splenomegaly; leukopenia and thrombocytopenia are also common findings in patients with splenic engorgement. Localized engorgement can result from splenic trauma and the accumulation of blood within the splenic capsule. Splenic engorge-ment can be observed in children with portal hypertension that is a con-sequence of hepatic disease, primary disease in the portal vein or splenic vein, or in patients with congestive heart failure.

Portal hypertension secondary to liver disease has many causes in pediatric patients. Diseases to consider in such circumstances include chronic hepatitis, cystic fibrosis, Wilson's disease, cirrhosis secondary to intrahepatic biliary atresia, and the consequences of ascending infection via the umbilical vein following catheterization in the neonatal period. In such circumstances, the presence of hepatomegaly, ascites, esophageal varices, internal hemorrhoids, and historical features of liver disease may be found. In patients with congestive splenomegaly as a result of portal vein thrombosis or obstruction to the splenic vein, diagnosis may often only be made with contrast studies of the portal circulation.

Acute splenic engorgement, the so-called "sequestration crisis," may also be observed in patients with sickle-cell anemia. In this circum-stance, for unknown reasons, the spleen rapidly fills with blood and the

Table 10-1. Characteristics of Niemann-Pick Disease

	Niemann-Pick Disease Type A	Niemann-Pick Disease Type B	Niemann-Pick Disease Type C	Niemann-Pick Disease Type D
Clinical onset (yrs.)	½	2–4	3–5	3–5
Life expectancy (yrs.)	<4	Unknown	<15	<20
Earliest manifestations	FTT*, HSmegaly, PM† deterioration	HSmegaly	PM deterioration, HSmegaly	PM deterioration, HSmegaly
Additional abnormalities				
Cherry red spot	+	−	−	−
Foam cells	+	+	+	+
Unique features	Reticular pulmonary infiltrates, vacuolated lymphocytes	Reticular pulmonary infiltrates		
Inheritance	Autosomal recessive	Autosomal recessive	Autosomal recessive	Autosomal recessive
Ethnic extraction	Often Jewish			Nova Scotian
Lipids accumulated	Sphingomyelin, cholesterol	Sphingomyelin, cholesterol	Sphingomyelin, cholesterol	Sphingomyelin, cholesterol
Enzyme deficiency	Sphingo-myelinase	Sphingo-myelinase	?	?

*FTT: Failure to thrive.
†PM deterioration: Progressive mental deterioration.
(From Sloan, H. R., and Breslow, J. L.: Foam cells. *In* Nathan, D., and Oski, F. (eds): Hematology of Infancy and Childhood. Philadelphia, W. B. Saunders, 1974.)

patient literally bleeds within himself. Such patients, usually children under the age of 5 years, may present with signs of profound hypovolemia and anemia. This complication of sickle-cell anemia is one of the primary causes of early death.

ENDOWMENT

This category is included for purposes of completeness but abnormalities in this category are rare causes of splenomegaly. Among congenital causes of splenomegaly may be included splenic hemangiomas, splenic cysts, and splenic cystic hygromas.

Table 10-2. Characteristics of Gaucher's Disease

	Gaucher's Disease Type I	Gaucher's Disease Type II	Gaucher's Disease Type III
Clinical onset (yrs.)	0–91	1/2	1–3
Life expectancy (yrs.)	Variable	<2	<30
Earliest manifestations	HSmegaly, thrombocyto-penia & bleeding	PM deterioration, HSmegaly	PM deterioration, HSmegaly
Additional abnormalities			
Cherry red spot	–	–	–
Foam cells	+	+	+
Unique features	Bony lesions, reticular pulmonary infiltrates	Head retroflexion, coughing, trismus, laryngospasm, abnormal facies, nystagmus	
Inheritance	Autosomal recessive	Autosomal recessive	Autosomal recessive
Ethnic extraction	Often Jewish		
Lipids accumulated	Glucosyl ceramide (GLIa)	Glucosyl ceramide (GLIa)	Glucosyl ceramide (GLIa)
Enzyme deficiency	GLIa-β-glucosidase	GLIa-β-glucosidase	?

(From Sloan, H. R., and Breslow, J. L.: Foam cells. *In* Nathan, D., and Oski, F., (eds.): Hematology of Infancy and Childhood. Philadelphia, W. B. Saunders, 1974.)

INVASION

Splenomegaly may accompany a variety of malignant processes. It is estimated that 50 to 60 per cent of children with leukemia may have splenomegaly at the time of diagnosis. Splenomegaly tends to be more common and of greater size in patients with myelogenous rather than lymphatic leukemia. Again, the other manifestations of the disease tend to dominate the clinical picture and it is extremely rare for the finding of isolated splenomegaly to be the sole historical or physical finding in a child with leukemia.

Table 10-3. Characteristics of G$_M$ Gangliosidosis and Other Storage Disorders

	G$_{M1}$ Gangliosidosis Type I	G$_{M1}$ Gangliosidosis Type II	Lactosyl Ceramidosis	Fabry's Disease	Krabbe's Disease
Clinical onset (yrs.)	Birth	1–2	1	5–20	¼–½
Life expectancy (yrs.)	<2	<10	<4	Variable	<2
Earliest manifestations	PM deterioration, FTT, HSmegaly	PM deterioration	FTT, PM deterioration, HSmegaly	Fever, joint swelling, peripheral pain and edema, telangiectasias	PM deterioration
Additional abnormalities					
Cherry red spot	+	–	–	–	–
Foam cells	+	Variable	+	Variable	–
Unique features	Bony lesions, abnormal facies, vacuolated lymphocytes, acid mucopolysaccharides in urine			Renal involvement	Optic atrophy
Inheritance	Autosomal recessive	Autosomal recessive	Unknown	Sex-linked	Autosomal recessive
Ethnic extraction				Often Scandinavian	
Lipids accumulated	Ganglioside G$_{M1}$	Ganglioside G$_{M1}$	Lactosyl ceramide (GL2a)	Trihexosyl ceramide (GL3), dihexosyl ceramide (GL2b)	Galactosyl* ceramide (GL1b)
Enzyme deficiency	G$_{M1}$-β-galactosidase	G$_{M1}$-β-galactosidase	GL2a-β-galactosidase	GL3-α-galactosidase	GL1b-β-galactosidase

*Extensive demyelination with relative increase of GL1b.
(From Sloan, H. R., and Breslow, J. L.: Foam Cells. *In* Nathan, D., and Oski, F. (eds.): Hematology of Infancy and Childhood. Philadelphia, W. B. Saunders, 1974.)

Lymphomas may also be associated with splenomegaly. In this circumstance, isolated splenomegaly may prove to be a source of real diagnostic confusion.

Splenomegaly is generally present in patients with histiocytosis, but this is rarely an isolated finding.

The spleen may be the site of metastatic disease. The most common pediatric tumor associated with metastases to the spleen is neuroblastoma.

The spleen may be the site of granuloma formation in diseases such as sarcoidosis, tuberculosis, and some of the systemic fungal infections.

Table 10-4. Characteristics of Metachromatic Leukodystrophies

	Infantile Metachromatic Leukodystrophy	Juvenile Metachromatic Leukodystrophy	Adult Metachromatic Leukodystrophy	Metachromatic Leukodystrophy, Multiple Sulfatase Deficiency Form
Clinical onset (yrs.)	1–2	5–10	19–46	1–2
Life expectancy (yrs.)	<10	<20	Variable	<12
Earliest manifestations	PM deterioration	PM deterioration	Dementia	PM deterioration
Additional abnormalities				
Cherry red spot	–	–	–	–
Foam cells	–	–	–	–
Unique features	Nonfunctioning gallbladder, optic atrophy	Optic atrophy		Acid mucopolysaccharides in urine, bony lesions, granulated lymphocytes
Inheritance	Autosomal recessive	Autosomal recessive	Autosomal recessive	Unknown
Ethnic extraction				
Lipids accumulated	Sulfatide	Sulfatide	Sulfatide	Sulfatide
Enzyme deficiency	Sulfatidase (arylsulfatase A)	Sulfatidase (arylsulfatase A)	Sulfatidase (arylsulfatase A) Arylsulfatase A, B, C	

(From Sloan, H. R., and Breslow, J. L.: Foam cells. *In* Nathan, D., and Oski, F. (eds.): Hematology of Infancy and Childhood. Philadelphia, W. B. Saunders, 1974.)

CONCLUSION

Because the causes of splenomegaly are so numerous, it is essential that a general attempt be made to fit the patient into one of the six categories just described before undertaking extensive diagnostic procedures. Usually a careful history, physical examination, routine blood count, and, on occasion, a bone marrow examination, are all that is necessary to reach a tentative assignment to a major pathophysiologic cause for the splenomegaly. After that decision has been reached, more specific tests can be employed to reach a precise diagnosis. Let the SPLEEN guide your thinking.

Table 10-5. Characteristics of Tay-Sachs Disease

	Tay-Sachs Disease Type I	Tay-Sachs Disease Type II	Tay-Sachs Disease Type III
Clinical onset (yrs.)	¼–½	¼–½	1–2
Life expectancy (yrs.)	<5	<4	<15
Earliest manifestations	PM deterioration, hypotonia, "hyperacusis"	PM deterioration, hypotonia, "hyperacusis"	PM deterioration
Additional abnormalities Cherry red spot Foam cells	+ –	+ –	– –
Unique features	Macrocephaly	Macrocephaly	
Inheritance	Autosomal recessive	Autosomal recessive	Unknown
Ethnic extraction	Usually Jewish		
Lipids accumulated	Ganglioside G_{M2}	GL4, ganglioside G_{M2}	Cholesterol, cholestanol
Enzyme deficiency	Hexosaminidase A	Hexosaminidase A & B	?

(From Sloan, H. R., and Breslow, J. L.: Foam cells. *In* Nathan, D., and Oski, F. (eds.): Hematology of Infancy and Childhood. Philadelphia, W. B. Saunders, 1974.)

BIBLIOGRAPHY

Boles, E. T., Jr., Baxter, C. F., and Newton, W. A., Jr.: Evaluation of splenomegaly in childhood. Clin. Pediatr., 2:161, 1963.

A review of the causes and diagnostic approach to splenic enlargement in the pediatric patient.

Sloan, H. R., and Breslow, J. L.: Foam cells. *In* Nathan, D., and Oski, F. (eds.): Hematology of Infancy and Childhood. Philadelphia, W. B. Saunders, 1974.

An extensive discussion of the biochemistry and clinical manifestations of the lipid storage disorders.

11

Abdominal Masses

Frank A. Oski, M.D.

The discovery of an abdominal mass requires an immediate orderly investigation to determine its precise nature. As is true with many signs and symptoms in pediatrics, the etiology of abdominal masses differs among infants and children of varying ages.

In the immediate neonatal period, the presence of an abdominal mass is generally a sign of a congenital malformation and in approximately one-half of all patients it reflects an abnormality of the genitourinary system. In older infants and children, neoplasms and complications of infectious processes are the more common causes of the presence of a palpable mass.

It is unfortunate that beyond the newborn period most masses are discovered by parents rather than physicians. In the examination of an otherwise healthy infant, the single most important portion of the physical exam is a careful palpation of the abdomen. After the initial exam of the newborn and the examination performed at 6 weeks of age, the routine physical examination of an asymptomatic, healthy infant generally discloses few or no abnormalities except for those that may be found in the abdomen. All too often, this portion of the examination may be most cursory.

The diagnostic considerations that accompany the finding of a mass are largely determined by the age of the patient, associated symptoms, and physical findings.

Many abdominal masses detected in routine physical examination ultimately prove to be fecal material, a distended urinary bladder, the abdominal aorta, or the pregnant uterus.

Fecal material in the colon is usually freely movable and easily compressed. If one suspects that the mass is fecal in nature and it cannot be confirmed by rectal examination, an enema should be given to the patient. Following the enema, the patient should be re-examined before proceeding to further diagnostic studies.

A distended bladder may be palpated in the newborn infant who has not voided within the first 24 hours of life. This may signify the presence of abnormalities of the urethra such as posterior urethral valves. Other causes of bladder distention include the use of anticholinergic drugs, spinal cord tumors, and abnormalities of the spinal cord. Bladder distention may also be observed in the comatose patient, during the immediate postoperative period, and as a result of bladder irritation produced by inflammatory lesions in the pelvis such as an appendiceal abscess. In these situations, the mass appears to originate at a point below the symphysis pubis and may extend as high as the umbilicus. Rectal examination usually confirms the presence of a distended bladder. If the child cannot be induced to void, catheterization may be required to confirm the diagnosis.

ABDOMINAL MASSES IN THE NEWBORN

The finding of an abdominal mass in the newborn most commonly signifies the presence of an abnormality of the genitourinary system. The major abnormalities detected during this period of life are listed below.

Abdominal Masses in the Newborn

Kidney
    Hypoplastic multicystic kidney, unilateral or bilateral
    Hydronephrosis secondary to distal obstruction
    Mesoblastic nephroma
    Solitary cyst
    Renal vein thrombosis

Liver and biliary tract
    Hematoma of the liver
    Hemangioma of the liver
    Solitary cyst of the liver
    Hepatoma
    Choledochal cyst
    Distended gallbladder secondary to cystic fibrosis

Gastrointestinal tract
    Duplication of the duodenum, jejunum, or ileum
    Mesenteric cyst
    Volvulus secondary to meconium ileus
    Leiomyosarcoma of the intestine

Female genital tract
    Ovarian cyst
    Hydro- and hematocolpos

Retroperitoneal teratomas

Adrenal hemorrhage

Neuroblastoma

It should be noted that malignant tumors are uncommon at birth. Although Wilms' tumor was previously believed to occur with some frequency during this period of life, it is now realized that most of these tumors are mesoblastic nephromas. This tumor is histologically distinct in its fibroblastic appearance and shows only minimal nuclear polymorphism and mitotic activity. Even though these tumors may grow large and show evidence of local extension, they do not appear to metastasize, and cure may be achieved with surgery alone. Mesoblastic nephromas may constitute as many as 50 per cent of the renal tumors of early infancy and may be responsible for the previous observation that children with Wilms' tumor under the age of 2 had a better prognosis than that observed in older children.

The finding of an abdominal mass in the newborn requires an immediate intravenous pyelogram and, ultimately, surgical exploration.

ABDOMINAL MASSES IN OLDER INFANTS AND CHILDREN

Gastrointestinal Masses

In the infant 3 to 6 weeks of age, the most commonly palpated mass is the "tumor" of *pyloric stenosis*. A history of vomiting, often projectile, of several weeks duration should alert the physician to this diagnostic possibility. This mass is best felt immediately after the infant has vomited. The mass is felt on deep palpation and is generally 1 to 2 cm. in diameter. It is usually located at the end of the stomach anywhere along the edge of the liver from the costal margin in the midline to the underside of the right lobe of the liver.

Another mass that is generally accompanied by symptoms of intestinal obstruction is that produced by the presence of a *duplication* of the alimentary tract. Symptoms may include pain, vomiting, and hemorrhage. Most duplications occur in the small bowel. Some of these cysts are of neuroenteric origin and may be associated with defects in the vertebral column. The mucosa of the cyst is usually well-preserved but need not correspond to that part of the gastrointestinal tract from which the duplication arises. Gastric mucosa is commonly present and occasionally these cysts may also contain pancreatic tissue.

In the infant 6 months to 3 years of age, symptoms of intermittent abdominal pain, often associated with vomiting, may indicate the presence of an *intussusception*. An intussusception may be initiated by enlarged mesenteric lymph nodes. In the young infant and child, the enlarged nodes are generally the result of an associated viral illness. In the child over 6 years of age, the enlarged lymph nodes should strongly suggest the presence of a lymphatic neoplasm.

Polyps, Meckel's diverticulum, and other anatomic abnormalities of the gastrointestinal tract may also serve as the leading point or initiator of the intussusception. Intussusception is also a well-recognized complication of Henoch-Schönlein purpura. Edema and hemorrhage of the bowel wall are responsible for the process. Although the cutaneous manifestations of this disorder are usually present at the time of the intussusception, this abdominal complication may precede the rash and thus produce diagnostic confusion.

The intussusception is a sausage-shaped tender mass that is usually palpable in the right lower quadrant. On occasion, the mass may travel up into the upper right quadrant leaving an empty right lower abdomen where no bowel is palpable (Dance's sign). An intussusception is usually accompanied by the presence of high pitched peristaltic sounds indicative of intestinal obstruction.

Painless abdominal enlargement, sometimes of several years' duration, should suggest the presence of a *mesenteric cyst*. The mass is freely movable in a lateral direction and sometimes a fluid wave or shifting dullness may be detected.

Inflammatory processes may be accompanied by abdominal masses. These include appendiceal abscesses and abscesses associated with fistulas in patients with granulomatous colitis. A history of fever, vomiting, irritability, diarrhea, and anorexia should arouse suspicion of this diagnostic possibility. The mass is tender and the white count is generally elevated.

Neoplasms

The most common abdominal tumors of childhood are Wilms' tumor and neuroblastoma.

Approximately three-fourths of Wilms' tumors appear before the age of 5 years and they are slightly more common in females. The presenting complaint is usually that of a palpable abdominal mass or asymptomatic abdominal enlargement. Fever, abdominal pain, and hypertension may also be present. Hematuria, considered a poor prognostic sign, may be present in approximately 20 per cent of children at the time of diagnosis.

The mass is generally large, firm, and non-tender. It may be palpable in either hypochondrium, extend to the midline and down into the iliac fossa. When present on the left, it may be confused with an enlarged spleen. Radiographic studies usually reveal a soft tissue mass that displaces the intestine to the opposite side. Calcification is uncommon in this tumor in contrast to the frequently speckled calcifications observed in neuroblastomas. Intravenous pyelograms may fail to visualize the affected kidney or may merely demonstrate the presence of an intrarenal mass. On occasion, the tumor may be bilateral at the time of initial diagnosis.

The tumor tends to spread locally but may also metastasize to liver, lung, brain, and, most uncommonly, to bone. The current prognosis for children with Wilms' tumor appears to be better than for any other malignancy of childhood. With surgery, radiation and chemotherapy, as many as 90 per cent of children may be cured.

Wilms' tumor occurs with increased frequency in children with sporadic (in contrast to familial) aniridia. It also occurs with increased frequency in children with congenital hemihypertrophy or with congenital macrosomia (Beckwith's syndrome).

Neuroblastoma is the second most common solid tumor of childhood (brain tumors are the most common). About 50 per cent of neuroblastomas manifest themselves during the first 2 years of life. In approximately one-half of the patients, the tumor arises in the abdomen, and in one-third, the neuroblastoma arises from the adrenal gland. In an additional 13 to 20 per cent of the patients, it arises from non-adrenal intra-abdominal sites. The mass is usually firm, irregular in outline, and nontender, and frequently crosses the midline. Although the most common initial presentation is that of a mass in the abdomen, the patient may also manifest symptoms and signs as a result of compression of other structures by the primary tumor or its metastatic deposits. Unfortunately, up to 70 per cent of patients may have signs of metastasis at the time of diagnosis. Skeletal lesions are common. Metastatic spread to the lung is very rare. Invasion of the retrobulbar soft tissues causes proptosis of the eye, as well as periorbital swelling and ecchymosis of the upper eyelid. Skin and nodal involvement may also be present.

Less commonly, the initial signs and symptoms are related to the catecholamine production of the tumor. These symptoms and signs may include skin flushing, perspiration, tachycardia, hypertension, paroxysmal headaches, and intractable diarrhea. Uncommon initial manifestations may include signs of encephalopathy or opsoclonus.

The prognosis for this tumor is very poor except for patients with well-encapsulated tumors or for patients under 1 to 2 years of age in whom the metastatic process is confined to skin, liver, and bone marrow.

Other tumors of intra-abdominal origin that may present as a mass in the pediatric patient include both Hodgkin's and non-Hodgkin's lymphoma, teratomas, ovarian neoplasms, hepatic tumors, and rhabdomyosarcoma originating from the muscles in the retroperitoneal area.

Kidney Masses

Renal enlargement as a result of multicystic or polycystic kidneys, multilocular cysts, and hydronephrosis may all present as abdominal masses. Frequently the signs of a urinary tract infection will accompany the process.

Liver Masses

Cystic disease of the liver, hepatic abscesses, hemangiomas, and hepatomas may all initially manifest themselves by abdominal enlargement and the detection of an abdominal mass.

DIAGNOSTIC APPROACH TO THE PATIENT
WITH AN ABDOMINAL MASS

As previously indicated, the diagnostic approach to an infant or child with an abdominal mass is generally dictated by the age of the patient, the location of the mass, and the associated physical findings and history. A list of the more common abdominal masses is presented below.

Abdominal Masses in the Older Infant and Child

Renal malformations
Hydronephrosis
Duplication cysts of the intestine
Volvulus of the gut
Intussusception
Periappendiceal abscess
Mesenteric abscess
Mesenteric cyst
Hepatic cyst or abscess
Choledochal cyst
Hepatoma
Hemangioma of the liver or spleen
Wilms' tumor
Neuroblastoma
Lymphoma
Ovarian cyst
Ovarian tumor

In general, initial evaluation should include a careful rectal examination, urinalysis, complete blood count, and flat plate of the abdomen. More precise studies will be dictated by these preliminary studies. Contrast studies of the kidneys are frequently performed first and then may be followed by radiologic examination of the bowel, scans of the liver and spleen, sonography, and computerized axial tomography.

BIBLIOGRAPHY

Arey, J. B.: Abdominal masses in infants and children. Pediatr. Clin. North Am., *10*:665, 1963.

An overview of abdominal masses in infants and children by an experienced pathologist.

Longino, L. A., and Martin, L. W.: Abdominal masses in the newborn infant. Pediatrics, *21*:596, 1958.

A surgeon's approach to the problem of masses in the abdomen of the neonate.

Sutow, W., Vietti, T. J., and Fernbach, D. J.: Clinical Pediatric Oncology. St. Louis, C. V. Mosby, 1973.

A comprehensive review of malignances that may be encountered in pediatrics.

12

Jaundice and the Liver

Robert Kaye, M.D.

Disease of the liver may be suspected by noting in history, physical or laboratory examinations any abnormality suggesting functional or structural pathology. These findings are grouped logically on the basis of their pathogenesis: impairment in the normal metabolic functions of the liver, circulatory abnormalities, response to infections, generalized metabolic disease or structural malformation involving the liver or its excretory ductal system. The principal abnormalities are presented in Table 12-1.

PHYSICAL EXAMINATION OF THE LIVER

In normal infants up to the age of 1 year, the liver edge may be palpable as much as 2 cm. below the costal margin in the midclavicular line. After this age, the liver edge is usually felt no more than 1 cm. below the costal margin. In children it is almost always possible to palpate the liver edge and thus know the position of its lower margin. Evaluation of liver size requires estimation of the position of its upper border by percussion, differentiating the resonance of the air-containing lung above and the liver dullness below. This will identify the liver that is pushed down below its normal position by over-inflation of the lungs due to airway obstruction. The consistency of the normal liver on palpation is comparable to that noted in the relaxed biceps muscle of the adult. A malignant or cirrhotic process may impart a "stony-hard" consistency resembling that noted when pressing the fingers against the dorsum of the wrist. Markedly enlarged livers are usually harder than normal. The chief exception to this is the hugely enlarged liver of glycogen storage disease which is felt to be of normal consistency.

Table 12-1. Abnormalities Suggestive of Liver Disease

Abnormalities	Significance
I. Impaired Metabolic Function A. Jaundice (bilirubin >1.0 mg./dl.)	
1. Indirect hyperbilirubinemia	Hemolysis, defective uptake or conjugation
2. Direct hyperbilirubinemia	Hepatocellular injury, ductal obstruction, defective transport within liver cells
B. Steatorrhea and itching	Reduced bile acid excretion into gut and systemic retention
C. Edema	Decreased albumin synthesis
D. Bleeding	Reduced synthesis of coagulation factors I, II, V, VII, XI and XIII
E. Non-glucose reducing substance in urine	Impaired metabolism of galactose or fructose
F. Hypoglycemia	Decreased parenchymal mass or gluconeogenic enzyme deficiency
II. Enlarged or indurated liver	Hepatocellular inflammation, bile duct obstruction, congestive circulatory failure, cysts, tumors, storage diseases, systemic metabolic disease.
III. Manifestations of portal hypertension	Intrahepatic portal obstruction: cirrhosis, fibrosis, cystic disease, storage diseases, systemic metabolic disease Extrahepatic portal obstruction: portal, splenic, hepatic vein thrombosis
A. Splenic enlargement	Impaired venous drainage
B. Hematemesis	Ruptured esophageal varix
C. Clubbing of nailbeds and spider nevi	Portal systemic shunting
D. Pancytopenia	Sequestration in engorged spleen

EVALUATION OF THE PATIENT

In the process of evaluation of the patient suspected of liver disease, a variety of biochemical, histologic, radiographic and isotopic techniques are available (Table 12-2). Because of its major role in metabolism, the

Table 12-2. Laboratory Aids in Evaluation of Liver Disease

	Normal Values	Significance
Bilirubin	0.2 direct, 1.0 total mg/dl	See text
Alkaline phosphatase	1–3 mos: 73–336 IU/L. 3–10 yrs: 57–151 IU/L. Puberty: 57–258 IU/L. 16 and older: 14–40	Increased: with complete or partial obstruction; biliary cirrhosis, tumors or inflammatory masses Decreased: with parenchymal injury; hepatitis
Transaminases SGOT	I.U./L. Infants 67–118 Older children 3–27	active hepatocellular injury; by infection or toxin
SGPT	0–54	SGPT more specific for liver
Sulfobromophthalein (BSP) excretion	95% clearance in 45 minutes of 5mg/kg	Hepatic excretory capacity; Impaired by reduced parenchymal function or impaired hepatic blood flow
Blood proteins Albumin and haptoglobulin		Reduced with parenchymal cell impairment
Electrophoretic alterations α and β globulins		Increased with infection and obstruction. Decreased with liver failure
Immunoglobulins		Increased with postnecrotic cirrhosis and chronic active hepatitis
Coagulation Factors		See text
α 1-fetoprotein		Presence associated with hepatoma
Bile acids and cholesterol		Elevated in obstructive and cholestatic processes
Hepatitis B antigen		Carrier state or present infection
Hepatitis B antibody		Past or present infection

liver will, when damaged, yield alterations reflecting impairment of one or more of its physiologic functions. Histologic material obtained by open or needle biopsy often provides useful information bearing on diagnosis and prognosis. Radiographic studies are of particular importance in delineating the anatomic abnormalities of the extra-hepatic biliary system and the hepatic vascular pattern which may yield evidence of an infectious or neoplastic mass. Nuclear medicine procedures yield information concerning the functioning mass of the liver, presence of masses and patency of the extra-hepatic biliary system.

Serum measurements of hepatic enzymes are useful in the study of liver disease as a consequence of their increased efflux to the circulation when the cell is injured or when excretion of an enzyme is blocked by obstructive processes.

BILIRUBIN METABOLISM

Bilirubin is a linear tetrapyrrole formed by cleavage of the cyclic tetrapyrrole, protoporphyrin. Protoporphyrin in its iron complex (heme) is the prosthetic group of hemoglobin and other hemoproteins. Bilirubin is readily soluble in organic solvents, but only slightly soluble in aqueous solutions at physiologic pH. It can be determined by coupling with diazotized sulfanilic acid (diazo or van den Bergh reaction). Unconjugated bilirubin reacts in aqueous solution only in the presence of accelerator substances, methanol or ethanol (indirect reaction) which are unnecessary for the reaction of conjugated bilirubin (direct reaction). After the newborn period, the total bilirubin in plasma does not exceed 1.0 mg./dl. with 0.2 mg./dl. reacting directly.

The conversion of heme to bilirubin involves cleavage of the ferroprotoporphyrin ring by microsomal heme oxygenase yielding biliverdin. The latter compound is reduced to bilirubin by biliverdin reductase.

The serum bilirubin concentration reflects an equilibrium between production and excretion. Bilirubin is derived from several sources. About 80 per cent of daily bilirubin production results from breakdown of senescent red blood cells, aged approximately 120 days. Studies with labeled precursors of bilirubin have revealed the label in the fecal bilirubin (urobilinogen) within 1–2 days. This material, representing 10–20 per cent of the daily bilirubin production, is referred to as the "early labeled" fraction. Its source is chromoproteins such as myoglobin, cytochromes, catalase and peroxidases as well as maturing red blood cells in the marrow. Each of these represents a potential source of over-production.

Understanding the metabolism of bile pigments is facilitated by recognition of the fact that unconjugated bilirubin is a potentially toxic, end-stage metabolite requiring elimination from the body.

Essentially all of the bilirubin in the circulation is tightly bound to albumin. In addition to conferring water solubility on bilirubin, the linkage with albumin restricts its transfer across cell membranes, thus protecting the cells from exposure to bilirubin toxicity. In competition with bilirubin for binding sites on albumin are free fatty acids, sulfonamides, thyroxine and salicylates. The displacement of bilirubin from its albumin linkage by these substances is of particular importance in the icteric newborn in whom bilirubin concentrations may rise to levels saturating the total binding capacity of albumin.

Hepatic Uptake and Conjugation

There are mechanisms within the liver cell which establish gradients for the movement of unconjugated bilirubin from plasma to cell and facilitate its clearance into the bile. Lipid-soluble unconjugated bilirubin is able to cross the lipid-containing cell membrane. There are two hepatic cytoplasmic acceptor proteins, Y and Z, capable of binding unconjugated bilirubin, preventing its back-diffusion from the hepatocyte and fostering further transfer of pigment from the plasma.

Another mechanism providing the liver with its unique capacity to remove bilirubin from the plasma is the conversion of the intracytoplasmic pigment to water soluble conjugates of glucuronic acid. The ionic nature and increased molecular size of the conjugates limit back diffusion across the plasma membrane and foster their excretion into the bile.

Glucuronic acid conjugation of bilirubin requires uridine diphosphoglucuronic acid which donates its glucuronic acid to the propionic acid side chains of bilirubin. The reaction is catalyzed by the microsomal enzyme glucuronyl transferase which may be induced by phenobarbital and other compounds.

The bacterial flora of the lower bowel reduces conjugated bilirubin to a group of chromogens designated urobilinogen. Urobilinogen is poorly reabsorbed from the bowel, about 100–200 mg./day is excreted in the stool of adults. Of the small amount reabsorbed, most is excreted by the liver with approximately 4 mg./day eliminated in the urine.

From the above considerations it will be clear that over-production of bilirubin by hemolysis, impaired hepatic uptake or glucuronide conjugation will result in increased concentrations of unconjugated (indirect reacting) bilirubin. Situations which permit bilirubin to gain access to the hepatocyte and undergo conjugation but interfere with its transport into the intestine (parenchymal cell injury, obstruction of the biliary tree or functional disorders of secretion into the bile) will lead to elevations of conjugated (direct reacting) bilirubin.

Stool color yields important clues to the origin of jaundice. Acholic stools are commonly seen during the early stages of hepatitis and in complete extrahepatic biliary obstruction.

Bilirubin Excretion in the Newborn (Physiologic Jaundice)

In the fetus and newborn there are special circumstances which modify the scheme of bilirubin metabolism described above. Unconjugated bilirubin formed by the fetus freely crosses the placenta and is excreted by the maternal liver. During the first week of extra-uterine life, hepatic function is inadequate to prevent its accumulation in plasma. This disability has been regarded as physiologic when limited to this age group and to a bilirubin concentration not in excess of 12 mg./dl. A pathologic process should be suspected and investigated when: (1) jaundice appears before 36 hours of age; (2) serum bilirubin concentration exceeds 12 mg./dl.; (3) jaundice persists beyond the eighth day of life; and (4) the direct reacting bilirubin exceeds 1.5 mg./dl.

A transient deficiency of gluconyl transferase observed in livers of newborn animals and recently expired premature infants was early proposed as an explanation for the impaired clearance of unconjugated bilirubin characteristic of this age. Impaired hepatic uptake of unconjugated bilirubin is observed in newborn animals and suggests an important role of the cytoplasmic acceptor proteins in physiologic jaundice. The Z protein reaches full concentration during fetal life while the major binding protein Y is almost absent at birth reaching mature levels during the second week of life. Decreased effectiveness of the intestinal component of bilirubin elimination is also important in the hyperbilirubinemia of the newborn. This is dependent on reduction by the intestinal flora of conjugated bilirubin to urobilinogen. The newborn infant with a relatively sterile bowel is disadvantaged in this process. Furthermore, glucuronidases present in the intestinal epithelium of the infant at birth are capable of regenerating free bilirubin from its conjugated form. Unconjugated bilirubin can be freely absorbed into the circulation and subjects ths neonatal infant to the superimposed burden of an enterohepatic recirculation of bilirubin. This phenomenon is exaggerated in infants with intestinal obstruction. As there is some bilirubin conjugation and excretion into the intestine beginning at 20 weeks of fetal life, this mechanism probably serves to protect the infant from accumulation of bilirubin within the intestinal lumen as a massive pigmented gallstone. Reabsorbed bilirubin traverses the placenta and is excreted by the maternal liver.

Early feeding of newborn infants serves to hasten bacterial colonization of the intestinal tract, thereby reducing the degree of unconjugated hyperbilirubinemia.

Also contributing to elevated levels of bilirubin in some newborns is continued patency of the ductus venosus which permits some portal blood to bypass the liver. Estrogens and progestins derived from maternal sources may play a role in physiologic jaundice through inhibiting bilirubin conjugation.

A variety of therapeutic approaches may increase the ability of the newborn to eliminate bile pigments. Phenobarbital can enhance bilirubin glucuronyl transferase activity and increase the concentration of the Y acceptor protein, thus increasing both uptake and conjugation of the pigment. The sedative properties of phenobarbital limit its clinical application. Cholestyramine combines with bilirubin and agar gels can sequester the pigment reducing the magnitude of the entero-hepatic recirculation. Phototherapy based on the photolability of bilirubin has been utilized to reduce elevated plasma bilirubin levels. The simpler pyrrole derivatives produced by the action of light (wave length 450 to 460 mn.) can be excreted in the bile and urine without prior conjugation. Light therapy will reduce but not eliminate the need for exchange transfusions.

Disorders of Bilirubin Excretion

There are a number of disorders which involve impairment in one or more of the steps involved in the sequence from bilirubin production to its excretion in the stool. It is helpful to group these on the basis of whether elevation of unconjugated or conjugated bilirubin predominates (Table 12-3).

Table 12-3. Disorders of Bilirubin Production, Hepatic Uptake, Conjugation and Excretion

I. Unconjugated hyperbilirubinemias	
A. Transient neonatal hyperbilirubinemia	
1. Delayed development of hepatic uptake and conjugating system	See above
a. Physiologic jaundice in full-term infant	
b. Physiologic jaundice in low-birth weight infant	More intense and prolonged
2. Inhibitors of conjugation	
a. Lucey-Driscoll syndrome	Serum inhibitors to conjugation of bilirubin
b. Breast-fed infant	Inhibitor, pregnanediol present in breast milk
3. Increased enterohepatic recirculation of bilirubin	
a. Gastrointestinal obstruction	Reduced hepatic blood flow with increased intra-abdominal pressure and increased reabsorption of bilirubin from gut
B. Over-production of bilirubin	
1. Hemolysis due to maternal-fetal blood group incompatibilities	
a. Rh and ABO systems	Antibody produced in mother to fetal red cell antigens leads to hemolysis in newborn
2. Deficiency of red cell enzymes	Glucose-6-phosphate dehydrogenase, fructokinase, glutathione peroxidase

Table 12-3. Disorders of Bilirubin Production, Hepatic Uptake, Conjugation and Excretion (*Continued*)

3. Other hemolytic disorders	
a. Congenital	Spherocytosis, Cooley's anemia, sickle cell disease
b. Acquired	Drugs, autoimmune disease
4. Shunt hyperbilirubinemia	Increased erythrocyte destruction in bone marrow
5. Drugs and chemical agents	Vitamin K, toluene phenacetin, lead
C. Mixed or undefined	
1. Septicemia	Hemolysis, toxic hepatitis
2. Hypothyroidism	Mechanism unknown
3. Drugs and chemical agents	See B5, red cell and hepatic injury
D. Persistent jaundice with defective conjugation	
1. Crigler-Najjar syndrome	
a. Type I	Death in infancy, decreased transferase activity, phenobarbital unresponsive, recessive inheritance
b. Type II	Adult survival, phenobarbital responsive, autosomal dominant
2. Gilbert's syndrome	Onset late childhood, more frequent in males, constitutional and G.I. symptoms, jaundice, phenobarbital responsive
II. Conjugated hyperbilirubinemia due to impaired bilirubin excretion	
A. Transient neonatal hyperbilirubinemia	
1. Following Rh isoimmunization	Hepatic injury or bile duct plugging
B. Chronic non-hemolytic jaundice	
1. Dubin-Johnson syndrome	Pigment in hepatic cells
2. Rotor's syndrome	Without pigment in hepatic cells, both show decreased BSP and cholecystographic agent excretion and G.I. symptoms
C. Benign familial cholestasis	Recurrent jaundice with itching, increased alkaline phosphatase, cholestasis on biopsy, benign course

Gilbert's syndrome is included under the designation of chronic non-hemolytic unconjugated hyperbilirubinemia with glucuronyl transferase deficiency. The enzyme deficiency in liver tissue has been demonstrated by Black and Billing. Certain features differ from those of the Crigler-Najjar syndrome and warrant its retention as a separate diagnostic category.

INFECTIONS

Neonatal Hepatitis

Hepatic inflammatory processes in the early weeks or months of life have several rather unique features. Chief among these, especially among familial cases, is a tendency to progression to post-necrotic cirrhosis and death with hepatic failure. The liver of the infant so affected responds to injury with the formation of multinucleated giant cells. This response may involve the entire hepatic parenchyma in a giant cell or syncytial transformation leading to use of the term "giant cell hepatitis" as a synonym for neonatal hepatitis.

Etiology. Among the viruses incriminated are those of serum hepatitis (hepatitis B), cytomegalic inclusion disease, herpes simplex, rubella and Coxsackie infections. The virus of infectious hepatitis has not proved to be a causative agent.

Hepatitis B antigen (HB Ag) positivity during pregnancy entails little risk to the fetus of a maternal carrier. However, acute infection in the mother, particularly in the third trimester of pregnancy or within 2 months postpartum, leads to a high incidence of infection in offspring. A high incidence of neonatal hepatitis and biliary atresia has been noted in infants with the trisomy 17-18 syndrome. This association has led to the suggestion that an *in utero* viral infection may be the basis for the trisomy and the hepatic lesions. Also, in infants with intra-uterine rubella, neonatal hepatitis and biliary atresia have been noted to occur at an increased rate. This coincidence supports the hypothesis that biliary atresia may be the consequence of an *in utero* viral infection in which the inflammatory reaction has been particularly localized in the biliary excretory apparatus.

The protozoan parasite toxoplasma has also been found in newborn infants with hepatomegaly and jaundice, usually as a part of a generalized infection involving the central nervous system, the eye and the heart.

Hepatic involvement may also be associated with such bacterial infections as septicemia, pneumonia, pyelonephritis and listeriosis. Though syphilis may be responsible for neonatal hepatitis, significant clinical evidence of hepatic dysfunction is not common. α-1-antitrypsin deficiency has recently been found to be a major cause of the neonatal hepatitis syndrome.

Clinical Manifestation and Diagnosis. Affected infants present with persistent jaundice due to increased conjugated bilirubin and often with the passage of acholic stools suggesting complete interruption of the excretion of bile pigments. The clinical pattern consists of a history of onset of jaundice in the second to third weeks of life, of initially normal-colored stools which become acholic, persistent conjugated hyperbilirubinemia and positive tests for urobilinogen in urine and stool. These suggest the presence of an acquired disease with partial obstruction; however, similar clinical findings have been noted in infants with proved extrahepatic biliary atresia.

The differentiation between these two conditions is made difficult by the frequency with which hepatitis leads to prolonged, essentially complete obstruction to the passage of bile and the imperfect correlation of tests for hepatic parenchymal damage and the underlying disease. Serial determinations of serum bilirubin in patients with hepatitis may exhibit initially high levels with a tendency toward an irregular decline with time. The infant with biliary atresia initially has lower values with a gradual increase.

A combination of percutaneous liver biopsy and determination of the 72-hour fecal excretion of ^{131}I-rose bengal will provide a definitive diagnosis in most cases. In hepatitis there is marked distortion of lobular architecture with prominent transformation of hepatocytes into membrane-enclosed multinucleated giant cells with distorted and diminished bile canaliculi. In contrast, the biopsy in excretory duct anomalies (atresia, stenosis, hypoplasia, choledochal cyst) reveals essentially normal lobular architecture with striking changes in the portal areas consisting of fibrosis and proliferation of bile ducts.

The rose bengal excretion test uniformly results in less than 10 per cent of the administered dye being recovered in the feces of patients with excretory duct abnormalities while 80 per cent of patients with parenchymal lesions excrete larger amounts.

A discrepancy between the biopsy and rose bengal study data may be resolved by administration of phenobarbital for 3 to 5 days. Patients with bilirubin excretory insufficiency on the basis of parenchymal injury will respond with an increased rate of secretion of the retained dye while those with excretory duct anomalies will not.

Persistence of HB Ag supports the diagnosis of neonatal hepatitis. If the studies suggest biliary atresia, operative intervention is undertaken promptly.

When a diagnosis of hepatitis is established and an additional period of a few weeks for observation shows no amelioration of jaundice, corticosteroid therapy should be tried for 4 to 6 weeks. It appears that prognosis for recovery varies inversely with the duration of disease and is more favorable in sporadic rather than familiar cases.

Viral Hepatitis

Viral hepatitis has its highest incidence, but lowest mortality, among children of school age.

Etiology. There are two well-characterized types of hepatitis, Type B (MS-2, long incubation, serum) and Type A (MS-1, short incubation, infectious). A serum antigen has been associated with serum hepatitis (HB Ag). Antigens have been identified corresponding to the surface and the core of the virus.

The antigen may appear during the incubation or prodromal stage and disappear from the serum prior to development of clinical symptoms. The corresponding antibody may remain detectable for many years.

Identification of the specific virus responsible for the initiation of the short incubation type hepatitis has recently been described. The technique utilizes immune electron microscopy in which particulate antigen (hepatitis A antigen) occurring in the feces during Type A disease is agglutinated by an antibody appearing in convalescence. By means of this procedure and application of techniques for identification of Type B disease, it has been established that other viral agents may cause hepatitis in man. There are probably two such non-A, non-B agents in addition to those of infectious mononucleosis and cytomegalovirus.

Clinical Manifestations. The incubation period of Type A hepatitis is approximately 14–40 days and 60–100 days for Type B. Type A hepatitis infection is usually marked by an abrupt onset with fever, an autumn-winter incidence peak and a predilection for children and young adults. Type B hepatitis usually exhibits an insidious onset with little or no fever and a year-round incidence without age preference.

In the first phase (pre-icteric), symptoms usually begin 4 to 5 days before the appearance of jaundice. Prominent are fever, malaise, mild headache, chilliness, signs of mild upper respiratory tract infection, arthralgia, anorexia, nausea and vomiting, upper abdominal distress and pain. Bile usually is present in the urine 1 to 3 days before the appearance of jaundice. Fever usually disappears with the onset of icterus, but anorexia continues, and severe prostration and vomiting may occur. Stools are light or clay-colored at this stage.

The second phase (icteric) usually continues 2 to 4 weeks with gradually increasing clinical and laboratory evidence of jaundice followed by a gradual diminution. There may be a further period of one to two months with malaise and fatigue.

The liver is commonly enlarged and tender. The spleen is palpable in up to 15 per cent of patients, and other evidence of adenopathy including cervical adenopathy may be present.

Diagnosis. Serum bilirubin values, predominantly direct reacting, may be as high as 10 mg./dl. or more. There is an increase in the urinary excretion of urobilinogen due to the inability of the damaged liver to excrete it. With complete failure of bile to reach the intestine, urobilinogen disappears from the urine. With partial resolution of hepatic injury there is resumption of excretion of bile into the intestine and urobilinogen is again formed and appears in the urine.

The serum glutamic oxaloacetic or glutamic pyruvic transaminases are elevated early in the course of the disease; their return to normal heralds the end of active disease and the beginning of recovery.

Differential Diagnosis. The diagnosis of viral hepatitis is dependent on the elimination of other causes of jaundice. The labial herpes, hemorrhagic exanthem, fever, leukocytosis, muscle pains and albuminuria occurring in leptospirosis serve to distinguish it clinically. Involvement of the liver, which may mimic that in infectious hepatitis, is relatively common in infectious mononucleosis.

In the early pre-icteric phase, symptoms may be suggestive of influenza or gastroenteritis. Abdominal pain may resemble that of pneumonia or acute appendicitis. Drug-induced or toxic hepatitis must also be considered.

Pathology. Similar pathologic changes in the liver occur in all types of hepatitis. The hepatic lobules show varying degrees of cellular necrosis, autolysis and thickening of the reticular fibers. Accompanying the hepatocellular necrosis is widespread infiltration with inflammatory cells. Proliferating bile ducts appear in the perilobular portal areas, and bile stasis is visible. With recovery, complete regeneration of the liver cells occurs without scarring. In fulminating and fatal cases the hepatic changes are typical of yellow atrophy.

Mild Anicteric Hepatitis

Mild anicteric hepatitis is apparently more common among infants than the icteric form of the disease. The symptoms are those of a mild gastroenteritis with anorexia, diarrhea and vomiting.

Hepatitis with Predominant Cholestasis

This disease is also referred to as "cholestatic hepatitis" and "cholangiolitic hepatitis," and is characterized principally by obstruction and dilatation of bile canaliculi with little evidence of hepatocellular necrosis. The clinical manifestations include jaundice with pruritis, bilirubinuria, pale stools with decreased fecal urobilinogen, and an enlarged, non-tender liver. Laboratory examinations show increases in alkaline phosphatase and 5-nucleotidase values in the serum with only slight increases in the serum transaminases. Hepatitis with predominant cholestasis is uncommon in children.

Chronic Hepatitis

Except in the very young infant, infectious hepatitis in childhood is usually a brief, self-limited illness. It is uncommon for children with an apparently typical bout of hepatitis to continue for months with hepatomegaly and biochemical evidence of continued hepatocellular injury. This type of course has been designated "prolonged or persistent hepatitis." Patients with this course may be expected to recover ultimately unless subacute hepatic necrosis progresses to postnecrotic cirrhosis. The unusual development of chronic active hepatitis is described below.

Treatment. Treatment is symptomatic during the interval required for immunologic defenses to eradicate the virus. Maintenance of a reasonable state of nutrition during the illness is beneficial and requires intravenous alimentation when vomiting or anorexia is prominent.

Prevention. Isolation precautions appropriate for patients with intestinal infections are indicated during the period of hospitalization. Gamma globulin prophylaxis is effective only in short incubation (or HB Ag negative) hepatitis. The use of high-titer anti-B serum for patients exposed to B-positive hepatitis is promising.

Fulminant Hepatitis

Fulminant hepatitis, or acute massive necrosis, is usually fatal within a few weeks after onset. Systemic manifestations during the preicteric phase are usually severe. Particularly prominent are high fever, abdominal pain and vomiting. Also indicative of an unfavorable outcome are rapid decrease in liver size, mental changes including lethargy, drowsiness and confusion, electroencephalographic changes of encephalopathy, and an increase in prothrombin time not corrected by parenteral administration of vitamin K. Transaminase levels may not be very high, reflecting failure of hepatic synthesis of the enzymes. Bleeding into the skin and mucous membranes, ascites and deep coma are among the terminal manifestations.

Liver Failure in Hepatitis

In viral and toxic hepatitis and in chronic liver disease, sufficient functional alteration or reduction in parenchymal cell mass may result in the critical syndrome of liver failure. Fluid retention and ascites may occur as a consequence of obstruction to hepatic circulation with increased lymph exudation into the peritoneal cavity. Impaired hepatic synthesis of albumin may contribute to the accumulation of ascites. Loss of extracellular fluid as ascites initiates hormonal changes that result in increased renal tubular reabsorption of sodium. Therapy is designed to reverse the positive sodium balance and includes rigid restriction of sodium intake combined with diuretics.

Decreased liver function and shunting of portal blood to the systemic circulation are the major underlying factors in hepatic encephalopathy.

Gastrointestinal bleeding is a frequent precipitating factor because of the impairment in circulation and increased nitrogenous burden which accompany it. By reducing blood volume and depleting potassium stores, diuretics may also contribute to hepatic encephalopathy. Cerebral metabolism may be altered by accumulation of ammonia and other nitrogenous compounds. Increased brain serotonin and neural catecholamine depletion have also been implicated. To reduce the intestinal production of ammonia, protein should be eliminated from the diet with adequate calories from carbohydrate limiting endogenous breakdown of protein. Bacterial breakdown of protein and ammonia formation are reduced by oral administration of a non-absorbable antibiotic such as neomycin. Lactulose given orally converts ammonia to the less well-absorbed ammonium ion and appears to be useful in limiting ammonia retention. Exchange transfusion is indicated in patients with acute, potentially reversible disease. The massive bleeding accompanying liver failure is best managed by the infusion of fresh frozen plasma. Vitamin K should be administered to all patients with prolonged jaundice.

CHRONIC LIVER DISEASE

Chronic liver disease may present as the principal clinical problem, e.g. the cirrhosis secondary to biliary atresia, or as an associated disability of a systemic disturbance, such as cystic fibrosis.

The term "cirrhosis" implies extensive destruction of hepatic parenchyma, with replacement by diffuse fibrosis and distortion of lobular architecture. When hepatic cells are destroyed new cells form from the cellular remnants. If cell death is confined to individual lobules, orderly restoration of histologic and functional relations is likely. Destruction of many adjacent lobules with collapse of intervening stroma leads to nodular regeneration. New blood vessels at the margins of growing nodules are compressed leading to dependence on hepatic arterial blood for nutrition as portal blood is shunted past. In conditions characterized chiefly by hepatic fibrosis, portal hypertension rather than parenchymal insufficiency may become the major clinical problem.

Acquired Hepatic Disease (Postnecrotic Cirrhosis)

In children, most instances of postnecrotic cirrhosis appear after recognized antecedent illness, e.g., neonatal hepatitis, or chronic active hepatitis. Children have fewer opportunities than adults to contact such hepatic toxic agents as carbon tetrachloride. Diagnostic efforts should be directed toward those diseases of childhood with which cirrhosis is associated, e.g., cystic fibrosis, Wilson's disease, neonatal hepatitis or α-1-antitrypsin deficiency.

Chronic Active Liver Disease

Chronic active liver disease (CALD) includes the following entities; plasma cell hepatitis, lupoid hepatitis, Kunkel's syndrome of hypergammaglobulinemia in young females, active juvenile cirrhosis and chronic active hepatitis. The etiology is often obscure but usually follows a bout of viral hepatitis.

Clinical Features. The peak incidence occurs in the 10- to 20-year age group with female predominance. The clinical course is prolonged and jaundice does not resolve at the expected time. The onset may be abrupt or insidious with malaise, fatigue, weight loss, anorexia and fever. Portal hypertension with bleeding esophageal varices or ascites usually occurs late. About 20 percent of patients have significant disease in other systems as the presenting complaint; hematuria, bloody diarrhea, acne, malar flush or amenorrhea in females. Clinical study may reveal the presence of nephritis, thyroiditis, myositis, arthralgia, colitis or hemolytic anemia. These multi-system symptoms may also develop during the course of the illness and suggest an "auto-immune" mechanism as etiologic or of importance in progression.

Laboratory Findings. Modest to marked elevations of bilirubin, serum transaminases and gammaglobulins are the usual biochemical changes. Serologic abnormalities, including LE phenomena, anti-nuclear and smooth muscle antibodies and positive Coomb's reaction are relatively common findings.

Pathology. Characteristically, the periolobular region shows degeneration and "piecemeal" necrosis of cells with lymphocytic and plasma cell infiltration. The limiting plate separating the portal tract and lobule is eroded. Varying degrees of fibrosis including features of multinodular cirrhosis can be seen as well.

Treatment. Over 80 percent of untreated patients die within 5 years. With treatment, improvement in early survival and quality of life is seen. The autoimmune mechanism hypothesis provides the rationale for corticosteroid and other immunosuppressive therapy which results in clinical, biochemical and histologic improvement in the majority of patients. It is not proven that survival is favorably effected by therapy, although complete resolution has been described.

Biliary Cirrhosis

In children, biliary cirrhosis develops after prolonged obstruction of the biliary system by extrahepatic atresia, stenosis or choledochal cyst. Less frequent causes in childhood are stones or sludge in the common bile duct, tumor and recurrent attacks of pancreatitis.

Vascular Obstruction

Cardiac failure is the principal cause of passive congestion of the liver. Long-standing pulmonary vascular disease with stasis in the right side of the heart will also engorge the liver. Constrictive pericarditis will produce passive vascular congestion as will myocardial or valvular disease. With continuation of the hyperemia, the liver cells surrounding the central vein undergo degenerative changes due to hypoxia and become atrophic.

There is a number of hereditary disorders affecting the liver which may lead to portal hypertension with or without cirrhosis (Table 12-4).

Table 12-4. Developmental and Metabolic Liver Disease Leading to Portal Hypertension or Cirrhosis

Disorder	Transmission	Pathology
Developmental Polycystic liver disease	Autosomal recessive Autosomal dominant	Multiple cysts in biopsy Usually with polycystic kidneys Wide bands of fibrotic tissue on biopsy
Congenital hepatic fibrosis	Autosomal recessive	Fibrous tissue in portal areas
Hereditary hemorrhagic telangiectasia (Osler-Rendu-Weber)	Autosomal dominant	Cirrhosis with immunologic impairment, discrete or massive hemangiomas
Metabolic Wilson's disease (Hepato-lenticular degeneration)	Autosomal recessive	Increased hepatic copper, decreased serum ceruloplasmin, cirrhosis, basal ganglia symptoms Kayser-Fleischer ring in cornea, treatment with penicillamine
Galactosemia	Autosomal recessive	Non-glucose reducing substance in urine, absent galactose-1-phosphate uridyltransferase, cirrhosis, cataracts, failure to thrive, treatment with galactose free diet
Cystic fibrosis	Autosomal recessive	Increased sweat chloride concentration, focal cirrhosis
Fructose intolerance	Autosomal recessive	Absent-fructose-1-phosphate aldolase, cirrhosis, hypoglycemia
Sickle cell disease	Autosomal dominant	Cirrhosis, hemachromatosis, diagnosis by hemoglobin electrophoresis
Glycogen storage disease Type IV	Autosomal recessive	Cirrhosis, deficiency of branching enzyme
Sphyngolipid and mucopolysaccharide storage diseases (Gaucher's, Niemann-Pick, Hurler's disease, etc.)	Autosomal recessive	Portal hypertension, deficiency of specific catabolic enzymes

(continued on overleaf)

Table 12-4. Developmental and Metabolic Liver Disease Leading to Portal Hypertension or Cirrhosis *(Continued)*

Disorder	Transmission	Pathology
Tyrosinosis	Autosomal recessive	Reduced p-OH phenylpyruvate oxidase, cirrhosis, rickets, renal tubular disorder, may present as neonatal hepatitis
Cystinosis	Autosomal recessive	Renal tubular dysfunction, rickets
Hepatic prophyria	Autosomal dominant	Abnormal prophyrins, post-necrotic cirrhosis
Hemachromatosis	Variable penetrance	Serum iron increased, saturation of iron binding protein
Progressive familial cholestasis	Autosomal recessive	Cirrhosis, steatorrhea, bile acid retention
α -1-antitrypsin deficiency	Autosomal recessive	May present as neonatal hepatitis decreased levels of α -l-antitrypsin in serum, cytoplasmic inclusions in liver

Inflammatory Bowel Disease

Involvement of the liver may take various forms in inflammatory bowel disease. Under-nutrition secondary to anorexia, anemia, and intestinal loss of protein are contributing causes. Pericholangitis may result from portal toxemia and bacteremia arising from the inflamed colon. It may be benefitted by prolonged treatment with a broad spectrum antibiotic.

ACUTE ENCEPHALOPATHY AND HEPATOMEGALY WITH FATTY INFILTRATION: REYE'S SYNDROME (ENCEPHALOPATHY AND FATTY DEGENERATION OF THE VISCERA)

This is an acute and frequently fatal syndrome. There is usually a preceeding mild viral illness which is followed by a rapid onset of vomiting and within hours by a change in the state of consciousness, which may progress through delirium to stupor and coma.

On examination, there is a mild to moderate hepatomegaly and central nervous system depression which may include signs of brain stem involvement, altered pupillary reflexes, and increased intracranial pressure. Marked increases in transaminases and ammonia are seen with little or no increase in the serum bilirubin. Bleeding may be a problem with reduction of the liver-dependent components of coagulation. Hypoglycemia occurs commonly and may be resistant to therapy. Spinal fluid is normal and only increased pressure is recorded.

Liver tissue obtained by percutaneous biopsy is pale and at times white. Microscopically, diffuse fatty vacuolization of the enlarged hepatocytes is seen. Ultrastructurally, mitochondrial swelling and pleomorphism are seen. Lipid stains are positive and chemical analysis of the liver tissue indicates large increases in triglyceride and fatty acid. Fatty degeneration of organs, such as the heart, pancreas, and kidney have been reported. The myocardial and renal tubular changes account for the occurrence of arrhythmias and aminoaciduria.

The etiology of Reye's syndrome remains obscure. Evidence of infection with influenza B, herpes simplex and varicella viruses have been found in some patients. Exogenous agents such as isopropyl alcohol, salicylates, and aflatoxins may be contributory.

Because the pathophysiology of this disease is poorly understood, specific therapy has not been found. The severe mitochondrial injury demonstrable by electron microscopy is accompanied by transient decreases in the levels of a number of mitochondrial enzymes with oxidative, gluconeogenic and urea cycle activities. First to be recognized were deficiencies of the urea cycle enzymes, carbamyl phosphate synthetase and ornithine transcarbamylase. Reduction in citrulline, the product of the enzymes, has been demonstrated and may account for the failure of conversion of ammonia to urea. Administration of citrulline may be effective in reducing hyperammonemia. Hypoglycemia is treated with infusions of glucose to support central nervous system metabolism and reconstitute glycogen stores. Acidosis should be corrected when present. Cerebral edema is managed by the infusion of mannitol and the administration of dexamethasone. Exchange transfusion may improve the survival rates and reduce neurologic sequelae.

HEPATIC DRUG REACTIONS

The liver may be injured by a variety of chemical agents. Some of these are hepatotoxins and the liver injury may be considered "predictable." With other compounds, hepatic damage is less frequent and may be considered "non-predictable" or of immunologic, allergic or idiosyncratic origin. Among the "predictable" agents are carbon tetrachloride, toluene and trichlorethylene in solvent "sniffers" and mitomycin in cancer therapy. These agents are generally toxic in animals, injurious after short exposure and produce characteristic hepatic lesions. In contrast, the "non-predictable" hepatotoxins do not produce lesions in experimental animals and usually exhibit evidence of hepatic toxicity after relatively prolonged use. Withdrawal of the offending agent is usually associated with reduction of the hepatic injury. Prominent among this group are chlorpromazine, isoniazid, antithyroid rugs, erythromycin estolate and oxyphenasetin, a component of some laxatives.

PORTAL HYPERTENSION

Etiology

In children, obstruction of the portal vein and cirrhosis are the leading causes of portal hypertension. Thrombosis may be secondary to neonatal omphalitis or to cannulation of the umbilical vein for exchange transfusion or other purposes. Sepsis in the umbilical region may spread along the umbilical vein to the portal vein where it may result in portal vein obstruction. Anomalies of the portal venous system are rare; obstructive valves in the portal vein, however, have been demonstrated. Obstruction of the portal vein by neoplastic invasion is uncommon.

Portal hypertension is a common sequel to cirrhosis secondary to extrahepatic biliary obstruction or to postnecrotic hepatocellular disease. Because of the poor prognosis for these conditions, documentation of the presence of portal hypertension is often of only academic interest.

Clinical Manifestations

In portal vein thrombosis, hepatic function is usually normal and the presenting signs are those resulting from portal hypertension. Hematemesis is common and is often accompanied by the passage of bright red blood by rectum. Collateral circulation between the portal and systemic vessels may be noted on inspection of the abdominal wall; such vessels radiating from the umbilical region are referred to as "caput medusae." Of the varicosities accompanying portal hypertension, those arising in the esophagus and stomach are the most important because of their tendency to bleed massively. Pancytopenia (Banti's syndrome) related to the enlarged spleen is common.

Diagnosis

Radiographic demonstration of esophageal varices is the simplest and safest means of establishing the presence of collateral circulation secondary to portal hypertension. Esophagoscopy with small, flexible fiberoptic esophagoscopes is now possible. Celiac arteriography can localize the site of thrombosis and delineate collateral circulation. Obstruction to the main hepatic veins by cardiac failure or constrictive pericarditis results in postsinusoidal extrahepatic portal hypertension.

Treatment

In infants and children with portal hypertension secondary to cirrhosis, the prognosis of the underlying liver disease is often so poor as to contraindicate surgical treatment. The surgical problems are more difficult in young children because of the small size of vessels available for portal to systemic vein anastomosis. The normal hepatic functions of patients with extrahepatic portal obstruction enable them to tolerate recurrent hemorrhages. Variceal bleeding may cease spontaneously after repeated episodes. These considerations make the delay of surgical intervention until at least 4 to 6 years of age or older a reasonable course in most instances. In emergency treatment of bleeding varices, transfusion of whole blood, preferably guided by measurement of central venous pressure, is indicated. Intravenous pitressin or esophageal tamponade with the Sengstaken tube will usually control bleeding.

CHOLECYSTITIS

Acute inflammation of the gall bladder is uncommon in childhood. It may accompany a variety of acute infections, including bacterial pneumonia, meningitis, peritonitis and typhoid fever. The symptoms are nausea, vomiting, fever, abdominal distention and pain in the right upper quadrant. The gall bladder may be palpable as a tense, excruciatingly tender mass. With advancing symptoms, surgery is advisable, although with treatment of the associated infection, symptoms and signs diminish rapidly.

CHOLELITHIASIS

Biliary calculi are infrequent in early life, but are more common than infection of the gall bladder. Cholelithiasis in childhood occurs frequently as a complication of the congenital hemolytic anemias and sickle-cell anemia. Calcium is deposited in some and a shadow may be visible radiographically. Pure pigment stones cast no shadow and are demonstrable only by the use of contrast medium. The treatment of symptomatic cholelithiasis is surgical. Dissolution of cholesterol gallstones by chenodeoxycholic acid in adults has been observed.

CHOLEDOCHUS CYST

Choledochus cyst, or cystic dilatation of the common bile duct, is generally considered to be of developmental origin. Cysts may grow to large dimensions; a capacity of 2 liters has been recorded. The clinical manifestations are upper abdominal pain, jaundice and abdominal tumor.

The liver may become enlarged and cirrhotic, and frequently there is cholangitis.

Prolonged obstructive jaundice associated with high serum alkaline phosphatase and cholesterol values is suggestive of choledochal cyst or other incomplete common bile duct obstruction by stenosis or tumor. Direct radiographic visualization by oral or intravenous cholangiography may be diagnostic. Demonstration of distortion or impression on the duodenal loop during barium contrast examination of the upper gastrointestinal tract are suggestive of obstruction of the common duct. Ultrasonography may yield diagnostic information. Treatment is surgical by anastomosis between the biliary system and intestinal tract. The results following operation are usually good, if cirrhosis has not developed and if cholangitis does not supervene.

ATRESIA OF THE EXTRAHEPATIC BILE DUCTS

Biliary atresia is generally thought to result from maldevelopment. In early fetal life the liver and its ductal system develop from a diverticulum of the ventral floor of the endodermal foregut. The ducts are initially patent, but become obliterated by epithelial proliferation to form solid cords. With further development the cords are recanalized. Failure of this last phase may involve all or part of the extrahepatic biliary tree. Biliary atresia may also result from intrauterine viral infection as described above.

Pathology

Histologically, there is little distortion of the normal architecture of the hepatic plates. The outstanding feature is the extensive fibrosis within the portal triads, in which proliferating bile ducts are embedded. With increasing fibrosis and the development of cirrhosis there is interference with hepatic circulation resulting in portal hypertension. The spleen becomes enlarged and during the second half of the first year of life esophageal varices, ascites and the hematologic changes of hypersplenism may appear. Osteomalacia develops with prolonged malabsorption.

Clinical Manifestations

Jaundice and indurated hepatomegaly are the most striking signs. The hyperbilirubinemia is predominantly conjugated and usually below 10 mg./dl. during the first 6 to 8 weeks of life, after which it steadily increases. Growth is impaired. Portal hypertension, hypoproteinemic edema, bleeding secondary to prothrombin deficiency and hyperammonemia occur during the latter part of the first year. The stools are pale and clay-colored. Small amounts of bile pigments on the surface of the stool are derived from intestinal secretions and epithelium. The urine is dark and contains large amounts of direct-reacting bilirubin. Urobilinogen is usually absent from the urine, but occasionally may be present in small amounts if bilirubin enters the bowel with intestinal secretions and desquamated cells and is subsequently absorbed and excreted in the urine.

There is moderate anemia and a steady increase in the conjugated hyperbilirubinemia. Transaminase values in the serum are elevated but usually remain below 400 units. Serum alkaline phosphatase is also moderately elevated. Prothrombin concentrations are maintained in the normal range in the early stages. When low values occur, correction is usually possible by parenteral administration of vitamin K until hepatic cellular failure has developed.

Diagnosis

Congenital malformation of the bile ducts must be differentiated from other causes of obstructive jaundice in early infancy. The principal problem is differentiation from neonatal hepatitis (see discussion above).

Treatment

When cholangiography determines that a portion of the extrahepatic biliary tree is patent, surgical correction of the obstruction is mandatory. Recently, a surgical procedure has been developed for treatment of those infants previously considered inoperable because of absent or atretic extrahepatic ducts. The procedure, introduced by Kasai, involves resection of a cone of liver tissue in the hilar area of the liver, thus opening up many small bile ducts. This is followed by suture of an intestinal pouch to the site. The procedure is temporarily effective in approximately one-third of infants if carried out at about 2 months prior to spontaneous obliteration of the lumen of the small bile ducts. Cholangitis or progressive sclerosis of the biliary ducts limits the long term effectiveness of the procedure.

ATRESIA OF THE INTRAHEPATIC BILE DUCTS

Intrahepatic atresia of bile ducts may be partial or complete and has been observed most often in association with atresia of the extrahepatic biliary system, especially in infants with an unusually long survival time. It is likely that, in some instances, the intrahepatic atresia represents an atrophy of disuse of structures deprived of their normal function. Atresia of the intrahepatic biliary system coexisting with patency of the extrahepatic bile ducts is possible in view of the separate origin of the two portions of the biliary system from the cephalad and caudate portions of the foregut diverticulum, respectively. The outstanding clinical features are prolonged survival, often to the end of the first decade, and hyper-lipidemia with prominent cutaneous xanthomas. Treatment is symptomatic, including that for pruritus. Cholestyramine increases the extra-hepatic excretion of bile salts and decreases the serum lipids. Recently acquired forms of intra- and extrahepatic biliary atresia have been recognized.

BIBLIOGRAPHY

Gartner, L. M., and Arias, I. M.: The liver. *In* Rudolph, A. M., Barnett, H. L., and Einhorn, A. H. (eds.): Pediatrics, 16th ed. New York, Appleton, Century Crofts, 1977.
Kaye, R., and Holtzapple, P. G.: The liver. *In* Vaughan, V. C., and McKay, J. R. (eds.): Nelson's Textbook of Pediatrics, 10th ed. Philadelphia, W. B. Saunders, 1975.

Both textbook articles provide more extensive coverage of the subject and good bibliographies.

Popper, H., and Schaffner, F. (eds.): Progress in Liver disease. New York, Grune & Stratton, Vol. 1 to Vol. 5.

This series offers excellent and complete reviews on selected topics related to liver physiology and disease. The fifth edition, 1976, includes chapters on "Neonatal Jaundice" by Gerard B. Odell and "Cryptogenic Liver Disease in Young Infants" by M. Michael Thaler. Both articles provide excellent summaries of these important areas of pediatric interest.

Schiff, L: Diseases of the Liver, 4th ed. Philadelphia, J. B. Lippincott, 1975.
Sherlock, S.: Diseases of the Liver and Biliary System, 5th ed. Oxford, Blackwell Scientific Publications, 1975.

These are general texts which provide authoritative and current discussions of the subject.

13

Abdominal Pain, Constipation and Melena

Ian S. E. Gibbons, M.D.

ABDOMINAL PAIN

Pathophysiology

Abdominal pain may arise in any of the tissues of the body from the skin to the spine. The causes of disease may range from an acute infection as in herpes zoster (shingles) to chronic degenerative change as in osteoarthritis of the spine leading to compression of nerves supplying the abdominal wall. The feature common to all of them is some disturbance of nerve fibers and end organs giving rise to the sensation of pain. Pain from mild disease in many intra-abdominal organs may be referred to the periumbilical region; but when an organ is more severely involved, symptoms tend to localize accurately over it.

Techniques of Study

A careful history and physical examination is an important part of the study. Hematologic, chemical, and infective agents must be looked for. Radiographic studies must be carried out according to the suspected diagnosis. If the focus is on the abdomen, then a plain film may be most useful. If a cerebral tumor is suspected, then a plain film of the skull may reveal calcification of a tumor. Other studies, including barium outline of the small and large bowel, may indicate abdominal masses, mucosal lesions, malrotation, and other conditions leading to intestinal pain such as duodenal bands and bowel atresias.

Radioisotope scan of specific organs is a rapidly advancing area where relatively innocuous techniques outline the liver, spleen, pancreas or brain and may assist in the diagnosis of lesions in these organs.

Biochemical Studies of Excreta. The stool may need to be examined for excessive fecal fat loss or for excessive stool sugars associated with disaccharidase deficiencies. It may also be examined for total nitrogen loss and pancreatic enzyme quantity and quality when pancreatic disease is suspected.

Stool Examination. Stools may carry ova or parasites associated with abdominal discomfort. Examination of two or three specimens of fresh stool may be helpful. Abnormal bacteria leading to invasive disease should be sought.

Ultrasound Techniques. Ultrasound has developed as a useful adjunct in looking for cystic masses and dilated ducts, particularly in the region of the liver, pancreas, and mesentery.

Computerized Axial Tomography. This technique has recently become available and is capable of producing a body scan showing a cross section of the body at various levels. Quite small masses or cysts may be detected by this technique.

Endoscopy. Various forms of endoscopy including sigmoidoscopy, colonoscopy, esophagogastroduodenoscopy, laparoscopy, and retrograde cannulation of pancreatic and biliary ducts may all be important in evaluating a variety of cases of abdominal pain.

Biopsy Techniques. The distal colon, the major part of the small bowel, esophagus and stomach are all accessible to various biopsy techniques without surgical operation. There are various instruments available that can be used with relative safety. Liver biopsy can be performed by a needle suction technique.

Manometrics. Pressure recordings of esophageal and sphincter function may be valuable in defining certain causes of abdominal pain. Spasm of the colon can be recorded by pressure-recording apparatus as well as by radiographic studies. These techniques are relatively simple, and cause little discomfort to the patient.

Electroencephalography. This may be important in looking for cerebral tumors or abdominal epilepsy. Computerized tomography has also been used in this area with success.

Examination of the Urine. Urinalysis is an important part of a search for the cause of abdominal pain. Infective and biochemical abnormalities may point to a diagnosis.

Intravenous Pyelography. This is an essential part of a search for organic causes of abdominal pain because genitourinary abnormalities account for half the organic causes of recurrent pain.

Differential Diagnosis and Symptoms

In determining any cause of abdominal pain in infancy and childhood, a well-organized and carefully pursued comprehensive history should be taken and put together with a well-executed physical examination. An examination of stool, urine and vomitus should be included. Many diseases can be diagnosed by these steps alone without introducing unnecessary, expensive, and painful laboratory studies.

There are two broad categories of pain to consider: acute and chronic.

Abdominal pain becomes chronic when episodes recur over a period of 2 to 3 months or more. In general the causes of acute pain are different from those causing chronic pain. This can be helpful in making an initial diagnosis and may influence the choice of the first steps taken in management of a patient's problem.

One way of approaching a diagnosis of pain is to consider various organ systems which may be involved. A knowledge of other symptoms and signs of disease together with examination of excreta will broaden the picture; extra help is obtained from the particular age group in which the problem presents. No attempt will be made to include all causes of abdominal pain but listed are some common disorders which should not be omitted in determining an initial diagnosis. Tables 13-1 and 13-2 contain some features of common disorders which may help in diagnosis, and name some of the rare causes of abdominal pain in childhood. In contrast to adults, peptic ulcer is not a common cause of pain in children.

When recording a history for abdominal pain, always ask the patient or parent what medications are being taken. Many substances prescribed by the physician as well as proprietory medicines bought by the patient or food fads followed by the family may be causes of pain.

Principles of Management

Acute Abdominal Pain. In most cases management revolves around a diagnosis that is usually followed by therapeutic steps leading to cure or dramatic relief of symptoms. If the whole episode is short-lived (1 to 2 weeks), there is little effect upon the family or child, provided the end result of the illness is satisfactory. If the end result is not good or the acute episode leads to chronic illness, then management emphasis must change. The physician should always be aware, even in the case of an acute illness, that certain children or their families may require in-depth studies and support, emotionally and physically, to help them through the crisis and to prevent an abnormal behavior pathway developing on the way to recovery.

Chronic Abdominal Pain. In this case, management also revolves around diagnosis, but the steps used in approaching this diagnosis are an important part of therapy and should be staged carefully. Usually the disease has existed for 2 to 3 months or more, and is likely to be present longer. Frequently, the underlying disease is not amenable to curative procedures and the physician, family and child are setting off together on a long road. Remember that therapy begins at the first sight of and with the first words spoken to the patient and family. The needs of emotional growth and development must be dealt with at the same time as diagnosis and therapy are started.

The struggle some children experience in developing emotional skills to cope with their environment may conveniently be called "adjustment

Table 13-1. Differential Diagnosis and Symptoms

System	Disease	Other major symptoms	Signs	Excreta
Gastrointestinal				
	Gastroenteritis, viral or bacterial	Vomiting, diarrhea	General abdominal tenderness	Bilious vomitus, watery diarrhea
	Appendicitis	Fever, vomiting	Right-sided tenderness	Fecal vomiting, constipation or diarrheal stool
	Mesenteric lymphadenitis	Fever, vomiting	Right-sided tenderness or diffuse tenderness	
	Hernia (strangulated)	Vomiting	Signs of distention	Fecal vomitus
	Volvulus	Vomiting	Signs of distention	
	Intussusception	Vomiting	Sausage-shaped mass, obstruction	Blood-tinged mucus
	Intestinal atresias	Constipation	Obstruction	Bile-stained vomitus
	Infectious hepatitis	Nausea, poor appetite	Tender liver	Pale stools, diarrhea
	Infectious mononucleosis	Nausea, poor appetite	Tender liver and spleen	Usually normal
	Inflammatory bowel disease			
	Ulcerative colitis	Weight loss	Tender colon	Bloody stools
	Crohn's disease	Short stature	Tender mass	Loose and bloody stools
Iatrogenic and poisons				
	Lead poisoning, drugs (steroids, iron, imipramine) antibiotics (tetracycline, ampicillin, lincomycin, erythromycin, etc.)			
Genitourinary				
	Infection	Dysuria, frequency	Tender renal angle	Urine may be cloudy or bloody
	Congenital abnormality	May be none	Abnormal facies or limbs	May be normal

Table 13-1. Differential Diagnosis and Symptoms *(Continued)*

System	Disease	Other major symptoms	Signs	Excreta
	Stone renal or ureteric	Frequency, dysuria	Tender kidney, ureter	Bloody urine
	Acute glomerulo-nephritis	Elevated blood pressure, swelling	Edema	Smoky urine
	Torsion testis	Testicular pain	Swollen testis	
	Twisted ovarian pedicle		Tender abdomen	
Respiratory	Streptococcal adenitis	Sore throat	Generally tender abdomen	Normal
	Pleurisy or pneumonia	Cough, fever	Abdomen—no findings	Normal
	Cystic fibrosis of pancreas	Cough, sputum	Simulate appendicitis or obstruction	Stool, bulky and foul-smelling
Hematopoietic	Sickle-cell anemia	Joint pain	Rigid abdomen	Normal
	Acute leukemia	Joint, bone pain	Tender spleen	Blood in stool and urine
	Infectious mononucleosis	Sore throat	Tender liver and spleen	Normal
	Septicemia	Weakness	Shock	Mostly normal
Metabolic	Diabetes	Vomiting, weight loss, diarrhea	Diffuse abdominal tenderness, dehydration, acidosis	Polyuria
	Hypoglycemia	Convulsions	Coma	Normal
	Porphyria (rare)	Skin rash	Diffuse abdominal tenderness	
	Alkaptonuria (rare)			Urine black on standing

(Continued on overleaf)

Table 13-1. Differential Diagnosis and Symptoms *(Continued)*

System	Disease	Other major symptoms	Signs	Excreta
Reticuloendothelial				
	Rheumatic fever	Painful joints	Diffuse, non-specific	Normal
	Henoch-Schönlein's purpura (rare)	Skin rash	Diffuse, non-specific	Urine and stool may be bloody
Cardiovascular system				
	Myocardial infarction (rare)	Chest pain, arm pain	Arrhythmias	Normal

reactions." These reactions to school, peers, family (including siblings and grandparents), and sexual awareness may sometimes be inappropriate. The persistence of an emotional struggle may lead to greatly increased abdominal symptoms; this is due to the well-known influence emotions have on the autonomic nervous system and intestinal motility. It is clear, therefore, that treatment should include appropriate medications and, at times, surgery, as well as informed, supportive psychotherapy for adjustment reactions. The primary physician should bridge the gap between physical and emotional requirements; he can allay fears about ups and downs in bodily symptoms while working with emotions in a supportive way. If emotional needs are left to the psychologist or psychiatrist (except when serious problems are present), they are placed in a very difficult position during supportive therapy if severe abdominal pain occurs. Treatment is less effective if the patient is caught between two different physicians who, unknowingly may be giving conflicting advice.

Management Steps for Chronic Abdominal Pain. 1. Establish a good relationship with your patient. If he or she is old enough (say 3 to 4 years or older) and can separate easily from the family, explain carefully what a history and physical examination involves. Then ask the parents to leave while you talk with and examine your patient.

2. Don't do painful procedures such as blood tests or rectal examinations on your first encounter unless they are absolutely essential.

3. Ask the parents in and send your patient out of the room to wait or play while you take a thorough history from the parents. (Always try to have both parents together.) The history should include current details of the patient and how he reacts to peers, school, family, emotional growth, fears, likes, dislikes, and other attitudes. The parents' approach

to and fear of the problem should be determined. When you have a well-rounded picture and have decided what you are going to do, invite your patient back in, explain the diagnosis in simple terms and indicate that you and the parents have agreed on a course of action. If the patient has irritable bowel syndrome (the most common cause of recurrent pain), reassurance that the child is safe is often sufficient to reduce symptoms. Sometimes a radiograph of the large and small intestine may be necessary to assure you and the family that no serious intestinal problem is present. Many children with irritable bowel syndrome will settle completely with this treatment.

4. If symptoms persist or signs indicate a serious problem, admission to hospital for investigation and treatment may be necessary. This provides a chance to know your patient and family by gathering data from both parents and patient. You can observe your patient away from home and get him to undergo difficult investigations as he develops confidence in you.

5. When you have a diagnosis (on the way to which you have kept the family informed about every step), arrange a separate and lengthy meeting with the parents to discuss all of the studies done, outline the diagnosis, and plan therapy. This provides an opportunity for parents to ask any questions, and especially allows them to express fears they may have. If you do not deal with these secret fears, therapy may not be effective.

6. Your patient should be interviewed separately at the time of discharge, his disease and therapy explained, and follow-up arranged. If necessary, you may have to contact school officials so they will be aware of treatment programs and will not unwittingly undermine any medical or supportive psychotherapy you have planned. Most school personnel are delighted to hear from a child's doctor and the teacher can be most helpful in keeping your patient in a normal school environment.

7. Sometimes an older brother or sister should be included in the understanding and counseling of your patient's disease.

8. Frequently repeated procedures should be avoided and reliance should be placed more on the history and progress of your patient (e.g., one should avoid frequent sigmoidoscopies in a child with ulcerative colitis).

Drug Therapy. The disease determines the medicine; at present, relatively few drugs are used in pediatric gastroenterology, but advances in understanding intestinal mechanisms are leading to the introduction of newer drugs.

In most cases, drug therapy can be minimal when a child has confidence in his doctor (Table 13-3). This principle applies to simple drugs such as Probanthine (for irritable bowel syndrome) as well as for potent drugs such as steroids and immunosuppressive agents for inflammatory bowel disease.

**Table 13–2. Chronic Recurrent Abdominal Pain:
Differential Diagnosis and Symptoms**

System	Disease	Other major symptoms	Signs	Excreta
Gastrointestinal				
	Irritable bowel syndrome	Headache, vomiting, blurred vision	Tender over colon and small bowel	Pellet stools
	Constipation	Poor appetite, soiling	Masses of feces in colon	Hard or soft stool, usually not inspissated
	Infantile colic	Poor appetite	Soft abdomen (hard during pain)	Normal
	Peptic ulcer	Poor appetite, weakness	Epigastric tenderness	Black stools or coffee-ground vomitus
	Crohn's disease	Weight loss, short stature	Tenderness	Loose stools and blood
	Ulcerative colitis	Anorexia, weight loss	Tender intestines	Loose bloody stools
	Ascaris lumbricoides	Anemia	Abdominal distention	Worms in stool or vomitus
	Disaccharidase deficiency, congenital or acquired	Diarrhea, weight loss, vomiting	Abdominal distention	Reducing sugars in stools
	Cystic fibrosis of the pancreas	Cough, Sputum	Palpable feces in right colon, enlarged liver and spleen	Fatty stools

Peutz-Jeghers syndrome (rare)

Superior mesenteric artery syndrome (rare)

Annular pancreas

Tumor gut or abdominal organs (Wilm's tumor) (rare)
Tuberculosis intestines (rare)
Pancreatitis (rare)
Meckel's diverticulitis (rare)
Cholecystitis and choledochal cyst (rare)

Genitourinary
(Accounts for half the "organic" causes of recurrent abdominal pain)

	Recurrent urinary tract infection	Dysuria	Loin tenderness	Cloudy, foul-smelling urine

**Table 13–2. Chronic Recurrent Abdominal Pain:
Differential Diagnosis and Symptoms *(Continued)***

System	Disease	Other major symptoms	Signs	Excreta
Central nervous	Congenital anomalies and obstructions	Other visible anomalies	Enlarged kidneys or ectopic organs	Urine may be normal
	Cerebral tumor	May be none	May be none or localizing cerebral signs	Normal
	Abdominal epilepsy	Transient impaired consciousness	None	Normal
Cardiovascular	Congenital heart disease with failure	Shortness of breath	Enlarged liver, cyanosis	Normal
	Coarctation of aorta	Cold feet	Diffuse non-specific tenderness	Normal

Table 13–3. Commonly Used Drugs

Drugs	Dose	Disease
Probanthine	7.5–15 mg./dose	Irritable bowel syndrome
Lomotil	2.5–15 mg./day	Loose stools with abdominal pain
Azulfidine (sulphasalazine)	3–5 g./day initially 2 g./day maintenance	Inflammatory bowel disease
Corticosteroids (prednisolone)	2 mg./kg./day initially 5–10 mg./day maintenance	Inflammatory bowel disease
Azathioprine (Imuran)	2 mg./kg. per day	Inflammatory bowel disease
Antibiotics	Appropriate dose	Infections
Antacids	Titrated by symptomatic relief	Ulcer disease, Esophagitis

CONSTIPATION
(FECAL RETENTION WITH OR WITHOUT SOILING)

Pathophysiology and Definition of the Problem

Definition. It is most useful to understand constipation as "a problem of elimination of feces with or without fecal soiling."

Pathophysiology. With normal anatomy, the basic mechanisms of an inability to eliminate feces are not well understood. Feces that remain longer in the large intestine undergo more water reabsorption, become inspissated, and are harder to pass rectally. This is the usual mechanism of simple constipation. However, many children who retain large amounts of feces but soil may fail to properly defecate for 3 to 4 months. Despite this, their feces can remain soft and even difficult to palpate abdominally. In place of passage of stools, fecal liquid material may leak out and cause anal soiling. This fact frequently leads to a mistaken diagnosis of diarrhea, which may be treated with agents to slow down colonic activity. The result is further retention of bowel contents.

Emotional stimuli can indirectly affect intestinal function. Many children become temporarily unable to defecate for several days after moving to a new environment such as school or summer camp. Others who become anxious and are emotionally immature may involuntarily withhold feces for many weeks or months at a time.

In abnormal anatomy, difficulty with bowel movements is usually self-explanatory. Conditions such as painful anal fissures, malrotation, imperforate anus or Hirschsprung's disease can be responsible.

The process of defecation is quite complicated. First, a colonic signal must be recognized, then, in addition to a massive propulsive colonic contraction, there must be closure of the glottis associated with a Valsalva maneuver, increased intra-abdominal pressure, reflex relaxation of the internal anal sphincter, and relaxation of the external anal sphincter and puborectalis sling. There is elevation of the pelvic floor as the bowel movement passes through the anus. If any one of these mechanisms is impaired (for example, congenital absence or weak abdominal musculature), defecation becomes difficult.

Another mechanism recently recognized involves incoordination of these maneuvers which is unrecognized by the patient; there may be contraction of the external anal sphincter during defecation that prevents easy passage of the bowel movement. This often persists until the colonic propulsive contraction ceases. Other patients develop a very high threshold of recognition of colonic propulsive activity (usually acquired) so that normal propulsive activity goes unrecognized and associated defecation maneuvers are not brought into play (e.g., the busy executive dealing with multiple daily crises or the busy child engrossed in play). Once acquired, this threshold allows more feces to accumulate and when large enough, normal rectal contraction and expulsion of the large stool becomes impossible. Soiling will frequently occur as a safety valve under these circumstances.

It is commonly believed that the primary mechanism (all too often the only one considered by many physicians in dealing with a toddler age group), is that related to a painful event such as fissure formation in the anus. This mechanism is represented schematically in Figure 13-1.

This form of constipation should respond quickly to simple remedies

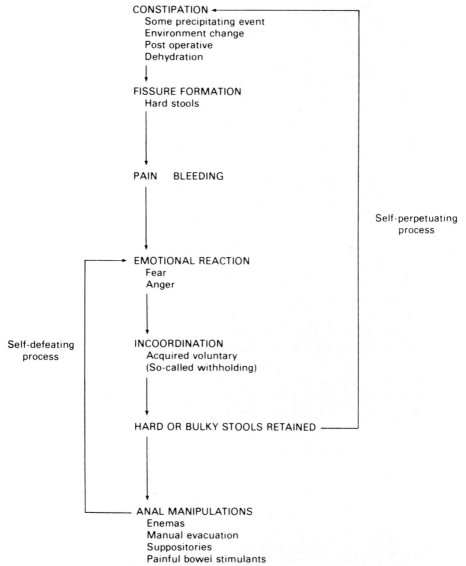

Fig. 13-1. A common series of events leading to chronic constipation.

such as lubricants or stool softeners, but, unfortunately, anal manipulations are frequently used to relieve the pain and crying of young children. These manipulations may become frequent without the physician or family realizing it. The result is the turning of a self-limited process into a prolonged problem. As seen in Figure 13-1, the emotional factors are reinforced, and a severe family emotional disturbance with ensuing behavioral abnormalities can develop in a child's formative years of emotional growth.

In summary, the mechanisms known for constipation in the absence of organic disease are as follows:

1. Simple constipation is a temporary event of inspissated feces without soiling, usually self-limited or responding to simple treatment.

2. Voluntary incoordination of the defecation process is usually acquired, for example, following a painful event like fissure formation or by conscious suppression of colonic propulsive defecation signals and consequent development of high colonic thresholds (usually in older children and adults). In general, these are short-term problems.

3. In involuntary incoordination of the defecation process, usually the stools are soft and bulky and paradoxical external anal sphincter squeeze may occur during defecation, always unrecognized by the patient and usually present in varying severity from birth.

This group emerges clearly through objective studies after 5 to 6 years of age, by which time the normal child should have developed full control of defecation. This problem can be falsely interpreted as withholding on an emotional basis and mistakenly treated psychiatrically after traditional simple methods of treatment fail. These patients respond poorly to psychotherapy, and in the past have been long-term problems persisting with symptoms into the late teens and early 20s. Categories 2 and 3 are a large group, accounting for 60 per cent of the patients who do not fall into category 1.

4. Coordinated processes of defecation by objective criteria, yet retention of feces with persistent soiling is usually associated with deep-seated emotional disturbances and requires full psychotherapeutic measures. Again, this group only emerges clearly when objective studies can be made at 5 to 6 years of age. Invariably, long-term therapy is required. They account for approximately 30 per cent of the patients who do not fit into the previous categories.

Organic Disease. Many disease states can have associated constipation on a temporary or long-term basis depending on the type of disease. Frequently when the disease is appropriately treated, the constipation will cease.

Techniques of Study

A careful history and physical examination should be done (Table 13-4).

Plain Film of the Abdomen. Feces frequently can be seen by radiograph. They may take the form of pellets or balls as in simple constipation, or may have a diffuse granular appearance throughout a large part of the colon even as far as the cecum. This is frequently seen in fecal retention with soiling.

Abnormal gas shadows of various types can be seen, and it is possible to diagnose obstruction, malrotation, a narrow rectum or short-segment Hirschsprung's disease, and many other conditions.

Barium Enema. In problems of elimination it is important to perform this study without the usual bowel preparations most radiology departments do routinely. We are interested in a problem of elimination, the

Table 13–4. Constipation: Differential Diagnosis and Symptoms

Disease mechanism	Symptoms	Signs	Soiling	Barium Enema	Sigmoidoscopy	Anal Tonometry
Functional						
Simple (any age)	Cannot defecate, pain	Hard feces in sigmoid (pellets)	None	Normal colon, pellet stools, normal post-evacuation film	Pellet stool, normal rectum	Normal
Voluntary incoordination	Cannot defecate, pain	Firm or soft feces in colon, fissures	Usually none	Large colon, inadequate evacuation	Hard or soft feces, dilated rectum	High colonic threshold, normal sphincter function
Involuntary incoordination	Cannot defecate, pain	Soft feces, whole colon	Present	Large colon, inadequate evacuation	Soft homogenous feces not adherent to mucosa dilated rectum, fluid feces at periphery	High colonic threshold, external sphincter squeeze during defecation
Coordinated	Cannot defecate, usually no pain	Soft feces, Present whole colon: Severe emotional disturbance	Present	Large colon, inadequate evacuation	″	Normal colonic threshold, normal external sphincter function, normal internal sphincter function

Other	Age Group	Cause
	Newborn	Anatomical obstruction Hirschsprung's disease Meconium plug Abdominal muscles (weak or absent) Anorectal stenosis
	Infancy and Childhood	Normal variations Insufficient milk, sugar or water 1. Vomiting, pyloric stenosis, esophageal reflux, toxemia. 2. Metabolic conditions associated with polyuria, hypercalcemia, adrenocortical hyperplasia, renal acidosis, diabetes insipidus. Hypothyroidism Congenital spinal palsy Hypotonia Lead poisoning

nature of the colon, the nature of the feces, and the propulsive capabilities of the colon, rectum, and sphincter under the circumstances of the illness. Very frequently when the bowel is cleaned out by preparation, much of this information is lost. The most important film of the barium enema is the film showing the post-evacuation capability of the colon and the presence or absence of retained feces.

Limited pictures can be taken, perhaps showing one overhead film outlining the whole colon to the cecum, anteroposter and lateral views of the rectum, and a post-evacuation film. It is important to avoid inserting a balloon-tipped catheter as this obscures information required about the rectum. The barium should be run in under gravity through an open-tipped catheter so that it is not too painful for the patient.

Intravenous Pyelogram and Urinalysis. A urinalysis is an important study. Some children—particularly girls—who have fecal retention with soiling may have chronic urinary tract infection.

Occasionally, the fecal material occupying the pelvis may cause compression of the ureters and may lead to dilatation of the renal pelvis and ureters. If this is the case, the management of that patient must be aimed vigorously at removing the fecal material so that hydronephrosis will not develop.

Sigmoidoscopy. This provides useful information not easily determined by finger rectal examination. It is possible to see an anal fissure when it may not be felt by an examining finger. The mucosa should be normal as feces usually do not adhere to the mucosal wall. The nature of the stool is important. In the child with simple constipation, the stool is pellet or ball-shaped or lies free in a vacuous rectum as a column. This column does not usually extend beyond 15 cm. In fecal retention with soiling, the feces are soft and the instrument can be passed readily into it. Frequently, such material will be present well beyond 15 cm. Spontaneous relaxation of the internal sphincter can be observed occasionally on insufflation of air into the rectum during sigmoidoscopy.

Anal Tonometry. The anal tonometer is a pressure-recording device consisting of three air-filled balloons supported on a thin metal introducer. Two of the balloons are placed in the anal canal, one at the level of the internal sphincter and one at the level of the external sphincter. These two are filled with a fixed volume of air while the third balloon, which is placed higher in the rectum or sigmoid, can be filled at will with varying amounts of air. This produces differing degrees of colonic stimulation (Fig. 13-2).

Variations in pressures recorded in the sphincter balloons reveal autonomic and voluntary sphincter responses to colonic distention. Normally, the resting tone maintained in both sphincters is such that they close the anal orifice and must be opened for the passage of a bowel movement. The internal sphincter has only smooth muscle controlled by the autonomic nervous system. The external sphincter is capable of both reflex and voluntary responses.

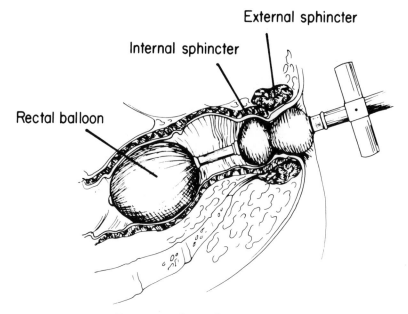

Fig. 13-2. The anal tonometer.

Normally when the rectum or sigmoid is stretched by the proximal balloon, there is a spontaneous relaxation of the internal sphincter and momentary constriction of the external sphincter (Fig. 13-3).

During normal defecation, the internal sphincter relaxes and the internal sphincter is not actively contracted. As a result, the instrument

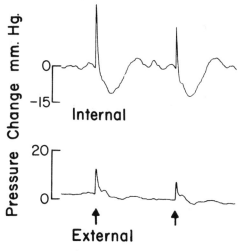

Fig. 13-3. Sphincteric responses to transient rectal distension. (Arrows indicate balloon distention.)

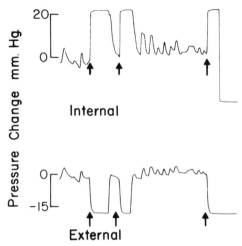

Fig. 13-4. Sphincter pressure responses during normal defecation. (Arrows indicate voluntary attempts to defecate.)

is pushed outwards through the anal canal and the pressure falls on the external sphincter balloon (Fig. 13-4). The increase in pressure recorded by the internal balloon is transmitted by intra-abdominal pressure from the Valsalva movement during defecation. These normal responses may be altered in various disease states (e.g., in Hirschsprung's disease where the internal sphincter will fail to relax normally).

Evaluation of Emotional Growth and Development. This is an essential part of any study of a patient with a problem of elimination and should go hand-in-hand with evaluation of the physical state.

Blood Tests. A number of disease states with alteration in chemical values in the blood may have associated constipation. Examples are: hypothyroidism, hypopituitarism, lead poisoning, or metabolic conditions such as hypercalcemia.

Management of Common Causes: General Principles

Evaluation of Emotional Growth and Development. Problems of elimination tend to be chronic and associated either primarily or secondarily with internal conflicts for the child and disturbed family relationships.

A psychological examination is often indicated and appropriate supportive action begun. Evaluation of the child's scholastic achievement or lack of it may be important and previously unrecognized problems must be faced. Emotional immaturity relating to self-image and peer relationships can be prominent difficulties. Differing opinions of siblings and parents in dealing with the problem enhance the child's internal conflicts and further confuse the normal process of defecation.

A child who has been manipulated by his family may discover that he can turn the tables and manipulate them by failing to defecate normally. This can be an unconscious skill and its unravelling may require psychotherapy if the problem has existed for many years.

As was shown in the section on pathophysiology, the emotional factors are important. If they are not reckoned with, they may become self-perpetuating and purely medical approaches will fail.

Management of Organic Causes. The underlying organic problem should be dealt with directly, if possible. Normal defecation will resume provided intrinsic mechanisms of intestinal function, abdominal musculature and sphincter control are intact.

Anal Manipulations. Repetitive anal manipulations should be avoided if at all possible; they produce temporary relief at best and may set up serious emotional reactions in the older child. The infant who has frequent enemas, suppositories or finger dilatations of the rectum may come to believe these are *necessary* for defecation and may not learn the normal process. It must be remembered that the entire process of defecation is *not* reflex and that some aspects (such as sphincter control and colonic signal recognition) have to be learned.

Dilatation of the anal sphincter in an infant who has constipation is not indicated. After stretching, a normal sphincter will rapidly return to its previous resting state, and only if fibers are torn will it return to a weaker resting tone. This may lead to involuntary soiling.

Impacted masses do occasionally require manual evacuation; if a fecal mass is compressing a ureter, it must be vigorously evacuated and prevented from reaccumulating.

Laxatives, Lubricants and Stool Softeners. Laxatives (such as milk of magnesia) may be useful in managing simple constipation but should be used sparingly. If the problem becomes chronic, investigation is needed to determine the mechanism of constipation.

Stimulant cathartics (cascara, senna, bisacodyl) are best avoided because they may cause frightening and severe abdominal cramps. Prolonged use (many years) may permanently damage the normal propulsive power of the colon.

Stool softeners (which act by inhibiting colonic reabsorption of water) can be effective in a young child who has hard stools. They may be given for quite long periods without harm until a regular pattern of defecation appears.

Lubricants (such as mineral oil) are most effective in patients who are attempting defecation when a pattern of fear has developed. Such children who have normal mechanisms of defecation may lose this fear when lubricants allow a less painful bowel movement. They are not habit-forming and are non-stimulating; used in reasonable doses in children, they do not lead to vitamin deficiency. Lipoid pneumonia will not occur unless the child is forced to swallow the lubricant.

Biofeedback. When the anal tonometer is used in diagnosis, there is usually a printed expression of pressure changes. If a child of 5 to 6 years of age or older is shown this, he can readily learn to control his anal sphincter in response to colonic distention. He can be taught to respond to progressively lower colonic stimuli by external anal sphincter squeeze and thus prevent soiling. If he has inappropriate external sphincter squeeze during defecation, he can see this on paper, associate it with physiologic sensation and be rapidly taught to reverse the phenomenon.

As with lubricants, softeners, and psychotherapy, biofeedback can be a useful adjunct in the management of these patients. However, the correct diagnosis must be established first.

Supportive Psychotherapy. As for abdominal pain, this involves a deep understanding of the child and family. It should be used in every case of chronic constipation. The principles depend upon: (1) the child being motivated to help himself with his problem and being actively involved in the process, and (2) the parents and siblings believing that their child or sibling is capable of normal function. They should show their confidence by their behavior and verbal and non-verbal communication. Disparaging the child should be avoided. Psychotherapy, if it is needed, should be directed at bringing about these two main objectives.

Finally, remember that children seldom grow into adulthood with fecal retention and soiling. Most learn to control bowel movement when their internal motivations have been developed and skills of bodily awareness are appropriately applied to restore normal function. The physician can be a helpful catalyst in bringing this about.

RECTAL BLEEDING
(MELENA)

Pathophysiology

The adage that children are not little adults applies particularly to the diagnosis and management of the child with gastrointestinal hemorrhage. Causes of rectal bleeding cover a wide range, from a simple anal fissure to failure to define any cause in a high proportion of cases. This is especially true in patients with transient bleeding. It is possible that previously unrecognized causes of gastrointestinal hemorrhage in the child may be revealed as modern instrumentation in skilled hands widens the scope of diagnosis. In general, melena indicates disease from the duodenum down but does not exclude bleeding from a higher source such as the stomach, nose, pharynx, or even the chest.

The age of the patient may help in diagnosis; for example, most diseases occur in any age group, but melena from swallowed maternal blood is confined to the newborn while melena from inflammatory bowel disease tends to occur most commonly in the older child.

The quantity of melena may help point out a possible source of bleeding. Profuse melena stool with shock, nausea or pallor more often suggests higher small intestinal bleeding or extensive inflammatory disease of the colon. Bright blood of smaller amounts in an otherwise well child is more suggestive of a rectal polyp or anal fissure.

The tarry stool color so often helpful in indicating a higher source of bleeding in adults is not as useful in the child. This is because intraluminal bleeding increases intestinal motility and speeds the rate of passage of the contents so that bleeding from the duodenum in a child may often produce bright red melena.

The location of the blood in relation to the stool is important. Blood spread or streaked on the outside of the stool suggests a lesion low down in the sigmoid or rectum. Similar low sources of bleeding together with anal fissures are commonly associated with several drops of blood following passage of both hard and soft stools.

The association of pain and abdominal cramps with melena may suggest a partial or complete obstructive lesion such as an intussusception, volvulus or pedunculated polyp.

Finally the question that should always be asked is: is it blood? Food colorings, beets, Kool Aid, gelatin desserts, ampicillin and lincomycin can all simulate rectal bleeding. The most simple test for blood is the hematest for hemoglobin.

Techniques of Study

A careful history and physical examination should be made and the bowel movement observed for appearance and odor. Do not rely entirely on the observation of others.

Rectal Examination. Observation of the anus for pigmentation, scars, fissures, polyps, skin tags, worms, hemorrhoids, asymmetrical folds and other local lesions is helpful. In children, examination with the finger for causes of bleeding will yield little information except for the nature and position of stool or a pelvic mass. Palpable rectal mucosal lesions causing bleeding (like cancer of the rectum in adults) are extremely rare in childhood. Occasionally, a polyp may be felt. However, a rectal examination should always be done and bimanual palpation included.

Sigmoidoscopy. Appropriately sized instruments are required. The procedure should always be done without general anesthesia; in only a few instances is sedation necessary. The older child should have each step of the procedure explained, and the infant must be properly held by trained assistants. The procedure should be considered early in the diagnosis of melena and the first time it is performed should be done without traditional colon cleaning procedures. Enemas and other preparations are holdovers from dealing with adults and their needs. These preparations may severely exacerbate disease (e.g., ulcerative colitis) and frequently cause terror in the patient who will refuse to cooperate for the subsequent sigmoidoscopy. This can lead to unnecessary general anesthesia and its potential complications. If the rectum is full, it is better to wait until the child has his next bowel movement and repeat the study immediately afterwards. When distal inflammatory bowel disease has been excluded by sigmoidoscopy, careful preparation of the colon is necessary before barium films are taken.

Colon Biopsy. If abnormal mucosa is seen during sigmoidoscopy, a suction colon biopsy should be taken from the abnormal area. This can be carried out safely with an all-purpose Rubin suction biopsy tube.

Plain Film of the Abdomen. Plain films may show abnormal thickening, distention, position of bowel shadows, soft tissue masses or a foreign body.

Barium Enema. When inflammatory bowel disease is not suspected, thorough colon preparation is required because small polyps may be missed if small amounts of feces are present.

Upper Gastrointestinal and Small Bowel Radiographic Series. Because high intestinal lesions may cause melena, this study is important. If colonic inflammatory bowel disease is present, the antegrade study followed through the colon is not likely to produce toxic megacolon as does a barium enema. Sufficient information about the colon can often be obtained in this way.

Technetium scan is a radioactive study in which the injected material will sometimes localize in the ectopic gastric mucosa of a Meckel's diverticulum and aid diagnosis.

Selective Angiography. If severe bleeding persists and no obvious cause is found, selective arteriography helps the surgeon localize a bleeding point in the gastrointestinal tract. This may avoid blind procedures of intestinal resection in an effort to stop catastrophic bleeding.

Upper Gastrointestinal Endoscopy. Fiberoptic instruments with excellent visibility, suitable for use in small infants, are available. Lesions not easily seen by radiographs (e.g., a Mallory-Weiss tear) can be detected. These instruments are being used more often to detect the cause of hematemesis and unexplained rectal bleeding.

Blood Tests. Abnormal bleeding tendencies or blood dyscrasias occasionally present as gastrointestinal hemorrhage. Liver disease with associated esophageal varices should always be looked for.

Chest Film. This should be done to exclude causes of hemoptysis in the young child who cannot spit up sputum and may be swallowing blood.

Diagnosis

Because high intestinal lesions may cause melena, the differential diagnosis should include causes of gastrointestinal hemorrhage.

Causes of Gastrointestinal Bleeding. The causes of gastrointestinal bleeding in children cover the same range as for adults, with certain differences. The more important causes of gastrointestinal bleeding in children are enumerated below. The causes of melena include all those of hematemesis, with the emphasis changing according to the age group (Tables 13-5, 13-6).

Principles of Management

Management for a first bleeding episode should begin conservatively unless bleeding is catastrophic and the hemoglobin drops to 6 g. or less in a shocked patient, or there is a complicating condition such as leukemia or congestive heart failure. As many as half of all episodes of gastrointestinal bleeding in children settle spontaneously and a specific cause may never be found, even after laparotomy. Furthermore, there may never be another episode.

The pediatric patient should *never* be sent to an adult intensive care unit. The patient should not be put into the pediatric intensive care unit if it can be avoided (in most cases of an initial bleeding episode this is possible). The atmosphere of strange noises, rapid movement, coming and going, physician anxiety and concern, other sick patients and their

Table 13-5. Differential Diagnosis and Symptoms of MELENA

Age	Disease	Other Major Symptoms	Other Signs
Newborn	Acute colitis (infective or inflammatory bowel disease)	Diarrhea	Frequent stools, blood, mucus in stools
	Disseminated intravascular (coagulation)	Overwhelming illness	Many bleeding sites
Infants	Anal fissure (any age)	Painful defecation	Fissure at anus, retained feces
	Infectious diarrhea	Vomiting, diarrhea, loss of appetite	Fever, weight loss
	Cow's milk allergy	May be none	Eczema
	Malrotation	Abdominal pain, vomiting	Abdominal distention
Preschool	Juvenile polyps	Painless, usually	Polyp may appear at anus
	Meckel's diverticulum	Abdominal pain	Tender abdomen, severe bleeding
	Intussusception	Abdominal pain	Sausage-shaped palpable mass, mucus mixed with blood
	Rectal prolapse	Frequent bulky stools	Prolapsed bowel seen
School age	Inflammatory bowel disease	Pain, anorexia, diarrhea	Poor growth, weight loss
	Peptic ulcer	Pain relieved by food	Epigastric tenderness
	Esophageal varices	Those of the primary disease	
	Esophagitis	Heartburn	May be none
	Malignancy	Multiple symptoms	Weight loss, fever

Table 13-6. Differential Diagnosis and Symptoms of HEMATEMESIS

Age	Disease	Other Major Symptoms	Other Signs
Intrauterine	Intestinal perforation	Postnatal vomiting	Tender distended abdomen
	Peptic ulceration	Postnatal vomiting	
Newborn	Swallowed maternal blood	Placental, vaginal bleeding	Hematemesis
	Swallowed hemoptysis	Respiratory distress	Abnormal air entry, pulmonary signs
	Iatrogenic (e.g., aspirin for fever)	Related to need for aspirin	Fever
	Hemorrhagic disease	Respiratory distress	Bruises, bloody urine, signs of CNS hemorrhage
	Congenital thrombocytopenic purpura	Depend on bleeding site	Purpura
	Hemorrhagic gastritis	Abdominal pain	Signs of infection or septicemia
	Pyloric outlet obstruction (stenosis, webs)	Avid hunger, projectile vomiting	Severe weight loss, visible gastric peristalsis
	Stress ulcer	Associated disease	Tender epigastrium, anemia
	Necrotizing enterocolitis	Pallor, weak suck reflex	Distended abdomen, shock
	Chalasia (severe)	Regurgitation of feeds	Aspiration pneumonia
	Hiatus hernia with esophagitis	Vomiting feeds	Failure to grow
	Esophageal, gastrogenic cysts	May be none	May be none
Any age group	Iatrogenic (e.g., aspirin)	Related to need for aspirin	Fever
	Esophageal varices	Cough (cystic fibrosis) Poor appetite (cirrhosis liver)	Malabsorption Enlarged spleen, hard liver, xanthomata
	Peptic ulcer (Zollinger-Ellison syndrome)	Abdominal pain	Anemia, tender epigastrium
	Telangiectasia	May be none	Skin telangiectasias
	Hemangiomatosis	Dependent on site	Consumption Coagulopathy
	Foreign body	Pain, dysphagia	Local or none

care, and the general hubbub will not help the patient and generally will make things worse. In particular, the sight of a half-naked elderly adult lying exposed and semiconscious with many tubes attached, is terrifying for children of all ages.

Family visits should not be restricted, no matter what one's opinion of the parents or the relatives may be. A much sounder approach than restriction is enlisting the support of the family in the management of their child and problem in a caring fashion.

Use of a nasogastric tube in the stomach for hematemesis is not recommended unless the patient is unconscious or there is a depressed cough reflex that makes aspiration a hazard. This procedure is not necessary for diagnosis or assessment of continued bleeding because a child may vomit blood from as high as the nose or as low down as the jejunum. A thorough physical examination and history-taking will serve the clinician just as well for diagnosis. Furthermore, placement of a nasogastric tube is extremely repugnant to most children; sometimes they will fight and pull out the tube, thus compounding the bleeding. The danger of a Mallory-Weiss lesion (tear of the esophageal mucosa) should preclude the indiscriminate placement of a nasogastric tube.

There should be no dietary restrictions for conscious patients unless the diagnosis indicates an acute surgical condition of the abdomen, esophageal varices, or Mallory-Weiss lesion. The diet should not be restricted because of infrequent vomiting episodes. It is appropriate to ask the family what the child's favorite foods are, and, if possible, provide them initially in accordance with a dietitian's advice.

It is prudent to avoid the insertion of an intravenous line; it is better for the child to be free to move and be held by relatives or nurses and go to the toilet normally. Frequently repeated venipunctures or fingersticks should be avoided, and all the specimens necessary for diagnosis should be obtained during the first venipuncture procedures. In addition, it is very important not to order *routine* repeated fingersticks (e.g., hemoglobin and hematocrit determinations two, three or four times a day). These tests should be done only when vital signs, history and physical examination indicate a further loss of blood. Children in certain age groups can be reduced rapidly to bundles of fear and apprehension, or can become violent fighters, by frequent, routine sticking.

It is not advisable to give blood in the face of a stable condition unless the hemoglobin is 6 g. or less, or unless the patient has a special need for increased oxygen exchange (e.g., cyanotic congenital heart disease, pulmonary insufficiency, or severe infections). Most children are resilient, and will manage with a hemoglobin of 6 g. without difficulty. Because of the risk of hepatitis or other disorders, blood transfusion itself can be more dangerous to the patient than a gastrointestinal bleed that has stopped at 5 or 6 g. and does not recur.

All too often the pediatric patient in a busy setting is physically restrained by having an arm or leg tied for an intravenous line, or because he wishes to move about. A child will govern his own movements depending on how he feels. The arm or leg should be tied down only if it is absolutely necessary to maintain a life-saving blood infusion.

Further Steps in Management

Vital signs such as pulse rate, respiration, and blood pressure are usually recorded every half hour. A gradual increase in pulse rate is the best indicator of continued bleeding. The blood pressure will fall if the patient has decompensated and is in shock, and it is not usually necessary to disturb a sleeping child to take frequent blood pressure recordings if the pulse rate remains steady.

The initial essential blood tests include determinations of hemoglobin, hematocrit, white blood cell count and differential, and sedimentation rate. Always incorporate a coagulation profile, ascertain the child's blood group, cross-match, and hold blood ready for transfusion. Other blood tests depend on the tentative clinical diagnosis.

Whole blood is best for replacing blood loss. Packed red blood cells should be used in long-standing chronic anemia or congestive heart failure. The amount of blood necessary can be based on 15 ml./kg. of whole blood. The rate of infusion will depend on the urgency of the patient's need.

Discussion

Without doubt it is true that children are different. They will reward the clinician with resilience, response, and recovery after confident, considerate management; this reaction is surprising when they are compared with adult patients. It is important to gain the child's confidence by talking with him on his own level. The nurses should be familiar with children and their specific needs, as well as being firm and sympathetic. All too often in adult units unaccustomed to children there is an overindulgence by adult patients and staff alike; this can be detrimental to a child's overall growth and development.

Schooling, play, peer interaction, and the presence of parents and siblings are of importance to a child. These needs should be given due consideration with any child with gastrointestinal bleeding, no matter how severe. The presence of familiar things will help the child to recover rapidly, and will reduce the apprehension that can only increase the risk of continued hemorrhage. It is not uncommon, after many transfusions, to see bleeding stop when the intravenous line is removed and a child is provided the right environment. When a child is restricted, venipunctured, frightened and transfused too often to increase the hemoglobin, he may continue to bleed; such patients may undergo laparotomy unnecessarily.

BIBLIOGRAPHY

Anderson, C. M., and Burke, V., (eds.): Pediatric Gastroenterology. London, Blackwell, 1975.
Gryboski, J.: Gastrointestinal Problems in the Infant. Philadelphia, W. B. Saunders, 1975.

Roy, C. C., Silverman, A., and Cozetto, F. J.: Pediatric Clinical Gastroenterology. St. Louis, C. V. Mosby, 1975.

These are good general tests of pediatric gastroenterology which focus on clinical aspects of diagnosis and treatment.

Davidson, M. (ed.): Clinics in Gastroenterology—Pediatric Gastroenterology. Philadelphia. W. B. Saunders, 1977.

A concise monograph, limited in scope, but which deals well with important common problems.

14

Vomiting

James A. Hallock, M.D.

Vomiting is one of the most common signs and symptoms in infancy and childhood. It may occur with any acute infection or emotional stress and is a sign of abnormality in either the gastrointestinal tract, urinary tract or nervous system. It is important to know the main etiologic factors and their variation in different age groups.

PATHOPHYSIOLOGY

The mechanisms responsible for vomiting depend upon stimulation of brain centers. The vomiting center is located in the medulla, near the tractus solitarius at the level of the dorsal motor nucleus of the vagus. The center receives stimuli from the visceral organs via the vagus or sympathetic afferent nerves. These stimuli may arise in any abdominal organ but the strongest stimuli arise from the stomach and duodenum. Following stimulation of the vomiting center, the act of emesis is transmitted through motor impulses via cranial nerves V, VII, IX, X, XII. This mechanism is responsible for the vomiting seen with gastrointestinal and renal disease. Vomiting with increased intracranial pressure also results from stimulation of this center.

Another mechanism involves stimulation of the chemoreceptor trigger zone (CTZ) which is located in the floor of the fourth ventricle above the area postrema. This area is sensitive to toxins and drugs such as apomorphine. The vomiting associated with infection is thought to be mediated via this mechanism.

The stimulus for vomiting in motion sickness arises from labyrinthine receptors. Impulses produced are transmitted either directly to the cerebellum or via the vestibular nuclei to the CTZ with emesis the result.

The chemical mediators involved with these mechanisms are unknown at this time.

Metabolic Changes Following Vomiting

Vomiting is followed by disturbances in fluid and electrolyte balance since there is loss of water, hydrochloric acid and electrolytes. As a result of these losses, clinical dehydration becomes evident with contraction of extracellular fluid volume and development of hypochloremic metabolic alkalosis.

The potential for dehydration should be considered in all cases of vomiting, especially in infants and small children. Documentation of fluid loss and ability to ingest fluids is a critical step in the evaluation of all children with vomiting. Further mention will be made of this in other discussions in this Chapter.

CHARACTER OF VOMITUS

The appearance of the vomited mateial is helpful in determining the significance of the vomiting and the level of involvement of the gastrointestinal tract (Table 14-1.)

Undigested or unchanged food suggests that the lesion is in the esophagus or stomach (e.g., esophageal atresia or stenosis). Digested food which is not bile-stained suggests a lesion proximal to the ampulla of Vater (e.g., pyloric stenosis). Bilious vomiting is suggestive of obstruction distal to the ampulla (e.g., small bowel obstruction). Fecal vomitus is an emergency suggesting distal gastrointestinal obstruction or peritonitis. Hematemesis is always pathologic and must be investigated thoroughly (see Neonatal Period).

Table 14-1. Character of Vomitus

Character of vomitus	Probable level of involvement	Example lesion
Undigested food	Esophagus	Esophageal atresia
Digested food, no bile	Proximal to ampulla of Vater	Pyloric stenosis
Bile-containing material*	Distal to ampulla of Vater	Jejunal atresia
Fecal vomiting*	Distal gastrointestinal tract	Peritonitis
Blood*	Upper gastrointestinal tract	Ulcer

*Should be initially approached as an emergency situation.

Table 14-2. Types of Vomiting

Type	Significance	Etiology
Projectile vomiting	Pathologic and Requires evaluation	Upper gastrointestinal tract Increased intracranial pressure
Vomiting without nausea	Pathologic and requires evaluation	Increased intracranial pressure
Vomiting with nausea	Common	Infection Toxicity

PATTERN OF VOMITING

The pattern of vomiting may be a clue to the diagnosis. Although each of the following patterns is suggestive, none is pathognomonic of a specific diagnosis (Table 14-2). Vomiting with nausea is a common sign of acute illness such as infection or ingestion of toxic material. Vomiting without nausea may be a sign of increased intracranial pressure and should be rapidly evaluated. Projectile vomiting also requires prompt evaluation and usually indicates the presence of gastrointestinal obstruction or increased intracranial pressure.

APPROACH TO DIAGNOSIS

The etiology of vomiting is usually considered in relation to the age of the child. The three age periods are: (1) neonatal period; (2) infancy through 2 years; and (3) childhood (after 2 years). In assessing a symptom such as vomiting, the history and physical examination are important keys to diagnosis. The vomiting should be categorized as acute or chronic since the approach varies depending on the duration of the vomiting.

Attention must be paid to the child's development. If growth and development are "normal" for age, this implies that the vomiting is not significant and that an extensive evaluation is unnecessary. If there is retardation of either growth or development, a search should be made for one of the causes of chronic vomiting listed for each age period below.

In each of the following discussions, an attempt will be made to demonstrate the most likely diagnosis and to present guidelines for evaluation.

Neonatal Vomiting

Vomiting is common (50%) in normal full-term newborns and is related to either swallowed amniotic fluid, swallowed blood or to faulty feeding techniques. If the baby is feeding well, gaining weight, and physical examination reveals no abnormalities, then no evaluation should be performed unless the vomiting is persistent. The evaluation of a vomiting neonate who appears ill is a critical situation. This is a symptom of a potentially rapidly fatal process and one which quickly leads to difficulty with fluid and electrolyte balance.

The signs and symptoms listed below are the ones associated with pathologic causes of vomiting in the newborn. Certain findings including dehydration, hematemesis, bilious vomiting, projectile vomiting, and abdominal mass, demand immediate evaluation since they indicate an emergency situation, surgical or medical. Maternal polyhydramnios, increased gastric contents (more than 25 ml.) at initial aspiration, abdominal distention, lack of meconium stools, decrease in feeding, lethargy, and irritability are signs or symptoms which demand close observation but not necessarily immediate evaluation. The appearance and physical

---

Signs and Symptoms of Disease Associated with Neonatal Vomiting

Dehydration—loss of 5–10% of birth weight

Hematemesis: This could be the presentation of upper GI bleeding or swallowed maternal blood. (An APT test with 10% NaOH should be performed to differentiate adult from fetal hemoglobin)

History of maternal polyhydramnios in this pregnancy

Increased gastric contents (>25 ml.) at initial aspiration after birth

Progressive abdominal distention

Lack of meconium stools

Bilious vomiting

Decrease in feeding

Lethargy

Irritability

Projectile vomiting

Abdominal mass

Differential Diagnosis of Vomiting in the Neonate

Gastrointestinal lesions (usually represent acute
   surgical emergencies in the neonate.)
   Esophageal atresia—tracheoesophageal fistula
   Duodenal, jejeunal or ileal atresia
   Annular pancreas
   Congenital bands
   Intestinal malrotation with volvulus
   Imperforate anus
   Toxic megacolon
   Meconium ileus (cystic fibrosis)
   Meconium plug syndrome
   Trauma to upper GI or respiratory tracts.
Infections (medical emergencies)
   Generalized sepsis
   Meningitis
   Urinary tract infection
   Pneumonia
Central nervous system
   Subdural hematoma
   Intracranial hemorrhage
Renal disorders
   Renal tubular acidosis
Metabolic (inborn errors)
   Galactosemia
   PKU
   Congenital adrenal hyperplasia
   Hypercalcemia
   Aminoacidurias
     Maple syrup urine disease
     Hyperglycinemia
     Citrullenemia
     Hypervalinemia
     Hyperammonemia
     Argininosuccinicaciduria

---

examination of the baby should be the major factor in evaluation. When indicated, this evaluation must be as rapid, thorough, and atraumatic as possible.

To rule out a surgical lesion such as intestinal obstruction, plain radiographs of the abdomen or radiographs using air as the initial contrast medium should be taken. Further radiological evaluation may include contrast enema and upper gastrointestinal films. If a surgical lesion is diagnosed, prompt stabilization and hydration should be accomplished prior to operation. These lesions are usually upper intestinal and include esophageal atresia with or without tracheoesophageal fistula, and duodenal obstruction secondary to atresia, anular pancreas or congenital bands.

If no surgical lesion is demonstrated, infection is the next major category to be considered. A blood culture, urine culture (suprapubic aspiration), lumbar puncture and other cultures must be performed if the baby appears ill with no obvious cause for vomiting. In this situation, antibiotic therapy is frequently initiated prior to culture results.

Further evaluation should be performed as indicated by the patient's status. The differential diagnosis is listed and can serve as a guide to most likely possibilities and studies needed. This is the presentation for many of the metabolic disorders listed.

Infancy

Most acute vomiting during this period is in conjunction with infectious diseases. Although any of the listed causes of chronic vomiting may start acutely, these are not thought of in the initial patient encounter unless some other factor is present. All normal infants "spit up" to some degree after feedings; here too, the history and physical examination are important in determining if the complaint of "vomiting" warrants further investigation.

In this period, infant regurgitation causes much maternal anxiety. Therefore, when you are presented with an infant 1 to 2 months of age, certain facts must be elicited. Probably all normal infants bring up some milk after feeding but the pattern is very important in deciding whether it is necessary or desirable to investigate for organic disease.

Since the child can give no history of nausea or abdominal pain, the physical examination frequently provides the answer. Each of the causes listed below must be considered and the likely ones ruled out by physical examination or appropriate laboratory study (e.g., urine culture in the case of suspected urinary tract infection). Also, during physical examination strict attention must be paid to fluid balance to ensure no problem with dehydration. Persistent or chronic vomiting associated with any of the following requires a more thorough investigation: projectile vomiting, decreased feeding, failure to grow and/or develop properly, bilious vomiting, hematemesis, abdominal mass, distention, and bloody diarrhea.

The two most important non-organic causes of chronic vomiting are: (1) Regurgitation or spitting-up. This represents the nonforceful expulsion of small amounts of food shortly after feeding. It may be related to

Causes of Vomiting During Infancy

Gastrointestinal lesions
  Pyloric stenosis (2-12 weeks)
  Intussuception*
  Malrotation with volvulus*
  Achalasia of esophagus
  Chalasia
  Hiatal hernia

Infectious problems
  Gastroenteritis*
  Urinary tract infections
  Meningitis*
  Pneumonia*
  Otitis media*
  Pertussis*
  Sepsis*
  Any URI*

Central nervous system
  Subdural hematoma
Hydrocephalus

Renal disease
  Nephrotic syndrome
  Renal tubular acidosis
  Polycystic kidneys
  Nephrogenic diabetes insipidus
  Uremia

Metabolic (inborn errors)
  Diabetes mellitus*
  Galactosemia
  Fructosemia
  Congenital adrenal hyperplasia*
  Aminoacidurias (as in neonate)

*A cause of acute as well as chronic vomiting in this age group (see text).

faulty feeding techniques or social/environmental factors. One- to 3-month old babies have this complaint which disappears when the baby begins to walk. These children have "normal" growth and development; this, together with a "normal" physical examination, supports the diagnosis. (2) Rumination is a rare but serious form of chronic vomiting with its onset during the latter half of the first year. The problem is psychogenic in origin due either to maternal deprivation or maternal inadequacy. There is usually associated failure to thrive. The child may be seen gagging himself but this frequently can be a difficult diagnosis to confirm.

Childhood Vomiting

As in the case with infants, this is not a variant of "normal" in children over the age of 2 years; therefore, all children with vomiting must be evaluated. The type of evaluation depends on whether the symptom is acute or long-standing.

Chronic Vomiting. The most common etiology for chronic vomiting in childhood is functional vomiting. When this complaint is made, the major thrust of evaluation should be a physical examination that includes blood pressure, and ocular fundi and visual field examinations. When evaluating this symptom, do not attempt a "full workup." The following are helpful indicators and should lead to a search for a specific diagnosis. Deterioration in health, weight loss, disturbance in growth pattern, urinary symptoms, neurologic symptoms, pallor, and unilateral abdominal pain. If the above are absent and physical examination is "normal," you are justified in following the child and observing the pattern.

Functional Vomiting. Usually this is made as a diagnosis of exclusion. However, an attempt must be made to gather historical data sufficient to support this diagnosis (e.g., evaluate school phobias or stresses in the child's environment).

Acute Vomiting. As with younger children, the most common association is with infections; these should be evaluated. In addition, ingestion of unusual substances gains in importance and must always be considered in any child with vomiting. The following is a list of some of the causes for acute vomiting in this age group.

Appendicitis. Special mention is made of this condition since in many reported series, more than half the children less than 6 years of age operated on for appendicitis have suffered a ruptured appendix. In order to prevent this, the diagnosis must be considered and made earlier.

SUMMARY

In any age group, the keys to proper evaluation are the history and physical examination. These should point to the diagnosis or provide the information to judge whether further studies are necessary. In addition, the history and physical examination should give a clear picture of the child's growth and development and how they are affected by the complaint of vomiting.

Vomiting in Childhood

Acute infection
Any infection may present with vomiting but it is most commonly
seen with:
    Gastroenteritis*
    Urinary tract infections (see below)*
    Pharyngitis*
    Pneumonia*
    Viral exanthems*
    Otitis media*
    Hepatitis*

Gastrointestinal
    Appendicitis*
    Small bowel obstruction*
    Meckel's diverticulum*
    Hiatal hernia
    Peptic ulcer
    Pancreatitis (rare)*

Renal
    UTI*
    Acute glomerulonephritis*
    Nephrosis
    Hypertension*
    Uremia

Intracranial disease
    Increased intracranial pressure
        Brain tumor
        Pseudotumor cerebri
        Hydrocephalus
        Others
    Migraine headaches
    Meningitis*
    Seizure disorders

Poisoning (drug ingestion)
    Lead*
    Salicylates*
    Most medications or drugs*
    Any toxin

Metabolic diseases
    Diabetes mellitus*
    Hypertension*
    Hyperlipidemia

*Acute or chronic vomiting in this age group. (See text.)

BIBLIOGRAPHY

Batzdorf, U.: The management of cerebral edema in pediatric practice. Pediatrics, *58*:78-87, 1966.

> This article deals with the management of cerebral edema, but also points out the recognition of vomiting as a manifestation of increased intracranial pressure and the evaluation of a patient for intracranial pressure.

Reinhart, J. B., Evans, S. L., McFadden, D. L.: Cyclic vomiting in children: Seen through the psychiatrist's eye. Pediatrics, *59*:371-377, 1977.

> This is a review of recurrent and repeated vomiting in childhood and delineates the multiple evaluation processes. Many of the children in this article underwent surgical exploration prior to their ultimate disposition.

Talbert, J. L., Felman, A. H., DeBush, F. L.: Gastrointestinal surgical emergencies in the newborn infant. J. Pediatr. 76:783-797, 1970.

> This is an excellent summary of all the findings present in newborns with intestinal obstruction and surgical emergencies and outlines diagnostic approach in evaluation of signs and symptoms.

Taneja, O. P., Taneja, S., Lal, A.: Intestinal obstruction in infancy and childhood. Arch. Surg., *97*:544-552, 1968.

> This article gives the statistical review of the causes of intestinal obstruction and an evaluation of children with intestinal obstruction.

Vulliamy, D. G.: Recurrent abdominal pain and vomiting in childhood. Br. Med. J., *1*:1113-1115, 1965.

> This article is an approach to nonorganic causes of vomiting and offers a good perspective on evaluating vomiting as a symptom in helping to decide if the problem is organic or inorganic.

15

Diarrheal Diseases

John I. Malone, M.D.

Diarrhea is not a disease but a symptom of a number of other disease processes that involve various organ systems including the gastrointestinal tract.

The term "diarrhea" is not precise. Thus it is important to have the patient or parent describe in other terms what they mean when using the word diarrhea. The medical definition is "an abnormally frequent discharge of *fluid* and *fecal material*." The exact meaning of "abnormally frequent" and its implication regarding the total amount of material lost continues to be vague and subjective, particularly at younger ages. Infants vary considerably in the number and consistency of normal stools passed per day. Four to six in a day may be normal for one infant, while one in two or even 3 days may be normal for another. Therefore, the definition of diarrhea must be modified to an increase in the frequency and looseness of stools beyond that which is common for a particular individual.

As the child grows older and the intestinal tract matures, the normal consistency and frequency of stooling becomes less variable. There is less response to variation in the components of the food stuffs (i.e., sugar, fat, protein) as the mechanisms of absorption mature, thus the "normal" stooling pattern of a person becomes more predictable with increasing age.

Acute diarrhea is commonly a self-limited aggravation for older children, adolescents and adults. This must be contrasted, however, with the life-threatening potential of acute diarrhea during the first year of life. Acute diarrhea during infancy has a much greater potential for massive fluid loss and resultant cardiovascular collapse than in older children.

Chronic diarrhea (more than 2 weeks duration), an even more life-threatening situation for an infant, also has significant morbidity and mortality for older children. This is due largely to the resultant malnutrition.

Diarrhea is a frequent and important problem in pediatrics. An understanding of the mechanisms that cause diarrhea may make its treatment more rational.

MECHANISMS OF DIARRHEA

Damaged Intestinal Brush Border Membrane

This is caused either by toxins or mechanical trauma. It results in impaired transport of water, electrolytes, and products of digestion in and out of the intestinal lumen.

Increased Intraluminal Unabsorbed Osmotically Active Substances

This may be the result of damaged intestinal brush border membrane or other causes. Drinking water that contains increased amounts of soluble sulfates is an example. The brush border membrane is unaffected, but the unabsorbed sulfate osmotically pulls extra water into the intestinal tract. Hereditary deficiency of intestinal enzymes (i.e., lactase, lipase, amylase) which break down ingested food to absorbable particles, results in increased intraluminal osmotically active substances. Certain antibiotics are believed to inhibit enzymes important for the absorption of digested food. Acquired enzyme deficiencies may occur secondary to certain antibiotics (ampicillin, tetracycline, erythromycin) or to the mechanical trauma of diarrhea.

Intestinal Microorganisms

These may cause diarrhea by mechanism of damaged intestinal brush border membrane by releasing an enterotoxin or by direct invasion of the epithelial lining of the mucosa. Another way that intestinal microorganisms cause diarrhea is by biotransformation of bile acids and saturated long chain fatty acids to substances that impair fat absorption and cause steatorrhea.

Bile Acids

Bile acids are normally absorbed in the ileum. Surgical resection of the ileum or anything that prevents this absorption allows for increased amounts of bile acids in the colon. Bile acids in the colon interfere with the absorption of water and electrolytes and induce the colon to secrete and increase the stool volume.

Diarrhea Due to Hydroxy-Fatty Acids

Deficient absorption of long chain fatty acids allows biotransformation by colon flora of these substances to hydroxy-fatty acids which are well-known cathartics.

Abnormal Intestinal Motility

Altered intestinal motility produces disturbances in digestion and absorption. Increased motility is the result of an excess of smooth muscle active substances such as prostaglandins and serotonin. It has been reported that the interaction of the pituitary polypeptide coherin with serotonin in mucosal receptors alters intestinal motor activity.

Decreased intestinal motility may occur in diabetes and scleroderma. This allows increased bacterial colonization which plays a role in the malabsorption and diarrhea observed in these patients.

Hypersecretory State

These are exudative enteropathies. This category varies from gastrin-induced gastric hypersecretion and hypersecretory states provoked by the chronic inflammation of ulcerative colitis and regional enteritis to intestinal lymphangectasia involving the loss of lymph and protein through the colon.

Unknown Mechanisms

The mechanisms responsible for the diarrhea of immune disorders, acrodermatitis enteropathica, and food intolerances, *are speculative at present.*

DISEASES CAUSING ACUTE DIARRHEA

Improper Feeding

This is the most common cause of acute diarrhea of infancy. Infants vary widely in their individual tolerance to both the quantity and the quality of food. A quantity of formula that is tolerated by one infant may cause diarrhea in a second. The commonly used infant formulas differ in the amount and types of protein, fat, and carbohydrate. Each of these components may affect the stool volume in variable ways. Stool volume and water content seem to vary directly with the fat and sugar content of the formula. Thus, babies on a formula high in polyunsaturated fats (Similac) have looser stools than those on a formula containing a greater percentage of saturated fats (SMA). Switching from one formula to another for nonspecific problems such as colic may result in a stool pattern interpreted as diarrhea. In a similar fashion, if the sugar content in a formula is much greater than 7.2 per cent weight per volume (W/V), the stools tend to become soft and watery. Some family feeding practices allow for the addition of honey to the proprietary formula to "enrich the formula." This usually loosens the stools. This type of intolerance decreases as the gastrointestinal tract matures and is, therefore, less apparent with increasing age.

Infections

Infections are the most common causes of diarrhea during infancy and childhood. Table 15-1 shows the clinical features useful in identifying the infectious diarrheas.

Infections outside the intestinal tract are frequently associated with diarrhea in younger children. This is called "parenteral" diarrhea. In such patients cessation or persistence of the diarrhea parallels the clearing or continuation of the primary infection. This suggests that parenteral diarrhea is associated with the response of the immature colon to non-gastrointestinal disease. This is supported by the observation that young infants are more sensitive than adults to the development of parenteral diarrhea. Diarrhea that results from the use of antibiotics, moreover, is much more common in children than adults and may have the same mechanism.

Protozoal infections cause both acute and chronic diarrhea. The onset is not likely to be sudden. The stools lack the odor and appearance of an infectious diarrhea. The mucus is white or yellowish, and the odor suggests an autolytic rather than a suppurative process. The children may have a variety of complaints that can be traced to the intestinal tract and appear to have a malabsorption syndrome such as celiac disease prior to the onset of diarrhea. The diagnosis requires reliable microscopic laboratory examination of several small quantities of stool.

Food Poisoning

Food poisoning as a cause should also be considered. This type of diarrhea is of acute onset and usually occurs in a large group of people within 4 to 6 hours of ingesting a specific food item. One type of food poisoning is called botulism and is caused by a toxin released by the *Clostridium botulinum*, an anaerobic spore-forming organism. The source of the organism is chiefly home-canned foods, especially underprocessed non-acid meat, fish, and vegetables. Some patients have acute nausea, vomiting, and abdominal pain. Central nervous system symptoms develop in 12 to 48 hours and are due to a curare-like action of the toxin on the motor end plate.

Some strains of staphylococci and streptococci produce an exotoxin that causes nausea, vomiting, abdominal pain, and acute prostration in addition to diarrhea, within 1 to 6 hours of ingesting contaminated food. Foods commonly infected are pastries, salads, chicken, ham, beef in hash, whipped cream and custards.

Table 15-2 lists some of the clinical features that are helpful in differentiating the non-infectious causes of diarrhea.

Table 15-1. Usual Clinical Features of Infectious Diarrheas

	Cholera	Enterotoxigenic E. coli*	Enteroinvasive E. coli*	"Enteropathogenic" E. coli	Shigella Diarrheic form	Shigella Dysenteric form	Salmonella	Reirus-like organism
Site of action	Small bowel	Small bowel	Large bowel	Small bowel?	Small bowel	Large bowel	Small and large bowels	Small bowel
Mechanism of action	Toxin	Toxin	Invasion	?	?	Invasion	?	?
Age	Any	Any?	Any?	<1 yr.	>2 yr.	Any	Any	<7 yr.
Diarrhea in household	++	?	?	0	++	++	+	+
Season	Epidemic	?	?	Fall	Fall	Fall	Any	Winter
Character of onset	Abrupt	Abrupt	Abrupt	Gradual	Abrupt	Gradual	Gradual	Abrupt
Vomiting	+ (Late)	++	0	+	++	+	+	++
Cramps	++	++	k++	?	0	++	+	?
Tenesmus	0	0	?	?	0	++	+	?
Fever >102° F.	0	0	++	0	++	+	0	0
Convulsions	0	0	0	0	++	0	0	0
Anal sphincter tone	Normal	?	?	Normal	Lax	Lax	Normal	Normal
Stool volume	Large	Large	Small	Moderate	Large	Small	Moderate	Large
Stool consistency	Watery	Water	Slimy	Slimy	Watery	Viscous	Slimy	Watery
Stool odor	Odorless	?	?	Musty	Odorless	Odorless	Foul	Odorless
Stool blood	0	0	++	+	0	++	0	0
Stool mucus shreds	++	++	++	0	++	0	0	0
Stool pus	0	0	++	+	0	++	+	0
Stool color	Colorless	Colorless	?	Green	Colorless	Bloody	Green/brown	Colorless/brown
Stool leukocytes	0	0	++	+	+	++	++	0
Bandemia	?	?	?	+	++	++	0	0
Duration (untreated)	3–6 days	5–10 days	?	7–14 days	2–3 days	7–14 days	3–7 days	5–7 days

(Table prepared by John D. Nelson, and J. Patrick Hieber, M.D. From Krugman, S., Ward, R., and Katz, S.: Infectious Diseases of Children. St. Louis, C. V. Mosby, 1977.)

*Based on observations in adults.

Key: ?, Insufficient data available; 0, usually absent; +, sometimes present; ++ commonly present.

Table 15-2. Clinical Feature of Acute Diarrhea (Non-Bacterial)

Clinical Feature	Overfeeding	Parenteral	Protozoal	Food poisoning
Age	0–2 years	Any	Any	Any
Well-being	Normal	ill	ill	Severely ill
Weight	Normal	Stable	Loss	Loss
Diarrhea in household	No	No	Variable	Yes
Vomiting	Variable	No	Occasionally	Yes
Fever	No	Variable	Occasionally	No
Abdominal discomfort	No	No	Variable	Yes
CNS signs	No	Variable	No	Yes
Stools				
Consistency	Loose	Loose	Watery	Watery
Odor	Normal	Normal	Variable	Variable
Blood	No	No	Yes	Variable

CHRONIC DIARRHEA

In infants and children, chronic diarrhea is often a diagnostic and therapeutic challenge. The clinical spectrum ranges from benign normal physiologic responses misinterpreted as problems to disorders which are life-threatening and frequently associated with severe nutritional deficiencies (Fig. 15-1).

Although novel techniques have been applied to the diagnosis of chronic diarrhea, a well-taken history (i.e., feeding history, stool description, general health) offers important clues which channel and identify priorities in the workup of such a patient. The physical exam must include an evaluation of the patient's growth and physical development. Normal growth and development are not likely to be associated with a process of a severe nature. Examination of the diarrheal stool is part of the complete physical examination on such a patient. The presence or absence of excessive mucus and water and their characteristics are very useful information. Purulent mucus suggests an infectious process, bloody mucus an ulcerative process. Disaccharidase deficiency results in

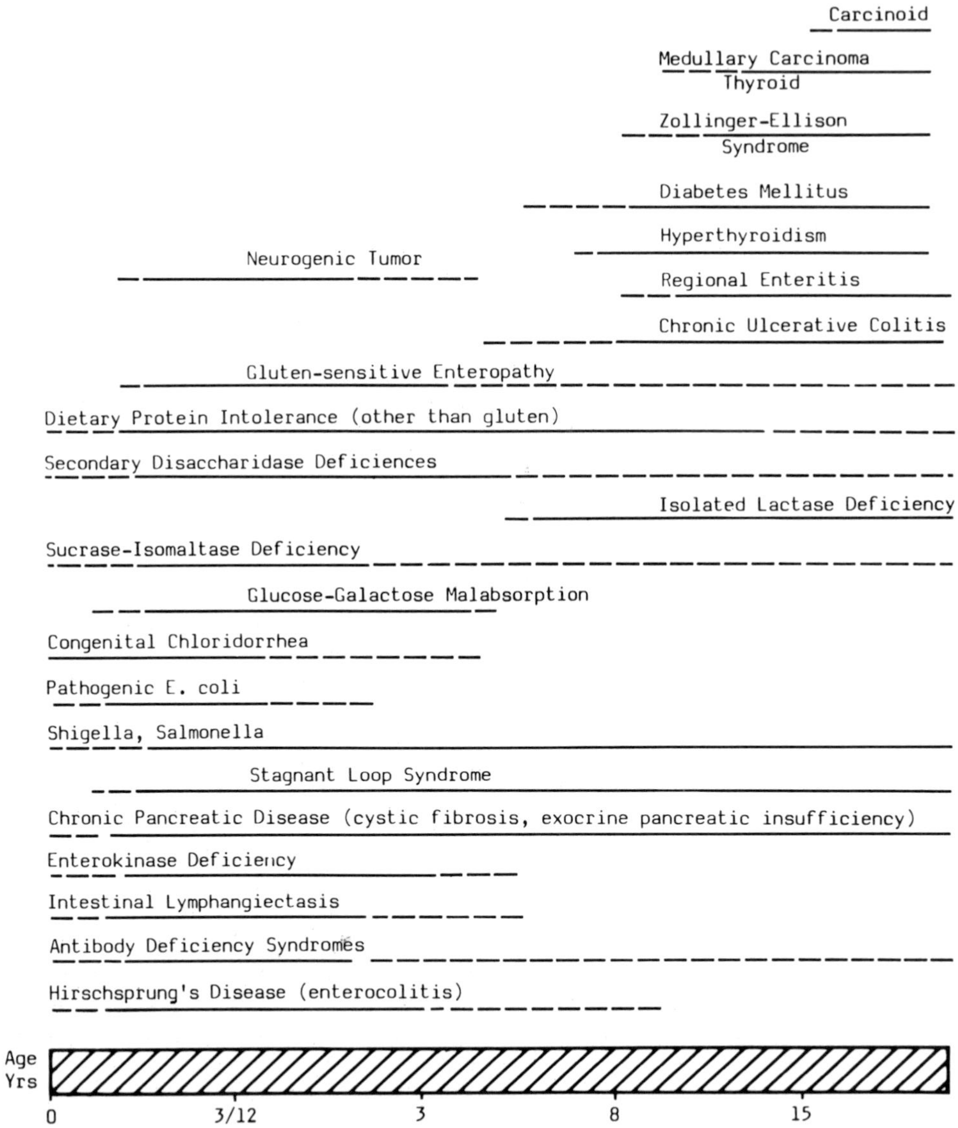

Carcinoid

Medullary Carcinoma
Thyroid

Zollinger-Ellison
Syndrome

Diabetes Mellitus

Hyperthyroidism

Neurogenic Tumor

Regional Enteritis

Chronic Ulcerative Colitis

Gluten-sensitive Enteropathy

Dietary Protein Intolerance (other than gluten)

Secondary Disaccharidase Deficiences

Isolated Lactase Deficiency

Sucrase-Isomaltase Deficiency

Glucose-Galactose Malabsorption

Congenital Chloridorrhea

Pathogenic E. coli

Shigella, Salmonella

Stagnant Loop Syndrome

Chronic Pancreatic Disease (cystic fibrosis, exocrine pancreatic insufficiency)

Enterokinase Deficiency

Intestinal Lymphangiectasis

Antibody Deficiency Syndromes

Hirschsprung's Disease (enterocolitis)

Age Yrs

0   3/12   3   8   15

Fig. 15-1. Relation of etiology to age of patient in chronic diarrhea in children. Solid lines: estimated greatest frequency of occurrence and/or diagnosis. Broken lines: possible occurrence or establishment of diagnosis at a younger or older age. (From Poley, J. R.: Chronic diarrhea in infants and children, Part I. South Med. J., 66:1050–1133, 1973.)

the excretion of large quantities of watery stool. In the absence of free water in the stool a disaccharidase deficiency is unlikely. The indirect tests used to make this diagnosis are the findings of an acid stool pH and the presence of unabsorbed sugar in the stool. In the absence of the intestinal disaccharide that hydrolyzes the sugar, it acts as an osmotically active substance which increases stool water. This same sugar is in turn metabolized by the enteric flora to produce lactic acid which lowers the pH of the stool water below pH 5. To test for reducing substance in the stool, one part liquid stool is mixed with two parts water. Fifteen drops of this mixture are then added to a test tube and a fresh clinitest tablet is added to the tube. The color chart for sugar in the urine (five-drop method) is employed. A reading of 0.5 per cent or greater is considered positive. If the stool water is missed and these substances are looked for in water in which the stool particles were emulsified many false negatives will occur.

While following the course of a patient with chronic diarrhea, daily weights must be noted. This is particularly important in untrained infants who may pass large quantities of fluid into the diaper with no solid material left as evidence. This can result in a significant fluid and weight loss during a time interval when the nursing observations indicate that the diarrhea has stopped.

The evaluation of poor fat absorption (steatorrhea) characteristically involves the measurement of the 24-hour excretion of fat in the stool. If consuming a diet of at least 50 g. of fat, a stool fat greater than 7 g. in 24 hours measured for 3 consecutive days, is considered normal. An easier indirect measurement of fat absorption is the level of the fat-soluble vitamins (A, D, E, K) in the serum.

There are several entities responsible for chronic diarrhea. These disorders are listed in Table 15-3 with several characteristic features that may help focus attention on the most appropriate etiology.

TREATMENT

The initial therapeutic approach to diarrhea is to make sure the patient is not in impending shock. If the patient is in shock, proper fluids and electrolytes must be administered immediately. Following that determination, the patient's diarrhea is then categorized as either mild, moderate, or severe. When making a decision about the seriousness of diarrhea, it is very helpful to know the daily weights of the patient. Therefore, a weight must be recorded on each visit of such a patient and may be the only objective evidence available during the clinical observations of a specific patient to determine the severity of the diarrhea (Table 15-4).

Table 15-3. Causes of Chronic Diarrhea: Features

Disease	Vomit	Stool			Red sub	Fat	Abd. dist.	Hered-itary	Acquired	Other
		H$_2$O	Mucus	pH						
Deficiency disaccharidase	N	+	N	<5	+	+	+	±	+	Renal calculi.
Glucose-galactose intol.	N	+	N	<5	+	N	N	+	N	—
Cystic fibrosis	N	N	N	6.5–7.5	N	+	±	+	N	Pulmonary disease
Pancreatic insufficiency	N	N	N	6.5–7.5	±	+	±	+	N	Cyclic neutropenia.
Giardiasis	N	+	N	6.5–7.5	N	+	±	N	+	Immune deficiency.
Blind loop syndrome	+	+	+	<5	N	+	+	N	+	—
A-beta lipoproteinemia	N	N	N	6.5–7.5	N	+	N	+	N	Acanthocytosis retinitis pigmentosis
Liver failure	N	N	N	6.5–7.5	N	N	+	N	+	—
Ileal resection	N	N	N	6.5–7.5	N	+	+	N	+	—
Proteolytic enzyme deficiency	+	N	+	6.5–7.5	–	–	+	+	+	Hypoproteinemia.
Intestinal lymphangectasis	N	N	+	6:5–7.5	N	+	+	–	–	Chylous ascities— hypoproteinemia.
Protein intolerance	+	N	+	6.5–7.5	N	N	++	±	±	Abdominal pain— eosinophilia.
Cows milk protein intol.	+	+	+ bloody	<5	+	+	+	N	+	Edema hypoproteinemia.
Gluten-sensitive enteropathy	N	+	+	6.5–7.5	+	+	+	+	+	Villous dystrophy.
Familial protein intol.	N	+	N	6.5–7.5	±	+	+	+	N	Hepatosplenomegally, rickets hyperammonia.
Ulcerative colitis	N	N	+	6.5–7.5	±	+	N	N	+	Skin, joint, and liver disease.

Table 15-3. Causes of Chronic Diarrhea: Features *(Continued)*

Disease	Vomit	Stool H₂O	Mucus	pH	Red sub	Fat	Abd. dist.	Hered-itary	Acquired	Other
Regional enteritis	N	N	Bloody	6.5–7.5	±	+	N	N	+	Fever, joints erythema nodosum
Ileal disease	N	±	+	6.5–7.5	±	+	N	N	+	B₁₂ deficiency.
Tumors catecholamines	N	±	N	6.5–7.5	+	+	+	N	+	Urinary VMA, cystathionine.
Antibody deficiency	N	±	N	6.5–7.5	+	+	+	+	±	Recurrent infections.
Hirschsprungs	N	±	N	6.5–7.5	−	−	+	N	+	Delayed passage of first stool.
Congenital chloride diarrhea	N	+	N	<5	N	N	−	±	−	Metabolic alkalosis.
Irritable colon	N	+	N	6.5–7.5	N	N	N	±	±	Pos. family history, self-limited. Ends 3–4 years.

N = Negative   + = Positive

Note: All of these disorders are associated with failure to thrive. The relationship of the etiology to the age of the patient is seen in Table 15-4.

Mild diarrhea is treated effectively by a modified fast that includes sweetened tea or apple juice offered only at the usual feeding times. This is continued for 12 to 24 hours depending on the response. The basic plan is to put the intestinal tract at rest. If this stops the diarrhea, the patient is gradually titrated back to a normal diet after 12 hours.

Moderate diarrhea differs from mild by having some degree of dehydration. Oral therapy may be successful, but close observation is required to be sure that intravenous fluids are not required to correct the dehy-

Table 15-4. Severity of Diarrhea Based on Weight Loss

Onset	Mild	Moderate	Severe
Acute*	3%	3–6%	> 6%
Chronic†	10%	10–20%	>20%

* Weight loss/24 hrs.
† Weight loss/2 wks.

Table 15-5. Treatment of Nonspecific Diarrhea

Therapy	Mild (hours)	Moderate (hours)	Severe (hours)
Correction of dehydration and acidosis with I. V. therapy	0	0–24	24–48 hrs
Trial of oral clear liquids	12–24	12–24	24 hrs
¼ strength milk (full liquids for older children)	0	0–12	24 hrs
½ strength milk (soft diet for older children)	12–24	12–24	24 hrs
Full strength milk (full diet for older children)	As desired		

Note: If diarrhea recurs, return to preceding step or step 2 and advance more slowly.

dration. Vomiting is frequently associated with more severe diarrheal conditions. This would preclude the use of oral fluids in the initial management.

Severe diarrhea merits hospitalization and intravenous fluid therapy. Then the patient should be maintained on appropriate intravenous fluids for 24 hours after the diarrhea stops while receiving no oral feedings.

Table 15-6. Etiologies of Treatment Failure

Problem	Mechanism	Solution
Damaged brush border membrane plus increased unabsorbed osmotically active substance	Damaged intestinal brush border membrane, increased intraluminal unabsorbed osmotically active substance	Dilute formula
Acquired lactase deficiency	Increased intraluminal unabsorbed osmotically active substance	Change from formula containing lactose to one with a different sugar
Steatorrhea	Intestinal microorganisms, diarrhea due to hydroxy-fatty acids, hypersecretory state	Use formula with medium chain triglycerides
Cow's milk protein intolerance	Unknown mechanisms	Change to milk that uses soy protein
Chronic idiopathic diarrhea	Unknown mechanisms	Hyperalimentation

After 24 hours, clear liquids should be offered by the method described above and the intravenous fluids discontinued when the oral feedings seem to be tolerated (Table 15-5).

The above routine is generally successful. However, diarrhea may again commence with realimentation. If this is so, possible mechanisms and solutions are suggested in Table 15-6.

BIBLIOGRAPHY

Nelson, J. D., and Haltalin, K. C.: Accuracy of diagnosis of bacterial diarrheal disease by clinical features. J. Pediatr., 78:519–522, 1971.

A discussion of clinical features useful for differentiating bacterial from nonbacterial diarrhea.

Poley, R. J.: Chronic diarrhea in infants and children: Part I. South. Med. I., 66:1035-1050, 1973.
———: Chronic diarrhea in infants and children: Part II. South. Med. J., 66:1133-1142, 1973.

A review of the diseases responsible for most chronic diarrheal syndromes with special emphasis on pathophysiology.

16

Dehydration and Fluid Replacement

John Curran, M.D.

Few entities in clinical pediatrics demand greater attention to detail than the management of infants with dehydration. Application of principles of rational fluid management tempered with a knowledge of fluid and electrolyte depletion states enable the physician to evaluate logically, investigate, and assemble a mode of therapy tailored to the individul patient. No single "cook book" approach to the dehydrated patient exists; however, sufficient latitude exists because of intrinsic lung, renal, and endocrine homeostatic mechanisms that mean values may be given as empiric guides to therapy.

Dehydration may perhaps be defined best as a net loss of body water and salts engendered by a pathologic or environmental state. Dehydration is never a primary disorder in itself. Salt loss is not only restricted to the major cations (sodium and potassium) but includes other cations such as calcium and magnesium in addition to anions such as chloride. Since most disease states leading to dehydration as a primary or secondary disorder produce their effect first on extracellular water and then upon intracellular fluid, greatest emphasis must be placed on three elements of dehydration—water, sodium, and potassium.

Pathologic states which frequently result in dehydration are listed in Table 16-1 along with the relative contribution of the three basic mechanisms.

EFFECTS AND TYPES OF DEHYDRATION

The effects of dehydration upon the patient and correlation with his chemical state can perhaps be appreciated by a consideration of the disturbances in the so-called internal environment. Basically, the disturbances are of five types which are listed in Table 16-2; the primary contribution is from the first two.

194

Table 16-1. Pathologic States Producing Dehydration

Disorder	Pathogenetic Mechanisms		
	↑ *Loss H₂O*	↑ *Loss salts*	↓ *Intake*
Diarrhea	+	+	±
Anorexia	0	0	+
Vomiting	+	+	+
Fever	+	+	±
Hyperventilation	+	0	0
High solute intake	+	±	±
Diabetes mellitus	+	+	±
Diabetes insipidus	+	+	− ↑
Adrenocortical insufficiency	±	+	±
Burns	+	+	+
Iatrogenica Pediatrica			
Hyperosmolal contrast media	+	+	±
Hypertonic bicarbonate, mannitol	+	±	0
Emetics	+	+	0
Induced hyperglycemia	+	+	±
Radiant warmers in neonate	+	0	±
Prematurity	+	0	+
Diuretic over usage	+	+	±

+ — positive effect
± — variable
0 — no definite effect

Table 16-2. Disturbances in Dehydration

1. Δ Volume (circulatory blood volume)→role in perfusion.

2. Δ Body fluid osmolality→profound effect on central nervous system, cellular integrity, and function.

3. ↑ (H+)→systemic acidemia and systemic effects.

4. Loss of intracellular ions—(K⁺), (Mg⁺⁺)→effect on neuromuscular contractility.

5. Δ Extracellular fluid ions ⇌ skeletal pool (predominantly Ca⁺⁺).

The major disturbances that require therapeutic assistance from the clinical practitioner are restricted to changes of volume and osmolality. Given correction of these disturbances, body homeostatic mechanisms will usually readjust the latter three except in pathologic states with lung, renal, or endocrine disease. Clinically, the disturbances in osmolality have given rise to classic types of dehydration disorders (Table 16-3).

Table 16-3. Clinical Class of Dehydration

Disorder	Ratio salt/water (relative to plasma)	Osmolality	Serum (Na+)
1. Isotonic	Loss salt/water - equal	Normal	Normal
2. Hypotonic	Loss salt>water	↓	<130 mEq/L
3. Hypertonic	Loss water>salt	↑	>145 mEq/L

Fundamental to understanding the occurrence of dehydration states is the principle that dehydration will only occur if intake (fluid + electrolyte) < output + insensible losses, i.e.:

Diarrhea
Anorexia
Vomiting
}
intake = output + insensible loss→normal state of hydration

intake < output + insensible loss→dehydration

intake > output + insensible loss→overhydration

Assessment of dehydration per se requires scrupulous attention to details of the antecedent history, physical findings, and objective measurements. Expertise is manifest by prompt recognition of the primary disorder causing dehydration, the magnitude, and judgment as to the type of dehydration from details of the history and physical examination. In this way prompt institution of an appropriate fluid and electrolyte therapy may be begun in the emergency room environment without undue dependence upon laboratory studies and results.

Basically, the three types of dehydration may be divided into two major groups which can be differentiated clinically prior to knowing electrolytes or osmolality values. Specific details are enumerated in Table 16-4.

Table 16-4 can be summarized by emphasizing that the signs of hypertonic dehydration are different from those of hypotonic or isotonic dehydration because of the relative preservation of circulating blood volume in the presence of hyperosmolarity. Thus, the extracellular and intracellular fluids are depleted of water via osmotic equilibria to support the plasma volume; this provides perfusion and avoids many of the signs

Table 16-4. Comparison of Clinical Findings

Symptoms & signs	Hypotonic (hypoosmolar)	Isotonic (isoosmolar)	Hypertonic (hyperosmolar)
History			
Fever	±	±	+ +
↓ intake	+	+	+
↓ urine output	+	+	+
Weight loss	+	+	+
Improper formula	Too dilute	−	Salt added or too little water
Physical examination			
Pulse*	↑	↑	± ↑ to normal
Respiration (if acidemic)	↑	↑	↑
Blood pressure*	↓ ↓	↓	Normal to ↓ late
Neurologic status*	Coma, lethargic	Lethargic	Irritable, restless
Seizures	May occur rarely	Uncommon	Usually occur late
Stiff neck	−	−	Common
Fontanelle	Sunken, soft	Sunken, soft	Not sunken till late
Skin*			
Color	Pallor	Pallor	May be flushed
Temperature	Cold	Cold	May be warm
Turgor	Creases, tenting	Tenting	"Doughy"
Mucous membranes	Slightly moist	Dry	Parched

+ = Present	↑ = Increased
± = Variable	↓ = Decreased

*Indicates major differential points between hyperosmolar dehydration and others

associated with the hypotension seen in the other types of dehydration. Nevertheless, it must be emphasized that children with hypertonic dehydration will rapidly pass into hypovolemic shock when body compensatory mechanisms have been exhausted.

With hypernatremia (hyperosmolar syndrome), circulation is not affected until late in the disease. Often there are neurologic symptoms, and hypocalcemic tetany can occur frequently with treatment. Renal tubular necrosis also may occur. If sodium is greater than 150 mEq/L. in

50 per cent of patients there may be hyperglycemia. Most patients have moderately severe metabolic acidosis if enteric disease is present. Metabolic acidemia (release of H+ from dessicated cells) is frequent.

The clinical estimation of the magnitude of dehydration can, of course, be easily assessed if a recent weight of the patient is known:

$$\frac{\text{Previous } \textit{recent} \text{ weight} - \text{Present weight}}{\text{Previous weight}} \times 100 = \% \text{ Dehydration}$$

Rarely is there such objective evidence so one must rely on the following clinical approximations for determining the severity of *acute* dehydration:

1. Mild—Early minimal signs (? dehydration): positive history, intake less than output and insensible loss and a less than 5 per cent decrease in body weight.

2. Moderate—Early circulatory impairment: classic signs (See Table 16-4) as well as a 10 per cent decrease in body weight.

3. Severe—Circulatory collapse: moribund and a 10–15 per cent decrease in body weight.

TREATMENT

Successful therapy of dehydration mandates consideration of the etiologic process(es) causing dehydration as outlined in Table 16-1. Dehydration is a secondary process preceded by one or more pathologic states. Correction of dehydration requires thorough understanding of normal daily fluid, electrolyte, and glucose requirements; estimation of deficits; and estimation of continuing losses. This can be exemplified by the therapeutic equation:

Fluid + electrolyte required =
maintenance + ongoing losses + replacement

Calculation of fluid requirements can be done in a number of different ways: per kilogram (varies with weight), per meter^2 (surface area), and by water requirements for each 100 calories metabolized. Each method has its advantages and disadvantages but the methods utilizing surface area and weight are more simple (Table 16-5).

Deficits of water and electrolytes may be estimated from Tables 16-6 and 16-7. In addition, the assessment of ongoing losses may necessitate consideration of the electrolyte content of various body fluids.

Therapeutic management of dehydration demands attention to three phases of correction: emergency, repletion, and recovery. Figure 16-1 is

Table 16-5. Maintenance Requirements*

Wt. in kg.	S.A. (m)²	H₂O(ml) Per kg	Per m²	Na⁺(mEq) Per kg	Per m²	K⁺(mEq) Per kg	Per m²	Glucose (g) Per kg	Per m²
3	0.20	100	1500	3	60	2	50	6–10	150
5	0.27	90	"	3	"	2	"	6–10	"
10	0.45	75	"	3	"	2	"	6–10	"
15	0.64	65	"	—	"	—	"	—	"
30	1.10	55	"	—	"	—	"	—	"
50	1.50	45	"	—	"	—	"	—	"
70	1.73	40	"	—	"	—	"	—	"

*Surface area may be approximated if a nomogram is not available by the equation S.A. (m)² = 0.1 + $\frac{\text{wt. in lbs.}}{60}$ for children.

an example of the approach to the dehydrated patient in the emergency phase.

Reassessment and Repletion

Hypernatremic Dehydration. After urine output has been re-established for 2 to 4 hours, start K⁺, 40 mEq/L. To determine the total fluid loss, calculate: deficit + ongoing loss + 2–3 days maintenance. Plan the total correction in 48–72 hours (if Na⁺>160 mEq/L correct over 72 hours or more) and administer fluids evenly throughout the entire 48–72 hours. These fluids should consist of Na⁺ 40–60 mEq/L, one-fourth as $NaHCO_3$,

Table 16-6. Deficits of Water and Electrolytes: Moderate Dehydration

Disorder	H₂O (ml.)	Per kg. body weight Na⁺ (mEq)	K⁺ (mEq)	Cl⁻ (mEq)
Fasting and thirsting	100–120	5– 7	1– 2	4– 6
Diarrhea Isotonic	100–120	8–10	8–10	8–10
Hypotonic	100–120	10–12	8–10	10–12
Hypertonic	100–120	2– 4	0– 4	−2 to −6
Pyloric stenosis	100–120	8–10	10–12	10–12
Diabetic acidosis	100–120	8–10	5– 7	6– 8

Table 16-7. Electrolyte Content of Body Fluids

Source	Na+ (mEq/L)	K+ (mEq/L)	Cl⁻ (mEq/L)
Gastric juice	20– 80	5–20	100–150
Pancreatic	120–140	5–15	90–120
Small intestine	100–140	5–15	90–130
Bile	120–140	5–15	80–120
Ileostomy	45–135	3–15	20–115
Diarrhea	10– 90	10–80	10–110
Sweat Normal	10– 30	3–10	10– 35
Cystic fibrosis	50–130	5–25	50–110
Burns	140	5	110

three-fourths as NaCl. Check calcium and if it has decreased, you may use 10% calcium gluconate, 1 ml./kg., slowly while the heart is monitored.

Isonatremic Dehydration. After the initial re-establishment of perfusion, give one-half the first day's fluid + electrolyte within 8 hours. The total should equal two times the maintenance for the first day as D5¼NSS, one-fourth as $NaHCO_3$ if acidosis is present. Potassium should be added only after voiding; give one and one-half to two times maintenance and do not exceed 40 mEq/L.

On the second day, give one and one-half times the maintenance volume of fluid. Usually this is given as D5¼NSS (40 mEq Na+/L). Follow closely the electrolytes, urine output, and urine-specific gravity.

Plan on total rehydration within 2 to 3 days. Usually oral realimentation can begin on the second day. Deduct 50 per cent oral intake from the day's I.V. orders if the fluids are given combined I.V. and P.O.

Hyponatremic Dehydration. After the initial stabilization of perfusion, continue with two times the maintenance volume, one-half in the first 8 hours of D5 ⅓–½NSS (Deduct the volume of plasma expander used from the total day's fluids.) Add K+, one and one-half to two times the maintenance volume. This should be added to fluids after voiding has been established. Follow the parameters listed under isonatremic dehydration so that total hydration will be established over 2 to 3 days. If seizures occur early in the disorder, use 3 per cent NaCl, 1 ml./min. intravenously up to a maximum of 12 ml./kg., until seizures stop.

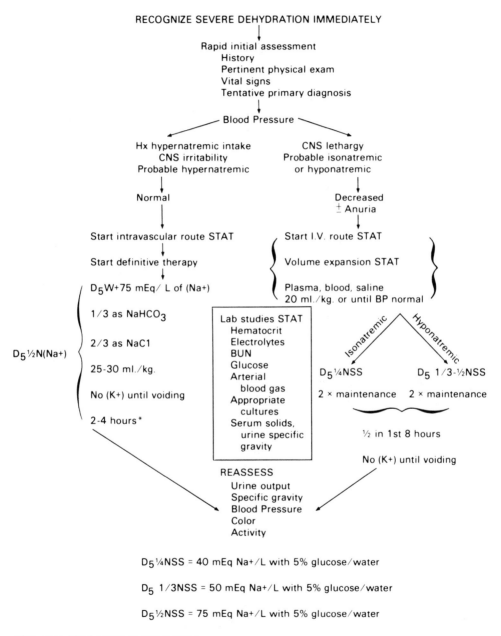

RECOGNIZE SEVERE DEHYDRATION IMMEDIATELY

Rapid initial assessment
History
Pertinent physical exam
Vital signs
Tentative primary diagnosis

Blood Pressure

Hx hypernatremic intake
CNS irritability
Probable hypernatremic

CNS lethargy
Probable isonatremic
or hyponatremic

Normal

Decreased
± Anuria

Start intravascular route STAT

Start definitive therapy

D_5W+75 mEq/ L of (Na+)

D_5 ½N(Na+)

1/3 as $NaHCO_3$

2/3 as NaC1

25-30 ml./kg.

No (K+) until voiding

2-4 hours*

Start I.V. route STAT

Volume expansion STAT

Plasma, blood, saline
20 ml./kg. or until BP normal

Lab studies STAT
Hematocrit
Electrolytes
BUN
Glucose
Arterial
blood gas
Appropriate
cultures
Serum solids,
urine specific
gravity

Isonatremic

Hyponatremic

D_5¼NSS

2 × maintenance

D_5 1/3-½NSS

2 × maintenance

½ in 1st 8 hours

No (K+) until voiding

REASSESS
Urine output
Specific gravity
Blood Pressure
Color
Activity

D_5¼NSS = 40 mEq Na+/L with 5% glucose/water

D_5 1/3NSS = 50 mEq Na+/L with 5% glucose/water

D_5½NSS = 75 mEq Na+/L with 5% glucose/water

*See page 199 for subsequent therapy.

Fig. 16-1. An approach to the dehydrated patient in the emergency phase.

Fluid and Electrolyte Calculation

As an example take the case of a hypotensive, 10 kg. infant with moderate to severe isonatremic dehydration:

Maintenance fluid/day $= 0.45^2 \times 1500$ ml./m^2 $= 675$ ml.
Deficit 10% depleted $= 1000$ ml., repair 2 days
Deficit Na$^+$ 80 mEq (10 kg $\times$ 8 mEq/kg.)
　　　　K$^+$ 80 mEq (10 kg $\times$ 8 mEq/kg.)
Maintenance Na$^+$ $= 27$ $(0.45 \times 60$ mEq/m$^2)$
　　　　　　K$^+$ $= 23$ $(0.45 \times 50$ mEq/m$^2)$
Plasma to expand 20 ml./kg. $\times$ 10 kg. $=$ 200 ml.
First day fluid total 675 + 500 ml.　　$= 1175$ ml.
Less 200 ml. plasma 　　　　　　　　　$\underline{-200}$
　　　　　　　　　　　　　　　　　　　975 ml.

Give one-half of this solution in the first 8 hours; this equals 61 ml./hr. $\times$ 8 hours for a total of 488 ml. The second half is administered during the next 16 hours. This equals 31 (30.5) ml./hr. $\times$ 16 hours for a total of 488 ml. The total for the 24 hours is 1176 ml.

The electrolyte content is determined by:

Maintenance Na$^+$　　$= 27$ mEq
$+$ ½ deficit Na$^+$　　$= \underline{40}$ mEq
　　　　　　　　　　67 mEq/1176 ml. $= 57$ mEq Na/L
Give ¼ as NaHCO$_3$ 　　　　　　　$= 14$ mEq NaHCO$_3$
　　　　　　　　　　　　　　　　43 mEq NaCl

Maintenance K$^+$ 　　　23 mEq
$+$ ½ deficit K$^+$ 　　　$\underline{40}$ mEq
　　　　　　　　　63 mEq/1176 ml. $= 53$ mEq K$^+$/L

But K$^+$ *cannot* exceed 40 mEq/L

Thus, the I.V. orders will read: 1000 ml. D$_5$W $+$ 14 mEq NaHCO$_3$ $+$ 43 mEq NaCl $+$ 40 mEq KCl to run at 61 ml./hr. $\times$ 8 hours, then 31 ml./hr. $\times$ 16 hours.

Much of the above cumbersome calculation can be avoided by simply figuring two times the maintenance fluid $+$ electrolyte as D$_5$¼NSS (40 mEq/L) during the first 24 hours in isonatremic dehydration. Thus the calculation becomes:

0.45 m^2 $\times$ 1500 ml./m^2　　$=$　675 ml.
2 $\times$ maintenance　　　　　$= 1350$ ml.
Less　　　　　　　　　　　　$\underline{-200}$ ml. plasma
　　　　　　　　　　　　　　1150 ml.

One-half in first 8 hours $= \dfrac{575 \text{ ml.}}{8 \text{ hours}} = 72$ ml./hr. $\times$ 8 hours

Second 16 hours $= \dfrac{575 \text{ ml.}}{16 \text{ hours}} = 36$ ml./hr. $\times$ 16 hours

Thus, the I.V. fluid is: 1000 ml. D_5W + 10 mEq $NaHCO_3$ + 30 mEq NaCl + 34 mEq KCl. The infusion rates are as above.

Principles to Remember

Certain principles should be followed if dehydration is to be treated successfully:

1. Treat hypotension aggressively.

2. Never give solute-free fluid.

3. Never give fluids rapidly to a patient with hypernatremic dehydration unless he is hypotensive.

4. Fluid and electrolyte administration to the dehydrated patient serves to restore body homeostatic mechanisms. Calculations are necessarily imprecise and follow more the "art" than the "science" of medicine.

5. Never give potassium before the patient voids, as serious arrythmia may result.

6. Never forget to reassess the patient frequently with a physical examination hourly or more frequently if need be.

7. Never base all treatment solely upon laboratory results but rather correlate them with clinical assessment of the patient.

There are a number of special fluid and electrolyte problems which do not fall into the framework previously outlined. These will be discussed. For brevity, they are presented in outline form.

A. Newborn infants (maintenance)

1. Premature infant > 1500 g.

a. Maintenance fluid: 90–100 ml./kg./day

Usually sodium and potassium not needed first day, 2nd and 3rd days add 20 mEq Na^+/L, 4th day and thereafter 40 mEq/L.

Begin maintenance K^+ (2 mEq/kg./day) 2nd day and thereafter.

b. Fluid may be D_5W or $D_{10}W$. If $D_{10}W$ is used, monitor for glycosuria or hyperglycemia, particularly in sick infants.

c. Increase fluids 1 ml./kg./hr. for infants under radiant heaters.

d. In infants receiving phototherapy and weighing > 1500 g. add 1.4 ml./kg./hr.

2. Premature infants < 1500 g.

a. Maintenance fluid—start with 100 ml./kg./day. Salt administration as previously noted above, but may need major increase if critical.

b. Always start D_5W, monitor as above and increase caloric content stepwise to $D_{10}W$ dextrose as per blood sugars and absence of glycosuria.

c. Infants under radiant warmers:

$$\left.\begin{array}{l} <1000 \text{ g. add up to } 50\% \\ 1000–1500 \text{ g. add } 25\% \end{array}\right\} \text{ maintenance fluid}$$

d. Phototherapy

<1500 g. add 1–2 ml./kg./hr.

  e. Attempt to establish urine flow ~ 2ml./kg./hr., Urine S.G. ~
   1.005
 3. Term infants
  a. Fluid D_5W or $D_{10}W$ with salts as above
  b. 70 ml./kg.   Day #1
   80 ml./kg.   Day #2
   90 ml./kg.   Day #3
   100 ml./kg.   Day #4

B. Dehydrated newborns—treat as previously outlined
C. Vomiting
 1. Volume and composition as previously outlined
 2. Replace volume of vomitus or nasogastric drainage as equivalent
  to physiologic saline as per Table 16-7.
D. Heat exhaustion
 1. Give fluids as D_5W glucose with 50–80 mEq Na^+/L. Volume as
  per dehydration.
E. Anuria
 1. Give 5%–10% DW at 400 ml./m² plus urinary losses.
 2. May be necessary to give fluid challenge prior to confirmation of
  diagnosis of anuria.
 3. Watch for hyperkalemia or hyponatremia. Appropriate therapy if
  present.
F. Inappropriate secretion of antidiuretic hormone—postoperative, with
 CNS disease, or trauma
 1. Establish diagnosis—hypo-osmolality with high urinary osmolality
  or specific gravity. Edema and overhydration may be present clinically.
 2. Treat with fluid restriction.
G. Cardiac disease with failure
 1. Clinical assessment (serial) with pharmacologic therapy and fluid
  restriction to less than maintenance until stabilized.
H. Fever: add 10% volume for each degree temperature elevation >101°.

SUMMARY

 The preceding presentation has demonstrated multiple facets of fluid
balance in disease states. Intrinsic to the outlined therapy is the maintenance of an adequate intravascular fluid administration route for acute
management of fluid and electrolyte deviations. One must never forget
that an intravenous route places the patient in potential jeopardy should
there be errors in medications, volumes, compositions, or rates of administration. Several axioms of intravenous maintenance must always be
remembered:

1. Always establish a *secure* intravascular route in hypotensive patients.

2. Always interpose a pediatric administration set between a large volume of fluid and the patient to prevent accidental, rapid administration of large volumes.

3. Always limit the maximum amount of fluid directly connected to a patient to an 8-hour supply.

4. Always write I.V. orders clearly, legibly, and include all desired components.

5. Number I.V.s consecutively.

6. Treat I.V. sites as areas of potential infection and prepare accordingly before venipuncture; sterile technique should be maintained.

7. Rotate I.V. sites to minimize phlebitis.

8. Scalp needles are preferred to intravascular catheters since there is less risk of infection.

9. Never mix sodium bicarbonate and calcium in I.V. fluid.

10. Check for drug incompatibilities before mixing in infusate.

These recommendations should be regarded merely as guidelines. The repeated clinical assessment of the individual patient may dictate deviation from these suggestions.

BIBLIOGRAPHY

Banister, A., and Hatcher, G. W.: Renal tubular and papillary necrosis after dehydration in infancy. Arch. Dis. Child., *48*:36-40, 1973.

> Describes renal complications of dehydration with gastroenteritis—case reports and discussion.

Barness, L. A., and Young, L. N.: A simplified view of fluid therapy. Pediatr. Clin. North Am., *11*:1091-1103, 1964.

> Older but excellent brief overview of fluid therapy.

Cooke, R. E.: Parenteral fluid therapy. *In* Nelson, W. E. (ed.): Textbook of Pediatrics. Philadelphia, W. B. Saunders, 1969; pp. 217-233.

> Excellent overview of dehydration, valuable tables.

Cornfield, D.: Post acidotic complications of diarrhea. Pediatr. Clin. North Am., *11*:963-969, 1964.

> Discusses treatment of post acidotic tetany.

Engelke, S. C., Shah, B. L., Vasan, U., and Raye, J. R.: Sodium balance in very low birth weight infants. Pediatr. Res., *11*:549 (Abst.), 1977.

> Unusually large sodium requirements for critically ill neonates are described.

Fanaroff, A. A., Wald, M., Gruber, H. S., and Klaud, M. H.: Insensible water loss in low birth weight infants. Pediatrics, *50*:236-245, 1972.

Insensible water loss in newborn infants.

Finberg, L.: Dehydration in infants and children. N. Engl. J. Med., *276*:458-460, 1967.

General discussion of dehydration.

Finberg, L.: Hypernatremic (hypertonic) dehydration in infants. N. Engl. J. Med., *289*:196-198, 1973.

Review of hypernatremic dehydration.

Kingston, N. E.: Biochemical disturbances in breast-fed infants with gastroenteritis and dehydration. J. Pediatr., *82*:1073-1081, 1973.

Large series studying special problems of dehydration in breast-fed infants.

Rosenfeld, W., de Romana, G. L., Kleinman, Q., and Finberg, L.: Improving the clinical management of hypernatremic dehydration. Clin. Pediatr., *16*:411-417, 1977.

Observations retrospectively from management of 67 infants.

Wu, P. Y. K., and Hodgman, J. E.: Insensible water loss in preterm infants. Pediatrics, *54*:704-712, 1974.

Recent evidence for increased water losses in very low birth weight infants associated with devices for modern intensive care.

17

Abnormalities of Urine

Lewis A. Barness, M.D.

The routine urinalysis is a test ordered for many conditions and is part of the complete pediatric physical examination. When abnormal findings in the urine are approached systematically, the routine urinalysis is a most useful aid in differential diagnosis.

Early in their careers students should develop a standard method of examining urine. Some prefer no centrifugation while others prefer spun urines. The advantage of learning to look at unspun urine is that the variance of centrifugation need not affect one's standard.

Elements of a Routine Urinalysis

Specific gravity
Protein
pH
Sugar-reducing substance
Acetone
Red cells (test for blood optional)
White cells
Casts
Ferric chloride
Color
Odor

ELEMENTS OF A ROUTINE URINALYSIS

Specific Gravity

Specific gravity in children ranges normally between 1.000 and 1.036 on random specimens, so a specific gravity in an isolated specimen is never abnormal. If the specific gravity is below 1.010 on several specimens, suspect that the child is deficient in a concentrating mechanism.

Among the causes of low specific gravity (hyposthenuria) are:

1. Low specific gravity is normal for infants less than 4 months of age.

2. Dilutional states e.g., water intoxication and psychological polydipsia.

3. Sickle-cell disease and sickle-cell trait. Usually the specific gravity in these cases may approach 1.015. The cause is uncertain, but it may be an allelic condition.

4. Diabetes insipidus—lack of antidiuretic hormone (ADH). This may signify a brain tumor or injury near the hypothalamus.

5. Renal tubular disease. This is a condition in which the tubules cannot reabsorb water (also called renal diabetes insipidus). Included are renal tubular acidosis, and certain inborn errors of metabolism, such as Detoni-Fanconi Syndrome.

6. Inappropriate secretion of ADH. This is common in brain injury or meningitis. Usually the patient does not excrete water normally, in spite of plasma dilution, and thus develops water intoxication. Occasionally, the opposite occurs. In spite of hypertonicity of serum, the patient excretes a dilute urine, and remains dehydrated.

7. Diarrhea in infants. This is perhaps a failure of secretion of ADH. In spite of dehydration, the patient excretes dilute urine.

If it is believed that one of the forms of diabetes insipidus exists, an evaluation of serum and urine osmolality after small doses of ADH usually indicates whether the lesion is in the hypothalamus (serum will become dilute and urine more concentrated), or is psychogenic or renal (no effect after ADH injection). Treatment of this deficiency includes injecting or sniffing ADH, regular doses of oral chlorpropamide or low protein diet. Psychogenic diabetes insipidus can usually be treated by counseling. Occasionally, renal diabetes insipidus, such as that which occurs in patients with pyelonephritis or renal tubular acidosis, can be improved with treatment of the underlying disease.

pH of the Urine

This varies normally from about 4.5 to 7.5, so that any isolated urinary pH is normal. Urine pH assumes significance in several clinical situations, the most important of which is obtaining a pH of 6.5 or higher when the pH of the blood is less than 7.2. This occurs when the kidney is unable to conserve base, renal tubular acidosis. The disease may be in the proximal or distal renal tubule. Hyperchloremia is a common accompaniment, particularly in distal tubular disease. An attempt should be made to return blood pH to normal with base.

The proximal tubule is concerned with the reabsorption of isotonic saline, glucose, amino acids, and phosphorus. Both proximal and distal tubules regulate pH by exchanging hydrogen ion for sodium in the tubule lumen, and by converting secreted ammonia to ammonium. It is helpful to know the distinctions between proximal and distal (see Table 17-1).

Table 17-1. Proximal and Distal Renal Tubular Acidosis

	Proximal	Distal
Presenting complaint	Failure to thrive Hyperchloremic acidosis Vomiting, constipation, dehydration	
Causes	Idiopathic Cystinosis Lowe's syndrome Wilson's disease Galactosemia Fructose intolerance Tyrosinemia Lightwood syndrome Poisons	Idiopathic Malnutrition Hyperparathyroidism Vitamin D intoxication Fabry's disease Hyperthyroidism Renal tubular necrosis Medullary sponge kidney Poisons
Inheritance of idiopathic	Mainly males	Autosomal dominant
Age of onset	0–2 years	2 years +
Bicarbonate requirement	>6 mEq/kg/day	<2 mEq/kg/day
Prognosis of idiopathic	Reversible	Permanent

Another clinically important use of urinary pH determination occurs in those children, particularly newborn or young infants, whose urinary pH persists at approximately 4.5 with a serum pH less than 7.2. It is normal for infants fed human milk or milk with less than 1.5 g. protein/dl. to have a urine pH of 6.5 or higher. If particularly low pH is found, it may be considered that the child has a metabolic error.

Lactic acid is a normal metabolic product in the glycolytic pathway. It accumulates in exercise but may become excessive, especially in states of anoxemia, or with decreases in perfusion, especially in shock. Hyperosmotic states, such as diabetic ketoacidosis, also produce lactic acidemia. Attention should be directed to the cause; treatment of lactic acidemia with sodium bicarbonate may increase hyperosmolality and worsen the patient. Because CO_2 (as carbonic acid) rapidly traverses the cerebrospinal fluid while HCO_3 enters more slowly, addition of bicarbonate in the presence of lactic acidosis causes a rise in serum pH but a fall in CSF pH and may be responsible for central nervous system deterioration during such treatment.

Other causes of resistant acidosis include: methylmalonic acidemia, propionic acidemia, maple syrup urine disease, lactic-pyruvic acidemia, isovaleric acidemia and others.

Since all of these may be amenable to treatment, specific diagnosis should be reached rapidly by identifying the acids in the urine or serum. Some patients with methylmalonic acidemia respond to vitamin B_{12}, some with propionic acid to biotin, and some with maple syrup urine disease or branched-chain amino aciduria respond to dietary management. Other patients with lactic-pyruvic acidemia may respond to thiamin, while those with isovaleric acidemia may respond to dietary management. Acidosis of metabolic cause should be accompanied by acid urine.

Occasionally, the urine pH will be found to be over 7 and the blood pH over 7.4. This type of alkalosis occurs with potassium deficiency and may be present in adrenal diseases with too low and occasionally too high serum potassium. It also occurs in diarrheal states with potassium depletion.

Protein

Normally, less than 30 mg. of protein/dl. is found in human urine. A greater percentage suggests renal disease. All of the following must be considered:

Nephritis. (See Hematuria.) All types develop proteinuria and may produce the nephrotic syndrome.

Nephrosis and Nephrotic Syndrome. The child with nephrosis usually presents in the first 3 to 4 years of life with an insidious onset of edema. Proteinuria may be massive; serum lipids are elevated and serum protein is decreased. Patients with lipoid nephrosis ("Nil" disease) have similar symptoms, as well as those due to other causes. Blood pressure in children with lipoid nephrosis is usually normal or low, and urine rarely contains many red blood cells. Measurement indicates that the amount of lost protein is small and constant, the cause of which is unknown.

Pneumococcal peritonitis may occur when the child is edematous. Edema and proteinuria usually decrease following the administration of prednisone (2 mg./kg./day). The dose is reduced to alternate day therapy when proteinuria disappears, and is discontinued after the patient is normal for 6 months. Some children who are resistant to steroid therapy respond to the addition of antimetabolites, e.g., cyclophosphamide 0.1 mg./kg./day orally for 2 weeks then 0.2 mg./kg./day for 6 weeks. A biopsy should be obtained before using antimetabolites. Prognosis is generally good.

Some other causes of the nephrotic syndrome are listed below. The prognosis for these is related to the prognosis for the underlying disease. Proliferating glomerulonephritis, a disease with poor prognosis, gives a similar picture and is distinguished from lipoid nephrosis by renal biopsy.

Congenital nephrosis is apparently inherited as an autosomal recessive disease. Proteinuria and edema begin in the first few weeks of life. Treatment is ineffective.

Renal Vascular Occlusion. Children with sepsis or kidney trauma, and in particular, infants born of diabetic mothers may develop proteinuria and the nephrotic syndrome. Usually an enlarged kidney can be felt. Renal arteriograms, umbilical aortogram, or intravenous pyelogram aid in diagnosis. Some resolve spontaneously, though removal of the kidney may be necessary. Some children with sickle-cell disease may develop the nephrotic syndrome probably secondary to renal vascular occlusion.

Polycystic Disease and Renal Dysplastic Disease. Anatomical kidney abnormalities, including varying degrees of renal agenesis, may present only with proteinuria. As the child gets older, serum proteins decrease and the nephrotic syndrome ensues.

Collagen-Vascular Diseases. (See Hematuria.) Children with these diseases may present with proteinuria and the nephrotic syndrome, but the urinary abnormality first noted is usually hematuria.

Obstructive Uropathy. Children with obstructive uropathy and hydronephrosis may develop proteinuria and abdominal masses. Frequently, a renal tumor is suspected but pyelograms lead to correct diagnosis. When infection or the nephrotic syndrome supervene, the diagnosis is usually more obvious. Occasionally, pyelonephritis alone may present as the nephrotic syndrome.

Metabolic Disease. Some children with diabetes develop severe renal disease (Kimmelsteil-Wilson disease) with the nephrotic syndrome.

Poisons. Multiple poisons, particularly heavy metals, cause tubular damage, protein loss, and the development of the nephrotic syndrome.

Structural anomalies of the kidneys may present with no urinary abnormalities and are detected only when signs of renal failure ensue. When other causes of proteinuria are not discovered, structural anomalies should be sought. These include polycystic disease, hydronephrosis, renal tumors and obstructive disease.

Renal Tubular Disease. (See pH.) Proteinuria is found in renal tubular acidosis and renal tubular necrosis.

Toxins. A variety of toxins cause tubular disease and result in proteinuria. This occurs in ingestion of heavy metals, papillary necrosis, and metabolic diseases, especially aminoacidurias and galactosemia.

Orthostatic Disease. Some children, particularly those with lordosis, develop proteinuria on standing, presumably because of renal venous congestion. The child should be tested after lying down and after exercise. Many otherwise normal children excrete protein after vigorous exercise. These children do not have renal disease.

Fever. Infants and children with fever and no renal disease may have 2 to 3+ proteinuria.

Heart Failure. Proteinuria in children with heart failure is apparently also due to renal venous congestion.

Hematuria. In the presence of hematuria, protein from the red cells results in a positive test for protein. Centrifuging the urine and testing the supernate gives a truer test for protein. Proteinuria without hematuria is much more likely to be benign than that associated with hematuria. Even more striking for prognosis, hematuria alone is more frequently a reversible finding than hematuria associated with proteinuria.

Summary. If the proteinuria is of short duration, the child should be tested for orthostatic proteinuria and observed for the possibility of febrile proteinuria. If the patient's condition is inconsistent with these, the diagnosis should be pursued. Most commonly the patient has an acute post-streptococcal glomerulonephritis with other urinary and physical findings that are consistent with this diagnosis: edema, hypertension, elevated antistreptolysin titre, hematuria, red cell casts.

If these are not present, intravenous pyelogram and renal biopsy may be helpful. The type of protein in the urine may help in prognosis of some diseases, e.g., if the protein is mainly albumin, a relatively small molecule, the tubular damage is generally less than that which produces globulinuria. Tests for type of protein require electrophoresis.

Reducing Substance

In pediatrics, any reducing substance in the urine is important. The testing papers containing glucose oxidase identify only glucose. Therefore, if a paper is used to determine pH, protein, acetone, sugar, and blood, the urine must be tested at least once to measure for reducing substances with clinitest or similar agents.

Glucose is the most common reducing substance. Excessive glucose ingestion may cause elevated blood sugar. When glucosuria is present, blood sugar should be determined. Glucosuria is found in the following conditions:

Diabetes Mellitus. Generally, a glucose tolerance test should be abnormal before making this diagnosis.

Poisons, Particularly Heavy Metals. History, specific tests for heavy metals and other urinary abnormalities should be sought. Glucosuria due to metal poisoning, like proteinuria, is due to tubular damage. Some poisons have specific antidotes; for example, copper can be chelated with penicillamine or lead with EDTA. Other poisonings can be reversed by removing the poison.

Increased Intracranial Pressure. The mechanism by which increased intracranial pressure causes glycosuria is poorly understood. It is usually associated with hyperglycemia.

Adrenal Cortical Excess, Cushings Syndrome. Cortisol is gluconeogenic and causes hyperglycemia.

Low Renal Threshhold. Usually renal tubules can reabsorb sugar when the blood sugar does not exceed 180-200 mg./dl. For unknown causes, in some children, maximal tubular reabsorption of glucose is decreased and glucosuria occurs at lower levels of blood sugar. Such children are usually normal otherwise, though some may fail to thrive due to caloric loss.

Renal Tubular Disease, Fanconi Syndrome. Any renal tubular disease may cause glycosuria. In the autosomal recessive disease cystinosis (Fanconi syndrome), cystine crystals are stored in the lysosomes of all tissues; in addition to glycosuria, infants develop polyuria, aminoaciduria, rickets, and renal tubular acidosis. The condition presents in adolescents as a milder disease and in adults with few symptoms. Cystine crystals appear in the corneas.

Reducing substances other than glucose include the following: galactose, which may be the first sign of galactosemia. The presence of lactose usually is due to excessive ingestion. The presence of pentose occurs as a recessively inherited condition with no known disease. The presence of ascorbic acid is due to excessive ingestion. Reducing amino acids such as in alcaptonuria may be present. Fructose in the urine may occur in children with fructose intolerance but usually this is due to excessive ingestion.

Any time reducing substances are found they must be identified and quantitated. Diabetes mellitus, of all the causes, must be considered first.

Ketonuria

Ketonuria is easily tested with nitroprusside-containing papers. This condition occurs whenever a considerable proportion of the child's energy needs are obtained from fat rather than from sugar. Likely causes of ketonuria are: diabetes with insulinopenia, persistent vomiting, starvation, reducing diet, heavy exercise, fever, lead poisoning, glycogen-storage disease, and hyperinsulinism with hypoglycemia. Sometimes in the very young, any of these causes may be present without ketonuria. The mechanism of the lack of ketonuria is obscure.

Aspirin poisoning may produce vomiting, dehydration and ketonuria. In addition, the breakdown products of salicylates may alter the color of the nitroprusside. If so, the urine may be boiled first, removing the acetone. It is better to test for salicylates with ferric chloride.

Hematuria

Normally 0–1 red cells may be present in a high power field. The presence of more than one red cell requires investigation for:

Acute Post-Streptococcal Glomerulonephritis. About 7–14 days after a streptococcal infection of the throat or skin, a child 2 or more years old may develop headache and hematuria. Edema, vomiting, fever, or abdominal pain may occur. In addition to hematuria, proteinuria is found. White cells may be present and usually occur in the recovery phase. Many children develop hypertension. Oliguria and renal failure may occur. At the onset, BUN, erythrocyte sedimentation rate (ESR), and streptococcal enzymes are elevated and C_3 complement is decreased. Complement and immunoglobulins can be found with immunofluorescence microscopy.

The complications in the acute period are those due to hypertension and they should be treated. Confining the child to bed alone may decrease the blood pressure. If the child is dehydrated due to previous vomiting and at the risk of causing edema, water loading of the child for 2 hours with the calculated water requirement of 6 hours may correct both the oliguria and the hypertension. If these measures fail, other treatments of hypertension should be instituted, and the child placed on a sodium-restricted diet.

Penicillin is usually prescribed during the acute phase. Bed rest is continued until the child's appetite returns. If hematuria does not increase on activity, activity is permitted. The ESR elevation and hematuria persist several months but do not indicate an unfavorable prognosis. Signs of overactivity include anorexia and tiredness. If these occur, the patient should be restricted. Almost 98 per cent of such children recover. When similar signs and symptoms are associated with pneumococcal, staphylococcal or viral infections, the prognosis is not as good.

Membranoproliferative Glomerulonephritis. This disease starts like acute post-streptococcal glomerulonephritis, but is progressive. Hematuria usually is accompanied by proteinuria. Serum complement is low and remains low. Hypertension and renal insufficiency develop.

Focal Glomerulonephritis with Recurrent Hematuria. Gross hematuria with respiratory infections followed by intervals of no or microscopic hematuria but no proteinuria is characteristic of this condition. Deposits of IgA are found in the kidney. It appears to be a benign condition, and is probably a variant of benign or essential hematuria in which microscopic hematuria without proteinuria appears to be consistent but nonprogressive. Hematuria may occur after exercise, and also seems benign.

Hereditary Nephritis. Alport's syndrome may be an autosomal dominant disease with variable penetrance or a sex-linked disease that, in addition to hematuria and proteinuria, which are found in the first decade in males and the third or fourth decade in females, is accompanied by progressive sensorineural deafness. Death in males usually is due to renal failure in the third decade. It is a much milder disease in females.

Chronic Nephritis. The causes of chronic nephritis are not always found, although frequently it is assumed that a preceding acute nephritis occurred. Kidney function may be reduced for a long time before any abnormalities, including those in the urine, are noted. Eventually, the child develops an inability to concentrate urine which is followed by oliguria. During the early phase BUN may be low or normal. Then, the BUN rises and the child may develop hypertension, headache, anorexia, pallor, anemia, acidosis, renal rickets, and bone pain.

When the glomerular filtration rate is 10 per cent of normal, the child should be observed closely. Blood pressure should be maintained as normal as possible, and the child should be investigated and treated for infections. As renal function decreases, dietary protein and phosphate are restricted. Sodium excretion is measured and salt supplied as needed. It may be necessary to use 1,25 dihydroxy-cholecalciferol or calcium to control serum calcium; dialysis may be necessary for the control of azotemia and electrolyte imbalance.

In acute renal failure, the cause should be sought and treated. The causes include dehydration due to vomiting or diarrhea, shock, or hypovolemia of any etiology. Pre-renal causes may be indicated by a urine osmolality greater than that of plasma with a very low urine sodium. Hemolytic uremic syndrome may cause acute renal failure, as may, rarely, acute glomerulonephritis, ingestion of poisons, and injuries. Drugs used for treatment of renal or other conditions can have toxic effects.

If the treatment of the underlying condition does not reestablish urine formation, fluid is restricted to maintenance levels with additional fluid allowed for urine formed. Electrolytes are carefully monitored, especially for the development of hyponatremia and hyperkalemia. If diuresis does not begin, mannitol (0.5 to 1 g./kg. I.V.) or furosemide (2 mg./kg. I.V.) should be given.

Pyelonephritis, Cystitis, Vaginitis, Urethritis. In both pyelonephritis and cystitis, pyuria is more common than hematuria. Hematuria occurs, particularly with tuberculous infections of the kidney, coliform or viral infections of the bladder. Pinworms or bubble baths, particularly in females, may cause vaginitis or cystitis. Foreign bodies also should be sought, especially in the urethra which should be observed for prolapse.

Neoplasms, Polyps, Bladder Tumors. Tumors anywhere in the urinary tract may cause hematuria. Investigation should first consider more common causes such as glomerulonephritis or pyelonephritis before diagnostic studies are used. These studies, such as cystoscopy, may hurt the child.

Trauma to any part of the urinary tract causes hematuria. Trauma may occur following a blow to the kidney or bladder area, or after introduction of foreign bodies. Children who have been battered may present with hematuria. If battering is suspected, the child should be admitted to the hospital and protective services notified. Investigation and treatment of the hematuria should be instituted, including a bone survey for fractures or other evidence of battering or neglect.

A psychosocial history should be obtained to determine methods of discipline, parent-child and parent-parent relationships, and parents' ability to escape temporarily from the child's needs. Psychiatric consultation should be obtained early. The battered child needs more frequent follow-up than most children, and the physician should participate in the decisions regarding disposition and care of the child before discharge. Placement of the child may be necessary.

Trauma to the kidney can result in rupture with extravasation or intrarenal bleeding. Bladder or urethral rupture can result in intra- or extraperitoneal bleeding. In addition to hematuria, there may be pain or palpable masses. Radiograms, including urograms, reveal the extent of injury or possible pelvic fracture.

Calculi, including renal stones and diseases in which crystals are formed can cause hematuria. Certain toxic substances including drugs such as sulfonamides cause crystal formation. In children with fever and dehydration, hematuria may occur that is possibly due to crystal formation by urates, phosphates, or oxalates.

Collagen-Vascular Disease. The collagen-vascular diseases are multisystemic; children develop joint pains, skin rashes, arthritis, and gastrointestinal and kidney involvement. Hematuria as part of the presentation may occur in children with any of these diseases.

In children with rheumatoid arthritis, fever and arthritis of one joint or of many joints may be the initial complaint. A fleeting salmon colored skin rash and painful subcutaneous skin nodules may occur. Some children develop iridocyclitis or pericarditis. Positive laboratory findings include elevated ESR and other acute phase reactants as well as the presence of histocompatibility antigen HLA B27. Antinuclear antibodies and rheumatoid factor may be present.

Treatment should be directed to maintaining and avoiding deformities. Aspirin, 60–130 mg./kg./day, usually controls symptoms though prednisone or other anti-inflammatory agents may be necessary.

In children with systemic lupus erythematosus, fever and skin rash are common. Arthritis and central nervous system and liver involvement may occur. Antinuclear antibodies, elevated ESR and elevated gamma globulins are found. Prednisone, 0.5–1.0 mg./kg./day, should be given until symptoms and signs disappear.

In children with other collagen-vascular diseases such as dermatomyositis, polyarteritis, or scleroderma, renal involvement with hematuria can also occur.

Henoch-Schonlein or anaphylactoid purpura, a non-thrombocytopenic purpura, may also be a collagen-vascular disease. Purpura is usually found on the lower extremities, with melena and hematuria. Joint swelling occurs. Other laboratory tests are usually normal. The disease is usually self-limited but intussusception or renal failure may occur. Prednisone (0.5–1 mg./kg./day) may be used for these complications. Urine should be examined periodically for proteinuria as well as hematuria, and if either is present, other anti-inflammatory agents may be tried.

Bleeding Diseases. Hematuria can occur in children with any bleeding diathesis.

Hemolytic Uremic Syndrome. Following sepsis, gastrointestinal infection, or other viral infections, some children develop hematuria, rapidly progressive renal failure, and encephalopathy. Platelets decrease and BUN is elevated. Red blood cells are crenated and fragmented in the peripheral blood, and prothrombin time is increased. Disseminated intravascular coagulation (DIC) occurs and treatment, if any, is for acute renal failure and DIC.

Infectious Diseases. Certain infections, particularly leptospirosis, scarlet fever, and occasionally infectious mononucleosis, are likely to be associated with hematuria. Children with subacute bacterial endocarditis almost always have hematuria, while other acute infections can produce hematuria. Prognosis is related to the successful treatment of the infection.

Sickle-Cell Anemia. Children with sickle-cell anemia or sickle-cell trait frequently develop microscopic hematuria, perhaps due to microthrombi or anoxia.

In diseases with hematuria with over 150 mg. of protein per dl., consider first upper urinary tract disease, when the concentration of protein is less, consider first cystitis of urethritis.

The cause of hematuria must be found. If other signs of acute glomerulonephritis exist (headache, hypertension, proteinuria, edema, or typical chest film) wait for the state to resolve. If this diagnosis seems unlikely, proceed with urine culture, intravenous pyelogram, voiding cystourethrogram, retrograde studies and renal biopsy.

If hematuria is found, the urine should then be centrifuged and the supernatant re-tested for protein. In this way, the amount of protein directly related to the red cells will not distort the estimation of protein. If available, also test for blood. This not only confirms the presence of red cells, but if the test for blood is much more positive than expected from the number of red cells, this is an indirect indication of hemolysis, either systemic or in the urinary tract.

White Cells (Pyuria)

Normally, 0–2 white blood cells may be seen per high power field. A greater number suggests urinary tract infection, and demands gram stain of sediment and culture of the urine.

Other causes of excess white cells in the urine include all the causes of hematuria.

Casts

Red cell casts, white cell casts, or casts from detritus occur more commonly with upper urinary tract disease than lower. Unfortunately, if many cells are present in the bladder, they may clump and appear to be casts similar to those formed in the renal tubules. Causes of casts are similar to causes of hematuria, pyuria, and proteinuria.

Crystals

Many urines, particularly concentrated ones, contain crystals. Most commonly, these are phosphates and disappear when the urine is re-warmed. Some crystals may be indicative of disease.

Cystinuria is a common cause of renal stones. Patients may also excrete lysine. High urine volume, alkalinization or penicillamine therapy prevent stone formation. The urine gives a positive test with nitroprusside-ferricyanide.

Oxalate crystals occur in oxaluria, which involves two enzymic errors. Pyridoxine may be helpful.

Calcium crystals following hypercalciuria are usually excreted with oxalate.

Urate crystals occur in children with hyperuricemia (e.g., Lesch-Nyhan syndrome). In this syndrome, the patients are self-mutilating and hyper-irritable; antihistamines may be beneficial. Gout occurs in older patients and may respond to xanthine oxidase inhibitors.

Crystals of administered medicines may appear.

Ferric Chloride

One the important urinary screening test is with ferric chloride. This reagent is stable on paper and in liquid as a 10 per cent solution. The urine should be tested fresh and poisonings or inborn errors of metabolism may be suggested by the change in color.

Among the causes of color change are: drugs or poisons (especially salicylates or phenothiazines), aminoacidurias, autosomal recessive diseases, such as phenylketonuria, tyrosinemia, histidinemia, Oasthouse disease, maple syrup urine disease, alcaptonuria and pyridoxine disorders. Tumors (e.g., melanin) may cause color changes, as may severe acidosis and other organic acids. When the test with ferric chloride is positive, exact identification of the substance is necessary.

Color

Urine is normally light yellow. Dark yellow or brown coloring of the urine suggests the presence of bile. This is usually due to excessive conjugated bilirubin, hemoglobin (especially in acute hemolytic states), myoglobin (as occurs with muscle breakdown), and dehydration due to concentration of pigment.

Red urine occurs in children with hematuria, hemoglobinuria and porphyria; it can be due to congenital porphyria or poisonings with excessive porphyrin production. Beeturia occurs in children with iron deficiency anemia when they eat beets. Dyes and serratia marcescens in the diaper of the newborn also cause color changes. Blue urine may be seen in infants with disorders of tryptophan metabolism and black urine is an indication of alcaptonuria or melanuria.

Odor

The urine frequently mimics body odor. For example, in diphtheria or phenylketonuria the urine smells "musty." The urine smells like fish in some patients with disorders of sulfur amino acid metabolism, and smells of maple syrup in children with disorders of branched-chain amino acids.

It should be remembered that almost no urine test is diagnostic. Urine tests are screening tests and indicate the direction for proceeding in further diagnostic work-up.

BIBLIOGRAPHY

Arneil, G. C.: The nephrotic syndrome. Pediatr. Clin. North Am., *18*:547, 1971.

> A comprehensive review of causes, diagnosis and treatment of various forms and presentations of children with the nephrotic syndrome.

Kincaid-Smith, P., Mathew, T. H., and Lorell Becker, E. (eds.): Glomerulonephritis, Morphology, Natural History and Treatment. New York, John Wiley, 1973.

> An extensive review of many forms of nephritis, particularly in children.

Roy, S., Pitcock, J. A., and Etteldorf, J. N.: Prognosis of acute poststreptococcal glomerulonephritis in childhood: Prospective study and review of the literature. Adv. Pediatr., 23:48, 1976.

> A compilation of the authors' long-term experiences with several hundred children initially diagnosed as having acute post-streptococcal glomerulonephritis.

18

Edema

Lewis A. Barness, M.D.

Edema results from an abnormal increase in the amount of extravascular extracellular fluid. It may be due to retention of water, salt and water, or to a shift of fluid between extracellular fluid and intracellular fluid.

Edema fluid is an ultrafiltrate of plasma. Its occurrence is usually accompanied by an excess of body sodium.

DETECTING EDEMA

Pressure over a part of the body which is larger than normal results in indentation, pitting edema. Measurement of the part, e.g. the leg, compared to normal indicates an increase in circumference due to an increase of volume. Similarly, measuring the circumference of the abdomen may indicate the progress of abdominal fluid, ascites. Nevertheless, the best method presently available for the detection and following the progress of edema in the child is determining the daily weight of the child and noting weight changes. Even in the newborn, lack of physiological weight loss in the first week of life may be the earliest evidence of abnormal water accumulation.

Edema accumulates usually in dependent parts and in easily distensible tissue. Thus, generalized edema may be present and distributed over the entire body but be detected only in the face or over the eyes in the morning, (periorbital edema), only to disappear as the child becomes upright when the fluid shifts to the scrotum and lower legs and feet in the afternoon. This is shifting edema and occurs in all cases, but is more marked in those with lesser amounts of edema fluid.

Localized edema and non-pitting edema may have special causes. These are discussed below.

MECHANISM OF EDEMA FORMATION

Edema is formed when those factors holding water in the intravascular space are unequal to those pushing fluid out of this space. Water and small solutes cross the capillary wall by diffusion. Larger molecules cross through clefts between endothelial cells.

Factors causing extrusion from intravascular space are:

1. Cellular dysfunction with equilibrium (e.g., death): Those mechanisms maintaining cellular integrity are lost. Sodium and water enter the cell. Potassium, phosphate, and water leave the cell.

2. Hydrostatic pressure changes: Increased intravascular pressure changes drive water and solutes into the intracellular spaces. For example, cardiac output decreases, leading to decreased renal perfusion; cardiac input decreases, leading to increased hydrostatic pressure; vascular constriction causes local increase in hydrostatic pressure; or venous obstruction causes an increase in hydrostatic pressure distal to the obstruction.

3. Osmotic pressure, regulated by osmoreceptors, located in the nucleus supraopticus and in the portal circulation: These regulate the release of ADH and perspiration. Osmotic pressure is caused by an increase of molecules on one side of a membrane compared to the other. Protein, especially albumin, is responsible for oncotic pressure. This is regulated by: formation, especially in the liver; nutrition, depending on protein and calorie intake; losses, especially through kidney (e.g., nephrosis); hypermetabolic states.

Osmotic pressure can be caused by electrolytes, the concentration of which is regulated by: intake; mineral corticoids which control sodium and chloride retention, (any state resulting in increased aldosterone secretion results in an increase in tubular reabsorption of sodium); changes in excretion, as in renal disease with decreased filtration (increased osmotic pressure) or decreased reabsorption (decreased osmotic pressure) as well as in heart failure with secondary decreased renal perfusion; and excess losses, (e.g., sweating, cystic fibrosis of pancreas).

Non-electrolytes, (e.g., urea, glucose) also cause osmotic pressure.

Diseases Associated with Edema Formation

Edema occurs in children with heart failure, with volume overload, kidney disease, diseases of the capillaries, improper fluid therapy, severe anemia or polycythemia, carcinoid, or any illness associated with low serum proteins.

Decreased blood volume on the arterial side occurs with left-sided failure; increased systemic venous pressure is termed backward failure. With heart failure edema fluid is a transudate, an ultrafiltrate of plasma. Protein content is less than 3 per cent and specific gravity less than 1.015.

Exudates, as occur with infections, contain more than 3 per cent protein and specific gravity is greater than 1.018.

Kidney Disease. Kidney diseases associated with decreased filtration, increased tubular reabsorption of electrolytes, or albumin loss include those diseases described in the proteinuria section.

Diseases associated with decreased oncotic pressure are due to decreased production or increased losses of proteins, particularly albumin and include: nephrosis and nephrotic syndrome: (see Proteinuria); and malabsorption syndromes. Any malabsorption syndrome may have such severe protein losses as to develop hypoproteinemia. These include: celiac disease, sprue, cystic fibrosis, the dysenteries, abetalipoproteinemia (though the carrier protein for fat is absent, protein is also lost), colitis (particularly ulcerative colitis), ileitis, and protein-losing enteropathy, which may be associated with anatomical or vascular anomalies of the intestinal tract.

Liver Disease. (see Chapter 12). In particular those with cirrhosis do not produce sufficient albumin. Some children with storage diseases or some with Wilson's disease where the copper in the liver is high, and some with cystic fibrosis develop this type of cirrhosis. Some chronic hemolytic anemias cause hemosiderosis and defective albumin production.

Hypothyroidism. Albumin production may be decreased or excessive albumin metabolized.

EVALUATION

In the patient with edema, first make certain that the child does not have congestive heart failure, not because this is the most common cause of edema, but because failure to recognize this cause early may lead to catastrophe. Look for: history of heart disease, history of fatigue, orthopnea, history of previous streptococcal infection, history of rheumatic fever and history of tuberculosis (? constrictive pericarditis). Look for these physical signs in those with edema: tachycardia, tachypnea, cardiomegaly (scratch percussion), hepatomegaly, rales, murmurs, cyanosis, hypertension, low pulse pressure and clubbing. Get a chest film to see if the heart is enlarged, small, or decreased cardiac motion. Take an EKG and measure hemoglobin levels and whether or not hematocrit is high or low. Finally, get an echocardiogram.

If heart disease is not present, eliminate kidney disease next as a cause of edema. Look for: history of previous infection (nephritis), familial kidney disease, deafness (Alport syndrome), oliguria, polyuria, polydipsia, history of hypertension, hematuria, headache, and exposure to poisons. The physical signs to check are: mass in abdomen, costovertebral angle; tenderness over bladder, costovertebral angle; or hypertension.

A urinalysis will measure: protein, specific gravity, hematuria (casts), reducing substance, white cells (casts), heavy metals, bacteria and culture. Check the blood for: anemia, urea nitrogen (creatinine), serum proteins and anti-streptococcal antibodies.

If the nephrotic syndrome is present, causes should be sought, as listed before.

Many of these diagnoses and others may be more specifically defined by renal biopsy. If these are not diagnostic, intravenous urography and voiding cystourethrogram may indicate an anatomical defect.

If the patient does not have heart failure or kidney disease but has generalized edema, suspect low serum proteins, particularly albumin. If this is the case, be sure to obtain: dietary history, social history, and history of jaundice, liver disease, or of chronic infection.

Physical examination may indicate only a large, tender, or hard liver. Then obtain: liver enzymes (e.g., SGOT), bilirubin, serum proteins (electrophoresis) and blood ammonia, urea (urea frequently decreased and ammonia elevated).

If liver tests are positive, test for specific liver causes, though cirrhosis may have no other abnormalities.

If dietary history is poor, first try the child on an adequate diet before doing extensive tests and making bizarre diagnoses. As his diet improves, the child may not gain weight for as long as 6 weeks, though serum proteins will increase and edema decrease.

If diarrhea is a problem, do a careful rectal exam looking for signs of megacolon. Then get: stool cultures, stool ova and parasites, stool blood, stool pH (pH below 5 suggests intestinal enzyme deficiency), stools for fat, sugar and protein, sweat test for cystic fibrosis, tuberculin test, and look at a blood smear for acanthocytes.

If these are not diagnostic, proceed with a GI series including barium enema and sigmoidoscopy. Specific malabsorption syndromes may be detected. If history suggests chronic infection, the sources of infection must be sought. These include cultures of: blood, urine, stools and perhaps ears, cerebrospinal fluid, and radiographs of sinuses.

If the source of edema is neither heart, liver, or kidney disease, or low serum proteins, look for diseases or states causing increased capillary permeability. Capillary permeability is probably the most common cause of localized edema and may be associated with generalized or localized edema. Diseases or states causing increased capillary permeability include: anaphylaxis or shock, allergies—angioneurotic edema, insect bites, measles, gonadal dysgenesis, hypothyroidism (get T4, T3, and TSH), scurvy, beriberi, rickets, poisons, position (e.g. facial edema in morning, obstruction to flow by crossing legs) and lymphatic obstruction (e.g. filariasis).

While the common causes are listed above, do not make a diagnosis of allergic or angioneurotic edema before examining the patient thoroughly (particularly for heart disease) and performing a urinalysis.

PRINCIPLES OF MANAGEMENT

In general, salt intake should be monitored or decreased in all patients retaining fluid. This is probably not as important in children with the nephrotic syndrome with normal blood pressure. More important for this group of children is *that* they eat rather than *what* they eat.

For children with heart failure, digitalis and diuretics are the basis of treatment. If anoxia is present, oxygen is helpful. For those with myocarditis, corticosteroids should be tried.

The usual renal disease causing edema is acute post-streptococcal glomerulonephritis. Penicillin therapy for several months usually suffices. If hypertension is present, salt should be restricted, the patient should be kept at rest, and antihypertensives such as phenobarbital, reserpine and hydralazine should be used.

If the diagnosis is nephrosis or the nephrotic syndrome, corticosteroids should be used for at least 4 weeks. For some of the poisonings, specific antidotes are available. Some children have surgically correctable kidney lesions; these should be corrected.

In children with hypoalbuminemia, suitable diets should be tried first. If these do not help, intravenous albumin may be necessary. Generally for those with allergy, antihistamines help.

HYPERTENSION

Hypertension results from increased salt retention, either dietary or due to excessive minerals, corticoids and aldosterone, or through the renin-angiotensin mechanism following renal stimulation of the juxtaglomerular apparatus. Other renal substances may also cause hypertension.

Hypertension in children is due most commonly to renal disease. Normal blood pressure is best obtained with a proper cuff size (see Chapter 1). Some children have elevated blood pressures only occasionally (labile hypertension); the relation of labile hypertension to true hypertension is unknown. Exercise and excitement cause sporadic hypertension and may be precursors of fixed hypertension. The most common cause of acute onset of hypertension in children is acute glomerulonephritis. Signs of hypertension include headache, vomiting, and bradycardia. Signs of hypertensive encephalopathy include papilledema, seizures, and retinal hemorrhages.

Evaluation

If there is a familial history of hypertension, renal or adrenal disease, direct the work-up to similar systems in the child. A history of excess ingestion of licorice which contains an aldosterone-like compound, or history of heavy metal exposure or of other drug ingestion may be obtained. Physical examination may reveal coarctation of the aorta. Hypertension will be found in upper extremities, hypotension in lower extremities, and femoral pulses will be absent.

In the absence of a leading history or physical finding, study the child's genitourinary system. Careful urinalysis may reveal abnormalities. Intravenous rapid sequence urogram may indicate intrinsic or destructive renal disease and is helpful in determining unilateral renal disease. Aortography and renal arteriography with differential renal vein renin levels, as well as renal scan, help delineate vascular or unilateral disease. Renal biopsy may also be helpful.

If all studies are negative, catecholamine-producing lesions such as neuroblastoma, pheochromocytoma, or carcinoid should be suspected. Urinary catecholamines, VMA, and cystathionine help distinguish these. Removal of a pheochromocytoma is complicated by paroxysms of hyper- and hypotension. Phentolamine should be given preoperatively and levarterenol should be available at operation for decreased blood pressure.

In the absence of specific cause of hypertension, a diagnosis of essential hypertension may be made. Organic cause of hypertension is much more commonly found in children than in adults.

Hyperthyroidism. Enlarged thyroid, tachycardia, hyperhidrosis, and tremor may be present.

Increased Intracranial Pressure. Many children with signs of meningitis, excephalitis, or brain tumor develop hypertension, usually with bradycardia. Sometimes it is difficult to distinguish signs of primary encephalopathy with hypertension from encephalopathy due to hypertension.

Obesity. Obese children may have hypertension. More commonly it is difficult to get an accurate blood pressure measurement in obese children.

Riley-Day Syndrome. Signs of familial dysautonomia such as absence of tears, decreased pain sensation, vomiting, and failure to thrive may indicate this syndrome.

Treatment

If signs of hypertensive encephalopathy are present, diazoxide 5 mg./kg. should be given rapidly and intravenously. This usually lowers blood pressure within a few minutes. For acute hypertension, reserpine 0.1 mg./kg. and Apresoline 0.1 mg./kg. is given intramuscularly. This dose may be repeated every 8 hours. For management of chronic hypertension, methyldopa 3—15 mg./kg. every 8 hours or propanolol 0.5 mg./kg. every 12 hours can be tried. Salt restriction is frequently helpful. If the patient is apprehensive, bed rest and small doses of phenobarbital should be tried.

BIBLIOGRAPHY

Ganer, O. H., Henry, J. P., and Behn, C.: The regulation of extracellular fluid volume. Ann. Rev. Physiol. 32:547, 1970.

A discussion of the physiological mechanisms involved in the regulation of body fluids.

Winters, R. W. (ed): The Body Fluids in Pediatrics. Boston, Little, Brown, 1973.

A thorough discussion of body fluids and their regulation, and a discussion of the diagnosis and treatment of errors in fluid balance.

Richard, G. A., Garin, E. H., and Fennell, R. S.: A pathophysiologic basis for the diagnosis and treatment of the renal hypertensions. Adv. Pediatr., 24:339, 1977.

A clear concise description of the steps necessary for the diagnosis and treatment of hypertension in children.

19

Disturbances of Growth

Allen W. Root, M.D., and Edward O. Reiter, M.D.

RETARDATION OF LINEAR GROWTH

Determinants of Growth

The most important factor that determines the linear growth of a person is the genetic potential for growth which the subject inherits from his ancestors. Genetic influences govern the rate of cell division and increase in cell size which are reflected ultimately as the patient's height. The genetic growth potential may be directly related to the growth of one or both parents or may reflect an inherited influence of more distant progenitors (grandparents, great grandparents, etc.). Superimposed upon the familial genetic potential for growth are internal and external factors which determine whether the person will realize his or her genetic growth potential.

Nutritional deprivation *in utero* may result in permanent retardation of growth. Fetal malnutrition due either to severe maternal malnutrition or more commonly to placental dysfunction of many sorts may permanently imprint a pattern of retarded growth upon the developing fetus by restricting cell division and cell size. A similar effect is observed if there is significant nutritional deprivation at puberty. In the latter instance sex hormone secretion in the nutritionally deprived state is associated with epiphyseal maturation and fusion without corresponding increase in chondrogenesis and linear growth. Malnutrition at other times of childhood probably does not permanently impair linear growth potential. "Catch-up" growth may ensue after many years of malnutrition if nutrition is improved. Specific dietary deficiencies of vitamins (A, D), trace elements (zinc, copper) and other dietary components may also impair growth.

Human pituitary growth hormone acting in part through induction of hepatic, renal and skeletal muscle synthesis of a group of proteins, the "somatomedins," which stimulate growth in diverse tissues (cartilage, fibroblasts, erythroblasts, etc.) plays a key role in cell division. Insulin is a fundamental growth hormone exerting effects not only upon carbohydrate metabolism but also stimulating amino acid transport, protein synthesis and cell division in a manner identical to that of the somatomedins. Thyroid hormone influences the rate of cell division and growth of cell size. Androgens increase the rate of cartilage cell division but accelerate epiphyseal maturation (calcification) to an even greater extent. Estrogens also stimulate chondrogenesis but advance epiphyseal maturation at an even faster rate. Glucocorticoids inhibit cell division in part by diverting amino acids from protein synthesis into gluconeogenic pathways. Other hormones such as glucagon, the enterohormones (gastrin, secretin, cholecystokinin-pancreozymin), parathyroid hormone and calcitonin also influence growth directly or indirectly by affecting the rates of cell growth and division.

Major diseases may temporarily or permanently impair the rates of cell division and cell growth. In the majority of instances termination of the disease state is followed by accelerated linear (catch-up) growth which is maintained until the pre-morbid growth channel is again achieved. The molecular and hormonal mechanisms of the accelerated growth following the termination of starvation or illness are poorly understood; thyrotropin and thyroid hormones are necessary for the recovery process.

Evaluation

An aberration of linear growth should be considered when the child's height falls more than three standard deviations below the mean height for age, when the patient's growth channel shifts from a higher to a lower position or when a patient is inappropriately small for family size. A decline in the linear growth velocity is the earliest sign of an abnormal growth pattern.

A precise history of the patient's growth pattern together with accurate past measurements of height (and weight) are needed. Past measurements may be obtained from parental baby books, school and summer camp physical examinations, or physician's records. The linear growth of a child is not steady. In order to define the child's growth velocity, measurements should be obtained at not less than 6 monthly and preferably yearly intervals. There may be a seasonable variation in growth acceleration observed during the spring and summer months.

One should determine when the decline in growth occurred and what symptoms and signs preceded, accompanied and followed the alteration in growth pattern. Maternal exposure to potential teratogens (drugs, alcohol) or complicating diseases (diabetes mellitus, infectious processes) at the time of conception and during gestation, the conditions of labor (analgesia, anesthesia, duration, fetal position), delivery (head position, umbilical cord position) and the early postnatal period (resuscitative measures) should be noted. Thereafter, the child's growth pattern, health and associated disease states, symptoms and signs until the interview are recorded in a chronologic manner. Historical data relative to the health and growth patterns of the parents, siblings, grandparents and other relatives are accumulated.

Measurements of height, weight, limb length, and head circumference are recorded in a uniform manner. Blood pressure and other vital signs are recorded. Thereafter, physical examination of the integumentory, musculoskeletal, cardiorespiratory, central nervous system and other systems is performed and the appropriate positive and negative findings recorded. Often the physical examination alone will provide diagnostic clues (e.g., of rickets, chondrodystrophy, hypothyroidism, congenital heart disease).

After completion of the historical review and physical examination, the height measurements are plotted; growth velocity should be calculated and plotted:

$$GV \left(\frac{cm.}{yr.} \right) = \frac{Ht_2 - Ht_1 \; (cm.)}{Time \; (yrs.)}$$

or

$$= \frac{Ht_2 - Ht_1 \; (cm.)}{Time \; (mo.)} \times 12$$

or

$$= \frac{Ht_2 - Ht_1 \; (in.)}{Time \; (mo.)} \times 2.5 \times 12$$

The height age (HA) is the chronologic age corresponding to the fiftieth percentile for the patient's height. The number of standard deviations the patient's height falls below the mean height for age can be determined (Table 19-1).

Linear growth potential may be assessed by determining the skeletal maturation or bone age (BA) of a person through roentgenograms of the epiphyseal centers appropriate to bracket both the patient's chronologic age (CA) and HA.

Assuming that the historical review and physical examination do not provide significant diagnostic probabilities, it is possible to classify the patient into one of three groups of patients with growth retardation (see outline p. 230):

Table 19-1. Means and Standard Deviations of Height (centimeters)

Age (years)	Males White Mean	SD	Males Black Mean	SD	Females White Mean	SD	Females Black Mean	SD
1	76.0	2.68	75.7	2.53	74.4	2.60	74.5	2.62
2	86.9	3.11	86.6	3.12	85.5	3.10	86.0	3.28
3	95.2	3.67	95.6	3.59	94.0	3.56	95.0	3.98
4	102.6	4.14	103.8	4.07	101.7	4.00	103.0	4.48
5	109.5	4.41	110.8	4.40	108.6	4.32	110.4	4.59
6	115.9	4.80	117.3	4.93	115.1	4.72	116.9	5.43
7	122.3	5.22	123.2	5.10	121.2	5.03	123.4	5.96
8	128.1	5.74	129.3	5.25	127.2	5.49	129.2	6.20
9	133.9	5.96	135.1	5.44	132.8	5.76	134.9	6.20
10	140.3		139.6		140.8		141.8	
11	145.7		145.7		147.3		149.2	
12	152.3	8.40	152.1	6.87	155.0	7.43	156.5	6.59
13	159.9	9.11	159.7	9.29	158.7	7.02	159.0	6.55
14	166.9	8.70	165.7	8.62	161.4	6.25	161.5	5.69
15	171.6	7.23	170.4	7.81	162.4	6.98	161.7	6.16
16	174.4	6.94	174.0	6.80	162.8	6.41	161.9	6.51
17	175.7	6.99	174.5	7.01	163.0	6.32	162.7	6.61

(Data adapted from: Ages 1–9: Wingerd, J., *et al.*: Pediatrics, *52*:555, 1973. Ages 10–11: Hamill, P. V. V., *et al.*: National Health Survey, Series 11, 1970. Ages 12–17: Hamill, P. V. V., *et al.*: National Health Survey, Series 11, 1973. National Center for Health Statistics, Public Health Service.)

Causes of Linear Growth Retardation

Genetic short stature
  Familial
  Intrauterine growth retardation (see page 232)
  Chromosomal anomalies
    trisomies 21,15,18
    gonadal dysgenesis—XO, XO/XX, XX pi . . .
  Chondrodystrophies
  Mucopolysaccharidoses
  Primordial
    Russel-Silver
    Seckel's bird-headed dwarf
    Cockayne's
    with advanced bone age

Constitutional delay in growth and development
  Malnutrition
  Psychogenic

Systemic disease
  Cardiorespiratory
    congenital cardiac malformation
    asthma

Gastrointestinal
  malabsorption
    celiac syndrome
    cystic fibrosis
  regional enteritis
Genitourinary
  renal tubular acidosis
  chronic renal insufficiency
  nephrogenic diabetes insipidus
Hematologic
  chronic anemia
Endocrinological
  hyposomatotropism
  hypothyroidism
  hypoadrenocorticism
  hyperadrenocorticism
  diabetes mellitus

Genetic Short Stature. (HA<BA=CA): The most common form of genetic short stature is familial. However, certain disease states are also characterized by genetic short stature, such as chondrodystrophies, chromosomal anomalies (Down's syndrome [trisomy 21], gonadal dysgenesis [XO and other aberrations of sex chromosome complement], trisomy 15-18) eponymic entities (Cockayne's dwarfism, leprechaunism, Seckel's bird-headed dwarf), intrauterine insults (rubella, placental insufficiency, maternal alcoholism, other drugs), storage diseases (mucopolysaccharidosis), central nervous system abnormalities, and others (see Causes of Small-for-Gestational-Age Births, page 232.)

Constitutional Delay in Growth and Adolescent Maturation. (HA = BA < CA): The growth pattern of children in this classification represents a normal variation in the timing of linear growth and sexual maturation. Growth velocity is normal; the HA and BA are usually similar and equally retarded behind (but more than 75 per cent of) CA.

Frequently this growth pattern is familial, the mother or father having been delayed in growth and sexual development. Suboptimal nutrition may also delay growth and sexual maturation, but these effects are potentially reversible with restoration of adequate caloric intake prior to the onset of puberty. Frequently, the suboptimal nutritional state reflects decreased appetite of the patient; this can be related to emotional problems, trace element deficiency or unknown factors involved in the regulation of appetite.

Chemical or radiographic studies do not positively identify the child with constitutional delay in growth and sexual development. This diagnosis is based upon the characteristic patterns of linear growth and skeletal maturation, family history, absence of detectable diseases and

---

Causes of Small-for-Gestational-Age Births

Placental insufficiency
    Maternal toxemia, cardiac disease, hypertension, ulcerative
      colitis
    Placental malformations, infarctions
    Twinning

Intrauterine infections
    Rubella
    Cytomegalic inclusion disease

Intrauterine drugs
    Narcotics
    Aminopterin
    Alcohol
Chromosomal anomalies
    Autosomal
      trisomies 21, 15, 18
    Sex chromosomal
      XO, XXXXY
    Chromosomal breakage
      Fanconi's anemia (pancytopenia, absent radius)
      Bloom's syndrome (telangectasis, broad thumbs)

Endocrine abnormalities
    Hypothyroidism (rare)
    Growth hormone insensitivity
    Human chorionic sommatomammotropin deficiency (?)

Primordial
    Russel-Silver
    Conradi
    Virchow
    Multiple congenital anomalies

---

the maintenance of the anticipated growth pattern during prolonged observation.

Systemic and Endocrine Diseases. Many systemic diseases and endocrinologic abnormalities may interfere with a child's linear growth, causing the patient's growth velocity to be abnormally slow. HA or BA are often less than 75 per cent of the CA.

Careful historical review and physical examination may provide the clues necessary to pursue the correct diagnostic pathways (e.g., skeletal deformities—rickets, chondrodystrophy, mucopolysaccharidosis; heart murmur or cyanosis—congenital or acquired abnormality of the cardiorespiratory system; hypothyroidism; frequent foul smelling, greasy stools with ravenous appetite—malabsorption syndrome, etc.). However, disorders of renal, (renal tubular acidosis, chronic renal insufficiency) gastrointestinal (regional enteritis) and pituitary (hyposomatotrophism) function may be occult.

It is necessary, therefore, to screen patients with suspected systemic or endocrine abnormalities. However, the majority of children screened does not have an identifiable disease process and represents more extreme examples of constitutional delay in growth and development than those identified by the criteria listed above.

In the authors' clinic the following screening studies are carried out on selected children: skull films, complete blood count, sedimentation rate, urinalysis (including pH and specific gravity), serum sodium, potassium, chloride, bicarbonate and calcium concentrations, thyroxine and triiodothyronine resin uptake, a screening test for growth hormone secretion, such as a brief exercise tolerance test. A buccal smear is obtained on all short girls and chromosomal karyotype is performed when there is clinical suspicion of gonadal dysgenesis. If any study is abnormal, appropriate diagnostic steps are pursued. If studies are normal, the patient is observed with periodic (6 month) measurements of height. Observation is continued as long as growth velocity is constant and additional signs and symptoms do not appear. With further deviation of growth pattern, additional investigative efforts are mandatory, including radiographic survey of the gastrointestinal tract and other measures appropriate to the situation.

Management

Management of the child with linear growth retardation depends upon accurate identification of the etiology of the growth pattern. The patient with familial genetic short stature cannot realize a height greater than the genetically determined growth potential. The rate of growth may be accelerated in such children by androgen administration, but this therapy is only used in specific instances. These children and their parents require explanation, reassurance and re-education of attitudes concerning the importance of height. Every effort should be made to emphasize the other talents and traits of the child that do not rely upon height.

In children with defined disease processes appropriate therapy should be undertaken. If the disease state can be identified and treated, the illness-induced impediment to growth can often be overcome and linear growth resumed. Patients undergoing treatment for hypothyroidism with thyroid hormone experience accelerated linear growth velocity, but skeletal maturation often advances still more rapidly. Human growth hormone administered to the patient with hyposomatotropism accelerates linear growth velocity to a greater extent than that of skeletal maturation. Appropriate treatment of the child with malabsorption syndrome or regional enteritis is followed by increased linear growth velocity. However, prolonged exposure to glucocorticoids, either therapeutically or, rarely, as a consequence of a glucocorticoid-secreting tumor, may permanently impair linear growth.

In the nutritionally deprived child, increased caloric intake, often extremely difficult to effect, accelerates growth (see below). A group of children with growth retardation attributed to psychogenic and nutritional factors are members of disturbed families characterized by discord, alcoholism, or infidelity. These children have bizarre behavioral and eating patterns (eating from garbage cans, wolfing loaves of bread and jars of mayonnaise, drinking from toilet bowls). There is decreased secretion of growth hormone and ACTH; after the child is removed from the home these levels return to normal and rapid growth resumes. The abnormal growth and endocrine patterns have been attributed to psychogenic factors but recent observations suggest that the basic abnormality may be severe nutritional deprivation.

Management of the boy with constitutional delay in growth and development requires reassurance and careful explanation of the normal variability of growth patterns. Prediction of adult height (range) may be helpful. The boy should be observed periodically to be certain that the anticipated patterns of growth and sexual maturation ensue. Occasionally these children are disturbed by the difference between their body image and that of their peers. Verbal reassurance may be insufficient and attempts to accelerate the rates of growth and development may be indicated. Testosterone (by intramuscular depot administration as the propionate or enanthate, or sublingually as methyltestosterone) or a synthetic derivative (fluoxoxymesterone or oxandrolone) may be administered for brief periods. In view of the potential hazards of androgen therapy, such a rapid acceleration of skeletal maturation and hepatocellular carcinoma, these drugs should only be administered under the supervision of experienced physicians.

In girls with constitutional delay in growth and development, therapy with androgens and estrogens is usually withheld unless there is an extreme degree of growth retardation and parental or patient concern. The decision to employ hormonal therapy in such children should be considered on an individual basis.

FAILURE TO GAIN WEIGHT

Etiology

Failure of a child to gain weight is a frequent maternal complaint. The causes of failure of weight gain are listed below. In the majority of instances inadequate weight gain reflects inadequate caloric intake. However, with the exception of underdeveloped countries, unavailability of food seldom accounts for decreased food intake. Inadequate caloric intake

Causes of Failure to Gain Weight

Caloric deprivation
  Inadequate nutrition (economic deprivation, protein-calorie malnutrition)
    marasmus
    kwashiorkor
    marasmic-kwashiorkor
    breast feeding
    zinc deficiency
    hypothyroidism
    hypercalcemia (subcutaneous fat necrosis, idiopathic
      hyperparathyroidism, vitamin A or D intoxication)
  Maternal deprivation
    psychosocial deprivation
    emotional deprivation
  Anorexia nervosa
Organic diseases
  Congenital anomalies
    cleft palate
    glossoptosis
    megacolon
    congenital cardiac anomalies
    biliary atresia
    obstruction of gastrointestinal tract
  Malabsorption syndromes
    cystic fibrosis
    disaccharide intolerance
    monosaccharide intolerance
    celiac disease
    parasitic infestation
    hypocalcemia
  Excessive utilization of calories
    hyperthyroidism—congenital or acquired
    narcotic addiction (maternal)
    infections
      urinary tract
      septicemia
    diencephalic syndrome
    neoplasia
  Failure to utilize calories
    renal insufficiency
    renal tubular acidosis (cystinosis)
    hypothyroidism
    hypopituitarism—hyposomatotropism
    hypoadrenalism
    galactosemia
    glycogen storage disease
    diabetes mellitus
    acrodynia
    CNS insult
    diabetes insipidus, central or renal

in the infant often reflects disturbance in the maternal-infant relationship which may be of a complex nature. Although generous quantities of foodstuffs are offered, the feeding period may be shortened because the mother is busy with other children, or there may be (unrecognized) conflict between the mother and child during mealtime. In children with genetic short stature and a fragile bony structure a small appetite seems appropriate for body size. Frequently, however, slow growth velocity and poor weight gain are due to a small appetite; in such patients a cause for the decreased appetite is usually not identified. Infrequently, low body levels of zinc may be associated with decreased sensations of taste and smell, leading to anorexia. Zinc supplementation may reverse these abnormalities and improve appetite in selected patients. The diencephalic syndrome secondary to a tumor in or near the third cerebral ventricle is characterized by anorexia and disproportionate happiness with inappropriate affect. These children may grow linearly but are emaciated; surgical or radiation therapy of the tumor may temporarily reverse these findings. Patients with anorexia nervosa are frequently females whose weight loss began with a self-imposed diet initiated because of actual or suspected overweight. Dieting continues to the point where appetite is lost and the thought, sight and smell of food become revolting. Frequently there is deep psychopathology, although vigorous interruption of the weight loss before it has progressed to the point of debility may reverse the process. Many disease processes (such as congenital heart disease, chronic renal insufficiency and diabetes insipidus) may be associated with anorexia; thus, children with these illnesses fail to grow, in part, because of decreased caloric intake. Electrolyte disturbances, particularly hypercalcemia, may be associated with anorexia.

Gastrointestinal malabsorption characterized by diarrhea and steatorrhea prevents normal absorption of food. These patients usually have large caloric intakes but poor linear growth and weight gain. Stools may be frequent, loose, foul smelling, or greasy. Certain foods may provoke these symptoms, particularly if the malabsorption syndrome is due to a specific intestinal enzyme deficiency. Hypermetabolic states such as hyperthyroidism, narcotic intoxication, diabetes mellitus and neoplasia may also be associated with weight loss or failure to gain weight despite excessive caloric intake.

Evaluation

Evaluation of the child who fails to gain weight normally begins with a thorough history and physical examination. A detailed dietary history may distinguish between the quantity of food offered and the amount actually ingested and retained, excluding food remaining on the plate, chair, floor, ceiling or bib. A description of the frequency, quantity and type of stool, and an extensive systemic review searching for clues to associated illness should be obtained. An attempt to define the maternal-child relationship should be undertaken. The interaction between mother and child during the examination and subsequent evaluation should be observed. In most children with inanition, the height is within the low normal range but the weight is below average for the height. Evidence of systemic illness is sought during the physical examination. Most frequently, both the historical review and physical examination are uninformative.

If the child with failure to thrive is hospitalized, the child's caloric intake should be measured. Every effort should be made to ensure sufficient calories for normal growth (approximately 150 calories/kg. body weight). If observation reveals that the child fails to grow or gain weight despite adequate caloric intake, then, depending upon the clinical findings, a more extensive evaluation is undertaken. Diseases of the cardiovascular, central nervous, gastrointestinal, genitourinary and endocrine systems should be eliminated. Studies should include the determination of skeletal maturation, radiographs of the skull, blood glucose, urea nitrogen, serum electrolytes, creatinine, calcium, pH, blood count, urinalysis and examination of stool for ova and parasites, pH, reducing substances and fat content.

Management

If a specific systemic disorder is identified, appropriate and rational therapy should be undertaken. Management of the child with failure to gain weight is difficult after treatable diseases or nutritional deficiencies have been eliminated as possible causes. Close supervision of the child in addition to frequent visits to the physician's office and frequent visits to the home by a visiting nurse, social worker or physician may reinforce the maternal-child relationship and permit more adequate nutrition of the child. Nevertheless, follow-up reports of infants in whom failure to thrive was clearly demonstrated to be due to decreased caloric intake indicate that at older ages these children are still considerably underweight for height. No appetite-stimulating medications are effective. Generally it is recommended that the children be offered substantial calories, but that no confrontation between child and parent over his food intake be permitted, as this is often a self-defeating action. The children should be encouraged to eat more, but not threatened to do so. A reward for weight gained and maintained may be considered in certain instances. Behavioral modification of the child with anorexia nervosa is often quite rewarding; these children are rewarded only for specific weight gain and must be made to earn even the most limited privilege by weight gain.

OBESITY

Etiology

Most frequently the obese child (weight more than 2.5 standard deviation above the mean or increased skin-fold thickness) presents a subject in whom caloric intake far exceeds caloric expenditure. Patients with exogenous (regulatory) obesity eat large meals (some state they miss breakfast), between-meals and before bed-time snacks. They eat frequently, even without hunger, and experience no feeling of satiety; this is a chronic pattern frequently beginning in early infancy and present for several years. It sometimes occurs in previously thin children following tonsillectomy. In addition to the large caloric intake, these children enjoy sedentary activities such as reading, watching television, knitting or model building. They sit stoically and immobile, conserving every possible calorie. The obese child is often a member of a family with obese parents and siblings. The Pickwickian syndrome is characterized by excessive and inappropriate somnolence secondary to hypercapnea, hypoxemia and right heart decompensation due to alveolar hypoventilation, a consequence of the relative immobility of the obese thorax.

Causes of Obesity

Excessive caloric intake
    Exogenous
    Emotional disorder

Organic diseases
    Hyperadrenocorticism
    Hypothyroidism
    Lawrence-Moon-Biedl-Bardet syndrome
    Pseudohypoparathyroidism
    Prader-Willi syndrome
    CNS injury
    Polycystic ovary syndrome

It is rare for children presenting with obesity to have a serious underlying disorder. The obesity may reflect an emotional problem; although the majority of obese children seem perfectly happy and content, this appearance often belies fundamental concern with body image, family strife or school performance. The possibility of a central nervous system hypothalamic lesion should be considered in children whose obesity begins after meningitis, encephalitis or head injury. Rarely is a patient with hypothyroidism confused with the obese subject. In general, the child with hypothyroidism presents with severe growth retardation. On occasion, however, the hypothyroid child may be seen shortly after the onset of the hypothyroid state; he is distinguished by the clinical symptoms (lethargy, fatigue, cold intolerance, constipation), physical signs (myxedema, delayed relaxation of deep tendon reflexes, bradycardia, low pulse pressure), and laboratory findings (low thyroxine, etc.) of hypothyroidism. The child with hypopituitarism may be slightly obese but is markedly short.

Although exogenously obese children often secrete excessive amounts of glucocorticoids, these levels are appropriate for the increased surface area. The child with Cushing's syndrome has a centripetal distribution of fat, violaceous striae, low-set hair line, increased eyebrow hair; these children are usually short. In early adolescent females with polycystic ovarian disease, obesity may be accompanied by hirsutism and irregular menses. Children with the Prader-Willi syndrome are characterized by severe hypotonia in the neonatal and early infancy periods which gradually improves thereafter; there is an initially difficult feeding pattern with poor weight gain followed at approximately 1 year of age by excessive weight gain and obesity along with hypogenitalism and hypomentia. The incidence of diabetes mellitus in these children is high. Patients with pseudohypoparathyroidism are characterized by classical phenotype (round facies, modest obesity, short stature, brachymetacarpals, brachymetatarsals, submentation) and biochemical abnormalities (hypocalcemia, hyperphosphatemia). Patients with the Lawrence-Moon-Biedl-Bardet syndrome are obese, short, and dull, with hypogonadism, polydactyly and retinitis pigmentosa.

Diagnosis

The diagnosis of exogenous obesity is established by historical and physical findings. The majority of children with regulatory obesity are excessively tall (HA>CA) with weight exceeding height (WA>HA); the bone age is advanced over chronologic age (BA>CA). Additional laboratory studies are not indicated unless other findings suggest the possibility of an underlying disease process.

Management

The management of the obese child is difficult. In the younger child whose diet is controlled by the family, decreased caloric intake may be possible, particularly if one eliminates from the household all foods inappropriate for the child (and usually the rest of the family). If continued rapid weight gain is prevented, the child's future growth will permit redistribution of mass and ultimate loss of obesity without actual weight reduction.

In older children who have achieved adult stature, weight reduction is most difficult to achieve. Dietary restrictions are successful only if the child is an active and willing participant in the prolonged therapeutic process. This requires a mature, thoughtful subject who believes that the long-term rewards of weight reduction are greater than the immediate gains of oral gratification and who is able to withstand the self-inflicted discomfort of decreased caloric intake. Stringent dieting may be accompanied by hyperuricemia which should be specifically monitored. The use of anorexigenic agents is usually without benefit, although these drugs occasionally may reinforce the will to forego immediate gratification for the future rewards of weight reduction. Older children benefit greatly by association with a peer group with similar problems, such as in professional weight reduction groups (Weight Watchers). In patients with the Pickwickian syndrome, immediate weight reduction is mandatory, as this is a life-threatening complication of obesity. Recent attempts at behavior modification by requiring strict recording of all dietary intake, prolonged and thorough mastication of food, and increased duration of meal time seem promising but will require more prolonged evaluation before their ultimate and long-lasting effects are known. Psychiatric counseling is of occasional benefit. In extreme instances, a bowel bypass operation has been recommended as a last resort.

GIGANTISM

Etiology

The mean adult height of males and females in America is increasing gradually due to improved nutrition and the absence of serious diseases during the periods of growth in infancy and childhood. Excessively tall stature is most frequently a consequence of genetic inheritance: tall children are often the offspring of tall parents. This is usually of no consequence to the male, but the excessively tall pre-teenage girl (and her mother) is often concerned about ultimate height. Modestly tall stature is also observed at diagnosis in children with obesity, hyperthyroidism and diabetes mellitus. Marfan's syndrome is an autosomal dominant disorder of mesodermal tissues, characterized by tall stature, long thin fingers and toes (arachnodactyly), subluxation of the lenses and aortic aneurysm. A similar phenotype occurs in patients with homocystinuria. Cerebral gigantism is a sporadic disorder characterized by excessive height and weight, macrocrania, high arched palate, large extremities and mental retardation. Normal sexual development occurs at the appropriate chronologic age. Bone age may be commensurate with chronologic or height age. Infants with the Wiedemann-Beckwith syndrome are large at birth and also have visceromegaly, omphalocoele and hypoglycemia. Rarely does excessive secretion of the pituitary growth hormone, usually associated with a pituitary tumor, cause gigantism and acromegaly characterized by excessive growth (increased deposition of membrane bone in the skull with coarse facial features, enlargement of hands and feet, cardiomegaly, visceromegaly, etc.). These patients are often sexually infantile.

Causes of Gigantism

Genetic tall stature
    Familial
    Obesity
    Hyperthyroidism
    Diabetes mellitus

Disorders associated with excessive stature
    Marfan's syndrome
    Homocystinuria
    Wiedemann-Beckwith syndrome
    Cerebral gigantism
    Growth hormone excess
    Primary hypogonadism
    Sexual precocity

In children with sexual precocity (see Chapter 20) there is excessive linear growth, but bones mature more rapidly than height increases; ultimately these children become short adults unless the process of sexual precocity is terminated. Some patients with primary hypogonadism (Klinefelter's syndrome) display long extremities (the eunuchoid habitus) and are of tall stature.

Diagnosis

The cause of tall stature is frequently apparent after historical review and physical examination. In the genetically tall subject, growth velocity is normal, physical examination is appropriate for age, and bone age is equal to chronologic age. In patients with disorders cited previously the clinical findings are usually sufficiently obvious to alert the examiner. The diagnosis of cerebral gigantism is established on the basis of clinical observations (prognathism, antimongoloid slant to the eyes, depressed nasal bridge, dolicocephaly), absence of a definable pituitary tumor and normal secretion of growth hormone. In patients with acromegalic gigantism, the sella turcica is enlarged and serum concentrations of growth hormone are elevated and often not suppressed by hyperglycemia. The diagnosis of Marfan's syndrome depends upon a positive family history and the presence of typical clinical characteristics. In patients with isosexual precocity, the bone age is markedly advanced and the urinary and plasma levels of gonadotropins and gonadal sex steroids may be elevated.

Management

Males with familial genetic tall stature are reassured as to their basic good health. Attempts to foreshorten excessively tall females by estrogen administration have been advocated. Estrogens accelerate the rate of bone age maturation to a greater extent than the attendant increase in linear growth velocity and height age. The efficacy of this therapy is questionable. In the authors' clinic the use of estrogens in such females is restricted to those whose predicted adult height is 6 feet or above. For greatest efficacy these medications should be initiated between 8 and 10 years of age and continued until the bone age has reached 14–15 years. The attendant hazards of such therapy (excessive vaginal bleeding and potential injury to the delicate hypothalamic-pituitary-ovarian axis) must be appreciated.

There is no specific treatment for patients with cerebral gigantism or Marfan's syndrome. Although neurosurgical removal of the growth hormone-secreting pituitary tumor has been advocated in patients with cerebral gigantism, the recent identification of hypothalamic growth hormone-release inhibiting factor (somatostatin) suggests that medical therapy for this abnormality may become feasible. Management of the child with sexual precocity or hypogonadism is discussed in Chapter 20.

BIBLIOGRAPHY

Brasel, J. A., and Blizzard, R. M.: The influence of the endocrine glands upon growth and development. *In* Williams, R. H. (ed.): Textbook of Endocrinology, 5th Ed. Philadelphia, W. B. Saunders, 1974; pp. 1030–1058.

> The authors present a comprehensive discussion of the influence of the endocrine system upon normal growth and illustrate the aberrations of growth which may occur in patients with varied endocrinopathies.

Green, M., and Richmond, J. B.: Pediatric Diagnosis, 2nd ed., Philadelphia, W. B. Saunders, 1962; pp. 230–235.

> This reference lists causes of aberrations of growth and the evaluation and management of these abnormalities with little descriptive text.

Root, A. W., Bongiovanni, A. M., and Eberlein, W. R.: Diagnosis and management of growth retardation with special reference to the problem of hypopituitarism. J. Pediatr., 78:737–753, 1971.

> This article discusses the problem of retardation of linear growth and presents clinical and laboratory data on patients with hypopituitarism.

Sobel, E. H.: Abnormal growth patterns in childhood. Organic disorders interfering with somatic growth. *In* Gardner, L. I. (ed.): Endocrine and Genetic Diseases of Childhood. Philadelphia, W. B. Saunders, 1969; pp. 60–76.

The chapter discusses the organic diseases which interfere with normal growth, presenting interesting clinical illustrations of potentially enigmatic problems.

Supported by National Foundation—March of Dimes Grants 1-323, C-199, and Basil O'Connor Starter Grant 5-71.

20

Normal and Abnormal Sexual Development

Mary L. Voorhess, M.D.

Sexual development in the human can be divided into two stages: (1) embryonic sexual differentiation and (2) pubertal sexual maturation. These two processes are usually uneventful, but abnormalities sometimes occur primarily because the sex primordia have the potential to differentiate into either male or female structures and because control of the onset and timing of pubertal maturation involves complex neuroendocrine control mechanisms. Human sexual anomalies may involve the gonads, the ductal structures or the external genitalia. We do not understand the pathogenesis of all the various defects.

EMBRYONIC SEXUAL DIFFERENTIATION

Embryonic sexual differentiation involves (1) differentiation of the primordial gonads, (2) differentiation and development of the gonaducts, and (3) formation of the external genitalia.

In man, the primitive gonad of both sexes is identical in appearance until seven weeks of embryonic life when testicular development begins under control of the Y chromosome. The H-Y histocompatibility antigen found in tissues of males may be the product of the Y chromosomal gene which induces testicular differentiation. Except in rare instances, two X chromosomes are required for ovarian differentiation which does not begin until about 12 weeks of gestation. The first follicles appear in the ovary after the sixteenth week of development.

Male and female genital ducts arise from duct primordia early in fetal life, and both are present together for a time in the embryo. Each is unipotential, and normal development involves persistence of the homologous pair and regression of the other except for vestigial structures.

244

In the male, Wolffian ducts form the vas deferens, seminal vesicles and epididymis, and the Mullerian ducts regress. In the female, the Mullerian ducts differentiate into the fallopian tubes, the uterus and the upper portion of the vagina, and the Wolffian ducts regress. Fetal testicular hormones are essential for differentiation of male sexual structures and for regression of the Mullerian ducts. There are two substances: (1) Mullerian duct-inhibiting factor secreted by the Sertoli cells which acts locally and causes regression of the Mullerian ducts, and (2) testosterone, secreted by fetal Leydig cells, which directly stimulates growth of the male gonaducts and is the prohormone for dihydrotestosterone. Conversion of testosterone to dihydrotestosterone is necessary for formation of male external genitalia. Female differentiation does not depend on the presence of a functioning fetal gonad, and it occurs, irrespective of chromosomal sex, when fetal testicular hormones are absent.

The external genitalia develop from the urogenital sinus and neutral primordia which give rise to homologous structures in both sexes. In the female, the genital tubercle gives rise to the clitoris, the urethral folds to the labia minora, and the labioscrotal folds form the labia majora. In the male, the genital tubercle develops into the corpora cavernosa and glans of the penis; the urethral folds form the perineal and penile urethra and the corpus spongiosum; and the labioscrotal folds fuse in the midline to form the scrotum and the ventral covering of the penis. Differentiation of the urogenital sinus and genital primordia in the male is a continuous process which begins posteriorly, extends anteriorly, and depends on the action of dihydrotestosterone. Fusion of the urethral and labioscrotal folds takes place before the twelfth week of fetal life while phallic enlargement occurs throughout intrauterine life under influence of androgenic hormones. In contrast, development of female external genitalia occurs when there is absence of androgenic stimulation. The female fetus may develop varying degrees of masculinization of the lower genital tract, however, when exposed to androgenic substances during critical periods of embryonic differentiation, but these compounds have no effect on differentiation of the gonaducts.

ABNORMALITIES IN SEXUAL DIFFERENTIATION

Abnormalities of sexual differentiation may result from a variety of factors, intrinsic and extrinsic, which interfere with one or another of the stages in embryonic development. Such factors include: (1) sex chromosomal abnormalities which affect gonadogenesis, (2) defects in testosterone and dihydrotestosterone biosynthesis, (3) end-organ insensitivity to action of androgenic hormones, (4) exposure of the fetus to androgens and progestogens from the maternal circulation, (5) defects in corticosteroid biosynthesis, and (6) unexplained causes.

There is no classification of abnormalities of sexual differentiation in the human which meets all needs, but it is convenient to group the disorders clinically into general categories on the basis of gonadal sex as listed in Table 20-1.

Female Pseudohermaphrodism

Individuals with female pseudohermaphrodism have normal ovaries and normal Mullerian duct differentiation (normal fallopian tubes, uterus and upper vagina). The abnormality in sexual differentiation is limited

Table 20-1. Abnormalities of Sexual Differentiation

Classification	Gonads	Sex chromatin	Sex chromo-somes	External genitalia	Gona-ducts	Secondary sexual development
Female pseudo-hermaphrodism due to						
Virilizing adrenal hyperplasia	Ovaries	Positive*	XX	Varying degrees of clitoral enlargement and fusion of labial scrotal folds	Female	Marked virilization if untreated
Maternal androgen or progestogen	Ovaries	Positive	XX		Female	Female
Other	Ovaries	Positive	XX		Female	Female
Male pseudo-hermaphrodism						
With female external genitalia	Testes	Negative	XY	Female with blind vaginal pouch. Occasional clitoral enlargement.	Usually male	Female with primary amenorrhea and sparse or absent sexual hair
With ambiguous or male genitalia	Testes or streak gonads	Negative	XY or XO/XY	Small to large phallus and variable fusion of scrotal folds	Variable	Male or female
True hermaphrodite	Ovary and testis or ovo-testes	Positive or negative	XX or XY or XX/XY	Ambiguous, male or female	Variable	Male or female
Syndrome of gonadal dysgenesis	Streak gonads	Negative or low percentage of positive†	XO, XO/XY XX/XO or other abnor-malities	Usually female. Slight clitoral enlargement rare.	Female	Infantile
Seminiferous tubular dysgenesis	Small testes	Positive	XXY, XXYY and other abnor-malities	Male	Male	Male with occasional gynecomastia and eunuchoidism

*20–35% of cells contain nuclear chromatin mass
†About 8–15% of cells contain nuclear chromatin mass

to the distal vagina and external genitalia when varying degrees of labioscrotal fusion and/or clitoral enlargement are found. In almost all cases, the disorder results from exposure of the female fetus to androgenic hormones, the degree of masculinization depending on the potency of the androgen and the stage of fetal development when exposure occurs. Labioscrotal fusion indicates that there was androgenic activity prior to 12–13 fetal weeks; by this time female differentiation of the external genitalia is completed. Often, this fusion extends anteriorly with enclosure of the urogenital sulcus so that there is a single perineal opening and the urethral and vaginal orifices are obscured. Clitoral hypertrophy results from androgen stimulation at any stage of intrauterine development or after birth.

Because congenital virilizing adrenal hyperplasia is the most common cause of female pseudohermaphrodism, it is appropriate, from a clinical point of view, to group the disorders into adrenal and non-adrenal causes. Adrenal includes congenital virilizing adrenal hyperplasia. There are three types of non-adrenal causes. The first is fetal virilization induced by maternal androgen: (1) when compounds with androgenic activity were administered to mothers during pregnancy; and (2) when there is a maternal virilizing tumor. The second and third types of non-adrenal causes are fetal virilization associated with abnormalities of the genitourinary and gastrointestinal tract, and fetal virilization of unknown cause.

Congenital Virilizing Adrenal Hyperplasia

This disorder is caused by a biochemical error in adrenocortical biosynthesis, the result being cortisol deficiency, an increase in ACTH production, adrenal cortical hyperplasia and overproduction of intermediary steroid metabolites and androgens. The most common form of the disorder is due to a deficiency of 21-hydroxylase enzyme with or without salt loss; a less common defect is deficiency of 11-hydroxylase enzyme. If the affected female fetus is exposed to excessive adrenal androgen before the twelfth fetal week, there are varying degrees of masculinization of the external genitalia manifested by labioscrotal fusion, a urogenital sinus and clitoral hypertrophy. The vaginal orifice and urinary meatus usually are found within the perineal opening of the urogenital sinus. Mullerian duct development is not influenced by adrenal androgen, so fallopian tubes, uterus and upper vagina are normal, as are the ovaries. Males with congenital virilizing adrenal hyperplasia have normal external genitalia, except in the very rare 3-beta-hydroxysteroid dehydrogenase deficiency where there is defective synthesis of fetal testicular hormones and, thus, incomplete masculinization of the urogenital sinus and neutral primordia.

Clinical Findings. The appearance of ambiguous genitalia at birth usually leads to prompt identification of females with congenital virilizing

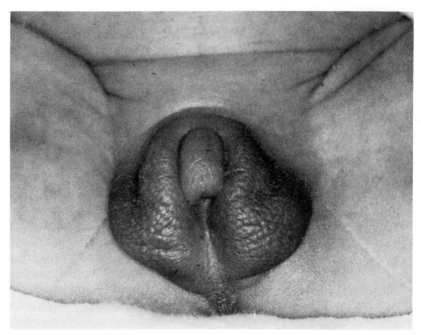

Fig. 20-1. External genitalia of a newborn girl with salt/losing congenital virilizing adrenal hyperplasia. (Reproduced with permission. From Schlegel, R. J., and Gardner, L. I.: Ambiguous and abnormal genitalia in infants. *In* Gardner, L. I. (ed.): Endocrine and Genetic Diseases of Childhood and Adolescence, ed. 2. Philadelphia, W. B. Saunders Co., 1975.)

adrenal hyperplasia. In severely affected individuals, virilization of the genitalia may be so marked that the newborn girls are mistakenly thought to be males with bilateral cryptorchidism with or without hypospadias. The enlarged phallus is similar to a penis and is bound down in chordee, the urogenital sinus resembles a perineal hypospadias, and the empty labioscrotal folds have the appearance of bifid scrotum with cryptorchidism (Fig. 20-1). Neonates with such external genitalia should have an immediate buccal smear to determine their sex chromatin pattern and a chromosome analysis. Individuals with two X chromosomes in their cells have a nuclear chromatin mass in 20–35 per cent of their cells and are said to be sex chromatin positive. When the pattern is positive, the diagnostic possibilities are limited to female pseudohermaphrodism or true hermaphrodism. Since the most common cause of female pseudohermaphrodism is congenital virilizing adrenal hyperplasia, immediate steps should be taken to establish a diagnosis to avoid the danger of an unrecognized salt-losing form of the disorder. No less urgent is the need to determine the appropriate sex assignment for the neonate.

Because their genitalia are normal at birth, males with non-salt losing congenital virilizing adrenal hyperplasia often are not suspected of having the disorder until they are several years old. By then, the excessive production of androgenic steroids has caused acceleration in the rate of somatic growth and progressive virilization with growth of sexual hair, enlargement of the penis, acne and deepening of the voice. The testes usually remain small, however.

Both male and female neonates with the salt-losing form of the disorder have difficulties early in life. Weight gain is poor. Vomiting and severe dehydration develop shortly after birth, and sudden death may occur unless prompt treatment is given. The symptoms resemble an Addisonian crisis.

Patients with the C-11 hydroxylase enzyme defect also have virilization, and they develop hypertension due to production of excessive amounts of desoxycorticosterone.

Diagnosis. Nearly all individuals with congenital virilizing adrenal hyperplasia excrete excessive amounts of 17-ketosteroids in their urine. In addition, the urine of patients with the 21-hydroxylase enzyme deficiency contains abnormally large amounts of pregnanetriol, and their plasma has a high concentration of 17-hydroxyprogesterone. Measurement of plasma 17-hydroxyprogesterone is a particularly helpful diagnostic test in identifying affected neonates since the analysis can be done rapidly without a 24-hour delay for a urine collection. In the hypertensive form of the disease, excessive quantities of tetrahydro compounds derived from 11-desoxycortisol appear in the urine. Following administration of cortisol, the excretion of these compounds falls to the normal range. Patients with the salt-losing form of the disease also have low serum sodium and high serum potassium levels before treatment.

Individuals with non-adrenal causes of female pseudohermaphrodism have normal urinary adrenocorticosteroid excretion and normal plasma 17-OH progesterone levels.

Treatment. The principle of therapy in congenital virilizing adrenal hyperplasia is to provide physiological doses of cortisol for the patient. This inhibits ACTH overproduction because of the negative feedback mechanism and prevents accumulation of steroid metabolites with androgenic and hypertensive properties. Patients with the salt-losing form of the disorder also must receive desoxycorticosterone to correct their electrolyte disturbance. Following treatment, the pattern of urinary adrenal steroid excretion becomes normal. Progressive virilization ceases, and the child grows normally.

In addition to steroid therapy, most affected girls need perineoplasty to correct the abnormalities of their external genitalia. Usually, a clitoridectomy or clitoral recession procedure is done during the first year of life together with exteriorization of the urinary meatus and vaginal orifice. Vaginal reconstruction may be necessary later in life. Because congenital virilizing adrenal hyperplasia is an autosomal recessive disorder, appropriate genetic counseling of the family is an important part of therapy.

Non-Adrenal Fetal Virilization

Maternal Androgen and Progestogen. Sometimes progestational steroids with androgenic activity are given to mothers during pregnancy to conserve the products of conception after threatened abortion or habitual abortion. Placental transfer of the androgenic compounds occurs, and varying degrees of masculinization of the external genitalia of the female fetus may take place, the severity depending on the dose of medication, duration of therapy and stage of pregnancy. If the drug is administered prior to the thirteenth week of fetal life, varying degrees of labioscrotal fusion occur. Clitoral enlargement may result from androgenic stimulation at any time during gestation. Steroids such as 17 a-ethynyl-19 nortestosterone (Norlutin), norethindrone with mestranol (Orthonovum), norethynodrel (Enovid) and testosterone have been implicated. It is rare for a virilizing ovarian tumor in a pregnant women to cause a similar picture.

When female pseudohermaphrodism is caused by maternal androgen, urinary steroid excretion of the infant is normal, and progressive virilization does not occur since the baby is separated at birth from the source of androgen. Surgical correction of the genital abnormalities may be necessary in selected cases.

Congenital Abnormalities. Some female neonates have ambiguous genitalia and varying congenital abnormalities of the genitourinary or gastrointestinal tract such as absent fallopian tubes, rudimentary uterus, rectovaginal fistula or absent vagina.

On buccal smear, 20–35 per cent of the cells contain a nuclear chromatin mass, the sex chromosome pattern is XX and adrenocorticosteroid excretion is normal. Abdominal laparotomy may be necessary to check the reproductive organs and define any structural abnormalities. The etiology of these disorders is obscure.

Male Pseudohermaphrodism

Affected individuals have gonads identified histologically as testes and varying abnormalities of the gonaduct system and external genitalia. Their sex chromatin pattern is negative, and their sex chromosomal constitution includes a Y chromosome. There may be unilateral or bilateral cryptorchidism, hypospadias, hypoplastic scrotum and penis, or the external genitalia may have a female appearance while the internal duct structures are male. The testes may be located in the pelvis, in the inguinal area or in the labioscrotal folds. The various abnormalities are due most likely to failure of the fetal testes to produce appropriate Mullerian duct-inhibiting factor, defects in testosterone or dihydrotestosterone synthesis or to impaired end organ response to fetal androgens.

There is no satisfactory way to classify the varieties of male pseudohermaphrodism. It is clinically practical to divide the patients into two general groups: (1) those with female-appearing external genitalia with or without clitoral enlargement, and (2) those with predominantly masculine or ambiguous external genitalia.

Female External Genitalia with or without Clitoral Enlargement

Individuals with this type of male pseudohermaphrodism (the Syndrome of Testicular Feminization) usually are not identified at birth because they have a female phenotypic appearance and are given a female sex assignment. Diagnosis is made later in life when testicular tissue is discovered in a hernial sac or when an XY sex chromosome pattern is discovered during evaluation of primary amenorrhea.

Clinical Findings. The external genitalia are female in appearance, but there may be some clitoromegaly and posterior fusion of the labioscrotal folds. Occasionally, testes are palpable in the inguinal region or in the labia. The vagina characteristically ends as a blind pouch. There usually is no cervix or uterus present. At puberty, estrogens, secreted by the testes, cause feminization of the body habitus, breast development and estrinization of the vaginal mucosa, but menarche does not take place. Pubic and axillary hair are sparse or absent.

Because affected patients have testes and a female phenotype, this disorder often is called the syndrome of testicular feminization. It is thought to be caused by a mutant gene that is transmitted as a sex-linked recessive or a sex-linked autosomal dominant; if this is so, more than one case may occur in a family. The syndrome results from a defect in the ability of testosterone and dihydrotestosterone to bind to the cytoplasmic receptor in the cell, so androgen action does not occur. Thus, there is failure of normal male differentiation of the external genitalia and failure of end organ response to testicular androgens at puberty. Most patients have plasma testosterone levels in the normal range for males. Urinary estrogen levels may be in the high normal range for males or in the female range. Since the hypothalamic feedback mechanism also is unresponsive to testosterone, luteinizing hormone (LH) levels are high, but follicle-stimulating hormone (FSH) concentration usually is normal.

Incomplete variants of the syndrome have been described with partial masculinization of the affected patient, presumably due to a partial defect at the cytoplasmic receptor. Varying degrees of clitoromegaly and posterior fusion of the labioscrotal folds are present in these cases.

Treatment. Malignant degeneration may occur in the gonads of patients with the syndrome of testicular feminization, but the true incidence is not known. It increases with advancing age, so most physicians

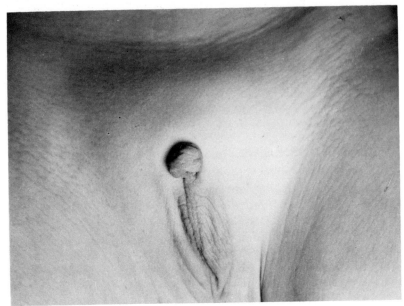

Fig. 20-2. Incomplete masculinization of the external genitalia in a 4½-year-old boy. The phallus and gonads are markedly hypoplastic.

recommend gonadectomy after the second decade of life. Prior to that age, there is no general agreement as to whether surgical removal of the gonads should be done at the time of diagnosis or after breast development has occurred at puberty. Subsequent to gonadectomy, breast atrophy and menopausal symptoms are treated with estrogen. Because there is end organ insensitivity to androgen, testosterone administration will not induce sexual hair growth.

Ambiguous or Masculine Genitalia

Clinical Findings. Usually, ambiguous genitalia bring these patients to medical attention. A variety of defects in development may be found, some resulting in mild hypospadias and a normal phallus while others are associated with such marked alteration in anatomical structures that sex assignment at birth is difficult (Fig. 20-2). Not only can the external genitalia be ambiguous, but some patients have complete Mullerian duct development with uterus and fallopian tubes while others have rudimentary genital ducts. Karyotype usually is XY, although XO/XY mosaicism has been described. Dysgenetic gonads or streak gonads may be present, and some patients have the somatic stigmata of Turner's syndrome.

Diagnosis. Male pseudohermaphrodism with anomalous development of the external genitalia may be found in association with: (1) disorders of testicular differentiation due to abnormalities involving the Y chromosome; (2) disorders of testicular function due to errors in biosynthesis of testosterone (17 α-hydroxylase, 20,22 demolase or 3 β-0H dehydrogenase enzyme deficiencies) and to disorders of Mullerian duct inhibiting factor; (3) abnormalities in testosterone metabolism such as reduced 5 α-reductase activity with resultant dihydrotestosterone deficiency; (4) other unidentified factors. Because some of these defects are transmitted as autosomal or X-linked traits, more than one affected member may occur in a family.

Injection of x-ray contrast media into the urogenital sinus and pelvic laparotomy usually are necessary to define the derivatives of the genital ducts. Detailed biochemical studies must be performed to define the various errors in steroid hormone synthesis and metabolism. Sex of rearing is determined by the functional capacity of the external genitalia.

Treatment. Reconstructive surgery of the external genitalia is performed appropriate to the sex assignment, and dysgenetic gonads are removed because of their malignant potential. Testosterone or other androgen therapy is prescribed as necessary to enhance masculine development. Extensive psychosocial counseling of parents and patients is an essential part of therapy from the onset whenever severe genital abnormalities are present. The obstetrician, pediatrician, surgeon, endocrinologist and psychological counselor should work closely as a team in providing for the needs of the patient and his family.

TRUE HERMAPHRODISM

These individuals have both an ovary and a testis or, more commonly, two ovotestes. Most have an ambiguous phallus with hypospadias or nearly normal-appearing male genitalia. Completely normal female external genitalia rarely are found. Breast development and menstrual periods may occur at puberty.

About two-thirds of true hermaphrodites are sex chromatin positive, and one-third are sex chromatin negative even though an XX sex chromosomal pattern in peripheral leukocytes is much more common than an XY constitution. Occasionally, a mosaic sex chromosome pattern is found.

After the sex of rearing has been selected, an effort should be made to preserve the appropriate gonad and remove the inappropriate one. The external genitalia should be reconstructed, as necessary, consistent with the sex assignment.

THE SYNDROME OF GONADAL DYSGENESIS

Clinical Findings

The first description of this disorder was reported in 1938 by Dr. Henry Turner and included seven short, sexually infantile girls with similar congenital anomalies including webbed neck and cubitus valgus deformity. Since then, a host of abnormalities has been described in affected individuals as listed below. The clinical features are so distinctive that diagnosis usually is suspected strongly before confirmation by chromosomal analysis (Fig. 20-3). This is particularly true in the neonatal period when lymphedema of hands and feet and extra skin folds in the neck are hallmarks of the syndrome of gonadal dysgenesis.

Typically, affected individuals have a short, husky build with broad shoulders. Pubic and axillary hair often appear at puberty, but there is lack of breast development and menarche because no true gonads are present. The external genitalia are normal but infantile in appearance. Fallopian tubes, uterus and vagina are present.

Clinical Features of the Syndrome of Gonadal Dysgenesis

Short stature
Low set ears
Hypoplastic mandible—high arched palate
Webbed neck
Low hair line, posteriorly
Shield chest—widely spaced nipples
Coarctation of aorta—20%
Renal anomalies—25% (especially horseshoe kidney)
Increased carrying angle—arms
Brachymetacarpelia
Lymphedema of hands and feet
Deeply set fingernails and toenails
Hypoplastic nails
Multiple nevi of skin
Mental retardation, 15–20%
Sexual infantilism

Diagnosis

The sex chromatin pattern usually is negative and chromosomal analysis reveals a total count of 45 with a single X chromosome. But sex chromosomal mosaicism, such as XX/XO, and structural abnormalities of the X chromosomes also may occur. In these cases, the phenotypic expression of the disorder is varied, and somatic abnormalities may be much less severe than those seen in monosomy X (Fig. 20-4). Sometimes a modest degree of feminization occurs during adolescence and, rarely,

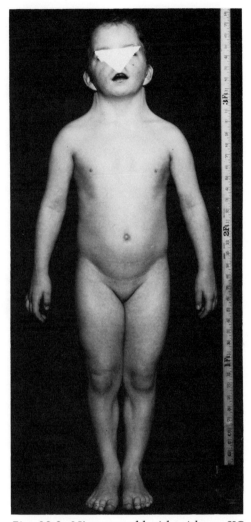

Fig. 20-3. Nine-year-old girl with an XO sex chromosomal pattern and gonadal dysgenesis including coarctation of the aorta. (Reproduced with permission. From Neu, R. L., and Gardner, L. I.: Abnormalities of the sex chromosomes. *In* Gardner, L. I. (Ed.): Endocrine and Genetic Diseases of Childhood and Adolescence, ed. 2. Philadelphia, W. B. Saunders Co., 1975.)

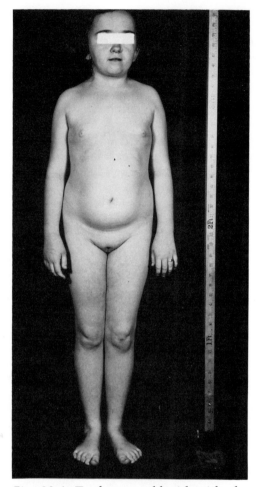

Fig. 20-4. Twelve-year-old girl with the syndrome of gonadal dysgenesis and XX/XO mosaicism. Buccal smear contained 14 per cent chromatin positive cells.

affected girls have menstrual periods. Patients with sex chromosomal mosaicism usually do not have a negative sex chromatin pattern but 8–15 per cent chromatin-positive cells on buccal smear. XO/XY mosaicism rarely is found, and this is associated often with abnormalities of the external genitalia as well as the stigmata described above. Before age 11–12 years, bone age is compatible with chronological age or slightly retarded. At the age of adolescence, pituitary gonadotrophins rise to high levels due to end organ (ovarian) failure. Estrogen levels are low, and adrenal steroid excretion is normal. Plasma growth hormone levels usually are normal.

Females with the somatic stigmata of Turner's syndrome who have a positive sex chromatin pattern, 46 chromosomes with an XX sex chromosome pattern and normal ovarian function (Noonan's syndrome), have been described. Congenital heart disease with atrial septal defect and/or pulmonic stenosis is common. The origin of this disorder is not known, but it may be transmitted as an autosomal dominant.

Treatment

Treatment of girls with the syndrome of gonadal dysgenesis includes correction of somatic anomalies, feminization with estrogen and progesterone at the age of puberty and psychosocial support. Sometimes, intermittent courses of anabolic steroids are prescribed in late childhood to enhance linear growth.

SEMINIFEROUS TUBULAR DYSGENESIS

In 1942, Klinefelter, Reifenstein and Albright described a syndrome in males which is characterized by small, firm testes, hyalinization of the seminiferous tubules with absent spermatogenesis but normal Leydig cells, increased secretion of follicle-stimulating hormone and gynecomastia. Affected individuals are said to have Klinefelter's syndrome. They usually have a eunuchoid build at puberty, subnormal virilization and a high incidence of mental retardation and emotional disturbance.

Approximately 75 per cent of patients have a positive sex chromatin pattern and a total chromosome count of 47 with an XXY or XY/XXY sex chromosome pattern. The extra chromosome is thought to arise from meiotic non-disjunction in either parent. Others with the Klinefelter phenotype are chromatin negative and have a normal XY sex chromosome pattern. The cause of the syndrome in these patients is not known.

Treatment

Where there is deficient virilization at adolescence, treatment with androgens is helpful. Cosmetic surgery may be necessary to correct severe gynecomastia and to improve body image. Psychosocial counseling of patients and parents is an important part of the medical care.

GUIDELINES TO DIAGNOSIS OF ABNORMALITIES OF SEXUAL DIFFERENTIATION

It is important that any abnormality of sexual differentiation be recognized and correctly diagnosed as soon after birth as possible so that the proper sex of rearing can be assigned and so that appropriate treatment is initiated. The etiology of an abnormality cannot be determined from

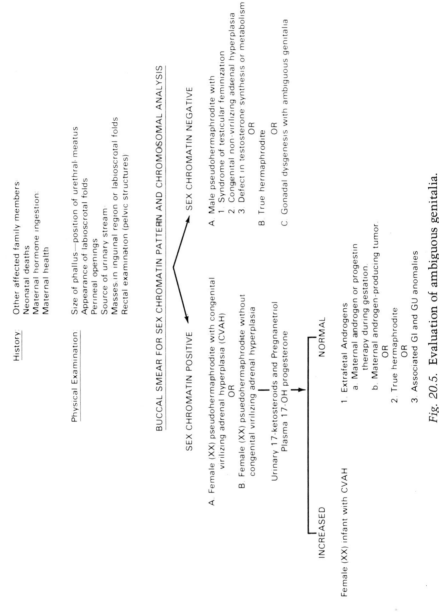

History:
Other affected family members
Neonatal deaths
Maternal hormone ingestion
Maternal health

Physical Examination
Size of phallus—position of urethral meatus
Appearance of labioscrotal folds
Perineal openings
Source of urinary stream
Masses in inguinal region or labioscrotal folds
Rectal examination (pelvic structures)

BUCCAL SMEAR FOR SEX CHROMATIN PATTERN AND CHROMOSOMAL ANALYSIS

SEX CHROMATIN POSITIVE

A. Female (XX) pseudohermaphrodite with congenital
   virilizing adrenal hyperplasia (CVAH)
   OR
B. Female (XX) psuedohermaphrodite without
   congenital virilizing adrenal hyperplasia

Urinary 17-ketosteroids and Pregnanetriol
Plasma 17-OH progesterone

INCREASED   NORMAL

Female (XX) infant with CVAH

1. Extrafetal Androgens
   a. Maternal androgen or progestin
      therapy during gestation.
   b. Maternal androgen-producing tumor.
      OR
2. True hermaphrodite
   OR
3. Associated GI and GU anomalies

SEX CHROMATIN NEGATIVE

A. Male pseudohermaphrodite with
   1. Syndrome of testicular feminization
   2. Congenital non-virilizing adrenal hyperplasia
   3. Defect in testosterone synthesis or metabolism
      OR
B. True hermaphrodite
      OR
C. Gonadal dysgenesis with ambiguous genitalia

Fig. 20.5. **Evaluation of ambiguous genitalia.**

history and physical findings alone. Diagnostic studies should be carried out. Some disorders such as the syndrome of testicular feminization and Klinefelter's syndrome often are not suspected until the adolescent years when normal pubertal development fails to take place.

An abnormality of sexual development should be suspected when the following situations are present: (1) ambiguous external genitalia, (2) phenotypical males with bilateral cryptorchidism, (3) phenotypic females with masses in groin or labia, (4) congenital edema of hands and feet and extra skin folds in neck of a newborn female, (5) primary amenorrhea in adolescent female with breast development and decreased or absent sexual hair, (6) gynecomastia and small testes in adolescent male, (7) phenotypic females with short stature and other stigmata of gonadal dysgenesis, and (8) sibling with a disorder of sexual differentiation.

Figure 20-5 outlines a plan for evaluating infants with abnormal external genitalia. It is particularly important to recognize female neonates with ambiguous genitalia and congenital virilizing adrenal hyperplasia to ensure appropriate assignment of sex and to avoid the risk of a salt-losing crisis. Determination of the sex chromatin pattern in cells from the buccal mucosa is an excellent screening test which can be performed quickly and which provides indirect information about the sex chromosomal constitution. Thus, a practical scheme can be based on classification of patients into chromatin-positive and chromatin-negative groups. Chromatin-positive patients with abnormal genitalia should be considered females with virilizing adrenal hyperplasia until proven otherwise.

A careful history from the parents and the obstetrician is an important aid in diagnosis. Since virilizing adrenal hyperplasia is an autosomal recessive disorder, the history may reveal that a sibling died early in infancy with dehydration and collapse (a possible salt-losing crisis), that siblings were born with abnormal genitalia, or that siblings had progressive virilization during childhood. Information about medications taken by the mother during pregnancy may suggest that virilization of the neonate is related to maternal hormone ingestion. It is rare for masculinization of a female offspring to be due to transplacental passage of androgen from a maternal tumor.

Systemic inspection and palpation of the external genitalia including a rectal examination are an integral part of the evaluation. Masses in the inguinal area or labioscrotal folds usually are testes or ovotestes that suggest a diagnosis of male pseudohermaphrodism or true hermaphrodism. Neonates with phallic enlargement, fusion of the labioscrotal folds, a single perineal opening and no palpable gonads most likely are female pseudohermaphrodites. Sometimes a uterus can be felt on rectal examination.

Determination of the sex chromatin pattern and chromosomal analysis will help distinguish male from female pseudohermaphrodites. Patients with virilizing adrenal hyperplasia have high urinary 17-ketosteroid and pregnanetriol excretion as well as increased concentration of plasma 17-OH progesterone. A history of maternal progestin ingestion during pregnancy does not negate consideration of a diagnosis of adrenal hyperplasia unless hormone levels are normal since pregnant mothers who are carrying babies with adrenal hyperplasia may have taken progestin.

Most patients with a chromatin-negative buccal smear and ambiguous genitalia will need to have a laparotomy to ascertain the pelvic contents and to biopsy the gonads. Urethroscopy and injection of contrast media in the urogenital sinus are necessary to help identify structures and abnormal communications.

GENERAL MANAGEMENT

Usually, chromosomal sex, gonadal sex, sex hormones, the gonaducts and the external genitalia are consistent with each other, and assignment of sex at birth is easy. When abnormalities are present, the physician has the responsibility to evaluate the problem carefully, make a diagnosis as soon as possible and be sure that the patient is assigned an appropriate sex of rearing. Then, serious psychosocial problems will be obviated for the patient and the parents.

Female pseudohermaphrodites should be reared as females, and the genital defects should be corrected, if necessary, by surgery during infancy. Patients with congenital virilizing adrenal hyperplasia need corticosteroid therapy as well.

Male pseudohermaphrodites should be assigned a sex of rearing appropriate to the functional capacity of the external genitalia. When the phallus is markedly hypoplastic or the external genitalia resemble female anatomy making reconstruction of male structures impossible, the individual should be reared as a female. The genitalia should be made to conform to the assigned sex as early in life as possible. If the gonads are not consistent with the expected secondary development at puberty, surgical excision will be necessary.

Psychosexual orientation is not due to chromosomal sex, gonadal sex or sex hormones but is the result of the gender role and life experiences of an individual. If the child is raised in the gender role for which he is best suited and there is no uncertainty in the mind of the parents and the physician about the sex assignment, there need be no psychosexual problems or abnormal sexual behavior.

PUBERTAL SEXUAL MATURATION

Puberty is that stage of development which is characterized by acceleration of somatic growth, appearance of secondary sexual characteristics and attainment of reproductive capacity. It involves maturational changes in the extrahypothalamic central nervous system, the hypothalamus, the pituitary, the gonads and the target organs for sex steroids.

ONSET OF PUBERTY

Much is known about the hormonal changes that accompany puberty, but relatively little is known about the control of its onset. Present evidence suggests that there is a change in sensitivity of the hypothalamic "gonadostat" to circulating sex steroids.[2] During the prepubertal years, small amounts of gonadotropins are secreted by the pituitary gland; the serum concentrations of estradiol and testosterone are low, and the negative feedback (inhibitory) effect of gonadal sex steroids on the hypothalamic-pituitary axis is active. Smaller amounts of estrogen and testosterone are required to suppress gonadotropin release than in the mature adult. As maturity takes place, there is decreasing sensitivity to circulating gonadal steroid feedback suppression, the result being an increase in the discharge of gonadotropin releasing factor, an increase in the secretion of luteinizing hormone (LH) and/or follicle stimulating hormone (FSH), and subsequent secretion of sex hormones by the ovary or the testis. As the quantity of gonadal steroids increases, pubertal development ensues. Finally, the gonadal hormones themselves are capable of further stimulating the hypothalamic-pituitary axis to secrete gonadotropins (positive feedback). This positive feedback control is particularly important in the female for ovulation.

The factor(s) which regulate the change in sensitivity of the hypothalamic "gonadostat" are not well understood in the human. Since a critical body weight and skeletal maturation correlate well with pubertal development, it is possible that somatic maturity influences the change in set point of the hypothalamic receptor sites. It is of interest that the female skeleton is somewhat more advanced than the male throughout childhood, and pubertal development occurs earlier in girls than in boys. Extrahypothalamic centers such as the cerebral cortex, amygdala, the pineal or the diencephalon and the chemical neurotransmitters (Dopamine, Norepinephrine, and serotonin) also may exert control on the timing of puberty.

CHANGES OF PUBERTY

FEMALES

As puberty approaches, the levels of estrogens increase and bring about development of the nipples and mammary ducts, stimulate growth of the uterus and vagina and enhance linear growth and skeletal maturation.

Production of adrenal androgens increases, and these compounds stimulate growth of pubic and axillary hair, contribute to oily skin and seborrhea and also accelerate the rate of linear growth and skeletal maturation. The mechanism that leads to this increased secretion of adrenal androgen is not precisely known, but it probably is mediated through the anterior pituitary since it is absent in children with hypopituitarism.

Menarche occurs when sufficient estrogen has been produced to cause proliferation of the uterine mucosa. The cyclic vaginal bleeding which occurs during the reproductive years is related to a cyclic pattern of gonadotropin and ovarian steroid production. Besides the negative or inhibitory feedback mechanism by which changes in the concentrations of circulating sex steroids cause reciprocal changes in secretion of gonadotropin-releasing hormones and gonadotropins, there is a positive or stimulating feedback mechanism in which a critical level of circulating estrogen results in synchronous release of LH and FSH. The negative feedback mechanism is functional in prepubertal children and adults, but the positive feedback mechanism does not appear until late puberty and continues during adulthood. It is this positive feedback that causes the LH surge which leads to ovulation.

There is considerable individual variation in the age of onset of secondary sexual characteristics, in the rate of progression of the changes of puberty and in the temporal relation of one event to another. In order to recognize an abnormal pattern of development, the physician must have a knowledge of the sequential changes which occur in healthy children. The stages of female breast development and pubic hair growth as classified by Tanner are listed in Tables 20-2 and 20-3 together with the estimated mean ages at which each stage was reached based on a study of 192 white British girls. The standards for breast development are shown in Figure 20-6, and the standards for pubic hair ratings are shown in Figure 20-7. The first sign of puberty (either breast or pubic hair growth) appeared between the age of 8.5 years and 13 years in 95 per cent of girls. The interval from the first sign of puberty to complete maturity varied from 1.5 years to over 6 years. The mean interval from the beginning of breast development to menarche was 2.3 ± 0.1 years, but the range observed was 6 months to 5 years, 9 months. Menarche occurred at mean age 13.47 ± 1.02 years. All the girls had passed the peak of their height spurt before menstruation began. Menarche was best correlated with skeletal maturation and occurred between bone ages 12.0 and 14.5. There was no apparent relationship between skeletal maturation and breast development, pubic hair growth or peak growth spurt.

The appearance of secondary sexual characteristics varies from population to population depending on many factors including inheritance, socioeconomic factors and geography. The trend toward earlier onset of maturity and an increase in adult height probably is due to improved

Table 20-2. Stages of Breast Development

Tanner stage	Mean age + S.D. in years at achievement of stage
1. Preadolescent; elevation of papilla only	Prepubertal
2. Breast bud stage: elevation of breast and papilla as a small mound, enlargement of areola diameter	11.15 ± 1.10
3. Further enlargement of breast and areola, with no separation of contours.	12.15 ± 1.09
4. Projection of areola and papilla to form a secondary mound above level of the breast.	13.11 ± 1.15
5. Mature stage; projection of papilla only, due to recession of the areola to the general contour of the breast.	15.33 ± 1.74

(Adapted from Marshall, W. A., and Tanner, J. M.: Variations in the pattern of pubertal changes in girls. Arch. Dis. Childhood, *44*:291–303, 1969.)

Table 20-3. Stages of Pubic Hair Growth in Girls

Tanner stage	Mean age + S.D. in years at achievement of stage
1. Preadolescent; no pubic hair	Prepubertal
2. Sparse growth of long, slightly pigmented, down hair, straight or slightly curled, appearing chiefly along labia	11.69 ± 1.21*
3. Considerably darker, coarser and more curled. Hair spreads sparsely over junction of the pubes.	12.36 ± 1.10
4. Hair adult in type but area covered is smaller than in adults. No spread to thighs.	12.95 ± 1.06
5. Adult hair distributed as an inverse triangle. Spread to medial surface of thighs.	14.41 ± 1.12

(Adapted from Marshall, W. A., and Tanner, J. M.: Variations in the pattern of pubertal changes in girls. Arch. Dis. Childhood, *44*:291-303, 1969.)
*Probably occurs earlier. See original article.

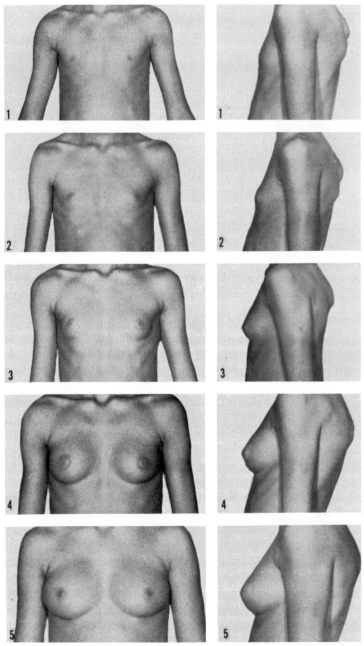

Fig. 20-6. Standards for breast development ratings. (Reproduced with permission. From Tanner, J. M.: Growth and endocrinology of the adolescent. *In* Gardner, L. I. (Ed.): Endocrine and Genetic Diseases of Childhood and Adolescence, ed. 2. Philadelphia, W. B. Saunders Co., 1975.)

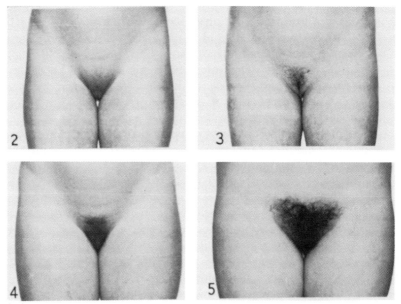

Fig. 20-7. Standards for pubic hair ratings in girls. (Reproduced with permission. From Tanner, J. M.: Growth and endocrinology of the adolescent. *In* Gardner, L. I. (Ed.): Genetic Diseases of Childhood and Adolescence, ed. 2. Philadelphia, W. B. Saunders Co., 1975.)

general health and nutrition. American girls have been reported to have onset of breast budding at a mean age of 143.0 ± 14.5 months, growth of pubic hair at a mean age of 142.5 ± 13.9 months and menarche at 151.8 ± 14.1 months. The relation between the events of puberty is more meaningful than the chronological age of occurrence, however. Primary amenorrhea in an 18-year-old girl who has stopped growing and who reached Stage 5 breast development 3 years previously warrants investigation. Primary amenorrhea in an 18-year-old girl who had onset of breast budding and appearance of pubic hair at age 14–15 years and who has shown progressive evidence of growth and development probably represents simple delayed adolescence.

MALES

At puberty, pituitary gonadotropin secretion increases and stimulates testicular maturation. LH acts on the Leydig cells causing them to secrete testosterone and estrogen while FSH acts on the seminiferous tubules to induce and maintain spermatogenesis. A negative feedback mechanism exists between testosterone and LH levels. The exact control mechanism between FSH and the seminiferous tubules is not clear. It may be a tubular secretion called "inhibin."

Testosterone and adrenal androgens stimulate growth of the penis and scrotum as well as facial and body hair, lowering of the voice and recession of scalp hair. They increase muscle mass and accelerate the rate of linear growth and skeletal maturation. Testosterone is necessary for full maturation of the seminiferous tubules and for growth of the prostate and seminal vesicles.

Marshall and Tanner have described the individual variation in the physical changes of puberty based on a study of 228 normal boys.[7] Pubic hair and genital growth were classified into five stages of development and are listed in Tables 20-4 and 20-5 together with the mean estimated ages at which each stage was reached. The standards for pubic hair growth and genital maturity are shown in Figures 20-8 and 20-9.

The genitalia began to develop between the ages of 9½ years and 13½ years in 95 per cent of the boys (mean 11.6 ± 1.07) and reached maturity at ages varying between 13 and 17 (mean 14.9 ± 1.10). On the average, the genitalia reached the adult stage three years after they first began to develop, but some boys completed this event as rapidly as 1.8 years while others took as much as 4.7 years. The maximum rate of growth occurred at a mean age of 14.1 ± 0.14 years; 95 per cent of boys did not reach peak height velocity until genitalia Stage 4 or more.

Table 20-4. Stages of Pubic Hair Growth in Boys

Tanner stage	Mean age + S.D. in years at achievement of stage
1. Preadolescent. No pubic hair	Prepubertal
2. Sparse growth of long, slightly pigmented downy hair, straight or slightly curled, chiefly at base of penis.	13.44 ± 1.09*
3. Considerably darker, coarser and more curled. The hair spreads sparsely over the junction of the pubes.	13.9 ± 1.04
4. Hair is now adult in type but area covered is still small. No spread to medial surface of thighs.	14.36 ± 1.08
5. Adult in quantity and type. Inverse triangle. Spread to medial thighs but not up linea alba.	15.18 ± 1.07

(Adapted from Marshall, W. A., and Tanner, J. M.: Variations in the pattern of pubertal changes in boys. Arch. Dis. Childhood, *45*:13–23, 1970.)
*Probably occurs earlier. See original article.

Table 20-5. Stages of Genital Growth in Boys

Tanner stage	Mean age + S.D. in years at achievement of stage
1. Preadolescent. Testes, scrotum and penis are same size and proportion as in early childhood.	Prepubertal
2. Scrotum and testes have enlarged and there is some reddening and change in texture of scrotal skin.	11.64 ± 1.07
3. Growth of penis has occurred, at first mainly in length but with some increase in breadth. Further growth of testes and scrotum.	12.85 ± 1.04
4. Penis further enlarged in length and breadth with development of glans. Testes and scrotum further enlarged.	13.77 ± 1.02
5. Genitalia adult in size and shape.	14.92 ± 1.10

(Adapted from Marshall, W. A., and Tanner, J. M.: Variations in the pattern of pubertal changes in boys. Arch. Dis. Childhood, *45*:13–23, 1970.)

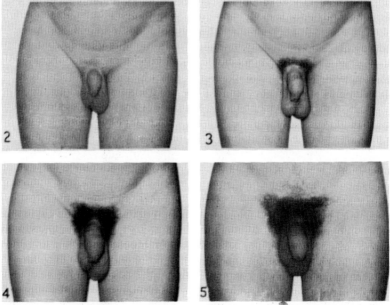

Fig. 20-8. Standards for pubic hair ratings in boys. (Reproduced with permission. From Tanner, J. M.: Growth and endocrinology of the adolescent. *In* Gardner, L. I. (Ed.): Endocrine and Genetic Diseases of Childhood and Adolescence, ed. 2. Philadelphia, W. B. Saunders Co., 1975.)

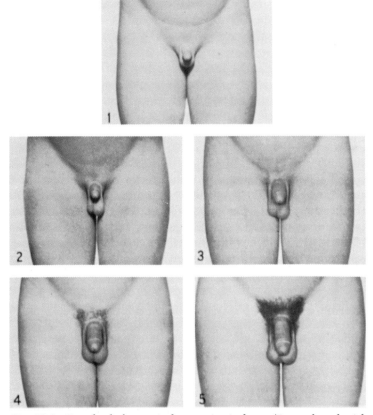

Fig. 20-9. Standards for genital maturity in boys. (Reproduced with permission. From Tanner, J. M.: Growth and endocrinology of the adolescent. *In* Gardner, L. I. (Ed.): Endocrine and Genetic Disease of Childhood and Adolescence, ed. 2. Philadelphia, W. B. Saunders Co., 1975.)

Figure 20-10 diagrams the sequence of events at puberty in relation to age in years for the average boy and girl. Girls begin their pubertal growth spurt early in the course of development of their secondary sexual characteristics while it is unusual for boys to reach their peak height velocity until their genitalia are quite well developed. Most girls have completed their linear growth at the age when boys attain their maximum adolescent spurt. Testicular enlargement usually is the first physical change indicative of pubertal development in boys; this suggests that testosterone plays a greater role in sexual hair growth and the growth spurt than adrenal androgen. Breast enlargement usually precedes other evidence of secondary sexual development in girls.

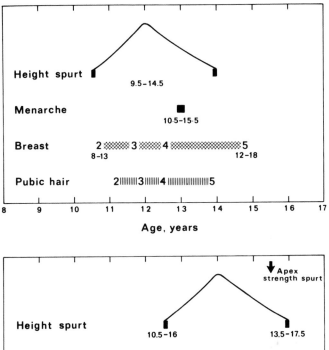

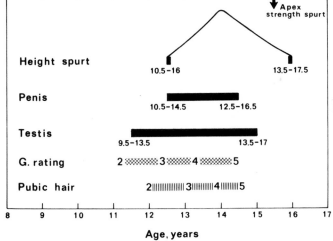

Fig. 20-10. Diagram of sequence of events at adolescence in girls and boys. An average girl and boy is represented; the range of ages within which each event charted may begin and end is given by the figures placed directly below its start and finish. (Reproduced with permission. From Tanner, J. M.: Growth and endocrinology of the adolescent. *In* Gardner, L. I. (Ed.): Endocrine and Genetic Diseases of Childhood and Adolescence, ed. 2. Philadelphia, W. B. Saunders Co., 1975.)

DISORDERS OF SEXUAL MATURATION

It is convenient, clinically, to consider disorders of sexual maturation on the basis of: (1) overproduction, (2) underproduction, and (3) normal production with increased or decreased tissue response of hormones involved in the various stages of pubertal development. Thus, the hypothalamus, the anterior pituitary, the gonads or the adrenals may play primary or secondary roles in the disturbance. Intrinsic factors of genetic, neural, infectious, metabolic or neoplastic origin and extrinsic factors such as environment and drugs may interfere with normal physiological processes, leading to overproduction or underproduction of hormones. The patient, in turn, may exhibit precocious, delayed, or absent secondary sexual development.

SEXUAL PRECOCITY

When secondary sexual characteristics develop at an earlier age than normal, the child has the syndrome of precocious puberty. Isosexual precocity refers to sexual development consistent with the phenotype of the individual, whereas heterosexual precocity implies development of sexual characteristics deviate from the phenotype of the person. In true precocious puberty, normal hypothalamic-pituitary-gonadal function is activated at an abnormally early age, whereas in pseudoprecocious puberty, secondary sexual characteristics develop because of abnormal production of estrogens or androgens without maturation of the gonads. True precocious puberty arises from dysfunction of the central nervous system and is characterized by an adult pattern of sexual function, i.e., menstruation in girls and testicular maturation and spermatogenesis in boys. Girls with pseudoprecocious puberty do not have ovulatory cycles, and spermatogenesis does not occur in affected boys because the disorder occurs without pituitary gonadotropic stimulation.

Precocious puberty is five to six times more common than pseudoprecocious puberty and occurs much more often in girls than in boys. About 80 per cent of prematurely developed girls have no demonstrable lesion of the hypothalamic-pituitary-gonadal axis or other identifiable etiology for their precocious development and are said to have "constitutional" or "idiopathic" sexual precocity. In contrast, more than 60 per cent of boys with precocious development have serious organic disease. When the only evidence of precocious development is breast enlargement, the disorder is called premature thelarche. When it is limited to early growth of pubic hair, it is called premature adrenarche.

Etiology

Causes of isosexual precocious puberty are listed below. Even though no etiology can be identified for the precocity in most girls and in some boys, a thorough study of each child must be done. A diagnosis of idiopathic or constitutional precocity should be made only after organic causes have been ruled out.

Causes of Isosexual Precocity

Central nervous system
  Idiopathic (more common in girls)
  Inflammatory disorders
    meningitis, encephalitis
  Congenital defects
    cyst, hamartoma, hydrocephalus
  Tumors
    glioma, astrocytoma, pinealoma
     (especially in boys), neurofibroma,
     craniopharyngioma
  Trauma
  Miscellaneous
    McCune-Albright syndrome
    hypothyroidism
    familial (occurs in boys)

Gonadotropin-producing tumors
  Teratoma, chorioepithelioma, hepatoblastoma

Gonads
  Ovarian and testicular tumors

Adrenal
  Feminizing tumor in girls and masculinizing
   tumor in boys
  Congenital virilizing adrenal hyperplasia
   in boys

Heterosexual precocity in girls is caused by abnormalities which result in excessive circulating androgens such as arrhenoblastoma of the ovary, tumor or biochemical defect in steroid hormone synthesis of the adrenal or ingestion of androgens. Heterosexual precocity in boys is rare and may be caused by excessive estrogen produced by a feminizing tumor of the adrenal or other estrogen-producing neoplasms as well as ingestion of estrogen.

Clinical Evaluation of the Patient

A carefully taken history is an important part of the initial evaluation of sexual precocity for it may provide clues concerning etiology. The physician should document the chronology of the sexual development and chart any growth data. The various stages of pubertal development may follow the usual sequence or occur in random fashion; sometimes vaginal bleeding is the first sign of precocity in girls. Acceleration of the linear growth rate usually starts at the onset of precocious development. Inquiry should be made about ingestion of drugs and vitamins as well as application of hormone-containing ointments. Signs and symptoms that can be referred to the central nervous system (visual disturbances, convulsions, behavior changes, polydipsia and polyuria, trauma and infection) are particularly important. A history of precocious development in relatives may be helpful in identifying familial male precocity or congenital virilizing adrenal hyperplasia.

The physical examination should include careful inspection for the pigmented areas, cafe-au-lait spots and asymmetrical growth which occur in the McCune-Albright syndrome and neurofibromatosis. Facial acne and increased hair growth suggest excessive androgen production. Breast, sexual hair and growth of genitalia should be rated according to the criteria of Tanner. Accurate measurements of head and chest circumference, length or height, arm span, lower segment, weight and blood pressure are obtained. Young children with a large head may have hydrocephalus, a congenital cyst or another expanding intracranial lesion. A detailed neurological examination including perimetry is essential. Visual field defects may occur before other signs of an intracranial lesion. Abdominal examination may reveal a mass in the suprarenal, hepatic or ovarian region. A careful search for evidence of virilization is an important part of the genital examination. Particular note is made of the size of the clitoris in girls and the penis and testes in boys. The clitoris and penis increase in size in response to androgens. Bilateral testicular enlargement indicates gonadotropin stimulation while unilateral increase in size occurs in the presence of tumor, adrenal rest cells or other localized pathology. Rectal examination is necessary to delineate adnexal anatomy and to check uterine size which is enlarged in response to estrogen and normal for age in virilization.

Diagnostic Studies

Both radiologic and laboratory studies may be necessary.

Radiologic. Skull radiographs may detect a change in the size of the sella turcica, intracranial calcifications or increased intracranial pressure. Patients with McCune-Albright syndrome often have sclerosis at the base of the skull as well as osteolytic lesions of polyostotic fibrous dysplasia.

Since androgens and estrogens accelerate osseous maturation, the bone age of children with progressive sexual precocity will be advanced except in the rare cases of hypothyroidism and isosexual precocity where osseous maturation usually is delayed.

When an intracranial abnormality is suspected, computerized axial tomography, brain scan and pneumoencephalography may be indicated.

After adrenal and testicular disease have been ruled out, these studies are recommended often in cases of precocity in males because of the high incidence of CNS disease in affected boys.

Intravenous pyelography, aortic arteriography, ultrasonography, computerized axial tomography, or pelvic pneumoperitoneography may be necessary in selected cases to define adrenal and/or ovarian masses.

Laboratory. Follicle stimulating hormone (FSH) and luteinizing hormone (LH) measurements are useful clinically only in situations where elevation of gonadotropins from extrapituitary sources, such as a trophoblastic neoplasm, are suspected. Marked elevation of human chorionic gonadotropins (which cross-react in the LH assay) is found in patients with chorionic gonadotropin-secreting tumors. Gonadotropin levels which are minimally elevated, normal or low for age do not provide other diagnostic information. It is preferable to obtain 24-hour or overnight urine specimens rather than single blood samples for gonadotropin assay because gonadotropins are released in pulsatile fashion from the pituitary. The concentration in one specimen may not accurately reflect hypothalamic-pituitary activity.

Cytologic examination of a vaginal smear or of urinary sediment cells may be used to indicate the presence of ovarian sex steroids. Plasma and urinary estradiol levels usually are markedly elevated in girls with granulosa cell tumors of the ovary. Urinary pregnanediol, the metabolite of progesterone, is elevated in thecomas as well as in cycling precocious girls during the luteal phase.

Urinary 17-ketosteroid, dihydroepiandrosterone (DHA) and pregnanetriol excretion is increased in children with congenital virilizing adrenal hyperplasia, and the levels fall to normal following dexamethasone suppression. The concentration of plasma 17-OH progesterone follows a similar pattern. In patients with adrenal tumors, steroid production is autonomous and not under ACTH control, so 17-ketosteroid and DHA levels cannot be suppressed by dexamethasone. Leydig cell tumors of the testis in boys also are androgen-producing neoplasms which function autonomously. Children with isosexual precocity of cerebral origin have levels of urinary 17-KS and DHA which are appropriate for their maturational ages or slightly elevated.

Treatment

Surgical removal of hormone secretory tumors of the ovary, adrenal gland or testis obviously is necessary. Unfortunately, tumors of the central nervous system rarely are amenable to curative surgery. Radiation therapy and chemotherapy may be helpful in selected cases.

The course of idiopathic isosexual precocity in girls is variable, sometimes remaining stationary, sometimes progressing slowly and other times moving rapidly to complete sexual maturation. Thus, it is necessary to observe the patient carefully for as long as one year or so after initial evaluation to determine the course of the sexual development. There is no satisfactory treatment to stop the process. Medroxyprogesterone therapy may be used to depress levels of gonadotropins and cause cessation of menses and regression of breast development. However, it usually has no effect on rate of linear growth or skeletal maturation.

Boys who have non-familial isosexual precocity of undetermined etiology must be followed very carefully because a central nervous system lesion can remain undetected for years.

Particular attention must be given to the psychological management of children with sexual precocity. Affected children appear much older than their chronological age because of their physical maturity, yet they have psychosexual development consistent with their chronological age.

DELAYED SEXUAL MATURATION

Delayed sexual development is much more common in boys than in girls, and a familial pattern sometimes exists. Puberty may be considered delayed in girls if breast development has not started by age 13 years or if more than 5 years have elapsed between onset of pubertal maturation and menarche. Boys may be considered to have delayed sexual maturation if testicular enlargemet has not begun by 13½–14 years or if more than 5 years have passed between the start and completion of genital growth. In neither boys nor girls is the time taken to pass through the various pubertal stages related to age of onset.

Etiology

Delayed adolescence may result from hypothalamic-pituitary dysfunction leading to gonadotropin deficiency, from intrinsic gonadal disease, or from a combination of both pituitary and gonadal hormone deficiency. Causes of delayed adolescence are listed below.

There may be isolated deficiency of gonadotropin, gonadotropin deficiency accompanied by lack of other pituitary tropic hormones (panhypopituitarism) or physiologic delayed adolescence. The deficiency may be caused by a disorder inhibiting synthesis and secretion of gonadotropin-releasing hormone in the hypothalamus or affecting pituitary hormones per se, such as tumor, trauma, infection or congenital defects.

The most common primary gonadal disorder in girls is the syndrome of gonadal dysgenesis which is usually associated with a sex chromosomal abnormality. Primary testicular dysgenesis is found in males with Klinefelter's syndrome. Other boys may have congenital hypoplasia or agenesis of the testes with or without associated somatic abnormalities. Occasionally, Leydig cell function is preserved so that virilization occurs, but the patients are sterile. In both cases, the gonads may lose function subsequent to trauma or inflammation.

Physiological or constitutional delayed adolescence is a common problem of unknown etiology characterized by a constant rate of linear growth until 11–12 years of age when deceleration occurs. Skeletal maturation is delayed and consistent with height age and the stage of pubertal development. Often there is a history of late adolescence in other family members.

Chronic diseases as well as malnutrition or significant weight loss from dieting often cause varying degrees of delayed sexual maturation. Primary amenorrhea rarely is caused by an imperforate hymen leading to hematocolpos or by absence of the uterus and/or vagina.

Causes of Delayed Adolescence

Central nervous system
    Congenital anomalies of hypothalamic-pituitary axis
    Constitutional (more common in boys)
    Inflammatory disorders
    Tumors (hypothalamus, pituitary)
    Trauma
    Miscellaneous
      suppression by exogenous hormone
      anorexia nervosa

Gonads
    Ovary
      Chromosomal abnormality (syndrome of gonadal dysgenesis)
      Tumors (requiring oophorectomy)
      Trauma (torsion, radiation)
      Inflammation
    Testes
      Chromosomal abnormality (Klinefelter's Syndrome)
      Hypoplasia or agenesis
      Tumor
      Trauma (torsion)
      Inflammation (mumps orchitis)

Chronic systemic illness—renal, gastrointestinal, cardiac, endocrine

Miscellaneous

Clinical Evaluation of the Patient

A historical review beginning with the obstetrical data is an essential part of the evaluation. Inappropriate birth weight and length for gestational age may indicate intrauterine growth failure. Babies who sustain cerebral anoxia during a difficult delivery and resuscitation sometimes grow poorly from birth as do those who have significant illness during the neonatal period. Malnutrition, chronic illness and endocrine disorders in childhood often cause deceleration in the rate of growth, delayed osseous maturation and delayed sexual development. Information about school achievement, psychosocial relations and family constellation provides clues to growth retardation due to emotional deprivation. Review of the family history may show that other members have had delayed growth and sexual maturation. All past measurements should be plotted on growth charts so that the pattern can be evaluated. Deceleration in the rate of linear growth usually indicates organic disease and requires thorough diagnostic evaluation, while children with constitutional short stature and delayed adolescence grow at a constant rate through the years to the age of puberty.

When partial sexual maturation has taken place, it is important to determine the exact chronology of the stages of pubertal development. A healthy 14-year-old boy who is prepubertal in development may have simple delayed adolescence, whereas a boy of similar age who has had Tanner Stage 4 genital development for 2–3 years except for small, prepubertal sized testes needs detailed evaluation.

General inspection of the patient at the outset of the physical examination provides useful clues. There may be no evidence of secondary sexual characteristics, or partial development may be present. A girl with gonadal dysgenesis may have pubic and axillary hair but no breast development. Boys with Klinefelter's syndrome may have gynecomastia, sexual hair and pubertal enlargement of the penis, but small testes. The physician should look for associated somatic abnormalities (see syndrome of gonadal dysgenesis). Accurate measurements of head and chest circumferences, height and weight, arm span and lower segment are made. Boys with a eunuchoid habitus and hypogonadism will have a long arm span and a decreased ratio of upper/lower body segments. On the other hand, the ratio is increased in hypothyroidism, and patients with hypopituitarism usually have normal body proportions. Examination for evidence of systemic disease is essential in patients with delayed maturation. A careful neurological evaluation including perimetry should be done. Since some patients with hypogonadism have anosmia, olfactory sensation should be checked.

Careful inspection of the genitalia in girls permits visualization of the hymen, and the uterine cervix can be palpated on rectal examination. In boys, particular attention should be directed toward the location of each testis and its size and consistency. The stage of sexual maturation of all patients should be assessed by the criteria of Tanner.

Diagnostic Studies

After the history, physical examination, and review of all available growth data, the physician must decide the appropriate diagnostic approach. Most often, particularly in boys, the lack of secondary sexual characteristics is due to constitutional delay in growth and development. The skeletal maturation of the patient is determined by x-ray examination of the hands and wrists. In addition, a buccal smear for sex chromatin pattern and a chromosomal analysis are obtained from girls with delayed sexual maturation and from boys with possible Klinefelter's syndrome to rule out a sex chromosomal abnormality. Children with constitutional delay are healthy persons who have had a constant rate of linear growth through the years at or slightly below the third percentile. Height age and bone age usually are equally delayed but they are more than 75 per cent of chronological age. Often there is a family history of delayed development. When these criteria have been met, it is appropriate to observe the patient and note his progress. Serial measurement of gonadotropins may be helpful in selected cases. Urinary gonadotropins increase before physical signs of sexual maturation in individuals with constitutional delay in development, and boys will have high nocturnal serum levels of LH.

When the linear growth rate has not been constant through the years, when there is interruption in the usual sequence of secondary sexual development or when subjects with suspected constitutional delay do not mature as expected, further evaluation is necessary. After non-endocrine systemic disease and chromosomal abnormalities have been ruled out, each component of the hypothalamic-pituitary-gonadal axis should be investigated in an orderly sequence.

Skull radiographs are obtained and visual field examination is done. When there is evidence of tumor or other expanding lesion, computerized axial tomography, electroencephalography, brain scan and pneumoencephalography may be necessary.

When hypogonadism is the result of hypothalamic-pituitary abnormalities, serum and urinary gonadotropin levels are low. After administration of synthetic gonadotropic-releasing hormone, the secretion of FSH and LH may remain abnormally low or increase to the normal range. Children whose delayed growth and development is on the basis of panhypopituitarism also will have low levels of growth hormone following provocative stimulation by agents such as insulin and arginine. Thyrotropin secretion can be evaluated by measurement of serum TSH and T4 levels. Function of the hypothalamic-pituitary-adrenal axis is assessed by determining plasma cortisol response to insulin-induced hypoglycemia and by the metyrapone test. Radioimmunoassay of serum ACTH is a difficult test which is not satisfactory for routine clinical use.

Children with primary gonadal disease have high amounts of gonadotropins in serum and urine. Estrogen levels of girls and testosterone levels of boys are low in serum and urine. The culdoscope may be used to visualize the ovaries and other pelvic structures in selected girls when ovarian agenesis is suspected. Boys with anorchia do not increase plasma levels of testosterone after human chorionic gonadotropin (HCG) stimulation in contrast to boys with cryptorchidism whose testosterone levels rise significantly.

Treatment

Patients with constitutional delay in growth and development should be followed regularly to be certain that maturation occurs and to reassure the patient and the parents. Many times, these individuals, especially boys, are subject to teasing by their age mates, and they may develop behavioral and school problems. All of them eventually will have normal secondary sexual characteristics without treatment. Rarely, when profound psychological problems arise, it is appropriate to give boys a short course of androgen therapy to enhance development. Some physicians use a short course of HCG to stimulate testosterone secretion. It is usually not necessary to treat girls who have constitutional delay. The physician must remember that gonadal steroid therapy has the potential to cause hypothalamic-pituitary suppression.

Patients with hypogonadotropic hypogonadism and primary hypogonadism may be given treatment with androgen and estrogen, as appropriate, to induce secondary sexual development. Individuals with deficiency of other pituitary hormones also may need treatment with growth hormone, thyroid hormone and hydrocortisone. In the future, treatment with gonadotrophic-releasing hormone or gonadotropins may be used routinely for primary hypothalamic-pituitary hypogonadism.

BIBLIOGRAPHY

Grumbach, M. M.: Abnormalities of sexual differentiation. *In* Rudolph, A. M.: Pediatrics, ed 16. New York, Appleton-Century-Crofts, 1977; pp. 1695–1712.

A well-written review of sexual differentiation for clinical use.

Grumbach, M. M., Roth, J. C., Kaplan, S. L., and Kelch, R. P.: Hypothalamic-pituitary regulation of puberty in man: Evidence and concepts derived from clinical research. *In* Grumbach, M. M., Grave, G. D., and Mayer, F. E.: The Control of the Onset of Puberty. New York, John Wiley and Sons, Inc., 1974; pp. 115–166.

Imperato-McGinley, J., and Peterson, R. E.: Male pseudohermaphroditism: The complexities of male phenotypic development. Am. J. Med., *61*:251–272, 1976.

A comprehensive description of the basic steps in human sexual differentiation, especially in the male.

Josso, N.: Fetal sexual differentiation in mammals. Pediatr. Ann., *3*:67–79, 1974.

Lemli, L., and Smith, D. W.: The XO syndrome: A study of the differentiated phenotype in 25 patients. J. Pediatr., *63*:577–588, 1963.

A clinical description of the findings in the XO syndrome.

Marshall, W. A., and Tanner, J. M.: Variations in the pattern of pubertal changes in girls. Arch. Dis. Childhood, *44*:291–303, 1969.

————: Variations in the pattern of pubertal changes in boys. Arch. Dis. Childhood, *45*:13–23, 1970.

The Marshall and Tanner texts are classic descriptions of normal pubertal development in girls and boys.

Nora, J. J., Nora, A. H., Sinha, A. K., Spangler, R. D., and Lubs, H. A.: The Ullrich-Noonan syndrome (Turner phenotype). Am. J. Dis. Childhood, *127*:48–55, 1974.

Root, A. M.: Endocrinology of puberty. I. Normal sexual maturation. J. Pediatr., *83*:1–19, 1973.

————:Endocrinology of puberty. II. Aberrations of sexual maturation. J. Pediatr., *83*: 187–200, 1973.

Zacharias, L., Wurtman, R., and Schatzoff, M.: Sexual maturation in contemporary American girls. Am. J. Obstet. Gynecol., *108*:833–846, 1970.

Zurbrügg, R. P.: Congenital adrenal hyperplasia. *In* Gardner, L. I. (Ed.): Endocrine and Genetic Diseases of Childhood and Adolescence, ed. 2. Philadelphia, W. B. Saunders Co., 1975; pp. 476–500.

Comprehensive review of congenital adrenal hyperplasia, its diagnosis and treatment.

21

Hypoglycemia

Charles A. Stanley, M.D., and Lester Baker, M.D.

The prevalence of hypoglycemia in the pediatric age group is still unknown, but the importance of hypoglycemia in the young infant is unquestioned. It has been accepted for many years that the brain depends exclusively on glucose for its metabolic needs. Although recent evidence indicates that the brain can utilize substrates other than glucose, particularly during prolonged fasting, it is still apparent that hypoglycemia can have both immediate and long-term adverse effects on the central nervous system. Seizures may be seen with acute hypoglycemia, and permanent brain damage may result from more prolonged hypoglycemic insults. It would also appear that the infant brain, during its phases of rapid growth and maturation, is particularly vulnerable to these insults; hypoglycemia can therefore be viewed as a potentially preventable cause of mental retardation.

Knowledge of the specific pathophysiologic derangements should lead directly to more rapid diagnosis and rational therapy. Since hypoglycemia in the child almost always occurs in the fasting state, the classification system must start with an analysis of the normal adaptation to fasting.

PHYSIOLOGY OF FASTING

In the early stage of fasting following the absorption of a meal, glucose is initially provided from hepatic glycogen stores. The small amount of liver glycogen (approximately 70 g. in a 70-kg. adult) is an important source of glucose only during the first 6 to 12 hours of fasting. Beyond this time glucose must be produced by the liver from circulating precursors (gluconeogenesis). The major source of precursors for new glucose formation is the amino acids in body proteins, the bulk of which are in skeletal muscle. Muscle protein is broken down and the amino acids are taken up by the liver for synthesis of glucose. Since all body proteins perform essential functions, the breakdown of protein for glucose formation during fasting must be limited. To reduce the need for glucose production, glucose utilization ceases in insulin-sensitive tissues (muscle and adipose tissue), and is limited primarily to the brain and red blood cell mass. Red blood cells oxidize glucose to lactate which can be reconverted to glucose by the liver. Therefore, during fasting, only that glucose which is consumed by the brain must be produced from the breakdown of body proteins.

During later stages of fasting, fuel for tissues other than the brain is derived from fat stored as adipose tissue triglyceride. This is broken down, and free fatty acids and glycerol are released. Glycerol is taken up by the liver and contributes to glucose production. Free fatty acids cannot be converted into glucose, but instead are used directly as a fuel by tissues such as muscle. Free fatty acids are partially oxidized in the liver to beta-hydroxybutyrate and acetoacetate, the ketone bodies. This provides the energy needed for hepatic gluconeogenesis and the ketones serve as an additional fuel for muscle. During prolonged fasting, the levels of ketones rise and the brain can then use beta-hydroxybutyrate as a fuel. This further reduces the requirement for glucose production and thus limits the need to break down essential body protein.

The processes involved in fuel production and utilization during fasting are shown schematically in Figure 21-1. Seven major systems can be identified which are required for fasting homeostasis. These can be divided into three groups: (1) those involved in glucose production: liver and muscle glycogenolysis, muscle protein breakdown, and hepatic gluconeogenesis (systems 1–4 in Fig. 21-1); (2) those involved in production of alternate fuels: adipose tissue lipolysis and hepatic ketogenesis (systems 5 and 6 in Fig. 21-1); and (3) hormonal regulation and integration (system 7 in Fig. 21-1, shown inhibiting glucose utilization by muscle).

Glucose Production

Liver Glycogenolysis. Glycogen is a branched-chain polysaccharide composed of glucose molecules connected through 1,4 linkages with branches attached by 1,6 bonds. It normally comprises 4 to 5 per cent of the weight of the liver. Two enzymes, glycogen synthase and amylo-(1,4→1,6)-glucantransferase (brancher enzyme) are necessary for glycogen synthesis. Two enzymes are also required for glycogenolysis: phosphorylase and debrancher enzyme. Approximately 8 per cent of the glucose in glycogen may be released directly as free glucose from branch points by debrancher enzyme. The remainder is released as glucose-1-P by phosphorylase and, after conversion to glucose-6-P, may be hydrolyzed by glucose-6-phosphatase to free glucose (Fig. 21-2).

Glucagon and epinephrine produce glycogenolysis by increasing adenyl

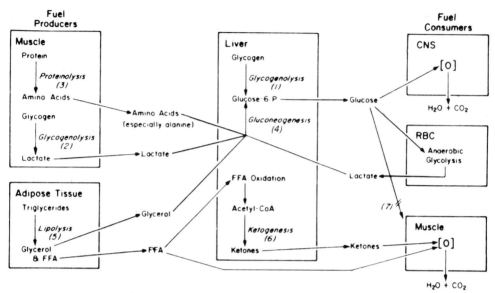

Fig. 21-1. Outline of fuel production and utilization during fasting. See text for details. (Adapted from Cahill, G. F.: Starvation in man. N. Engl. J. Med. *282*:668, 1970.)

cyclase activity which elevates the intracellular concentration of cyclic-AMP. This, in turn, acts through a series of protein kinases to stimulate glycogen breakdown by reciprocally increasing phosphorylase and decreasing glycogen synthetase activities. Glycogenolysis is suppressed by insulin.

Muscle Glycogenolysis. Since muscle lacks glucose-6-phosphatase, muscle glycogen cannot be released as free glucose. Instead, it is broken down to lactate and pyruvate which may be used by the liver for gluconeogenesis (Cori cycle). The total store of glycogen in muscle is about twice that contained in the liver. Muscle glycogen is mobilized during exercise or anoxia. Its contribution to glucose production in fasting is not known. Disorders of muscle glycogenolysis such as deficiencies of phosphorylase (McArdle's disease) or phosphofructokinase are not associated with hypoglycemia.

Muscle Protein Degradation. Amino acids in the muscle represent the largest source of substrate in the body for glucose production. During fasting there is a net breakdown of muscle protein. The various amino acids are largely converted to alanine. Alanine, released by muscle, serves as a major substrate for hepatic gluconeogenesis. Pyruvate, generated by glycolysis, may combine with ammonia released by oxidation of amino acids to synthesize alanine. Thus, alanine also serves to transport carbon skeletons derived from glucose back to the liver for resynthesis of glu-

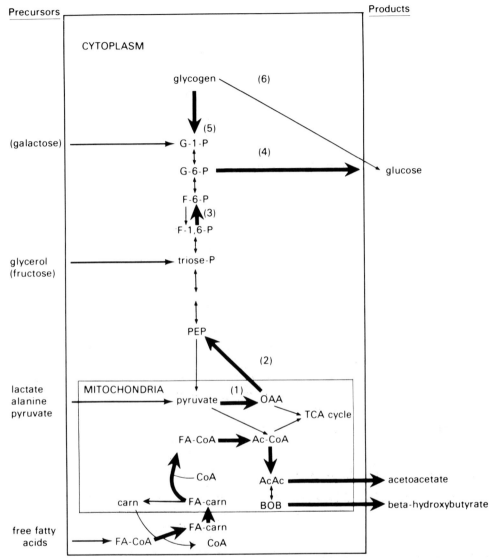

Fig. 21-2. Liver metabolism during fasting. Shown are the major steps in gluconeogenesis and ketogenesis. The heavy arrows indicate irreversible or dominant pathways. Dietary sugars which require the presence of enzymes of gluconeogenesis for conversion to glucose are shown in brackets. The numbers identify reactions catalyzed by enzymes of gluconeogenesis: (1) pyruvate carboxylase, (2) phosphoenolpyruvate carboxykinase, (3) fructose diphosphatase, (4) glucose-6-phosphatase; and glycogenolysis: (5) phosphorylase, (6) debrancher enzyme. Abbreviations: FA (fatty acid), CoA (coenzyme A), carn (carnitine), AcCoA (acetyl CoA), AcAc (Acetoacetate), BOB (beta-hydroxybutyrate), OAA (oxaloacetate), PEP (phosphoenopyruvate), triose-P (triosephosphates), F-1,6-P (fructose-1,6-diphosphate), G-6-P (glucose-6-phosphate), G-1-P (glucose-1-phosphate).

cose. This has been called a glucose-alanine cycle, and is analogous to the Cori cycle.

The liver has a large capacity for gluconeogenesis. Glucose synthesis is controlled primarily by the rate of substrate delivery to the liver. Therefore, the rate of muscle protein degradation is the major determinant of glucose production during fasting. It should be emphasized again that there is no "spare protein," so that regulation of this process is essential. Little is known about the mechanisms which govern muscle protein breakdown, but it is presumed that insulin plays an important role.

Hepatic Gluconeogenesis. As shown in Figure 21-2, to bypass the irreversible steps in glycolysis, four enzymes are required for gluconeogenesis: pyruvate carboxylase (PC), phosphoenolpyruvate carboxykinase (PEPCK), fructose-1,6-diphosphatase (FDPase), and glucose-6-phosphatase (G-6-Pase). About 90 per cent of the glucose released from liver glycogen requires G-6-Pase. These enzymes are also involved in the formation of glucose from dietary sugars. As shown in Figure 21-2, the fructose portion of sucrose requires the presence of FDPase and G-6-Pase, while the galactose moiety of lactose requires G-6-Pase.

The activities of the four gluconeogenic enzymes in the liver are increased in concert by glucagon, cortisol and fasting, and are suppressed by insulin. However, as noted above, the rate of substrate delivery to the liver primarily determines the rate of glucose synthesis during fasting.

Alternate Fuels

Lipolysis. Fat is stored in adipose tissue as triglyceride, which is composed of three fatty acid molecules linked to a glycerol backbone. Decreased insulin levels or activation of adenyl cyclase by epinephrine and other hormones cause hydrolysis of the triglyceride via a hormone-sensitive lipase. Free fatty acids and glycerol are released. Free fatty acids are transported in plasma bound to albumin. They may be oxidized directly by muscle. In the liver free fatty acids may be partially oxidized to ketones.

Hepatic Fatty Acid Oxidation and Ketogenesis. As shown in Figure 21-2, plasma free fatty acids taken up by the liver are activated to form coenzyme A esters in the cytoplasm. During fasting, these fatty-acyl esters are transported from the cytoplasm into mitochondria by a shuttle involving carnitine. In the mitochondria fatty acids are oxidized to acetyl-CoA, with production of ATP. A portion of the ATP is used to provide the energy for gluconeogenesis. Some of the acetyl-CoA is oxidized in the Krebs cycle; the remainder is condensed by specific enzyme steps (the hydroxymethylglutaryl CoA [HMG-CoA] pathway) to acetoacetate and beta-hydroxybutyrate.

Ketogenesis is stimulated by glucagon and suppressed by insulin. The mechanisms by which these hormones act have not been entirely worked out. Control of liver carnitine levels appears to be an important site for regulation. In the fasting state, hepatic carnitine levels increase and fatty acids are directed across the mitochondrial membrane for oxidation and ketogenesis.

Hormonal Integration

Efficient balance of fuel production and consumption during fasting requires an intact endocrine system. The primary controlling hormone is insulin, which has widespread effects on the fasting systems outlined above. In the liver, insulin promotes glycogen synthesis, inhibits glycogenolysis and gluconeogenesis, and suppresses ketogenesis. In muscle, insulin stimulates glucose and amino acid uptake, and protein synthesis. In adipose tissue, it stimulates glucose uptake and triglyceride synthesis and suppresses lipolysis.

During fasting, an initial decrease in glucose level leads to a fall in insulin levels. This inhibits glucose utilization by muscle and adipose tissue, allows for accelerated protein breakdown, and promotes glycogenolysis and gluconeogenesis. Further reduction in insulin levels promotes lipolysis and ketogenesis with elevation of free fatty acid and ketone body levels. Continued secretion of insulin at low levels (5–10 μU/ml.) is necessary to control fuel production and to prevent runaway diabetic ketoacidosis.

Other hormones which oppose the action of insulin in various tissues are also required for successful adaptation to fasting. These include glucagon, epinephrine, cortisol, growth hormone, and thyroxine. With insulin, glucagon is probably an important factor in regulating the switch in hepatic metabolism from the fed to the fasted state. Hypoglycemia may occur in infants and children with growth hormone or cortisol deficiency and in panhypopituitarism.

CLINICAL ASPECTS: DEFINITION AND SYMPTOMS

The generally accepted definition of hypoglycemia in infants and children is a true blood glucose level less than 40 mg./dl. This is a clinical definition, derived from the clinical observation that symptoms are rarely seen when the blood glucose is above this level. For the newborn, a statistical definition of hypoglycemia has been derived, setting as the lowest normal limit the mean minus two standard deviations. This figure is 30 mg./dl. for the full-term, normal weight newborn; for the small for gestational age newborn, it is 20 mg./dl. Whether what is statistically normal is also physiologically healthy (particularly with relation to brain function) is a subject of continuing controversy, especially in the newborn (see the section on neonatal hypoglycemia).

It should be remembered that the values cited are those of true blood glucose. Any method which measures reducing substances other than glucose may give a false reading. In addition, many current methods measure serum or plasma glucose, which, because of the different distribution of glucose between cells and serum, gives values approximately 15 per cent higher. The specific techniques and methods used within a given institution should be checked in order to relate these to the values found in the literature.

Symptoms related to central nervous system dysfunction dominate the picture produced by hypoglycemia; seizures and coma are the most dramatic of these. More subtle manifestations may be seen as irritability, confusion, headaches, bizarre behavior, and hypothermia. The classic symptoms associated with an autonomic nervous system response to a falling glucose, such as tachycardia, pallor, cold sweat and nervousness, are often not found, even in the older child. The newborn infant in particular tends to respond to hypoglycemia in a relatively nonspecific manner. Symptoms of hypoglycemia in the neonate can be poor feeding, high pitched cry, cyanosis, lethargy, or irritability, all of which may be present prior to an overt seizure.

Since the symptoms of hypoglycemia are not specific, it is necessary to document that symptoms are truly related to hypoglycemia. This is done by having at least one, preferably two, glucose values which are in the hypoglycemic range at the time of symptoms, accompanied by the demonstration that there is relief of symptoms when the blood glucose is raised.

General Classification of Hypoglycemic Disorders in Childhood

Hypoglycemia as a major feature
  Defect in glucose production
    Hepatic glycogenolysis
      Debrancher deficiency
    Gluconeogenesis
      Glucose-6-phosphatase deficiency
      Fructose diphosphatase deficiency
      Phospho-enol pyruvate carboxykinase deficiency
      Pyruvate carboxylase deficiency
    Deficient substrate
      Ketotic hypoglycemia
      Starvation
  Defect in alternate fuel production

    Ketogenesis
      Defect in ketogenesis
   Hormonal
    Hyperinsulinism
      Organic
        Islet adenoma
        Beta-cell adenomatosis
        Nesidioblastosis
        Infant of diabetic mother (transient)
        Beckwith syndrome
      Exogenous cause
        Insulin reactions in diabetics
        Oral hypoglycemic agents
    Deficiency of other hormones
      Panhypopituitarism
      Growth hormone deficiency
      Cortisol deficiency
  Miscellaneous
    Neonatal
    Reactive hypoglycemia (rare)
Hypoglycemia associated with other disorders
   Inborn errors
    Galactosemia
    Hereditary fructose intolerance
    Maple syrup urine disease
    Tyrosinemia
   Sepsis
   Toxins
    Jamaican vomiting illness
    Ethanol
    Aspirin
   Liver Failure
    Cirrhosis
    Reye's syndrome

A general classification of the hypoglycemic disorders seen in childhood is outlined above. It is obvious that this list could be expanded several times. In terms of actual experience at a referral center, Table 21-1 presents the causes of hypoglycemia in infants and children at the Children's Hospital of Philadelphia over a 10-year period, 1965–1975. The children included in this table are those in whom hypoglycemia was the major feature of the clinical presentation. This list does not include newborns with transient hypoglycemia, or those who were infants of diabetic mothers. Also excluded are patients in whom hypoglycemia was a relatively minor part of the presentation, as in Reye's syndrome.

Table 21-1. Causes of Hypoglycemia in Infants and Children at the Children's Hospital of Philadelphia, 1965–1975.

Cause	All ages		Onset <1 year	
	No.	%	No.	%
Hyperinsulinism	29	30	26	55
(with hypopituitarism)	2		1	
Hypopituitarism	5	5	5	11
Ketotic hypoglycemia	50	51	5	11
Hepatic enzyme deficiencies:	12	12	11	23
Glucose-6-phosphatase	7		7	
Amylo-1,6-glucosidase	3		3	
Fructose-1,6-diphosphatase	1		1	
Defective ketogenesis	1			
Classification uncertain	2	2	—	—
Total	98		47	

NEONATAL HYPOGLYCEMIA

It has been known for many years that low levels of plasma glucose are not uncommon in newborn infants. The significance of this was recognized in 1959 by Cornblath and co-workers; it is now acknowledged that hypoglycemia in newborn infants may be a major cause of brain damage. Infants who have symptoms (such as seizures) in association with hypoglycemia have a much worse prognosis for normal development than infants who are asymptomatic.

The overall incidence of symptomatic neonatal hypoglycemia is estimated to be about 4.4 per 1000. Depending on the definitions used, the incidence of chemical hypoglycemia is much higher. Lubchenko and Bard estimated that 11 per cent of all newborns could be expected to have plasma glucose levels below 30 mg./dl. between birth and a first feeding at 6 hours of age. As shown in Fig. 21-3, the risk of hypoglycemia is particularly high in infants who show signs of intrauterine malnutrition (small-for-gestational-age infants), in premature and in large-for-gestational-age infants.

Hypoglycemia in newborns is usually a transient problem which is most often seen before feedings are begun and is usually resolved within a few days. The symptoms of hypoglycemia in neonates are very nonspecific and infants may show no obvious symptoms even with plasma glucose levels of 10–20 mg./dl. Symptoms which may be seen include irritability, apathy, tremors, hypothermia, cyanosis, and seizures. Similar

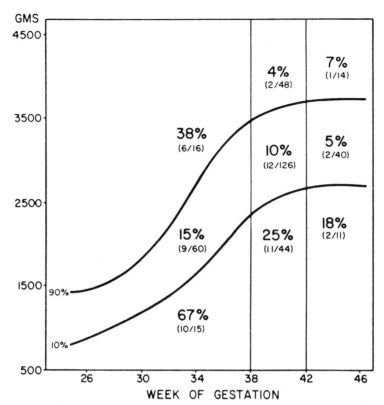

Fig. 21-3. Incidence of hypoglycemia (plasma glucose < 30 mg/dl.) prior to first feedings at six hours of age in newborn infants grouped by birth weight and gestational age. The normal range of birth weights is shown by the 10th and 90th percentile lines. The large figures give the percentage and the small figures the number of infants with low plasma glucose in nine groups: term—SGA, AGA and LGA; post-term—SGA, AGA and LGA; and pre-term— SGA, AGA and LGA. SGA: small for gestational age; AGA: appropriate for gestational age; LGA: large for gestational age. (From Lubchenko, L. O., and Bard, H.: Incidence of hypoglycemia in newborn infants by birth weight and gestational age. Pediatrics, 47: 831, 1971.)

symptoms may occur in other disorders such as sepsis, congenital heart disease, CNS lesions, and hypocalcemia. The risk of hypoglycemia is increased in these disorders. Therefore, hypoglycemia must be suspected in any newborn who does not appear normal; conversely, the possibility of an underlying disease must be considered in any infant with hypoglycemia.

Clinically, it is useful to classify transient neonatal hypoglycemia into three groups: (1) infants of diabetic mothers, (2) hypoglycemia associated with other disorders such as sepsis or asphyxia, and (3) the hypoglycemia found in small-for-gestational-age infants and less often in normal weight neonates. Recurrent, usually severe, hypoglycemia may also occur due to early presentation of metabolic-hormonal disorders. Only in the case of infants of diabetic mothers is the mechanism of the hypoglycemia understood. Unless there is placental insufficiency, infants of diabetic mothers may be exposed *in utero* to excessive maternal levels of glucose. This may lead to islet hyperplasia and hyperinsulinism that stimulates fetal weight gain. At birth, these infants are markedly obese and may develop hypoglycemia due to hyperinsulinism within 1 or 2 hours. The hyperinsulinism usually resolves within a few days. All large-for-gestational-age newborns should be suspected of being infants of diabetic mothers. Plasma glucose should be monitored closely and feedings begun early. If hypoglycemia occurs, intravenous glucose infusion at concentrations as high as 15–20 per cent may be necessary. The plasma glucose should be maintained in a low normal range (50–60 mg./dl.) to avoid further stimulation of insulin secretion. In difficult cases, the addition of glucocorticoids may be helpful.

Transient hypoglycemia seen in other newborns may be considered a manifestation of a temporary inability to tolerate fasting after birth. At delivery, the supply of nutrients from maternal circulation abruptly ceases; the mechanisms for maintainance of plasma glucose during fasting are called into play for the first time. In the small-for-gestational-age newborn, brain size is normal while liver glycogen, adipose tissue and muscle protein mass are lower than normal. It has been suggested that this discrepancy between brain demands for glucose and reduced fuel stores might be responsible for the hypoglycemia. An alternative possibility is that there may be a delay in maturation of one or more of the systems required for adaptation to fasting. Evidence for a transient defect in one of the fasting systems has recently been provided by Haymond and co-workers. They noted that levels of gluconeogenic precursors (lactate, pyruvate, and amino acids) were higher in small-for-gestational-age infants who had fasted than in normal infants, and suggested that there may be a delay in maturation of capacity for gluconeogenesis. It should be pointed out that hypoglycemia is not uncommon in normal weight newborns (Fig. 21-3), and that all infants may be born with a relative defect in one of the fasting systems. Further investigations of the integrity of all the fasting systems at birth may provide an explanation for transient neonatal hypoglycemia.

There is continuing controversy over what level of blood glucose should be used to define hypoglycemia in the newborn period. Since low levels of glucose are observed so frequently in normal infants, it has been suggested that hypoglycemia exists when glucose concentrations are below 30 mg./dl. in normal weight infants, and below 20 mg./dl. in low birth weight infants. If these values are accepted, treatment is only necessary for those infants who are symptomatic or who are found to have hypoglycemia by this definition on two determinations. Other workers have pointed out that these limits only define a statistical norm for blood glucose values under a given regimen of nursery care. The critical question of whether levels of blood glucose which are normal by this definition are also physiologically appropriate for the brain in newborn infants remains unanswered. Until information is available on whether the brain of the newborn infant requires a lower level of blood glucose, it would be wise to assume that the newborn requires at least the same level of blood glucose as older infants and children. Therefore, hypoglycemia in newborn infants should be defined by a blood glucose less than 40 mg./dl.

Hypoglycemia should be suspected in the smaller infant of a set of twins, in all small-for-gestational-age infants, and in all infants who have suffered unusual stress during delivery. Plasma glucose levels should be monitored closely in these infants and feeding begun as early as possible. Plasma glucose levels should be determined in any infant who displays symptoms suggestive of hypoglycemia. If a plasma glucose level below 40 mg./dl. is found, intravenous glucose (0.5 g./kg.) should be given immediately. An infusion of 5 or 10 per cent glucose with appropriate electrolyte, given at maintainance rates, should then be started to maintain plasma glucose levels above 40 mg./dl. This may be discontinued when normal feeding patterns have been established and plasma glucose levels remain above 40 mg./dl.

INBORN ERRORS RESULTING IN HEPATIC ENZYME DEFICIENCY

Given the central position of the liver in energy balance, it is not surprising that, as a group, hereditary deficiencies of key hepatic enzymes account for the second most common cause of hypoglycemia in the infants that are under one year of age. These hepatic enzyme deficiencies will be discussed under the broad categories of those affecting hepatic glycogen and hepatic gluconeogenesis.

Hepatic Glycogen

Deficiency of Glucose-6-Phosphatase. (Type I glycogen storage disease). The enzyme is not directly involved in glycogen synthesis or degradation, but its absence does cause an increased storage of glycogen. Its clinical manifestations so closely resemble those of a defect in gluconeogenesis that it is discussed with that group.

Deficiency of Debrancher Enzyme. (Type III glycogen storage disease). Children with debrancher deficiency present with massive hepatic enlargement, growth retardation and fasting hypoglycemia. The hypoglycemia is often severe and symptomatic, and is attributed to the fact that glycogen can only be degraded to the outer 1,6-branch points; the inner branches of glycogen are thus not available with hypoglycemia the result. These patients respond to glucagon with a rise in serum glucose in the postabsorptive state when the outer branches of glycogen are intact (e.g., 2 hours after a meal). Glucagon will not elicit a rise in serum glucose if administered after more prolonged fasting when the outer branches have been degraded. This differential response to glucagon is no longer considered diagnostic. Failure of serum glucose to rise following glucagon stimulation at a time of hypoglycemia could be related to exhaustion of glycogen stores (as is seen in defects of gluconeogenesis and in ketotic hypoglycemia), as well as to a defect in the actual process of glycogen breakdown. The specific diagnosis is made by enzyme analysis of liver and muscle. Assays of enzyme activity in leukocytes, erythrocytes and cultured skin fibroblasts may be helpful. The disease is inherited in an autosomal recessive manner.

Considering the role of hepatic glycogen in fasting adaptation, it is surprising that a defect in hepatic glycogenolysis should result in episodes of hypoglycemia which are frequent and severe. Lipolysis and ketogenesis are intact; these alternate fuels can be made available. Gluconeogenesis is also intact, and administration of amino acids such as alanine at the time of hypoglycemia results in a glycemic response. That these systems do not respond to prevent hypoglycemia suggests a disturbance in hormonal regulation. Thus far, it has not been possible to pinpoint the specific endocrine signal which may be inappropriate in the switch from the fed to the fasting state.

Patients with debrancher enzyme deficiency often exhibit a remission at puberty, with disappearance of the massive hepatic enlargement and improved growth. The explanation for this is unclear.

Deficiencies in the Hepatic Phosphorylase System. No longer considered a single entity, these may be a deficiency of either liver phosphorylase or of one of the activating steps of the phosphorylase kinase system. One variety of phosphorylase kinase deficiency is inherited as an X-linked defect.

Hypoglycemia in these patients is usually absent or extremely mild. The infants most often present with asymptomatic liver enlargement and mild growth retardation. The adaptation to fasting is normal as is the response to glucagon. Leukocytes of affected patients show the deficiency and can be used for diagnosis.

As in patients with debrancher deficiency, the liver enlargement and growth retardation disappear after puberty.

Deficiency of Glycogen Synthase. In this disorder, the absence of the key enzyme in the synthesis of glycogen leads to inadequate stores. The small amount of glycogen is rapidly depleted during brief fasting, with the result being hypoglycemia. The disease is rare, and has been described in only a few families. In the patients originally described by Spencer-Peet, frequent feeding proved effective in eliminating hypoglycemia.

Hepatic Gluconeogenesis

These diseases are all characterized by life-threatening lactic acidosis, hypoglycemia which may be asymptomatic, massive hepatomegaly, and presentation within the first months of life.

Deficiency of Glucose-6-Phosphatase. The absence of this enzyme effectively eliminates the liver as a source of glucose. Shortly after gut absorption ceases, the level of glucose falls. There is a reciprocal rise of lactate. Although the source of this lactate is not completely clear, much of it is apparently derived from hepatic glycogen and recycled gluconeogenic precursors from the periphery. The rise in lactate may provide brain substrate, and the hypoglycemia is frequently asymptomatic. The acidosis can be lethal, and probably accounts for the 50 per cent mortality seen in some reports. Chronic lactic acidosis may also be responsible for the growth retardation and osteoporosis seen in these children. Other clinical abnormalities include hyperuricemia, hyperlipemia, and clotting defects. The hyperuricemia is the result of both purine overproduction and decreased excretion of uric acid in the presence of high concentrations of lactic acid.

The disease is inherited in an autosomal recessive manner. Massive hepatomegaly, hypoglycemia, and a metabolic (lactic) acidosis suggest the diagnosis. The clinical diagnosis can be made on the basis of the glucagon stimulation test performed after a meal at the time when hypoglycemia is not present. In these patients, there is no rise in glucose concentration, but a significant increase in lactate levels. The definitive diagnosis is based on liver biopsy and determination of the enzyme.

The realization that many of the clinical and biochemical abnormalities are secondary to events that occur when the blood glucose falls and the anabolic effects of insulin are reduced has led to a regimen designed to keep blood glucose levels normal at all times. Frequent starch feedings during the day and a continuous intragastric glucose infusion through the night have been utilized. With this treatment the chronic acidosis disappears, the levels of lactate, urate and lipids return toward normal, there is a decrease in hepatic size, and there is rapid catch-up growth followed by normal linear growth.

Fructose-1, 6-diphosphatase Deficiency. The symptoms are almost identical with those seen in glucose-6-phosphatase deficiency. The onset of hypoglycemia in these patients is not as rapid as in glucose-6-phosphatase deficiency since the ability to mobilize hepatic glycogen is normal. Chronic acidosis does not occur in these children, but episodes of acute lactic acidosis can be life-threatening.

Fructose diphosphatase deficiency is inherited in an autosomal recessive manner. It should be suspected in a young infant with hepatomegaly, lactic acidosis, and hypoglycemia. The clinical diagnosis can be made by the demonstration of a normal rise of blood glucose following the infusion of galactose, but no rise or a fall in glucose levels following the administration of any gluconeogenic precursor which enters below the triosephosphate level (this would include alanine, glutamate, glycerol and fructose). This disease should also be distinguished from hereditary fructose intolerance. Patients with hereditary fructose intolerance demonstrate a drop in blood glucose following the infusion of fructose, similar to that seen in fructose diphosphatase deficiency. However, patients with hereditary fructose intolerance show a normal rise in glucose following the infusion of glycerol or alanine. Clinically, the two diseases differ: hereditary fructose intolerance is not associated with hypoglycemia upon fasting, and patients do not develop lactic acidosis. The definitive diagnosis, is, of course, made on hepatic biopsy.

Treatment for this disease is both simple and physiologic. These patients cannot perform gluconeogenesis; therefore, they should never be allowed to depend upon gluconeogenesis. In practice, this means that the young child, during intercurrent illnesses, is required to have a constant source of glucose. The patient is given a supply of dextrose to be used at home. In addition, sucrose and fructose are eliminated from the diet.

Deficiency of Pyruvate Carboxylase. Hypoglycemia, severe lactic acidosis, and psychomotor retardation have been reported in an infant with a deficiency of hepatic pyruvate carboxylase activity. Treatment with thiamine apparently ameliorated the tendency to acute bouts of lactic acidosis, presumably by shunting pyruvate into the pyruvate dehydrogenase pathway. In view of the key role of pyruvate carboxylase in generating oxaloacetate, it may be necessary to supplement the diet in such patients in order to provide additional sources of oxaloacetate.

HYPERINSULINISM

Until very recently, hyperinsulinism was considered an extremely uncommon cause of hypoglycemia in the pediatric age group. This was because clear-cut clinical or even pathologic evidence of hyperinsulinism could very rarely be demonstrated. Most patients who would now be recognized as having hyperinsulinism were therefore placed in nonspecific diagnostic categories such as idiopathic hypoglycemia of infancy or leucine-sensitive hypoglycemia. As shown at the Children's Hospital of Philadelphia (Table 21-1), hyperinsulinism was found to be the single most common cause of recurrent hypoglycemia in infants under 1 year of age.

Many of the infants who present with hyperinsulinism in the first year have abnormally high birth weights. This resemblance to infants of diabetic mothers suggests that, in some cases, hyperinsulinism may have begun before birth. There may be a history of hypoglycemia in the newborn period; usually, hypoglycemia is not recognized until 3 or 4 months of age. The symptoms are the same as those seen in hypoglycemia due to other causes, with seizures predominating. The physical examination is normal, except for large size. Plasma glucose levels are very unstable in these patients and hypoglycemia may occur after brief fasts of only 2 to 6 hours. Infusions of hypertonic glucose solutions may fail to prevent hypoglycemia. This evidence of rapid glucose utilization may provide a clue to the diagnosis of hyperinsulinism.

The usual approach to the diagnosis of hyperinsulinism has been to demonstrate abnormally high fasting insulin levels or to show abnormal insulin and glucose responses to various insulin secretogogues. These traditional approaches have not proved entirely satisfactory, particularly in the infant. Although the diagnosis can be made when elevated insulin levels are found at times of hypoglycemia, frequently insulin levels are not clearly abnormal.

Tolbutamide and leucine have been the secretogogues most commonly used to document hyperinsulinism. Both agents stimulate insulin secretion and cause a fall in plasma glucose in normal patients. In patients with hyperinsulinism, the fall in glucose may be more pronounced and prolonged and the peak insulin level may be higher. It is frequently impossible to perform the tests because plasma glucose levels are too unstable in patients with hyperinsulinism. Therefore, the leucine and tolbutamide tolerance tests cannot be recommended for routine use in the diagnosis of hyperinsulinism in infants and children.

Because of the difficulty in reliably documenting hyperinsulinism by the measurement of insulin levels, it has been necessary to develop an approach based on secondary evidence of the physiologic effects of excessive insulin secretion. In hyperinsulinism there is over-utilization of glucose, as insulin-sensitive tissues are unphysiologically permitted during fasting to continue consuming glucose. Glucose production by the liver is suppressed and there is inappropriate conservation of liver glycogen. In addition, adipose tissue lipolysis and hepatic ketogenesis are suppressed so that concentrations of alternate fuels are maintained at low levels. These physiologic markers of hyperinsulinism, and particularly the demonstration of suppression of lipolysis and ketogenesis, are helpful indicators of the diagnosis of hyperinsulinism when clearly elevated insulin levels cannot be demonstrated.

In our experience, a rapid and efficient method of making the diagnosis of hyperinsulinism in infants and children is to begin by observing the pattern of metabolic fuels and hormones present at the time of fasting hypoglycemia. If levels of free fatty acids and ketones are elevated at the time of hypoglycemia, hyperinsulinism is clearly excluded. If the levels are suppressed at the time of hypoglycemia (free fatty acids less than 0.5

mM and beta-hydroxybutyrate less than 1.1 mM) and the level of plasma insulin exceeds 12 μU/ml., the diagnosis of hyperinsulinism is clearly established. If the level of plasma insulin is not diagnostically elevated, hyperinsulinism should be suspected, but other possible causes of low free fatty acids and ketones should be excluded. This essentially entails ruling out the possibility of panhypopituitarism. The diagnosis of hyper-insulinism can be further confirmed by demonstrating a glycemic response to glucagon at the time of hypoglycemia (inappropriate conservation of liver glycogen) or by showing a rapid glucose disappearance rate following the intravenous administration of glucose (over-utilization of glucose).

Presently, two choices for the treatment of hyperinsulinism are available: long-term medical management with diazoxide which suppresses insulin secretion, and pancreatic surgery. The choice of treatment depends on the nature of the lesion most likely to be found in the pancreas. Table 21-2 shows the distribution of lesions associated with hyperinsu-linism in infants and children at the Children's Hospital of Philadelphia from 1965 to 1975 and from 1950 to 1975. It can be seen that the lesions may be localized, such as an islet adenoma, or there may be widespread involvement of the entire pancreas as in beta cell adenomatosis or ne-sidioblastosis (neo-formation of beta cells from ductal epithelium). In infants under 1 year of age with hyperinsulinism, diffuse lesions are most common, while in older children localized islet adenomas are more likely to be found. Only localized lesions have the potential to be cured by surgery. Therefore, the first choice of therapy in young infants is treatment with diazoxide and the first choice in older children is surgery.

Table 21-2. Pathologic Lesions Found in Infants and Children With Hyperinsulinism at the Children's Hospital of Philadelphia.

	1965–1975 (age at onset)		1950–1975 (age at onset)	
	< 1 year	> 1 year	< 1 year	> 1 year
Localized lesions				
Islet adenoma	3	2	3	2
Adenomatosis of uncinate process	2	—	2	—
Diffuse lesions				
Nesidioblastosis	4	—	12	—
Beta cell adenomatosis	1	—	1	—
Islet hyperplasia	—	1	2	1
Totals	10	3	20	3

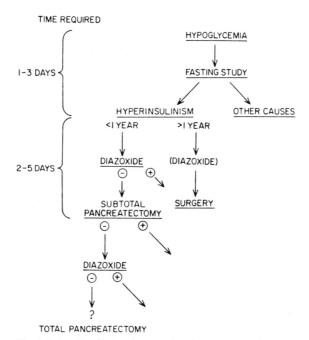

Fig. 21-4. Outline of steps for diagnosis and treatment of hypoglycemia due to hyperinsulinism. The response to therapy is indicated by + (good control of hypoglycemia) and − (poor control). (From Stanley, C. A., and Baker, L., Hyperinsulinism in infants and children. *In* Barness, L. A. (ed.): Advances in Pediatrics, vol. 23. Copyright © 1976 by Year Book Medical Publishers, Inc., Chicago. Used by permission.)

Neither diazoxide nor surgery alone can be expected to give good control of hypoglycemia in all patients. Diazoxide appears to be effective in 60–80 per cent of infants with hyperinsulinism, and subtotal pancreatectomy is effective in about 50 per cent of cases. Therefore a combination of therapy may be necessary. Figure 21-4 shows a recommended sequence of steps for the management of hyperinsulinism in children under and over 1 year of age. It should be possible to make the diagnosis of hyperinsulinism rapidly. In children over 1 year of age, an islet adenoma should be suspected, and surgery is the preferred treatment. Diazoxide may be used to control hypoglycemia preoperatively and again if surgery fails to control the hypoglycemia. Diazoxide should be tried first in infants under 1 year of age in whom diffuse lesions are more likely. If diazoxide gives good control of hypoglycemia, it should be continued until 4 to 6 years of age at which time some patients no longer require therapy. As shown in Figure 21-4, if diazoxide fails to control hypoglycemia, surgical exploration and subtotal pancreatectomy should be performed, followed by a second trial of diazoxide if necessary. If these measures fail to control hypoglycemia, total pancreatectomy may have to be considered. With the sequence outlined (Fig. 21-4), it should usually be possible to make a diagnosis and adequately control hypoglycemia in patients with hyperinsulinism within a week to 10 days. This is important in preventing possible brain damage due to hypoglycemia.

KETOTIC HYPOGLYCEMIA

As shown on page 288, ketotic hypoglycemia is the most common form of hypoglycemia in childhood. It is likely that this is not a single entity, but will prove to be a syndrome of varied causes.

Clinically, the disorder is seen most commonly between the ages of 1½ and 4 years, although occasional cases may present in the latter part of the first year of life. There is frequently a history that the infant was small for gestational age at birth, and there may have been difficulties with hypoglycemia in the neonatal period. Males are affected more frequently than females. The children are usually below the 25th percentile for height and weight, with weight being more affected than height. Eye abnormalities (usually cataracts) are found more frequently than explicable by chance alone. The hypoglycemic episodes almost invariably occur in the morning, and one can often elicit the fact that breakfast was delayed or that dinner or the usual bed-time snack was omitted or poorly eaten. Hypoglycemic episodes occur relatively infrequently (approximately three to five times per year); the children are in good health between episodes. It is frequently stated that a spontaneous remission of symptoms occurs around the age of 7 to 9 years.

The diagnosis should be suspected in a child of the appropriate age who presents with symptomatic hypoglycemia and who has a large amount of ketone bodies in his urine. Complete caloric deprivation (fasting) is a simpler method than a high fat hypocaloric diet for study and diagnosis. Ketonuria usually develops 6 to 12 hours prior to the fall in glucose to hypoglycemic levels. Glucagon stimulation at the time of hypoglycemia fails to cause a rise in plasma glucose concentration, while glucagon stimulation causes a normal rise of plasma glucose during a period when the child is adequately fed.

In terms of the physiologic model of the normal adaptation to fasting, the clinical evidence strongly suggests that the basic defect must lie outside the liver. Hepatic glycogen can obviously be synthesized and released. The high levels of ketone bodies indicate normal hepatic fatty acid oxidation and ketogenesis. Insulin concentrations at the time of hypoglycemia are appropriately low. Infusion of alanine or lactate at the time of hypoglycemia causes a rise in glucose concentration, thus providing further evidence that the hormonal "set" of the liver is appropriate for the performance of gluconeogenesis, and that the hepatic enzymes of gluconeogenesis are intact.

Pagliara and co-workers have suggested that ketotic hypoglycemia represents a substrate deficiency disease. Specifically, they have pointed out that plasma alanine concentrations are significantly lower during fasting in children with ketotic hypoglycemia than they are in normal children of similar age. The importance of alanine as a gluconeogenic substrate and as a rate-limiting factor in gluconeogenesis has recently been emphasized by Felig and co-workers. Attractive though this hypothesis may be, it is still not completely clear that hypoalaninemia is the primary cause of ketotic hypoglycemia. The rise in serum glucose following alanine infusion is not specific, since infusion of lactate or glycerol will produce similar results. Recent studies have shown that abrupt elevation of ketone concentrations (produced by the infusion of beta-hydroxybutyrate) causes a specific lowering of plasma alanine concentration. It is thus conceivable that the low alanine levels may be secondary to the increased ketone concentration, rather than being a primary and causal event. In addition, ketotic hypoglycemia as a substrate deficiency syndrome rests on the premise that there is decreased protein breakdown in these children during fasting. The elevated plasma concentration of the branched chain amino acids in children with ketotic hypoglycemia, however, argues strongly in favor of normal protein catabolism during fasting.

Among the many unanswered aspects of ketotic hypoglycemia, there are two questions which appear to be particularly important: (1) Is this a true disease, or is it an expression of the decreased tolerance to fasting of all children, and therefore an extreme variant of normal? (2) Why should these children have such marked symptoms at a time when the elevated ketone concentrations should provide adequate fuel for the brain?

Despite reservations about ketotic hypoglycemia as a specific syndrome, it is still important to make the diagnosis in any individual patient. By definition, it will require the exclusion of any disease that could be diagnosed and treated more specifically (see the section on diagnosis). The diagnosis of ketotic hypoglycemia also allows the physician to suggest therapy and to offer support to the family concerning prognosis and natural history. The parents should be told to monitor urinary acetone at any time when the child is not in his normal pattern (e.g., during intercurrent illnesses, when highly excited because of visitors, or when more active physically than is usual—all of these may be associated with decreased caloric intake). Carbohydrate supplementation is recommended if acetonuria is observed. A late-night snack as part of the daily regimen is also suggested. With this approach, hypoglycemic attacks usually disappear completely. If a child diagnosed as having ketotic hypoglycemia has more than two episodes of symptomatic hypoglycemia per year, complete re-evaluation should be performed, searching rigorously for other possible causes. The parents may be told that a complete remission of symptoms is often observed by the time the child reaches eight or nine years. The nature of this remission is unknown. It may relate to relative changes in central nervous system glucose requirements vs. the supply of gluconeogenic precursors.

DIAGNOSTIC APPROACH TO THE PATIENT WITH HYPOGLYCEMIA

Because there are many disorders that can cause hypoglycemia, a systematic approach to the evaluation of a patient with hypoglycemia is necessary. As noted previously, essentially all of the disorders found in infants and children involve fasting hypoglycemia. It is helpful, therefore, to base the approach to a given patient on an evaluation of fasting adaptation. This can be used not only to document hypoglycemia but also to identify which of the systems required for fasting adaptation is abnormal.

Some clues to the cause of hypoglycemia may be obtained from the history, physical examination, and routine laboratory studies (see outline below). If the patient is under 1 year of age, hyperinsulinism should be suspected, while ketotic hypoglycemia is suggested if the child is between one and five years of age. Hypoglycemia occurring within a few hours of meals may suggest hyperinsulinism, an inborn error of gluconeogenesis or glycogenolysis, or panhypopituitarism. Hypoglycemia occurring after 12 or more hours of fasting would suggest the possibility of ketotic hypoglycemia, cortisol deficiency or growth hormone deficiency. In infants with hyperinsulinism there may be a history of an exacerbation of symptoms in association with an increase in dietary protein. A family history of previous unexplained deaths in infancy may suggest the possibility of an inborn error of gluconeogenesis.

On physical examination, the finding of an enlarged liver may suggest the possibility of an inborn error of glycogen metabolism or gluconeogenesis. Hyperinsulinism should be suspected in infants with a large birth weight and rapid weight gain. Deceleration of growth rate or an unusually small penis in a male infant should raise the possibility of hypopituitarism.

Routine laboratory studies should include a urinalysis and measurement of serum electrolytes. Ketonuria at the time of hypoglycemia would direct attention away from hyperinsulinism. Evidence of lactic acidosis would suggest the possibility of a defect in gluconeogenesis.

While the data base of history, physical examination and routine laboratory studies may suggest the cause of the hypoglycemia, usually a

---

Major Features of Hypoglycemic Disorders in Infants and Children

Hyperinsulinism
  Onset during the first year of life
  Brief fasting tolerance
  Severe difficulty in maintaining normoglycemia
  Glycemic response to glucagon

Ketotic hypoglycemia
  Onset between 1 and 5 years of age
  Symptoms occur after overnight fast
  Ketonuria present at time of symptoms
  No response to glucagon

Cortisol and growth hormone deficiency
  Clinical picture similar to ketotic hypoglycemia

Panhypopituitarism
  May resemble hyperinsulinism

Inborn errors of glycogenolysis and gluconeogenesis
  Onset during the first year of life
  Hepatomegaly
  Positive family history
  Severe metabolic acidosis

---

more general approach is needed. The study of fasting adaptation (described below) has proven to be an efficient initial study.

Fasting Study

In preparation for this study, the patient should be given an adequate diet for 2 to 3 days. The fasting is usually begun after an 8 p.m. bedtime snack. If hypoglycemia is expected to occur in less than 12 hours, the fast may be started after a morning meal. During the fast the patient is encouraged to drink water. An indwelling venous needle should be maintained for obtaining blood samples and to provide a route for the administration of glucose if severe hypoglycemia occurs. The level of plasma glucose should be monitored every 2 hours and more frequently as it falls towards 40 mg./dl. Results must be available within a few minutes to avoid provoking severe hypoglycemia. Dextrostix may be used for this purpose. However, because the results are often unreliable, instruments such as the Beckman Glucose Analyzer are preferred. The fast is ended after 24 to 36 hours or when the plasma glucose level falls below 40 mg./dl. At the end of the fast, blood is drawn for determination of glucose, gluconeogenic substrates (lactate, pyruvate, alanine and glycerol), alternate fuels (free fatty acids, beta-hydroxybutyrate, and acetoacetate), and key hormones (insulin, growth hormone, cortisol, and glucagon). If desired, samples may also be taken at intermediate time points for these assays. The fast is ordinarily ended with a glucagon stimulation test.

This study provides information on five of the seven systems involved in fasting adaptation: hepatic gluconeogenesis, glycogenolysis, lipolysis, hepatic ketogenesis, and hormonal adjustments. After a 24- to 36-hour fast in normal infants and children the following results are observed: glucose, greater than 40 mg./dl.; lactate, 1 to 2 mM; pyruvate, 0.1 to 0.2 mM; glycerol, 0.1 to 0.3 mM; alanine, 0.2 to 0.4 mM; free fatty acids, 0.5 to 3 mM; beta-hydroxybutyrate, 1 to 5 mM; acetoacetate, 0.5 to 2 mM; and insulin, less than 12 μU/ml. The observed responses may depend more on the level of plasma glucose than on the duration of fasting. As plasma glucose approaches and drops below 40 mg./dl., levels of alanine fall toward the lower limit, and levels of free fatty acids, glycerol and ketone bodies rise towards the upper limits of the ranges given. Under the stress of a fall in plasma glucose to below 40 mg./dl., levels of growth hormone above 6 ng./dl. and cortisol greater than 20 μg/dl. are usually seen.

The levels of circulating fuels and hormones found at the time of hypoglycemia can be compared with the normal response to assess the integrity of the systems required for fasting adaptation. Normal levels of lactate indicate that hepatic gluconeogenesis is intact. Elevations of lactate and other gluconeogenic precursors suggest a defect in gluconeogenesis. Low levels of free fatty acids and ketones point to an inappropriate suppression of lipolysis and ketogenesis, as seen in hyperinsulinism. Appropriate elevation of free fatty acids with inappropriately low levels of ketone bodies is seen in defects in hepatic ketogenesis. Normal levels of lactate with elevation of free fatty acids and ketones provide evidence that lipolysis, hepatic gluconeogenesis, and ketogenesis are intact and that there is appropriate suppression of insulin secretion. Normally, there should be little response to glucagon after prolonged fasting or at a time of hypoglycemia. A rise in plasma glucose after glucagon administration during hypoglycemia suggests abnormal conservation of liver glycogen as is seen in hyperinsulinism. As shown in Figure 21-5, the information on the fuel response to fasting hypoglycemia allows for a marked reduction in the number of disorders which must be considered. These few disorders can then usually be easily distinguished by the use of appropriate tests which evaluate specific fasting systems. Some of these tests are described below.

TESTS

Tests of Specific Fasting Systems

Hepatic Glycogenolysis: Glucagon Stimulation Test. Glucagon (1 mg. I.M.) is given and levels of plasma glucose are determined every 10 min-

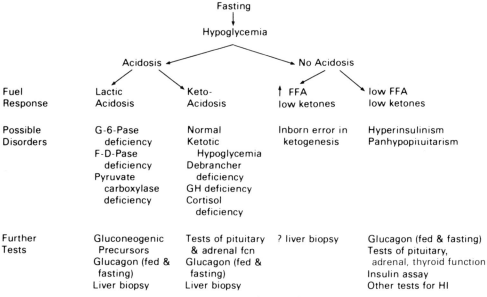

Fig. 21-5. See text for explanation.

utes for an hour. Normal persons demonstrate an increase of 25 mg./dl. or more in plasma glucose after a brief fast. If liver glycogen is depleted appropriately by prolonged fasting or during hypoglycemia, little or no response is seen. Patients with debrancher deficiency (Type III glycogen storage disease) show a normal response after a meal, but no response after 4 to 5 hours of fasting when the terminal branches of glycogen have been released. Patients with hyperinsulinism inappropriately conserve glycogen during fasting and continue to show a glycemic response to glucagon even when hypoglycemic.

Gluconeogenesis. *Glucose precursors* such as alanine, lactate, glycerol, fructose, and galactose may be given during fasting to test hepatic gluconeogenesis. After administration of the test substance, fasted normal persons show a rise in plasma glucose of 20 mg./dl. or more. Since these precursors enter the pathway of glucose synthesis at different levels, selected portions of the pathway may be tested. Patients with glucose-6-phosphatase deficiency fail to respond to any precursor. Patients with fructose diphosphatase deficiency respond to galactose, but not to lactate or alanine. Fructose and glycerol produce hypoglycemia in these patients. Since alanine stimulates glucagon secretion, a glycemic response to alanine may reflect glycogenolysis as well as gluconeogenesis.

Liver Biopsy. Definitive diagnosis of glycogen storage disease and inborn errors in gluconeogenesis depend on histologic and biochemical analysis of liver tissue. The analysis should include assay of glycogen content (4–5% in normals; up to 8–12% in debrancher and glucose-6-

phosphatase deficiency) and activity of the enzymes of glycogen metabolism and gluconeogenesis.

Hormonal System. *Tests for Hyperinsulinism.* As noted in the description of hyperinsulinism, it is sometimes difficult to demonstrate clear elevations of plasma insulin levels. It is necessary, therefore, to rely on physiologic markers such as inappropriate suppression of lipolysis and ketogenesis. An inappropriate glycemic response to glucagon at a time of hypoglycemia also serves as a marker for hyperinsulinism. Other tests for hyperinsulinism include intravenous glucose tolerance, leucine tolerance and tolbutamide tolerance.

1. Intravenous glucose tolerance test: Glucose (1 g./kg.) is infused rapidly over 1–2 minutes. Plasma glucose levels are measured at 0, 2, 5, 10, 15, 20, 30, 40, and 60 minutes. These values are plotted semi-logarithmically; the initial linear segment is used to estimate the disappearance rate, K_G. A high K_G (greater than 4) indicative of rapid utilization of glucose provides physiologic evidence of hyperinsulinism.

2. Leucine tolerance test: Leucine is one of several amino acids which stimulate insulin secretion. Normal subjects show a drop in plasma glucose of less than 25 mg./dl. after oral leucine administration (150 mg./kg.). Some patients with hyperinsulinism show a greater fall in plasma glucose level. Very often patients with hyperinsulinism cannot be tested because their plasma glucose levels are not stable. Great care must be taken to avoid causing profound hypoglycemia. Because of these drawbacks, the leucine tolerance test can rarely be performed in infants and children.

3. Tolbutamide tolerance test: Normal subjects show a drop in plasma glucose of less than 50 per cent, with a rapid return toward the baseline after tolbutamide (20 mg./kg.) is given intravenously. Patients with hyperinsulinism may show a greater and more prolonged fall. Insulin response is maximal at 2 to 5 minutes after the start of infusion, and may exceed 100 μU/ml. in patients with hyperinsulinism. The tolbutamide tolerance test has the same drawbacks as the leucine tolerance test and cannot be recommended for routine use in the diagnosis of hyperinsulinism in infants and children.

Tests of Other Hormones. Many hormones are involved in opposing insulin action, but only growth hormone, cortisol and thyroxine need be considered in infants and children with hypoglycemia. Thyroid function can be assessed by measuring T_4 levels. Cortisol and growth hormone secretion are stimulated by hypoglycemia and it is convenient to include them as part of the fasting study. Cortisol levels greater than 20 μg./100 ml. and growth hormone levels greater than 7 ng./ml. suggest adequate adrenal and pituitary function. Glucagon assays are available but there have been no fully documented reports of hypoglycemia due to deficiency of glucagon.

Miscellaneous Tests. (1) Oral glucose tolerance test: this test is mentioned here only to emphasize that it has no place in the evaluation of fasting hypoglycemia. (2) Ketogenic provocative diet: as discussed in the section on ketotic hypoglycemia, this test has been replaced by simple fasting.

BIBLIOGRAPHY

Cahill, G. F., Jr.: Starvation in man. Clin. Endocrinol. Metab., 5:397, 1976.

> This review of the physiology of fasting in adult man provides a basis for understanding the hypoglycemic disorders.

Cornblath, M., and Schwartz, R.: Disorders of Carbohydrate Metabolism in Infancy. 2nd ed. Philadelphia, W. B. Saunders, 1976.

> This book provides extensive coverage of hypoglycemia in the pediatric age range and provides more details on the topics discussed in this chapter. It is a good source of references.

Haworth, J. C.: Carbohydrate metabolism in the fetus and the newborn: Neonatal hypoglycemia. *In* Gardner, L. I. (ed.): Endocrine and Genetic Diseases of Childhood and Adolescence. 2nd ed. Philadelphia, W. B. Saunders, 1975.

> This textbook chapter provides a more extensive discussion of neonatal hypoglycemia.

Huijing, J. F.: Glycogen metabolism and glycogen-storage diseaes. Physiol. Rev., 55:609, 1975.

> This article reviews glycogen metabolism and the glycogen storage diseases.

McGarry, J. D., and Foster, D. W.: Hormonal control of ketogenesis. Arch. Intern. Med., 137:495, 1977.

> This review discusses the control of the hepatic pathways of fatty acid oxidation and ketone body synthesis.

Pagliara, A. S., Karl, I. E., Haymond, M., and Kipnis, D. M.: Hypoglycemia in infancy and childhood. J. Pediatr., 82:365, 82:558, 1973.

> This is an excellent review which provides both a good background discussion and an analysis of some specific disorders which cause hypoglycemia in children.

Sauls, H. S.: Hypoglycemia in infancy and childhood. *In* Kelly, V. C., (ed.): Metabolic, Endocrine and Genetic Disorders of Children. New York, Harper and Row, 1974.

> This textbook chapter is also a good review of disorders of hypoglycemia in pediatrics.

Stanley, C. A., and Baker, L.: Hyperinsulinism in infants and children: Diagnosis and therapy. Adv. Pediatr., 23:315, 1976.

> This article reviews in more depth the diagnosis and therapy of hyperinsulinism as a cause of hypoglycemia in infants and children.

22

Juvenile Diabetes

Robert Kaye, M.D.

The onset of diabetes in children is usually accompanied by the classic symptoms of polyuria and polydipsia. If untreated the disease progresses with weight loss, ketoacidosis, dehydration, coma, peripheral circulatory failure and death. The fully developed manifestations are the consequences of an essentially complete deficiency of insulin production by the pancreas possibly compounded by an excess of glucagon.

INCIDENCE

Estimates of the prevalence of diabetes in children under the age of 15 years range from 1/600 to 1/1200. Sampling techniques indicate that there are approximately 85,000 children with diabetes in the United States at the present time. It is the most common childhood endocrine disorder. Of the entire diabetic population approximately 4 per cent are children, 0.5 per cent of whom experience the onset under 1 year of age. A recent survey reports the female to male ratio as 5:3. The average age of onset is 10–11 years, although the disease has appeared as early as 11 days of life.

Diabetes occurring in children has been characterized as "juvenile diabetes," "growth-onset diabetes," "ketosis-prone diabetes," and "insulin-dependent diabetes." These designations have served to emphasize certain differences between the disease (Table 22-1) as it occurs in the child and in the adult ("maturity-onset" or "adult diabetes").

The manifestations of childhood diabetes do not always occur abruptly. Children with impaired glucose tolerance are being identified prior to the exhibition of frank diabetic symptoms. The largest group of such subjects are asymptomatic siblings of children with known diabetes, ap-

Table 22-1. Differential Features of Juvenile and Adult Onset Diabetes

	Juvenile Diabetes	Adult Diabetes
Exogenous insulin	Required for long-term management	Usually not
Ketosis	Prone	Resistant
Obesity	Not characteristic	80%
Response to caloric restriction alone	Poor, leads to cachexia	Often restores glucose tolerance to normal
Oral hypoglycemic agents	Effective only in partial remission	Usually effective
Insulin response to glucose	Decreased or lacking	Delayed and reduced magnitude
Life expectancy reduction	Approximately 30%	Less with advancing age
Quality of control	Labile	Stable
Brittleness or hyper-lability	Common	Rare

proximately 20 per cent of whom exhibit impairment in glucose tolerance without apparent symptoms of diabetes (chemical diabetes). Chemical diabetes will also be detected in some of the children studied because
of symptoms suggestive of hypoglycemia. In these subjects, fasting glucose concentrations are normal but 1- and 2-hour values are elevated. A
rapid fall to low normal or hypoglycemic levels occurs between the third
and fifth hours of the glucose tolerance test.

Genetic Considerations

The predisposition to diabetes is genetically determined. There is an
increased frequency in some families compared to the general population
and in monozygotic compared to dizygotic twins. Genetic data best fit
a multifactorial inheritance pattern—a number of genes on separate loci
which contribute equal and additive effects to the development of the
characteristic. Pyke has observed among identical twins that almost all
twin pairs are concordant for diabetes when the onset of the disease
occurred over the age of 40. Concordance was only 50 per cent when the
index case appeared earlier. Such observations suggest the presence of
environmental in addition to genetic factors in the causation of diabetes.
Heterogeneity in the clinical and genetic aspects of diabetes in young
people is apparent in the group of diabetics studied by Tattersall and
Fajans. These subjects exhibited a milder diabetic state than is usual for

juvenile diabetes and were characterized as "maturity onset diabetes in the young" (MODY). A different inheritance pattern was noted in these cases; approximately 85 per cent of the parents had diabetes in contrast to only 11 per cent of the parents of the patients with typical juvenile onset diabetes. These observations are compatible with a dominant mode of inheritance. Of further genetic interest is the finding that juvenile diabetes is highly associated with certain histocompatibility loci, DW3 and DW4.

Environmental Factors

Possible causative or contributing factors to the development of juvenile diabetes can be related to environment. Observations that two diabetic parents do not always produce diabetic offspring and that identical twins were not necessarily concordant for diabetes pointed to a role of non-genetic factors in the etiology of diabetes. Viral infection has been considered a possibility in this regard. Evidence indicates that Coxsackie B virus infection appears more frequently in diabetic children than in the normal population. Diabetes has been observed in young children affected by the intrauterine rubella syndrome; outbreaks of mumps among children have been followed in several years by an increase in the incidence of diabetes in children living in the area. Several viruses are capable of producing inflammatory changes in the pancreas of experimental animals associated with insulin deficiency and clinical diabetes. An interplay of genetic factors is suggested by species specificity in susceptibility to viral diabetes.

Immunologic components in some cases of diabetes are suggested by the finding of a 30-fold increase in the frequency of antibodies against thyroid, adrenal and gastric antigens in diabetic compared to normal children. In addition, antibodies against isolated pancreatic islet tissue have been detected in the sera of juvenile diabetics. These observations suggest that a means of preventing some cases of diabetes may be developed by the use of vaccines or anti-viral drugs.

DIAGNOSIS

The possibility of diabetes as the cause of polyuria and polydipsia is usually considered by parent or physician prior to the development of profound ketoacidosis. The suspicion leads to appropriate testing of urine for glucose, and if positive to determination of blood glucose concentration. The random blood glucose concentration of symptomatic children with glycosuria will usually exceed 250 mg./dl., which is diagnostic of diabetes mellitus.

In the preverbal or non-toilet trained infant increased thirst and urine

**Table 22-2. Levels of Blood Glucose Diagnostic of Diabetes Mellitus
in Oral Glucose Tolerance Testing**

Fasting	>110 mg./dl.
1 hour	>180 mg./dl.
1½ hours	>160 mg./dl.
2 hours	>140 mg./dl.

output may not be noticed and diabetes is more likely to progress to ketoacidosis. The child with brain damage may fail to sense the need for increased water intake to compensate for polyuria; extremely high blood glucose concentrations and dehydration may lead to the development of hyperglycemic, hyperosmolar non-ketotic diabetic coma.

Other symptoms suggesting diabetes mellitus are: enuresis in a child previously toilet trained, vulval pruritis due to monilial infection, and an abrupt onset of disturbances of visual acuity. The latter is attributable to changes in the lens of the eye as the result of hypertonicity of the extracellular fluid. It is exceptional for recurrent skin infections to be associated with underlying diabetes.

If glycosuria is observed and the random blood glucose concentration is normal or borderline, a glucose tolerance test should be performed. Oral glucose tolerance testing is more sensitive in revealing impaired carbohydrate disposal than is the intravenous test. Table 22-2 presents the values for blood glucose which are diagnostic of diabetes mellitus. Recommended glucose dosage levels are given in Table 22-3.

The glucose tolerance test is often useful in excluding diabetes in patients with findings such as asymptomatic glycosuria. It is also valuable in evaluation of patients with symptoms suggestive of reactive hypoglycemia: pallor, dizziness, anxiety or confusion occurring in the postprandial period. In a significant number (perhaps 30% of these individ-

Table 22-3. Glucose Dosage for Oral Glucose Tolerance Testing

Age	Grams glucose/kg.
0–18 mos.	2.5
1½– 3 years	2.0
3–12 years	1.75
7–12 years	1.25 (maximum 100 g.)

uals) chemical diabetes is present often with a rapid drop after the third hour substantiating reactive hypoglycemia.

There are a number of situations in which non-diabetic hyperglycemia may be encountered: (1) Carbohydrate deprivation followed by glucose loading; (2) Stress (physical, emotional or infection); (3) Drugs (epinephrine-like compounds, thiazide diuretics, oral contraceptive agents, diphenylhydantoin); or (4) Excessive production of anti-insulin hormones (growth hormone, catecholamines—neuroblastoma, pheochromocytoma, adrenal glucocorticoids, ACTH, thyroid, aldosterone).

Starvation is accompanied by an appropriate suppression of insulin secretion which serves to protect against hypoglycemia. The pancreas abruptly challenged with a glucose load may be unable to respond with a sufficient output of insulin to dispose of this load. Patients with head injury or intracranial infection may develop hyperglycemia secondary to central stimulation of alpha-adrenergic neurons inhibitory to insulin secretion. Insulin-antagonistic hormonal concomitants of stress—growth hormone, cortisol and catecholamines—may also be involved.

The epinephrine-like compounds may exhibit diabetogenic effects by suppression of insulin secretion, enhanced lipolysis, glycogenolysis and gluconeogenesis. Thiazide diuretics exert hyperglycemic effects by inducing potassium deficiency, and in the case of diazoxide by suppressing insulin secretion. Oral contraceptive agents containing estrogens and progestins vary in their capacity to reduce glucose tolerance. Their use may be associated with the induction of insulin resistance as shown by an increased insulin response to glucose in spite of concomitant hyperglycemia.

TREATMENT

Fundamental to an understanding of the difficulties encountered in the treatment of the diabetic child is the fact that juvenile diabetes is associated with a reduced or almost absent endogenous secretion of insulin. Present methods of insulin treatment sustain life and well-being for long periods but are not adequate replacements for the rapidly responding homeostatic system involving insulin and its counter-regulatory hormones operative in the normal subject. In health, insulin release is stimulated in seconds by increments of blood glucose (about 10 mg.) and falls to basal values when the glucose level is restored to normal. In the diabetic patient, insulin is administered peripherally rather than intraportally in anticipation of rather than after nutrient ingestion. Maintaining blood glucose levels within normal range in the majority of juvenile diabetics is beyond the capability of current treatment regimens. The metabolic lability of the juvenile diabetic, while primarily due to inadequate endogenous insulin, is compounded by variations in nutrient intake, physical activity, growth and maturation and in some instances by emotional arousal. These considerations should temper the degree of metabolic control demanded of a partially unphysiologic system inherently lacking in the rapid and precise adjustments characteristic of the metabolic-homeostatic hormone complex in the normal subject.

Hospitalization

Under most circumstances hospitalization of the newly diagnosed diabetic child is indicated. Some degree of emotional upset is usual at this time making it difficult for the family to assimilate the considerable body of new information requisite for the supervision of their child's illness. It is comforting to them to delegate temporary management of the child to the physicians, nurses and dietary staffs of the hospital. During hospitalization, the essential elements of diabetic management are explained to the parent and older patients. These include the role of diet, physiologic functions of insulin, recognition and treatment of hypoglycemia, pathogenesis of ketosis, management of vomiting episodes, and adjustment of insulin dosage on the basis of glycosuria. Also presented are the goals of therapy: maintenance of well-being, normal physical and emotional growth, and age-appropriate assumption of responsibility for self-management by the patient.

Diet

Opinion varies concerning the relative merits of "free" in contrast to "prescribed" diets in the management of diabetic children. Proponents of both recommend a diet conforming to acceptable nutritional practices for all children with appropriate response if the diet proves to be excessive or fails to lead to satiety and satisfactory weight gain. If a free diet is used, parents are helped by initial prescription of the quantity and composition of the diet, with the explanation that it is an estimate that may be modified according to their child's individual requirements. It is physiologically sound to permit some flexibility in the daily caloric intake. It should be assumed that the non-obese diabetic child possesses the normal homeostatic mechanisms which balance caloric intake and expenditure. Increased physical activity requires an increase in caloric intake, and hunger is often a manifestation of hypoglycemia. Caloric requirements are listed in Table 22-4.

General Principles of Treatment

It is helpful if the physician states clearly his standards of control. These should include the primary goal of fostering satisfactory physical and emotional development as well as the provision of adequate amounts of insulin to avoid the return of diabetic symptoms. In spite of our acknowledged inability to maintain normoglycemia, the family is assured

Table 22-4. Caloric Requirements

Age in years	K cal./kg./24 hr.
½–1	120–100
1–3	100– 90
5–6	90– 80
7–9	80– 70
10–12	70– 60
13–15	60– 50
16–18	50– 40

Calories/m.^{2} may be approximated as 1800 or 1000 + age in years × 100 (From Kaye, R.: Juvenile diabetes. *In* Shirkey, H. C. (ed.): Pediatric Therapy, ed. 5. St. Louis, C. V. Mosby, 1975.)

that a continuous effort will be made to limit glycosuria. Avoidance of repeated hypoglycemia and a rigidity in management that is almost certain to adversely affect the emotional adjustment of the child and the family is also of paramount consideration in structuring the plan of treatment.

The need of the adolescent to achieve a growing sense of independence and to identify with his peers leads to conflict when diabetes is superimposed on the characteristic stresses of this period of life. The physician should attempt to foster in the diabetic child a graded, age-appropriate sense of responsibility for his welfare by establishing a direct relationship with the child, rather than working solely through the parents. If the physician has a relatively relaxed attitude toward diabetic management, excessive parental concern may be avoided; this concern often culminates in serious strains between parent and child that focuses on the diabetic regimen. When strained relationships appear, it is often helpful to discuss with parents and child the full scope of their mutual dissatisfactions. Refractory situations with serious ramifications in relation to diabetic control will often be greatly improved by psychiatric therapy.

INSULIN TREATMENT

Insulin Biosynthesis and the Dynamics of Insulin Secretion

The insulin molecule is made up of two polypeptide chains, A and B, joined by a pair of disulfide bridges. A single chain polypeptide precursor, proinsulin, has been identified that includes in its structure both the A and B chains of insulin. Proinsulin is synthesized in the microsomal fraction of the pancreatic beta cell, actively transported to the Golgi apparatus and processed into granules; there it is transformed into insulin by an enzymic cleavage of the connecting peptide, C-peptide. Proinsulin exhibits less biologic activity than insulin and no biologic effect of C-peptide has been shown. C-peptide measured in blood or urine serves as a marker for continued insulin secretion.

Insulin secretion in response to glucose stimulation follows a biphasic course. The initial secretion achieves a maximal rate in 2–3 minutes and then falls with a nadir 10 minutes later. There is a subsequent gradual increase in secretion which persists as long as hyperglycemia is maintained. This pattern is altered in the diabetic with a decreased or absent initial peak of insulin secretion. The later phase of the insulin response is also reduced, delayed or almost lacking. Essentially flat insulin responses to glucose predominate in juvenile diabetes. As a consequence of a decrease in the number of insulin receptors on the cell surface, obese subjects show an increase in fasting insulin levels and a hyperresponsiveness to elevated levels of blood glucose that is indicative of insulin resistance. The obese adult diabetic, while exhibiting higher basal and glucose-stimulated insulin levels than the non-obese, non-diabetic individual, responds with a lower insulin output than the obese non-diabetic control. These observations indicate that the diabetic whether obese or not secretes less insulin in response to a glucose challenge than does the appropriate control subject.

Glucose is the most potent stimulus for release of insulin. In addition, other nutrients, certain hormones, and drugs have stimulating properties. These include proteins and amino acids, medium and short chain fatty acids and ketones, glucagon, ACTH, beta adrenergic agents, gastrointestinal hormones and some sulfonylureas.

Immunoassay for Insulin

The procedure originally described by Berson and Yalow has contributed greatly to our understanding of clinical diabetes and of the physiologic mechanisms of insulin biosynthesis, secretion, transport and utilization. The assay requires an antibody to insulin and it is fortunate that the antibody produced in the guinea pig is adequate for measurement of insulin levels in man. In most assay methods, a trace of radioiodinated insulin is added to the reaction mixture and its conversion to labelled hormone-antibody complex is used to determine the insulin content of the sample.

Metabolic Effects of Insulin

Insulin plays the major role in regulating the blood glucose level as it is the only hormone that decreases the entrance of glucose and augments the outflow of glucose from the extracellular space. Its action permits the body to conserve the excess of nutrients absorbed following meals by stimulation of glucose transfer across cell membranes into skeletal and cardiac muscle and adipose tissue and subsequent conversion to glycogen and triglyceride. It also fosters the intracellular transport of amino acids and their conversion to protein. These actions increase the rate of glucose removal from the blood and decrease the supply of gluconeogenic metabolites, amino acids and glycerol to the liver. In the liver, insulin promotes glycogen formation, and suppresses glycogenolysis and gluconeogenesis. The hepatic effects of insulin are mediated through the adenyl cyclase system leading to a decrease in the intracellular concentration of cyclic AMP.

During fasting, when exogenous nutrients are unavailable, partial suppression of insulin release is appropriate. Low levels of insulin limit lipolysis and thereby provide free fatty acids for the body's energy needs at a rate that does not result in an accumulation of excessive quantities of ketone bodies. Fasting levels of insulin do not stimulate glucose uptake by skeletal muscle, glucose is then available to meet the obligatory requirements of the brain, formed elements of the blood, and the renal and adrenal medullas. Suppression of insulin secretion during fasting further ensures an adequate supply of glucose to the brain by increasing the availability of gluconeogenic substrates (amino acid and glycerol) with the mediation of glucagon, cortisol and catecholamines. Concommitantly there is increased glycogenolysis and hepatic glucose output, facilitated by glucagon and catecholamines.

The metabolic sequence set in motion by insulin deficiency (diabetes mellitus) can be regarded as an exaggeration of the physiologic suppression of insulin release during fasting. The primary effects of insulin deficiency are: (1) decreased peripheral uptake of glucose, (2) increased gluconeogenesis and hepatic output of glucose, and (3) uncontrolled lipolysis leading to ketosis. These metabolic changes are the key features in the pathogenesis of diabetic ketoacidosis and are illustrated in Figure 22-1.

Polyuria and polydipsia, symptoms suggesting diabetes, are the result of hyperglycemia and its consequent glycosuria. As the concentrating ability of the kidney is exceeded, marked glycosuria obligates an increase in renal excretion of water that is compensated by an increase in intake. Uncontrolled lipolysis leads to accumulation of the strong acids, beta-hydroxy-butyric and acetoacetic, which augment the body's hydrogen-ion pool and require neutralization chiefly by the bicarbonate buffering mechanism. In health, ketone bodies are oxidized via the Krebs cycle to yield carbon dioxide and water. In diabetics, the decreased activity of the pathway is a consequence of reduced peripheral uptake of glucose.

The solute diuresis accompanying hyperglycemia augments the acidosis as dehydration and decreased renal perfusion compromise renal excretion of hydrogen ions derived from fatty acid and protein catabolism. Solute diuresis also contributes to dehydration by decreasing renal reabsorption of sodium and potassium. Compensatory hyperventilation initiated by metabolic acidosis also adds to the deficit of body water. As acidosis and ketonemia progress, nausea and vomiting occur and reduce

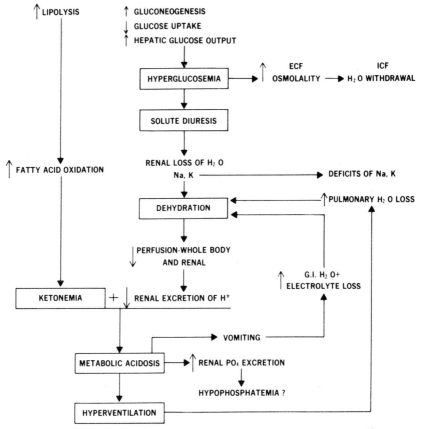

Fig. 22-1. Pathogenesis of diabetic acidosis. (From Kaye, R.: Juvenile diabetes. *In* Shirkey, H. C. (ed.): Pediatric Therapy, ed. 5. St. Louis, C. V. Mosby, 1975.)

water and electrolyte intake; the development of acidosis, dehydration and hypovolemic shock are accelerated.

With hyperglycemia in untreated diabetes, the extracellular fluid becomes hypertonic and osmotic shifts of water from the intra- to the extracellular compartment take place. The intracellular deficit of potassium is increased by its movement to the extracellular fluid consequent to metabolic acidosis. The process can be reversed by appropriate treatment with insulin, water, electrolytes and glucose.

Symptomatic diabetes mellitus in children always requires insulin therapy in the initial and later phases of treatment. A small group (perhaps 5% of patients) may experience a period of weeks or months of improved carbohydrate tolerance in which blood glucose levels remain in the normal range without the administration of exogenous insulin. It is important to explain that the remission will be temporary and insulin therapy will again be required.

Table 22-5. Some Properties of Currently Used Insulins

Type of Insulin	Onset (hr.)	Peak (hr.)	Duration (hr.)	Intensity of peak
Rapid-acting				
Crystalline zinc (insulin injection, USP) ("regular" insulin)	½	2–4	6–8	Marked
Semi-Lente (prompt insulin zinc suspension, USP)	½	2–4	10–12	Marked
Intermediate-acting				
Globin (globin zinc insulin injection, USP)	2	6–10	12–18	Moderate
NPH (isophane insulin suspension, USP)	2	8–10	18–24	Moderate
Lente (insulin zinc suspension, USP)	2	8–12	20–26	Moderate
Prolonged-acting				
Ultralente (extended insulin zinc suspension, USP)	6	18–24	36+	Mild
Protamine zinc (PZI) (protamine zinc insulin suspension, USP)	6	14–20	24–36	Mild

(From Kaye, R.: Juvenile diabetes. *In* Shirkey, H. C. (ed.): Pediatric Therapy, ed. 5. St. Louis, C. V. Mosby, 1975.)

A number of types of insulin are available and grouped conveniently on the basis of rapidity and duration of action (Table 22-5). A mixture of regular and NPH insulins are used for the treatment of most of our patients. Rapidly acting regular insulin facilitates utilization of the breakfast calories and also quickly reverses the inhibition of insulin action present in the fasting state when free fatty acid levels are elevated. In about 50 per cent of patients the combined use of NPH insulin will permit utilization of calories ingested during the balance of the day.

The lente insulins have the theoretical advantage of being free of the foreign protein, protamine, present in NPH and protamine zinc insulins. Ultralente insulin is sometimes useful in limiting excessive overnight glycosuria when intermediate-acting insulins fail to do so. In many instances, ultralente will not accomplish this purpose. Therefore, approximately one-half of children will require a second injection of an intermediate-acting insulin that is approximately 20 per cent of their morning dose; it should be given 45 minutes before dinner. A clear-cut indication for instituting the additional dose is nocturia and acetonuria in the prebreakfast specimen in a patient who is aglycosuric in the afternoon and therefore cannot be safely given an increased amount of intermediate-acting insulin in the morning. A less clear indication for a second dose is the patient who exhibits asymptomatic but marked glycosuria overnight.

A more highly purified insulin preparation designated "Single Peak" has been introduced for routine use. It is available only in a concentration of 100 units/ml. (U100) as regular, NPH, semi-lente, lente and ultralente. There are indications that this preparation produces less subcutaneous atrophy than the previously available products and often corrects insulin lipoatrophy when injected directly into affected sites.

Initial Insulin Treatment

In addition to the patient's weight, one must consider the severity of the existing metabolic disturbance; this disturbance correlates highly with the degree of insulin resistance likely to be encountered in an individual patient. Insulin resistance of diabetic acidosis is the result of acidosis that appears to decrease insulin receptors and elevations of stress-induced hormonal antagonists of insulin. These factors combine to yield an initial insulin requirement that may vary tenfold in patients of the same size who show equal amounts of glycosuria. There have been several recent reports of successful treatment of diabetic acidosis; utilizing small quantities of regular insulin, 0.1 units/kg./hr, administered intravenously by constant infusion. In this method a bolus injection of approximately 0.1 units/kg. is given prior to the constant infusion. Insulin levels of 40 to 120 μunits per ml. are achieved which are comparable to the insulin levels observed following glucose tolerance testing. These findings do not support the concept that diabetic acidosis is associated with significant insulin resistance; further studies are necessary before the current "high dose" therapy for severe diabetic acidosis is abandoned.

To establish an estimate of the initial insulin requirement, it is useful to classify the patient's condition on admission into progressive grades of severity on a scale of I to IV following the criteria indicated in Table 22-6.

Improvement with treatment is accompanied by increasing sensitivity to insulin and progress of the patient's diabetic state through successively milder grades. As shown in Table 22-6, improvement is reflected in a decrease in quantity and frequency of insulin injections.

In most instances, grading can be achieved on clinical grounds and examination of the urine for glucose and acetone. Clinical impression should be supported by determination of blood glucose, CO_2 content of the serum, and semiquantitative determination of plasma acetone; in the severely ill child grading should be determined by measurement of sodium, potassium, chloride, pH, and BUN as well.

The first two insulin injections are given in the quantity and at the time intervals specified in Table 22-6; subsequently, the patient's general condition and insulin sensitivity will have improved sufficiently to permit the insulin schedule to follow that for the next less severely affected grade. Usually, in 12–24 hours the patient's clinical status will have progressed to Grade IIb. At this time, fruit juices or carbonated drinks in small amounts can be tolerated.

Table 22-6. Initial Treatment Based on Clinical State

	Grade				
	IV	III	IIa	IIb	I
↓ Consciousness	+	−	−	−	−
Hyperventilation	+	+	−	−	−
Dehydration	+	+	−	−	−
↓ CO_2 content	+	+	+	+	−
↑ Serum ketones	+	+	+	+	±
4+ glycosuria	+	+	+	+	±
Acetonuria	+	+	+	+	±
Vomiting or nausea	+	+	+	−	−
Route of fluid therapy	IV	IV	IV	0	0
Initial insulin dose, (units/kg.)	1–2*	1	0.5	0.25	0.2
Subsequent dose (units/kg.)	0.5–1	0.5	0.25	0.25±50%	0.2±50%
Frequency of insulin injections (hr)	1–2	2–4	4	4–6	6

*Half intravenously and half intramuscularly. (From Kaye, R.: Juvenile diabetes. *In* Shirkey, H. C. (ed.): Pediatric Therapy, ed. 5. St. Louis, C. V. Mosby, 1975.)

The majority of patients in recent years has presented for treatment with findings characteristic of Grade IIb or Grade I. These patients may be offered a regular diet *ad libitum* until the dietary prescription can be put into effect. Regular insulin is given 15 minutes before the major meals and at bedtime. Subsequent doses are modified, usually within a 50 per cent range, depending on the effectiveness of the preceding dose. On succeeding days the basis for dosage estimate is the effectiveness of the quantity of insulin administered prior to the same meal on the preceding day. As tolerance returns and freedom from glycosuria is achieved, insulin dosage is reduced in steps of about 20 per cent. When reduction of insulin dosage results in re-establishment of glycosuria, the approximate insulin requirement of the patient has been established; it is then feasible to attempt control with a single injection of a mixture of short- and intermediate-acting insulins administered 15 minutes before breakfast. This stage is usually reached 6–10 days after admission.

When the patient's requirement for insulin has been determined as described above, short-acting insulin (regular) is administered in an amount equal to 75 per cent of the prebreakfast dose, and intermediate-acting insulin (NPH) in a quantity equal to 75 per cent of the sum of the regular insulin dosages administered before lunch, dinner, and at bedtime on the previous day. Further adjustments are made in approximately two-unit amounts for short-acting insulin, based on the glycosuria after breakfast, and for intermediate-acting insulin, based on the glycosuria during the balance of the day.

GENERAL PRINCIPLES OF TREATMENT
OF DIABETIC KETOACIDOSIS

Diabetic ketoacidosis can be viewed as the advanced stage of insulin deficiency. The process is initiated by hyperglucosemia and ketonemia and prgresses to metabolic acidosis, dehydration and coma (Fig. 22-1).

Treatment is aimed at reversal of these metabolic derangements by provision of insulin, water and electrolytes. Appropriate treatment accomplishes this purpose and avoids cetain undesirable side-effects which may accompany rapid correction of hyperglycemia and its associated hyperosmolarity and acidosis.

Hyperosmolarity

As ketoacidosis develops, the rise in blood glucose increases the osmolality of the extracellular fluid by 10 mOsmol/liter for each increment of blood glucose of 180 mg./dl. The extracellular hyperosmolarity draws water from the intracellular compartment including the brain. As the blood glucose level is reduced with insulin treatment, the movement of water is reversed and the potential then exists for the development of cerebral edema and increased intracranial pressure. This sequence can be avoided by maintaining the blood glucose at moderately elevated levels during the first 16–18 hours of treatment (approximately 250 mg./dl.) by the infusion of glucose-containing solutions when the above level is approached.

The initial intravenous infusion should consist of an isotonic or near isotonic solution of NaCl or $NaHCO_3$, free of glucose. Solutions with this concentration of sodium will also increase more effectively intravascular volume and peripheral perfusion. They will also serve to replace the loss of water from the vascular compartment that results from osmotic shifts as blood glucose levels are reduced.

Correction of Acidosis

Conservative use of alkali is indicated for the following reasons: (1) administration of glucose and insulin stops further ketogenesis and permits oxidation of preformed ketones to CO_2 and H_2O, thereby regenerating HCO_3; and (2) increased serum HCO_3 and extracellular pH suppress respiratory minute volume causing a rise in blood pCO_2. As cells including the blood-brain barrier are freely permeable to CO_2 but not to HCO_3 and other anions, rapid increase in extracellular bicarbonate results in a fall in intracellular pH as CO_2 enters cells in which HCO_3 remains low. Decreasing blood glucose and increasing serum HCO_3^-, which usually indicate recovery from diabetic acidosis, have occasionally been associated with alarming deterioration of the patient's condition with signs consistent with cerebral edema. This situation may be due in part to the changes in osmolarity and central nervous system pH described above.

A further basis for conservative use of $NaHCO_3$ in diabetic acidosis is that the acidotic state is associated with a "shift to the right" of the hemoglobin - O_2 dissociation curve. This shift is beneficial permitting the delivery of more O_2 to the tissues at a given O_2 tension and compensating in part for the decreased tissue perfusion consequent to dehydration. Rapid correction of blood pH to normal eliminates this adjustment. This undesirable effect is compounded as acidosis also leads to reduced levels of certain organic phosphate compounds in the red cell, 2, 3 - diphosphoglycerate (2, 3 - DPG) and adenosine triphosphate (ATP) which decrease O_2 release to the tissues and persists for some time after acidosis is corrected. Thus, rapid correction of acidosis is associated with two phenomena which diminish release of O_2 to the tissues at the time when decreased tissue perfusion is still present.

The above considerations suggest that HCO_3 administration to patients with diabetic ketoacidosis should be avoided. There are, however, circumstances in which its use is appropriate and perhaps life-saving; these involve the effects of reduced blood pH on respiratory minute volume and myocardial contractility. Little stimulation of ventilation occurs until arterial pH falls to 7.2. Below this level, there is a rapid increase in minute volume which declines at pH levels of approximately 7.1 and below. The fall in minute volume decreases the effectiveness of the respiratory compensation for metabolic acidosis and may lead to a potentially lethal increase in acidosis. It has also been documented that adverse effects on myocardial contractility occur at pH values of 7.1 or below. It is therefore good practice to avoid the use of exogenous alkali in patients with blood pH values above 7.15 or serum HCO_3 levels above 8 mEq/liter and to administer $NaHCO_3$ solutions to those with values below these levels. As current methods for estimating the base deficit in diabetic ketoacidosis tend to exaggerate its magnitude, an arbitrary dose of 2.0–2.5 mEq/kg. is appropriate for this purpose.

Patients who are dehydrated or nauseated will require administration of H_2O and electrolyte by the intravenous route (Grade IV, III and IIa). All will require maintenance amounts of water, sodium and potassium (Table 22-7) with additional allowances for dehydration, if present, and for increased urinary water losses due to continued glycosuria. Approximate deficits in the moderately dehydrated patient are given in Table 22-8.

Administration of Water. All patients receiving parenteral fluids will require maintenance amounts of water (1500–1800 ml./m.²/24 hrs. The deficit of H_2O is approximately equally divided between the intra- and extracellular body water compartments. The rate of repair of the intracellular water deficit is limited by the rate of cellular uptake of potassium which occurs against a concentration gradient and is therefore limited

Table 22-7. Maintenance Requirements by Body Weight and Surface Area

Wt (kg.)	Surface area (m.²)	H₂O (ml.)		Na (mEq)		K (mEq)		Glucose (g.)	
		kg.	m.²	kg.	m.²	kg.	m.²	kg.	m.²
3	0.20	100	1500–1800	3	60	2	50	6–10	150
5	0.27	90	1500–1800	3	60	2	50	6–10	150
10	0.45	75	1500–1800	3	60	2	50	6–10	150
15	0.64	65	1500–1800	—	60	2	50		150
30	1.10	55	1500–1800	—	60	—	50		150
50	1.50	45	1500–1800	—	60	—	50		150
70	1.73	40	1500–1800	—	60	—	50		150

*These quantities of H_2O, Na, and K will be approximated by using Butler's solution (concentrations in mEq/liter: Na, 40; K, 35; Cl, 40; HCO_3, 20; and P, 15) in the above specified quantities. Another suitable solution is provided by saline in one-fourth of physiologic concentration supplemented by appropriate amounts of a K concentrate (1 mEq/ml.). (From Kaye, R.: Juvenile diabetes. *In* Shirkey, H. C. (ed.): Pediatric Therapy, ed. 5. St. Louis, C. V. Mosby, 1975.)

even in the presence of marked intracellular deficits. As a result, repair of only a portion of the estimated water deficit is indicated in the first 24 hours of treatment, i.e. 70 per cent or 70 ml./kg. It is also necessary to consider that estimates of maintenance requirements for water are based on a urinary water excretion of about 800 ml./m²/24 hrs. The continued solute diuresis of diabetic acidosis necessitates an adjustment of estimates of renal water requirements. Urinary water excretion in excess of the usual output requires the addition of an equal amount to meet maintenance requirements. It is prudent to administer intravenous fluids at a rate that provides half of the estimated 24-hour quantity in the first 6–8 hours of treatment.

Administration of Sodium. NaCl in isotonic solution, 20–30 ml./kg. is administered initially to expand blood volume and improve whole body and renal perfusion. This quantity may be administered safely in 1½–2 hours. If pH is depressed below 7.15, 2.0–2.5 mEq of $NaHCO_3$ may be substituted for an equivalent amount of NaCl. The total amount of sodium required for maintenance (60 mEq/m.²) plus repair of deficit (10

Table 22-8. Water and Electrolyte Deficits in Diabetic Coma

Water	Total	per kg. body weight
Water	5–11	100 ml.
Sodium	300–700 mEq.	7–10 mEq.
Chloride	350–500 mEq.	5–7 mEq.
Potassium	200–700 mEq.	5–10 mEq.

*Approximate. Based upon retention of water and electrolyte during treatment of ketoacidosis. (Modified from Bradley, R. F., and Rees, S. B.: Water, electrolyte and hydrogen ion abnormalities in diabetes mellitus. *In* Bland, J. H. (ed.): Clinical Metabolism of Body Water and Electrolytes. Philadelphia, W. B. Saunders Co., 1963; p. 448.)

mEq/kg.) can be provided in the appropriate amount of water; one-third of the total fluids in isotonic strength, one-third at one-half normal and the balance at one-fourth normal concentrations.

Potassium Administration. Serum potassium concentrations are usually elevated or normal at the onset of treatment; for this reason, its administration should be delayed for 2–4 hours and until urine flow is established. As the rate of cellular uptake is limited, no effort should be made to restore the entire estimated deficit in the first 24 hours of treatment. The recommended dosage is 3.5 mEq/kg., recognizing that this amount may not be adequate to prevent hypokalemia and additional amounts may be required. Parenteral potassium should be given in a concentration usually not in excess of 40 mEq/liter.

Administration of PO_4. Hypophosphatemia may be associated with diabetic acidosis as a consequence of increased H^+ excretion, solute diuresis, tissue protein catabolism and intracellular movement with restored glucose utilization with insulin treatment. Hypophosphatemia leads to impaired O_2 release from hemoglobin and to the development of rigid red cells which are readily hemolyzed. It is appropriate, therefore, to administer phosphate parenterally. This can be done by administering half of the parenteral potassium as $K_2 HPO_4$.

The progress of therapy is indicated by clinical response and by serial examinations of blood and urine for glucose and acetone. A progressive decline in serum and urine acetone concentrations with maintenance of a modest hyperglycemia and glycosuria are factors determining satisfactory treatment.

INFECTIONS

During upper respiratory infections of average severity, mild ketosis is common and may require an increase in insulin. Ten per cent of the total daily dosage is given as regular insulin before each of the main meals, and at bedtime if acetonuria is present.

During episodes of gastroenteritis accompanied by nausea and vomiting, treatment is designed to provide enough insulin to prevent uncontrolled lipolysis and ketogenesis, adequate carbohydrate to permit oxidation of fatty acids mobilized from fat depots, and to prevent hypoglycemia. This can be accomplished usually by administering 80 per cent of the usual dose of insulin along with quantities of carbohydrate-containing liquids—citrus fruit juices, or carbonated drinks adequate for fluid maintenance (Table 22-7). As the tolerance for food returns, additional carbohydrate-containing foods (toast with jelly, stewed fruits, etc.) can be offered to avoid ketosis and hypoglycemia.

SURGERY

Surgery does not usually require an increase in insulin dosage. One-half of the patient's total daily dose is given as intermediate acting insulin prior to the operation, with the balance given at 6-hour intervals as regular insulin if hyperglycemia indicates the need for additional insulin. Adequate carbohydrate and NaCl will be furnished by provision of the child's water requirement as 10 per cent glucose in one-fourth strength physiologic saline.

PATHOGENESIS OF LATE COMPLICATIONS

The consensus of studies designed to gain an understanding of the late complications of diabetes has tended to implicate hyperglycemia in the pathogenesis of lesions of the peripheral nervous system, lens of the eye and capillaries throughout the body. Increased activity of the polyol pathway consequent to hyperglycemia may play a role in the development of diabetic cataracts, neuropathy and in lesions of major arteries. Polyols are organic compounds containing multiple alcohol groups derived from sugars by reduction of the terminal aldehyde or ketone group. Sorbitol is the polyol derived from glucose. The reaction is catalyzed by aldose reductase which has a high Km for glucose, the rate of the reaction varying directly with increasing glucose concentration permitting sorbitol to accumulate in tissues in hyperglycemic states. Sorbitol accumulation has been demonstrated in lenses of human diabetics where its osmotic activity can result in increased water content as well as interference with the sodium and potassium "pumps" regulating the intracellular concentration of these ions. Similar mechanisms may be of pathogenic significance in the metabolism of the Schwann cell contributing to the development of diabetic neuropathy and in the wall of the aorta where edema may interfere with the diffusion of O_2 and other nutrients to the deeper portions of the blood vessel wall.

The microangiopathic lesions of diabetes consist of thickening of the basement membrane which surrounds the capillaries of all tissues. This alteration is particularly important in the kidney where it involves both the glomerular capillary loops and mesangial regions leading to an impairment in the function of the glomerulus as a selective filter. Similar changes have been shown in the capillaries of the retina, skin, nerves and muscle. These changes may result from alterations in chemical composition of glycoproteins of the basement membrane secondary to hyperglycemia.

The prevalence and magnitude of thickening of the basement membrane of muscle capillaries increases with the duration of the disease. Some workers believe that this alteration can be observed in prediabetic subjects and may be a genetic marker for diabetes mellitus. It would seem more reasonable that the electron microscopic changes described are related in some way to the metabolic alterations of diabetes and that the mechanisms described above contribute to these anatomic findings. Basement membrane thickening is not present in diabetic children under the age of five but involves the majority of diabetics by age twenty.

It is tempting to utilize the data incriminating hyperglycemia in the pathogenesis of diabetic vascular injury as an argument supporting attempts to rigidly control the level of blood glucose in diabetic patients. It is likely, however, that present treatment methods are incapable of accomplishing this end in most cases of juvenile diabetics.

Pathology

Hyalinization of the islets of Langerhans is characteristic of the findings in the pancreas of the older diabetic patient. In the juvenile diabetic, the lesions are more subtle. Gepts has described autopsy findings in subjects developing diabetes under the age of 21 years. In 22 individuals who died less than 6 months after onset, the number of beta cells was found to be reduced to less than 10 per cent of normal. Lymphocytic inflammatory infiltrates in or around the islets were prominent and fibrosis was evident. The inflammatory changes noted are compatible with an infectious or toxic origin and also suggest the possibility of an autoimmune mechanism being of etiologic importance in some cases.

COMPLICATIONS AND PROGNOSIS

Ketoacidosis as a cause of death in diabetic children is fortunately relatively uncommon. Sepsis is no longer a significant threat to the survival of the young diabetic.

Vascular injury remains the most important cause of late morbidity and mortality in juvenile-onset diabetes. Priscilla White has reported that large vessel calcifications occur between the ages of 10–19 in about 6.5 per cent of juvenile diabetics. These changes lead to significant impairment of health. Among 30-year survivors of childhood diabetes, 4 per cent experienced cerebral vascular accidents and 19 per cent suffered myocardial infarctions. Retinopathy is the earliest of the microangiopathic lesions to occur. These have been classified into exudative, angiopathic and proliferative types. Angiopathy includes dilated venules, microcapillary aneurysms, hemorrhages and neo-vascular formation. Retinal lesions that threatened vision occurred in 3 per cent of patients after 15 years of diabetes; this figure rose to 46 per cent by 30 years, at which time 8 per cent of patients were blind.

Nephropathy, while second in frequency of microangiopathy, is first as a cause of morbidity and mortality. It is present in 18 per cent of patients by 15 years and 44 per cent by 30 years of disease. The prognosis of diabetic renal disease correlates best with elevation of blood urea nitrogen. Sustained elevation to 25 mg./dl. is associated with an average life expectancy of 6 years. Duration of life is adversely affected by the occurrence of diabetes in childhood. A youngster becoming diabetic at age 15 has a life expectancy of 56 years in contrast to 73 years for his non-diabetic peers. It is hoped that more effective methods of treatment such as pancreas transplantation will improve the present unsatisfactory prognosis.

BIBLIOGRAPHY

Diabetes Mellitus, 4th edition, 1977.

> This volume provides an up-to-date summary of the major topics of pathophysiology and treatment of diabetes. It is issued periodically by the Committee on Professional Education of the American Diabetes Association, Inc., 600 Fifth Avenue, New York, N. Y. 10020.

Ganda, O. P., and Soeldner, S. S.: Genetic, acquired, and related factors in the etiology of diabetes mellitus. Arch. Intern. Med., *137*:461, 1977.

> An excellent review of genetic, viral and autoimmune factors in diabetic etiology.

Kaye, R.: Diabetic ketoacidosis—the bicarbonate controversy. J. Pediatr., *87*:156, 1975.

> A brief review of considerations for and against the use of bicarbonate in the treatment of diabetic ketoacidosis.

Marble, A., White, P., Bradley, R. F., and Krall, L. P.: Joslin's Diabetes Mellitus, ed 11. Philadelphia, Lea and Febiger, 1971.

> An excellent reference book dealing comprehensively with physiologic and clinical aspects of diabetes.

23

Respiratory Signs and Symptoms

Douglas S. Holsclaw, M.D.

The diagnosis, assessment and management of pediatric pulmonary diseases require an understanding of the normal structure and an appreciation of the major presenting signs and symptoms of deviations from the normal. The history and physical examination are of primary importance, laboratory studies of lung function less so. Most of the pulmonary function tests used for adults are difficult for younger children to perform, and few of the available tests are critical for the diagnosis of the majority of clinical conditions in pediatrics.

Rather than dwell on a detailed review of respiratory physiology, an approach has been chosen to integrate structure of the respiratory tract with function and introduce some of the terms and symbols used in the assessment of respiratory physiology. Since deranged pulmonary function is expressed in the child by certain symptoms which are usually the reason for the patient being brought to the physician's attention, consideration of the major presenting signs and symptoms and their implications for certain disease processes follow.

Principles of clinical evaluation applicable to a broad spectrum of lung diseases conclude the chapter.

PULMONARY STRUCTURE AND FUNCTION

The main function of the lung is to enable air to come into close proximity to the red blood cells flowing through the pulmonary capillaries. In this way oxygen (O_2) can diffuse into the blood and carbon dioxide (CO_2) can diffuse out.

Several structural adaptations are needed to produce this functional relationship. Included are the development of the right ventricle and the pulmonary vascular system, by means of which all blood returning to the heart is pumped through a vast array of thin sheets infolded into a relatively small space, and an airway system that can deliver a large volume of air at almost zero velocity when it comes into contact with these sheets of blood. The large internal surface area of the adult human lung—approximately 1 m.²/kg. body weight at 75 per cent of total lung capacity (TLC)— is not related to the act of distributing air into the lung (ventilation, V). Instead, it fulfills the need to distribute a large quantity of blood (perfusion, Q), into a very fine film such that:

1. The capillary transit time, during which gas exchange occurs, is long enough to permit equilibration.
2. The tissue phase of gas diffusion is minimized.
3. The resistance to flow in the pulmonary vascular bed remains low.

The structures that allow this to take place are discussed with particular reference to the function of each segment involved.

AIRWAYS

There are about 25 generations or branches of the airways that can be classified longitudinally into three groups: the cartilaginous airways (trachea and bronchi) generations 0 to 7; the membranous airways (bronchioles) generations 8 to 22; and the gas exchange airways (respiratory bronchioles and alveolar ducts) generation 23 to 25.

Cartilaginous Airways

Structure. Cartilaginous airways include the trachea and all its branchings down to the small bronchi (approximately 0.1–0.3 cm. in diameter when the lung is fully inflated). The main structural supports for the bronchi are C-shaped cartilaginous rings and plates supporting their anterior and lateral walls connected by a strong fibrous layer. The cartilaginous plates become smaller and fewer in number with each successive branching of the bronchial tree. Within this framework is a layer of circularly arranged smooth muscle whose motor innervation is the parasympathetic branch of the autonomic nervous system (vagus nerve). This smooth muscle is also capable of being contracted, thus narrowing the airway by direct stimulation.

The mucous membrane is pseudostratified, ciliated epithelium. Interspersed between the ciliated cells are mucus-secreting goblet cells in, roughly, a 1 to 5 ratio. A distinctive feature of the large cartilaginous bronchi is the presence of bronchial glands situated deep within the submucosa connecting to the surface through ducts. These glands contain both mucus and serous-secreting elements and may be stimulated to secrete via the vagus nerve. The bronchial glands are particularly dense in the medium-sized bronchi, decreasing in number and size distally, finally disappearing altogether near the transition from cartilaginous bronchi to membranous bronchioles.

The mucosal surface of the cells is covered by a thin blanket formed by continuous serous and mucus secretion of the airway epithelium and glands. In a normal adult, the mucous membrane of the tracheobronchial tree secretes about a half liter of fluid in a 24-hour period. This blanket is propelled continuously upward through the airways to the pharynx, (the mucociliary escalator) pushed along by the constantly beating cilia (1000 strokes/minute). Two hundred cilia are on each ciliated cell, each cilium being 4–6 μm. long).

The sensory innervation of the large airways is by vagal nerve fibers whose receptor endings appear to be adjacent to the surface epithelial layer. These fibers are sensitive to irritation and appear to be identical to cough receptors that are particularly abundant in the trachea and largest bronchi.

The blood supply of the bronchi is via the bronchial circulation arising from the aorta (systemic circulation).

Function. The cartilaginous airways are the conduits through which gas enters and leaves the respiratory gas exchange areas of the lung. Since these airways do not allow gas exchange across their walls, they contribute to that portion of the freshly inspired breath that does not undergo gas exchange—the dead space. Indeed, the cartilaginous airways, together with the nose and throat, account for almost all the anatomical dead space volume. In addition, because of the air flow through this system of branching and narrowing tubes, the cartilaginous airways contribute to a large portion of the total resistance to breathing. Resistance to gas flow in the bronchi can be increased by reflex or local stimulation of the smooth muscles which causes narrowing of the airways. Both inert particles impinging on the airway surface and chemically active agents may stimulate the irritant constrictor mechanism.

The cartilaginous airways also aid in the warming and humidification of incoming air, particularly during mouth breathing when the nasal mechanism is bypassed.

Inhaled particles in the size range between 2 and 10 μm usually settle or impact onto the mucociliary surface layer during inspiration, and are transported out of the airways to the pharynx where they are swallowed. This remarkable mechanism, which propels particles at a rate of 1.0 cm./min. in the upper airway, is dependent on stable temperature and humidity and can be temporarily inactivated by noxious substances such as cigarette smoke. Highly soluble gaseous materials (sulfur dioxide) are very efficiently scrubbed out of the inspired air; none reaches the distal delicate gas exchange surfaces.

Chronic irritant stimuli appear to cause hypertrophy of the mucus-secreting elements and glands of the upper airway with a parallel increase in the production and secretion of the airway mucus.

Membranous Airways

Structure. The bronchioles, direct continuations of the airways, end in the terminal bronchioles which are approximately 0.4 mm. in diameter. The chief difference between them and the bronchi is the absence of both the fibrocartilage framework and the secretory glands. The patency of the bronchioles is greatly influenced by the negative intrapleural pressure.

Structural support of the bronchioles comes from their being directly imbedded into the connective tissue framework of the lung. They contain a continuous circular layer of smooth muscle whose innervation is believed to be similar to that of the bronchi.

The mucosa is continuous with that of the bronchi. The epithelial layer consists of low ciliated columnar cells which gradually become more cuboidal as the terminal bronchiole is approached. Interspersed with the ciliated cells is a decreasing number of goblet cells which normally disappear completely at the terminal bronchiole.

Blood supply to the bronchioles is also from the bronchial artery. Sensory innervation consists mainly of undifferentiated fibers in the subepithelial portion of the mucosa.

Function. The functional difference between small bronchi and large bronchioles is not as sharp as the anatomical description suggests; there is a gradual transition. Although the bronchioles contribute to the dead space and airflow resistance, normally this contribution is considerably less than that of the bronchi. The bronchioles are affected by lung volume since these airways are imbedded in the lung tissue and are passively dilated during lung inflation and, conversely, narrowed in lung deflation (expiration).

Edema of the bronchiolar mucosa, mucus accumulation or active contraction of the circular smooth muscle by reflex or by local irritation can greatly increase the resistance to airflow through these very small tubes.

The mucociliary blanket in the terminal bronchioles is mainly a watery fluid, but it gradually accumulates mucus as it moves up the airways. With chronic irritant stimulation, the mucus-secreting goblet cell population in the bronchioles may markedly increase.

Gas Exchange Airways

Structure. The respiratory bronchioles and alveolar ducts are the final branchings of the airways. They are continuous with the terminal bronchioles. Chief distinguishing feature of these gas exchange airways is the presence of alveoli, an estimated 300,000,000 in number, in whose walls the pulmonary capillaries are distributed and where the O_2 and CO_2 exchange occurs.

All the gas exchange airways are approximately the same diameter (0.05 cm.), and, like the bronchioles, receive their structural support from the connective tissue framework of lung tissue. There is an interrupted circular layer of smooth muscle whose motor innervation is probably similar to that of the bronchioles; however, this is not clearly defined. The mucosa of the respiratory bronchiole is a single layer of low cuboidal epithelial cells some of which contain cilia. The Clara cell, recently discovered and believed to secrete a surfactant-like material, is interspersed. There are no goblet cells. Sensory nerves in the mucosal layer are of the undifferentiated type, similar to those seen in the bronchioles, but much less numerous.

The blood supply to the gas exchange airways comes via the pulmonary circulation, not the bronchial circulation.

Function. The gas exchange airways serve to distribute the inspired gas by bulk flow within the terminal respiratory units. Because of their blood supply via the pulmonary circulation, the smooth muscle of these units (particularly the respiratory bronchioles) may be selectively influenced by agents present in the pulmonary blood. These airways dilate and narrow with changes in lung volume. They account for approximately one-third of the total alveolar gas exchange volume.

PULMONARY CIRCULATION

Structure

The quantity of blood flowing through the lungs is equal to that flowing through the systemic circulation. The muscle wall of the right ventricle is only one-third as thick as that of the left ventricle, yet the right ventricle pumps as much blood as the left at much lower pressure. The entire output of the right ventricle enters the pulmonary artery and is distributed to the lungs through the pulmonary arteries. These branch out with the airways down to the respiratory bronchioles. Thus, at all levels the pulmonary arteries are adjacent to the airways. The branches of the pulmonary artery are all very short and accommodate very small quantities of blood in comparison with the relatively large amounts that can be stored in the systemic arterial system. The average blood pressure in the pulmonary artery reaches 22 mm. Hg during systole and falls to 8 mm. Hg during diastole with a mean pressure of about 13 mm. Hg. If it were not for the extreme distensibility of the thin pulmonary arteries, the pulmonary arterial pulse pressure would have to be greater than it is. Larger pulmonary arteries are of the elastic variety, whereas the smaller ones that accompany the terminal bronchioles are described as muscular. The pulmonary arteries are richly innervated from the sympathetic branch of the autonomic system.

Pulmonary microcirculation consists of an extensive capillary network which some investigators believe behaves more as a sheet of blood than as individual channels. The pulmonary capillaries are somewhat larger than systemic capillaries. The capillary network originates in short pre-capillary vessels branching at right angles from the small arteries. Each capillary network is continuous over several alveoli before condensing into the pulmonary venous system.

The pulmonary venous system is not closely related to the airways and, in fact, lies as far from the airways as anatomically feasible. The pulmonary veins drain into the left atrium. The venous system contains smooth muscle and is well innervated, presumably via the sympathetic branch of the autonomic nervous system.

Function

The pulmonary vascular bed is highly distensible and has a low resistance to blood flow. All the right ventricular output passes through the pulmonary vascular bed at a driving pressure that is about one-seventh that of the systemic circulation. Pressure in the pulmonary capillaries is about 5 mm. Hg when measured by catheterization. Blood passes through the pulmonary capillaries in about 0.8 of a second. This allows time for the red cells to remain in contact with the gas phase and is sufficient for O_2 and CO_2 equilibration under all except the most severe conditions, such as heavy exercise while breathing low oxygen tensions.

With a normal increase in cardiac output into the pulmonary circuit, this transit time remains at about 0.8 of a second. The increased blood flow is accomplished by a reserve of capillaries which normally remain collapsed, but which open up to accommodate increased blood flow.

Since the pulmonary circulation is a flow-through system, there is no dead space comparable to that in the airways. Because all venous blood passes through the pulmonary microvascular bed before entering the systemic circulation, the pulmonary capillaries act as a filter for removal of embolic material and as a site of inactivation of certain chemical substances in blood.

Because the pulmonary arteries are adjacent to the airways, inflammatory airway disease may cause scar tissue to encompass the adjacent pulmonary artery, thereby affecting the distribution of blood flow to the distal segment.

The smooth muscle of the pulmonary microvascular bed, particularly the small muscular pulmonary arteries, is sensitive to the partial pressure of oxygen in the surrounding airspaces (PaO_2). Breathing low oxygen concentrations (which results in hypoxia) stimulates the smooth muscle to constrict.

The endothelium of the pulmonary microvascular bed forms a substantial component of the tissue structure of the alveolar walls (approximately 30% by volume). There are data to suggest that the endothelial cells are more sensitive than other cells to damage by toxic substances such as high levels of oxygen and endotoxins.

THE TERMINAL RESPIRATORY UNITS

Structure

Beyond the last membranous airway (terminal bronchiole), the airways contain alveoli, in whose walls the pulmonary capillaries course and where the exchange of O_2 and CO_2 occurs. The respiratory bronchiole, the alveolar duct and the alveolar sacs constitute the terminal respiratory unit (TRU). The basic functional structure of the lung is that of a very large number (100,000 in man) of TRUs arranged in parallel. Each of these units receives ventilation through a terminal bronchiole and perfusion through a pulmonary arteriole.

At the end of a normal expiration, the total volume of gas in all the TRUs is the functional residual capacity (FRC) of the lung. In the normal adult, the FRC is approximately one-third of the maximal possible volume that all the TRUs can hold (total lung capacity: TLC).

The principal cellular structures of the alveolar epithelium are the broad pavement cells that cover 95 per cent of the alveolar surface (Type 1 cells), granular pneumonocytes, which are smaller, more numerous and more active-appearing cells (Type 2 cells), and alveolar macrophages. Type 2 cells contain peculiar, dense granules thought to be the precursors of alveolar surfactant. Found in varying numbers, alveolar macrophages are migratory phagocytic cells submerged in the extracellular lining of the alveolar surface. There is general agreement that alveolar macrophages originate from stem cell precursors in the bone marrow and reach the lung through the blood stream, presumably as circulating monocytes. Alveolar macrophages are of considerable interest because they constitute the chief mechanism for clearance of bacteria and particles deposited in the terminal respiratory units. Deficiencies in their function undoubtedly contribute to the pathogenesis of pulmonary infections.

As mentioned in the section on pulmonary circulation, the capillary endothelium accounts for some 30 per cent of the non-blood portion of the alveolar walls, making it a large tissue in its own right.

On the surface of the alveolar epithelium, separating the gas phase from the epithelial cells, is a thin film of fluid on whose surface is distributed a monomolecular phospholipid film (alveolar surfactant). Surfactant is believed to be actively secreted by Type 2 alveolar cells.

The respiratory membrane is between 1 and 4 μm in thickness, and is composed of three layers: the endothelial cells of the capillary wall, the epithelial cells of the respiratory epithelium, and the interstitial layer. The capillaries are about 8 μm in diameter, so the red blood cells, which are a little over 7 μm, actually squeeze through the pulmonary capillaries. The surface membrane of the red blood cell contacts the walls of the capillaries, and oxygen traverses very little plasma before it enters the red blood cells. These narrow clearances facilitate rapid oxygen uptake by the red blood cells.

To recognize the magnitude of the blood-air interface at the respiratory membrane and the capability for rapid, thorough exchange of gases, imagine a wall 20 ft. high and 30 ft. long, 85 to 95 per cent of which is covered with pulmonary capillaries. In the normal adult about 60 to 100 ml. of blood occupy the pulmonary capillaries at one time. A third of a billion red blood cells are exposed over a 600 ft.² respiratory membrane surface at any instant. This area of surface contact is 40 times greater than that of the body's external skin. Within 0.8 of a second the alveolar gases and pulmonary capillary blood of a normal man are in close equilibrium.

As well as having an important but passive role in gas and liquid exchange, the capillary endothelium is thought to be the site of active biochemical events, such as the inactivation of polypeptides, prostaglandins and amines that have important physiologic functions.

Function

Current evidence indicates that the entire TRU expands and contracts proportionately with breathing, but over the range of the lung volume from FRC to TLC the alveoli remain inflated.

In breathing, the gas exchange airways receive the bulk of fresh air flow coming down the airways, whereas the alveoli receive the air that was in the gas exchange airways and dead space at the end of the previous expiration. Aerosol particles, in the size range from 0.3 to 2 μm in diameter, do not impact or settle in the conducting airways and, therefore, reach the respiratory bronchioles and alveolar ducts by bulk flow. Gases and particles less than 0.3 μm in diameter diffuse from the gas exchange airways into the alveoli themselves and are generally exhaled with a subsequent breath.

The phospholipid monolayer at the alveolar air-liquid interface has the special property of varying surface tension with TRU volume. Its most important attribute is to decrease surface tension to nearly zero as TRU volume decreases during expiration, thus avoiding the collapse of the alveoli.

The surfactant film is critical to normal breathing. It decreases the work of breathing, permits alveoli to remain inflated at low distending pressures, and reduces the net forces causing tissue fluid accumulation (pulmonary edema). Changes in alveolar surface area with breathing causes movement in the surface film with loss of some surfactant material and replacement by new molecules. Movements of the alveoli cause the surface film to flow over alveolar walls to the central airway (first order respiratory bronchiole) of the TRU. Alveolar clearance of surfactant and entrapped particles is predominately by macrophage ingestion or, alternatively, by penetration through the alveolar epithelium and clearance through the interstitium via lymphatics.

Fresh air ventilation of the TRU is only useful if it is matched by a proportionate blood flow through the pulmonary capillaries of that unit.

The relationship of alveolar ventilation ($\dot{V}$) to blood flow ($\dot{Q}$) for each TRU is called the ventilation/perfusion ratio ($\dot{V}/\dot{Q}$). The ventilation/perfusion ratio averaged from all the TRUs of the lung is the overall ventilation to perfusion ratio of the lung and determines the arterial O_2 and CO_2 pressures by which the efficiency of the gas exchange process is judged. Within limits, each TRU can regulate $\dot{V}/\dot{Q}$ through changes in respiratory bronchiole and pulmonary artery smooth muscle tone. The earliest manifestation of uneven $\dot{V}/\dot{Q}$ is a fall in PaO_2, while $PaCO_2$ is essentially normal if overall $\dot{V}$ is normal.

The extremes of $\dot{V}/\dot{Q}$ unevenness are zero (blood flow without ventilation) and infinity (ventilation without blood flow). The former is an anatomic or physiologic shunt; the latter is wasted ventilation also known as physiologic dead space. That process by which oxygen penetrates from the gas phase of the TRU into the red blood cells in the capillaries is called diffusion. Ordinarily there is rapid diffusion of O_2 and CO_2 within the gas phase of the TRU. Within the alveolar wall tissues, however, the low solubility of oxygen tends to limit its transport. This is not a problem for CO_2. Fortunately the distance over which O_2 molecules have to diffuse to reach the red blood cells does not exceed half the width of the alveolar wall—1–4 μm.

The force (pressure difference between inside and outside of the lung or transpulmonary pressure) necessary for lung expansion during breathing is normally quite small. The distensibility of the lung as measured by the change in lung volume for each unit change in transpulmonary pressure is called lung compliance. In diseases in which the alveolar structure is destroyed, the units may be more easily inflated and even remain distended during expiration. In diseases leading to fibrotic changes, the lung may resist changes of volume and is then said to be stiff or have a low compliance.

CLINICAL EVALUATION OF RESPIRATORY DISEASE

Of necessity, clinical evaluation of the child with respiratory disease begins with an accurate and thorough history. Careful attention should be paid to the onset of symptoms and any associated signs. In cases of acute illness, the family may be able to easily elicit the beginning of respiratory distress. This may be accompanied by fever, cough, vomiting and chest pain. The degree and character of all of these should be noted. The nature of the cough, if present, should be carefully described: e.g., dry, loose, productive, spasmodic. The presence of noisy breathing, wheezing or grunting should also be noted.

The onset of chronic respiratory illness may be much more difficult to determine. Subtle events such as occasional cough, decreased appetite, slow weight gain and fatigue may herald the presence of more serious respiratory disease.

Family history may also be helpful in establishing a diagnosis. The health of the family should be investigated, as there may be direct or indirect associations between it and the patient's disease. Familial disease may be explained by a common genetic background or by exposure to a common group of infectious or physical agents.

Physical Examination

Careful pulmonary evaluation must include a thorough general physical examination. With this information, plus the knowledge obtained from historical and objective data, one is able to formulate a differential diagnosis. Laboratory diagnostic studies may be helpful in pinpointing a specific diagnosis, but none is as important as careful clinical evaluation and judgment.

Physical examination begins with quiet observation of the undisturbed child. Respiratory rate should be counted and the depth of the efforts noted. Look for dyspnea or labored breathing and the character and location of retractions should be noted. It should be noted whether or not other accessory muscles are used such as occurs with flaring of the alae nasi and head bobbing. Any chest abnormalities should be noted; if present, the distribution and degree of cyanosis should be ascertained.

In addition to the respiratory rate, several objective measurements can be performed that are helpful in the clinical evaluation of a child with pulmonary disease. Height and weight should be compared with normal values as an indication of the adequacy of nutrition and growth. An obstetrical caliper and a tape measure can be used to measure the anteroposterior and lateral diameters of the thorax. The thoracic index can be calculated from this by dividing the anteroposterior diameter by the transverse diameter. As obstructive airway disease increases, the chest shape becomes more circular and the thoracic index approaches 1.0. Another measurement, useful in patients with chronic respiratory illness, is the quantitation of digital clubbing if it is present. By means of either a plaster finger cast or a shadowgraph, the distal phalangeal depth (DPD) and the interphalangeal depth (IPD) are measured with a micrometer. Values of DPD/IPD greater than 1.0 at all ages are considered indicative of clubbing. All of these objective measurements are helpful in clinical evaluation, but none can approach the diagnostic importance of a careful physical examination.

Evaluation of respiratory diseases requires particular attention to the upper airway, lungs and cardiovascular system. The patency of the nose should be determined and the nature of the nasal mucous membrane noted. The pharynx should be inspected for hypertrophied tonsils, malformations and evidence of secretions. The tracheal position should be palpated. The thorax should be lightly percussed. Dullness to percussion is often noted with pneumonia, atelectasis and pleural effusion. Hyperresonance may be noted with pneumothorax, emphysema and in patients with chronic obstructive pulmonary disease and air trapping.

Auscultation

Auscultation can be performed satisfactorily with either the bell or the diaphragm as long as it fits over the interspace. A knowledge of bronchopulmonary segments and lobes is necessary to record accurately the location of auscultatory findings. Breath sounds should be described as vesicular, tubular or bronchovesicular. Vesicular sounds are normal and are heard over most of the upper chest and axilla. In this area, inspiration is a normal, high-pitched sound that is longer than expiration, which may be imperceptible. Tubular breathing is normally heard over the trachea, larynx and upper sternum where the expiratory phase is longer. Tubular (bronchial or tracheal) sounds are louder and more high pitched and may be heard in parts of the lung affected by pneumonia, atelectasis and effusion.

Rhonchi are continuous loud musical expiratory sounds produced by air moving past a fixed obstruction. This obstruction may be secretions, a foreign body or a bronchospastic area. Rhonchi usually indicate problems in the upper airways rather than in the lung parenchyma itself. Rales are discontinuous, non-musical crackling sounds produced by air bubbling through fluids in the lungs. They may be described as fine or coarse depending on the quality of the sound. Moist rales may be heard in pneumonia, atelectasis, pulmonary edema, bronchiectasis, and tuberculosis.

Another sound heard frequently is wheezing which can be localized or diffuse. This high pitched whistling sound can be heard in inspiration, expiration or both. It is characteristic of bronchoconstriction from asthma, foreign body and any other partial airway obstruction.

The role of pulmonary function tests should be kept in perspective. They are rarely a key factor in making a definitive diagnosis. Rather, the various patterns of impaired function overlap disease entities. While the tests are often valuable for following the progress of a patient with continuing or progressive lung disease and in assessing the results of treatment, in general it is far more important for the student to understand the principles of how the lung works than to concentrate only on the numerical results of lung function tests.

Although the number of different pulmonary disorders is immense, the number of presenting complaints of the pediatric patient (or those presented for him by parents, etc.) is relatively few. The most common of these include cyanosis, rapid breathing (tachypnea), labored breathing (dyspnea), audible breathing (stridor), wheezing and cough.

CYANOSIS

Cyanosis refers to a bluish color of the skin and nailbeds, attributable in most cases to the presence of an abnormally large amount of reduced hemoglobin in the capillaries and is indicative of arterial oxygen unsaturation.

Physiology

Cyanosis appears when the absolute amount of reduced hemoglobin in the capillaries reaches 5 g./dl. An anemic patient with less than 5 g. of hemoglobin cannot become cyanotic. If a patient had exactly 5 g. of hemoglobin/dl., it would be necessary for 100 per cent of his hemoglobin to be in the reduced form in the capillaries to produce cyanosis, a situation incompatible with life. With 10 g. of hemoglobin/dl. of blood, 50 per cent of the hemoglobin would be required to be in the reduced form in the capillaries to cause cyanosis. If a patient had 15 g. of total hemoglobin/dl., only 33 per cent of this hemoglobin in reduced form would be required in the capillaries. Thus, cyanosis appears less often in the anemic patient.

There are four primary factors that serve as the basis for a working classification of cyanosis:

1. The amount of hemoglobin unable to become fully saturated in the lung because of a variety of conditions interfering with ventilation.

2. The amount of hemoglobin unable to reach the lung, passing in reduced form through veno-arterial shunts from the right side of the heart to the arterial blood.

3. The amount of hemoglobin converted to the reduced form in the capillaries, i.e., the extent of deoxygenation in the capillaries.

4. The amount of hemoglobin in abnormal or reduced form passing through normally aerated portions of the lung.

Clinical Evaluation

Cyanosis is first apparent and most evident in areas where the epidermis is thin and capillaries are numerous: the tips of the fingers and toes (nail beds), the ear lobes, the tip of the nose, the lips and buccal mucous membrane, and, most reliably, the tip of the tongue. It may at times be difficult to ascertain clinically the presence of cyanosis, especially in darkly pigmented persons. The color of true cyanosis disappears if the blood is expressed from the capillaries by blanching pressure. Cyanosis is not necessarily accompanied by dyspnea or distress.

The distribution and duration of cyanosis should be determined. Cyanosis may be central or peripheral. The central type is characterized by cyanosis of the skin as well as the mucous membranes of the mouth and the conjuctivae. Peripheral cyanosis results from blood stasis, is usually not seen in the oral and conjunctival membranes, and the systemic O_2 saturation is normal. In a newborn with immature peripheral vascular responses or the chilled child who has been swimming in cold water too long, for example, the cyanosis is transient and has little cardio-respiratory significance. Lasting cyanosis, however, almost always indicates a hemoglobin or cardio-respiratory abnormality and may demand emergency treatment.

The clinical assessment of oxygenation is hazardous because poor peripheral circulation may result in peripheral cyanosis when the arterial blood is well oxygenated. The amount of light available for inspection, the room temperature, age of the patient and the effect of various medications all contribute to the difficulty of accurately determining cyanosis by inspection alone. Comparison of the patient with normal controls is essential. When there is frank central cyanosis, arterial PO_2 almost always is below 45 mm. Hg, depending on hemoglobin content and arterial pH. This is dangerously close to the level at which cell enzyme systems stop functioning normally. This is depicted in Figure 23-1.

Thus, the most reliable estimate of the oxygen content of arterial blood

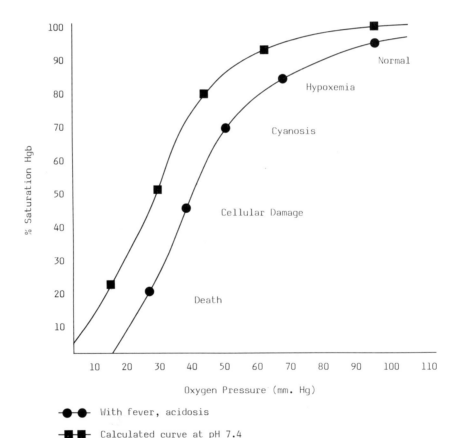

Figure 23-1.   A plotting of the oxyhemoglobin dissociation curve showing the effects of fever and acidosis compared to the curve at normothermia and pH 7.4.

requires direct measurement since both hypoxemia and hyperoxemia cannot be reliably assessed by clinical observation.

Of the four primary factors potentially responsible for cyanosis, the specific cause in the individual patient should be determined first. An accurate etiology for the cyanosis can usually be established by a careful history, physical examination and available laboratory techniques.

Cyanosis Because of the Inability of Hemoglobin to Become Fully Saturated in the Lung. A variety of conditions leads to inadequate alveolar ventilation resulting in an increased amount of hemoglobin in reduced form passing through the lung back to the left side of the heart. On a developmental basis, there may be upper airway obstruction to adequate air entry as in atresia of the posterior nasal choanae; combinations of small jaw and large tongue (Pierre Robin syndrome); infants with poor neuromuscular control of the tongue (which becomes easily displaced posteriorly); compression of the trachea by a large mass such as a congenital goiter; laryngeal webs or cysts; tracheal stenosis; subglottic hemangiomas and vascular rings compressing the trachea inside the thorax.

Acquired airway obstruction is vastly more common. The most common cause of inadequate upper airway ventilation is the accumulation of nasal mucus in the young infant who is normally an obligate nose breather. Another common condition is partial obstruction because of enlarged tonsils and adenoids. Infections such as epiglottitis and acute bronchiolitis are important as well as common. Episodes of sudden onset such as angioneurotic edema and a foreign body in the larynx or trachea must always be considered and require emergency treatment.

A variety of lower airway conditions interfere with the ability of adequate air to reach the alveoli. Acute bronchial asthma, smoke inhalation, bronchopneumonia and cystic fibrosis are examples of inflammatory conditions causing intrinsic lower airway obstruction, while atelectasis, lobar emphysema and acute pneumothorax are examples of extrinsic obstruction.

The inability of the alveoli to function properly is seen earliest in the hyaline membrane disease of the newborn. Aspiration pneumonitis, drowning, parenchymal pneumonia, pulmonary alveolar proteinosis, pulmonary fibrosis, pulmonary hemosiderosis and pulmonary edema all effectively block the diffusion of oxygen across the alveolar membrane.

Lastly, the pulmonary pump may be unable to deliver an adequate volume of air to the alveoli through normal airways. Paralysis of the diaphragm, bulbar polio, advanced muscular dystrophy, cervical cord lesions, impairment of the respiratory center—in short, any neuromuscular dysfunction may lead to alveolar hypoventilation.

It should be apparent that almost all of the above conditions are contributors to cyanosis dependent only on the degree to which they are expressed. Few are absolutely causative of cyanosis, as are some of the cyanotic congenital heart lesions discussed next.

Cyanosis Due to Inability of Hemoglobin to Reach the Alveoli. In this category, normal hemoglobin remains in the reduced form due to shunting from the right side of the heart to the arterial blood. This results in an increased level of unsaturated arterial blood distributed to the periphery of the body. Blood that does pass normally through the lungs becomes normally oxygenated and is mixed in the left side of the heart. Thus, administration of oxygen to these patients will cause only a slight decrease in the degree of cyanosis observed because the portion of hemoglobin that does pass through the lungs is normally oxygenated.

The location of the veno-arterial shunting is almost always intracardiac. There are some rare extracardiac locations (e.g., pulmonary arteriovenous fistula and portopulmonary anastomoses) found in some cases of chronic hepatic disease with portal hypertension. The degree of cyanosis in the extracardiac lesions depends upon the size and number of the shunts.

As mentioned, the intracardiac shunts that produce cyanotic congenital heart disease are by far the most common cause of cyanosis in this general category. This finding of often intense cyanosis gave rise to the popular term "blue-babies." The timing of the appearance of cyanosis can vary with the lesion, some appearing at birth, some appearing later. Factors which lead to the later appearance of cyanosis include the closure of the ductus arteriosus, the presence of a patent foramen ovale, the start of exercise or exertion and the degree of pulmonary hypertension.

Examples of conditions underlying severe cyanosis typically present from birth are: complete transposition of the great vessels, tricuspid atresia, pulmonary atresia with a ventricular septal defect and aortic atresia. Later appearance of cyanosis is found in cases of tetralogy of Fallot, truncus arteriosus, pulmonary stenosis with patent foramen ovale, the Eisenmenger complex and total anomalous pulmonary venous return.

Generalized cyanosis in the presence of polycythemia causing capillary stasis may be a secondary cause of cyanosis in patients with certain forms of congenital heart disease.

Increased venous pressure with resulting stasis may also produce generalized cyanosis. This is most commonly seen as a result of hard crying by an infant and may also occur during a grand mal seizure. A variety of heart disorders may also contribute, most notably constrictive pericarditis. Patients with cardiac failure resulting from rheumatic mitral valvular disease, left-to-right shunts, myocarditis, endocardial fibroelastosis and infantile coarctation of the aorta may develop generalized cyanosis due in part to the increased venous pressure and stasis.

Cyanosis Dependent upon the Extent of Deoxygenation in the Capillaries. Here, normal hemoglobin is converted to the reduced form while passing from the arteries to the veins. The oxygen saturation of the arterial blood is generally normal and the cyanosis is due to capillary stasis. Oxygen therapy does not reduce this form of cyanosis.

The most common clinical expression of this is the local cyanosis observed while an extremity is constricted by a tourniquet. Cyanosis of the face, hands and feet in the first few hours after birth is another common example of local cyanosis. In older children head and neck cyanosis because of obstruction of the superior vena cava is a rare example.

This form of cyanosis can also be generalized. Chilling of the skin from a variety of causes is the most common example. Shock, especially that associated with dehydration, is a major serious cause of capillary stasis. This may occur with severe diarrhea, acute adrenal insufficiency and sepsis. A mottled or grey cyanosis may result from peripheral vascular collapse and pooling of blood in the skin.

Abnormal Hemoglobin Passing through Normally Aerated Lung. The most common abnormal form of hemoglobin is that found in methemoglobinemia. This condition requires spectrophotometry for diagnosis. Methemoglobinemia can be congenital, due to a deficiency of the enzyme hemoglobin reductase, inherited as either a recessive or dominant form. The ingestion of well water high in nitrates, of aniline dyes, old wax crayons, phenylhydrazine, acetanilid, primaquine phosphate, and benzocaine ointment or rectal suppositories can produce methemoglobinemia. Sulfhemoglobin is another abnormal form of hemoglobin attributed to sulfonamide administration. Since carboxyhemoglobin, resulting from carbon monoxide exposure, is bright red, it produces a reddish rather than a bluish or cyanotic discoloration of the skin. Since CO has 210 times more affinity for hemoglobin than oxygen, it is important to note that PO_2 may be normal in CO poisoning, while oxygen content is markedly reduced.

DYSPNEA

Dyspnea is a sympton, not a disorder. It can be defined as breathing that is perceived as difficult or labored accompanied by an unpleasant feeling of discomfort or distress. This may be visibly evident or may be a subjective feeling expressed by the patient or by his parents on his behalf.

Apnea is the absence of respiratory movement. Bradypnea is slow respiration; tachypnea is a rapid or an increased rate of breathing as is polypnea; hypopnea is shallow and hyperpnea is an increase in the depth of respiration. Hyperventilation is breathing in excess of the body's needs. It should be emphasized that dyspnea is *not* the same as tachypnea, hyperpnea or hyperventilation.

It is important to be familiar with normal respiratory patterns and rates of different ages in order to recognize the abnormal states. For example, short apneic episodes and irregularity of respiration, grave signs in older children, may be normal findings in a small premature infant.

There are patterns of breathing that are related to position and to dyspnea. Orthopnea is a preference for a sitting position because the dypsnea is much less than that felt in the recumbent position. Children with severe dyspnea and orthopnea often find the most comfortable position is to sit cross-legged in bed leaning far forward over a couple of pillows or a bed table. Trepopnea is the preference for one lateral recumbent position over another, seen in tension pneumothorax and pleural effusion.

Physiology

The causes of dyspnea are very complex and not well understood. Awareness of the behavior of one's lungs and of the act of breathing is derived from several sources. These include vision, hearing, the sensation of movement and temperature change in the upper respiratory tract, sensations from vagal irritant and cough receptors, and sensations of chest wall movement.

Dypsnea occurs, in part, when the muscles of respiration perform either an unusual amount or an unaccustomed type of work. This includes all cardiopulmonary conditions in which the work of breathing is definitely increased. During normal respiration, 1.3 per cent of the total oxygen consumption of the body is accounted for by diaphragmatic and intercostal muscles. With dyspnea, oxygen consumption by the respiratory muscles increases to 9 per cent. This increased oxygen need may in itself contribute to a continuing respiratory distress.

Conditions in which there is an increased airway resistance commonly cause dyspnea. A normal person in whom bronchial obstruction is induced experimentally by histamine inhalation, for example, does not experience any respiratory symptoms until airway resistance is increased 3-fold or more. Severe dyspnea may not result until airway resistance is increased 5- to 15-fold.

In general, it seems likely that the sensation of dyspnea may be caused by any one or a combination of mechanisms: increased respiratory work, reduced ventilatory capacity, increased stimulation of receptors, and increased subjective sensitivity.

Clinical Perception

The sensation of dyspnea is a subjective one; therefore evaluation by the clinician is as difficult as the evaluation of other sensations, such as pain, hunger, thirst, feeling cold, etc.

Patients may use a variety of words to describe the sensation of dyspnea: shortness of breath, "unable to get my breath," tightness, panting, wheezing, fullness, constriction, etc., are but a few terms commonly used.

A history of difficult breathing should first suggest airway obstruction. Note should be made of any relation to time of day, exercise, meals, posture, etc. Is the dyspnea of relatively short term but steadily becoming worse, as in bronchiolitis, or does it seem to come and go as in asthma? Is there a seasonal variation? diurnal? (Both of these suggest asthma.) Is the onset sudden as in a previously well child who is found coughing and dyspneic with peanuts in his mouth? Has the child always had labored breathing, as with anomalies of the lungs or heart? Paroxysmal nocturnal dyspnea is associated classically with left ventricular failure. Exertion, if marked enough, will cause dyspnea in anyone; thus a grading system for the assessment of "dyspnea on exertion" must be used and must be age appropriate. Infants may become dyspneic while feeding from a bottle, which constitutes exercise for the infant, while an older child may develop dyspnea as a result of exercise-induced bronchospasm brought about by a vigorous game of soccer. On a +1 to +4 scale, a +1 might be the ability to keep up with peers during normal activity but inability when strenuous exercise is involved. A +4 might be shortness of breath and dyspnea at rest.

Clinical Conditions

At best, any classification of conditions that give rise to dyspnea is an arbitrary one. The following is a general outline that may be practical:

1. Mechanical factors: These inhibit or restrict the normal respiratory mechanisms.
   a. Upper airway obstruction, (congenital, foreign body, inflammation, bronchospasm)
   b. Painful breathing, pleurisy, rib fracture
   c. Body casts
   d. Pleural effusion, hemothorax, pneumothorax
   e. Flail chest (rib fractures and/or costochondral junction separation)
   f. Thoracic dystrophy
   g. Elevation of diaphragm by abdominal fluid or masses
   h. Extreme obesity
2. Tissue hypoxia: Conditions other than those of primary alveolar or cardiac origin that result in an insufficient supply of oxygen to the tissues.
   a. Anemia
   b. Overexertion
   c. High altitude
   d. Carbon monoxide exposure
3. Pulmonary insufficiency: Conditions at the alveolar level that result in inadequate ventilation.
   a. Atelectasis (intrinsic-obstructive or extrinsic-compressive)
   b. Alveolar flooding (aspiration, near-drowning, bleeding)
   c. Alveolar interference (hyaline membranes, alveolar proteinosis)
   d. Pulmonary edema and interstitial edema
   e. Interstitial fibrosis (alveolar-capillary block)

      f. Diseases of the pulmonary parenchyma due to inflammation
      g. Decreased pulmonary distensibility
      h. Obliterative bronchiolitis
4. Cardiac and vascular insufficiency
      a. Cardiac failure
      b. Congenital cyanotic heart disease. Depending on the degree of hypoxia associated with the cardiac lesion, dyspnea on exertion may range from mild to severe. Children, especially those in whom pulmonary stenosis is severe, may experience attacks of paroxysmal dyspnea. During these spells, the cyanosis becomes much more intense, the patient gasps for breath and may become unconscious for a time. These spells may occur spontaneously or be precipitated by feeding, crying or defecation. Older children learn to interrupt these spells by assuming a squatting position.
      c. Pulmonary congestion
      d. Pulmonary hypertension
      e. Decreased pulmonary circulation (congenital, embolism, thrombus)
5. Neuromuscular
      a. Unilateral or bilateral paralysis of the diaphragm
      b. Polio
      c. Guillain-Barré syndrome
      d. Muscular dystrophy
      e. Myasthenia gravis
      f. Hypopotassemia
6. Central nervous system
      a. Acidosis
      b. Drugs (salicylates, heroin)
      c. Immature respiratory center
      d. Encephalitis, meningitis
      e. Inappropriate response to hypoxia (familial dysautonomia, narcolepsy)
7. Emotional-functional

STRIDOR

Stridor is a harsh sound caused by obstruction to breathing in the larynx or trachea. Derived from the Latin, *stridulus*, meaning creaking, whistling or grating, it is predominantly an inspiratory sound but there is often a softer expiratory element, particularly if obstruction is in the subglottic area or trachea. In some tracheal lesions, the expiratory element resembles a wheeze.

Stridor is an important indication of respiratory obstruction and should never be disregarded. To produce stridor means that somewhere between the inlet to the respiratory tract and the outlet from the bronchi to the lungs lies a partial obstruction.

In minor degrees of narrowing, breathing may be quiet at rest, but with increased physical activity and consequent increased velocity of air flow stridor may develop. In lesions causing narrowing at the level of the vocal cords or above, the stridor is predominantly inspiratory, but in some infants with subglottic lesions (particularly if there is involvement of the lower trachea as well) prolonged expiratory stridor is marked.

Pathophysiology

Stridor is produced by turbulence of airflow and increased velocity of air brought about by the narrowed or partially obstructed airway. A greater negative intratracheal and intrathoracic pressure must be generated to overcome the obstruction, resulting in a dynamic compression of the extrathoracic trachea during inspiration. In younger children the larynx and trachea are relatively soft and compressible, thus dynamic compression occurs more readily than in an adult and is an important secondary factor in the production of inspiratory stridor.

Three normal anatomical features lead to a greater incidence of acquired stridor in infants compared to older children and adults: (1) the small size of the infant larynx; (2) the presence of loose submucosal connective tissue in the supraglottic and subglottic regions; and (3) rigid encirclement of the subglottic area by the cricoid cartilage.

The triangular glottic opening of the infant larynx is approximately 77 mm. in length and 4 mm. in width at the base. In infants, edema produces a reduction in the size of this opening and signs of respiratory obstruction, but a similar degree of edema in the adult results only in hoarseness. The laryngeal mucosa is loosely fixed anteriorally to the epiglottis and laterally along the aryepiglottic folds. Collection of edema fluid in these supraglottic spaces in association with inflammatory processes leads to downward pressure on the epiglottis and to laryngeal obstruction. A similar process may occur in the narrow subglottic area with swelling of the submucosal tissue and acute respiratory obstruction. Since this area is completely encircled by the cricoid cartilage, swelling due to edema must impinge upon the airway.

History

If the condition has been present since birth, the underlying cause may well be a congenital abnormality or birth trauma. In general, disorders of structure tend to be more noisy when the tissues are relaxed (e.g., when the child is asleep). Disorders of function, e.g. paralyses, tend to produce more noise when the child is awake and active.

Any difficulty in breathing in the newborn may be accompanied by a difficulty in feedings. If the underlying cause of the breathing difficulty is a paralysis of the vocal cord there may be paralysis of one side of the cricopharyngeal sphincter that leads to a failure of relaxtion during peristalsis. This causes food to "bounce back" from the projecting shelf of unrelaxed muscle and to spill over into the tracheobronchial tree. Secondary pneumonic consolidation is not uncommon therefore, and often recurs during the early months of life.

It is a common experience in pediatrics to find several abnormalities in the same patient. Troubles rarely come singly, and the presence or absence of a second abnormality should always be kept in mind. An interval between birth and the onset of the noise suggests that the cause has been acquired. In young children common conditions which give rise to acquired stridor are inhaled foreign bodies and respiratory tract inflammation. Therefore, it is important to ask what the child was doing when the noise was first noticed; if he was playing with a toy, part of which is missing, or if he was eating, then it is wise to offer a tentative diagnosis of inhaled foreign body and to proceed with radiographic and endoscopic studies without delay.

Physical Examination

The child should be examined in a warm room because the clothes must be removed in order to observe the movements of the chest and respiratory muscles. As a consequence of increased negative intrapleural pressure during inspiration, retraction of the suprasternal tissues, sternal, costal cartilages and intercostal spaces may occur. By applying a stethoscope to the side of the patient's neck, the position of the noise in the respiratory cycle is noted. If the noise is loud on inspiration the cause should be sought in the larynx; if the noise is loud on expiration the cause lies in the bronchial region; if the noise can be heard clearly in both phases of the respiratory cycle the obstruction lies below the vocal cords and above the bronchi. Some examiners claim to distinguish the brassy noise of subglottic stenosis, the pure tone of congenital laryngeal stridor, and the wheeze of the impacted foreign body. In certain instances the obstruction may be moved by changes of posture. In the Pierre Robin syndrome, the noise will disappear altogether if the child is placed in the prone position. This provides a clue to the diagnosis and an indication as to how the child may be managed. Children in whom infection has narrowed the respiratory pathway are often more comfortable when nursed sitting up.

Tachycardia, apprehensiveness, increase in respiratory rate and use of the accessory muscles of respiration indicate progression of the obstruction. Restlessness is an early indication of hypoxia and occurs before overt cyanosis. Increasing restlessness in an infant or child with respiratory obstruction may indicate the need for a tracheostomy. Since sedatives may mask the manifestations of lack of oxygen and inhibit needed accessory respiratory efforts, such medications should not be given in these instances. With establishment of an adequate airway, restlessness is followed dramatically by deep sleep.

Diagnosis

After the clinical examination is complete it is necessary to assess the degree of narrowing and the cause of the obstruction. Almost invariably, the child must have an endoscopic and radiological examination of the airways. The only exception to this rule is when the pediatrician is certain that infection is the cause and certain too that endoscopy represents a greater hazard to the child's life than the infection.

Some conditions can be determined by direct examination, such as the passage of a soft catheter through the nares to detect choanal atresia or the visualization of the cherry red epiglottis characteristic of acute epiglottitis.

Anteroposition and lateral films of the neck and of the chest are essential to the diagnostic evaluation. The patency of the upper airway can be estimated, looking for such signs as ballooning of the supraglottic airway, compression from the retropharyngeal space, a large swollen epiglottis, subglottic narrowing or an opaque foreign body, to name but a few patterns. The column of air in the airway can be used as a contrast medium. At times, fluoroscopy and films in both full inspiration and expiration may be helpful. The inability of one lung to empty when placed uppermost in the lateral recumbent position is very suggestive of an aspirated foreign body.

Fluoroscopy or cineradiographic studies of a barium swallow may be helpful in outlining an area of compression or displacement as might be seen with certain vascular rings or a variety of mediastinal cystic structures.

Bronchography is generally not required since the avenue of most direct diagnostic evaluation is by laryngoscopy and bronchoscopy. Only if the cause of the stridor cannot be identified in the supraglottic and glottic regions is bronchoscopy indicated.

Direct visualization of the larynx before using a general anesthesia is most important so that the movement of the vocal cords can be assessed. Accurate diagnosis of the two most common causes of stridor present since birth—congenital laryngeal stridor and paralysis of the vocal cords—can only be made by direct laryngoscopy. In children this should be done by someone who is familiar with the characteristics of the normal infant larynx and airway and who has the necessary specialized instruments.

Etiology

Since the affected sites are hollow, the lesion responsible for stridor may lie in the lumen, in the wall, or outside the wall of the airway.

Obviously, there are many causes of stridor in infancy and childhood.

For our purposes, they are best divided into those of acute or acquired origin, and those that are congenital, persistent or recurrent.

Acute, Acquired. These are mainly caused by infection and are discussed in more detail in the section dealing with infectious diseases.

1. Croup, infectious croup, acute laryngotracheobronchitis. The etiologic agent is most often viral, usually the para influenza viruses.

2. Acute spasmodic croup. The etiology is uncertain but may be viral, allergic or psychological.

3. Acute epiglottitis. Usually caused by *H. influenza.* This is a potentially fatal disease and is a true medical emergency.

4. Infectious mononucleosis. Often the edema and swelling of the tonsils and adenoidal tissue can nearly occlude the airway.

5. Angioneurotic edema

6. Laryngospasm

7. Foreign bodies. The presence of a foreign body in the respiratory tract should be considered in the differential diagnosis of respiratory obstruction and of unexplained chest lesions in children.

Congenital, Persistent, Recurrent. There are a number of conditions in this category, the three most common of which are discussed in some detail.

(1) Congenital Laryngeal Stridor. (Laryngomalacia, infantile larynx, inspiratory laryngeal collapse.) There is no satisfactory term for the most common cause of persistent stridor in infancy. The condition has been termed simply "congenital laryngeal stridor" but this describes a symptom rather than gives any indication of underlying pathology.

The term "laryngo-malacia" is commonly used in North America, and suggests a pathological cause; but as the condition is rarely fatal there is no good evidence that the cartilage of the larynx is abnormally soft. "Inspiratory laryngeal collapse" is a descriptive term which simply draws attention to the mechanism of the production of the stridor. "Infantile larynx" is probably the most acceptable name because the larynx, particularly the glottic region, appears disproportionately small for the child's size. Further, it does not presume to give the pathological basis of the lesion which has yet to be determined.

The larynx is small and placed anteriorly. The epiglottis is long and omega shaped, the aryepiglottic folds long and floppy with prominent arytenoids, and the interarytenoid cleft is deep but does not extend to the cord level. During inspiration the epiglottis, the aryepiglottic folds and arytenoids collapse into and over the glottic orifice leaving a slit-like opening. These floppy tissues intermittently obstruct the entrance of air and vibrate, thus causing stridor. During expiration the positive pressure of air from below blows them apart. The glottis is normal in size and there are no special dangers to be expected here unless an acute respiratory infection supervenes, in which case relief of the obstructed airway is urgently required.

The onset of the stridor usually occurs within the first 4 weeks of life, most often in the first week; it may even be noted within hours of birth. Occasionally parents do not become aware of the noise until the baby develops a respiratory infection as late as 6–8 weeks. Stridor is predominantly inspiratory, but in about 20 per cent of patients there is a definite expiratory element. The inspiratory stridor varies considerably in intensity, being loudest with increased ventilation associated with crying or excitement. The sound varies in pitch, is often coarse and jerky or interrupted during inspiration, and varies considerably from breath to breath and when the baby is held in different positions. In some infants little or no air is heard entering the lungs during some inspiratory efforts. The cry and cough are normal.

It is rare for babies with infantile larynx to develop respiratory obstruction of sufficient degree to require an artificial airway. The stridor is more often an annoyance than a problem. If severe obstructive episodes occur in a baby in whom a clinical diagnosis of infantile larynx has been made, further investigation to determine the cause is essential.

The stridor usually becomes less after the age of 12 months and may be heard only when the infant is upset or has intercurrent respiratory infections. By the age of 2½–3 years or before it usually disappears completely. A uniformly good prognosis can be given to parents of babies with this type of laryngeal malformation, provided it is the only lesion present.

(2) Paralysis of the Vocal Cord. Inspiratory stridor, respiratory distress and feeding difficulties are the common symptoms of bilateral or unilateral vocal cord palsy. Bilateral palsy usually results from severe malformations of the central nervous system, most commonly of the Arnold-Chiari type. The stridor becomes more obvious with the development of hydrocephalus, but when the intracranial pressure is controlled it may disappear. Bilateral palsy occasionally occurs as an isolated anomaly and spontaneously improves by 2–3 months of age.

Unilateral palsy may occur as an isolated anomaly, in association with major malformations of the heart and great vessels, or with other neurological disease. The lesion associated with cardiac malformations is almost invariably left-sided because of compression of the recurrent laryngeal nerve. In some babies with isolated palsy there is a history of difficult labor.

These children have feeding difficulties, too, and patchy consolidation of the lungs frequently results from inhaled milk. They will be slow to gain weight, therefore, and may have to be weaned early to solid food because it is swallowed more easily. In children with paresis or paralysis, more than one direct laryngoscopy may be required in order to assess progress or resolution of the causative lesion. It is not unusual for the paralysis to clear completely, although the voice may be husky or normal. The diagnosis of cord palsy, particularly unilateral, may be difficult to establish by laryngoscopy. It is best to examine the larynx without general anesthesia. In older children, indirect laryngoscopy can be used.

(3) Subglottic Hemangioma. It is probably more common than reported figures suggest, as the diagnosis may be difficult to establish during life and also at post mortem. The epithelium covering the hemangioma may mask its vascularity during life, and after death it may contract so much that it can only be identified by microscopic examination.

The clinical pattern is surprisingly constant. The principal features are variable inspiratory and prolonged expiratory stridor and respiratory difficulty, a croupy or brassy cough and normal cry. The symptoms are not present at birth but develop either insidiously or more abruptly between the ages of 1–3 months. There is usually progressive increase in severity of the stridor and respiratory difficulty during the ensuing few weeks or months. During the period when the symptoms are most marked, the infant usually fails to grow. Only in mildly affected patients is normal growth maintained.

The stridor and respiratory difficulty are much worse when the baby cries or struggles due to engorgement from obstruction of venous drainage. In infants with small hemangiomas the symptoms may be minimal when the child is breathing quietly, as when asleep. Upper respiratory tract infections aggravate the symptoms.

Other congenital, persistent or recurrent causes of stridor are:
    Nasal polyps
    Nasal foreign body
    Laryngeal webs
    Laryngeal cysts
    Subglottic stenosis
    Tracheal stenosis
    Laryngeal papilloma
    Extrinsic airway obstruction
        Thyroglossal duct cyst
        Micrognathia with glossoptosis
        Macroglossia
        Retropharyngeal abscess
        Cystic hygroma
        Congenital goiter
        Mediastinal masses
        Vascular rings
            Double aortic-arch
            Right aortic-arch with left ligamentum arteriosum
            Anomalous innominate artery
            Anomalous left common carotid
            Aberrant subclavian artery
            Anomalous left pulmonary artery

Neurogenic
    Palatal control
    Tonic contractions of base of tongue and posterior pharynx in pa-
    tients with cerebral palsy.

WHEEZING

Wheezing is an audible, high-pitched sound associated with breathing. It is heard during expiration, but there may be an associated sound during inspiration, either stridor or a rattle, depending on the origin of the wheeze. It is frequently associated with obvious expiratory effort. Wheezing is not synonymous with bronchospasm and can result from causes of airway obstruction other than bronchospasm.

Pathophysiology

Normal breathing is not audible because, even at the maximum rate of air flow in the normal subject, the linear velocity of air flow in the tracheo-bronchial tree is too slow to provide a sound. Breathing only becomes audible when there is an increase in the linear velocity of air flow resulting from narrowing of the air passages.

Wheezing is produced by diseases that cause a direct or indirect narrowing of the trachea and major bronchi. The linear velocity of air flow in the smaller airways is far too low to cause any audible sound even when these are narrowed.

Narrowing of the trachea and major bronchi sufficient to produce an audible sound can occur in two types of disease processes. In the first there is dynamic narrowing of the trachea and major bronchi when the pressure outside the airways exceeds the pressure inside during expiration because of widespread obstruction of the medium and small airways. In the second there is a localized obstruction of either the trachea or a major bronchus.

In diseases which cause obstruction in the medium and small airways, a wheeze is heard only during expiration. During inspiration the pressure inside the trachea and major bronchi exceeds that outside. An inspiratory rattle may be associated with the expiratory wheeze if there is mucus in the trachea or major bronchi. The inspiratory noise has a different quality from a wheeze.

Focal narrowing of the trachea or of a major bronchus can cause an expiratory wheeze. There is an increase in the linear velocity of airflow past the obstruction and this may produce a wheeze. If the obstruction is in the intrathoracic portion of the airways there may also be dynamic compression of the airways downstream from the obstruction if a positive pleural pressure develops during expiration. This occurs if the ob-

Table 23-1. Causes of Wheezing in Children

Obstructive Disease of the Small Airways
    Acute
        Acute viral bronchiolitis
        Hydrocarbon ingestion
    Recurrent or Persistent
        Asthma
        Hypersensitivity pneumonitis
        Aspiration bronchitis
        "H" type tracheoesophageal fistula
        Subacute and chronic infective bronchitis
          cystic fibrosis
          immune-deficiency disorders
          non-specific infective bronchitis
        Alpha-1-antitrypsin deficiency
        Obliterative bronchiolitis
        Congenital heart disease with pulmonary hyperperfusion

Obstructive Lesions of the Trachea or Major Bronchi
    Acute
        Foreign body in trachea, bronchus or esophagus
    Recurrent or Persistent
        Foreign body in trachea, bronchus or esophagus
        Vascular rings
        Mediastinal lymphadenopathy
        Mediastinal cysts and tumors
        Tracheal webs, tracheal stenosis, bronchial stenosis
        Tracheomalacia

structing lesion causes a significant rise in the airway's resistance. An inspiratory stridor may also be heard if the rate of inspiratory airflow and the degree of obstruction are sufficient. The stridor heard when there is an obstructing lesion in the trachea or major bronchus is higher pitched than that produced by a laryngeal lesion, and may resemble a wheeze in quality.

In both types of obstruction wheeze may be absent during quiet breathing but it develops when the patient increases ventilation as a result of activity. With hyperventilation the linear velocity of air flow increases; if there is airway obstruction the expiratory pleural pressure becomes more positive. In many asthmatic patients exercise-induced bronchospasm occurs, but in a patient with moderate airway obstruction the development of a wheeze after exercise may be due to increased air flow velocity without any alteration in airway resistance.

Etiology

Chevalier Jackson is credited with the commonly quoted aphorism "All that wheezes is not asthma, and not all asthma wheezes." The important causes of wheezing in childhood fall into two main groups (Table 23-1): (1) Obstructive lesions involving the smaller bronchi and bronchioles; and (2) Obstructive lesions in the trachea or major bronchi.

Acute Viral Bronchiolitis. Infants with bronchiolitis, usually due to respiratory syncytial virus, have marked tachypnea, dyspnea, expiratory wheezing and grunt; they may have cyanosis. These symptoms are associated with generalized obstructive emphysema. The differentiation between acute bronchiolitis and infantile asthma may be difficult and is discussed in greater detail in Chapter 26.

Hydrocarbon Ingestion. Hydrocarbons such as turpentine, gasoline, lighter fluid, etc., are examples of substances which, if aspirated, cause an acute inflammatory response of the bronchial mucosa with resultant cough and bronchospasm.

Asthma. Asthma is by far the most common cause of wheezing in infancy and childhood. Obstruction occurs mainly in the medium and smaller airways as a result of smooth muscle spasm, mucosal edema and hypersecretion of mucus. Wheezing in asthma is typically recurrent but some children develop chronic airway obstruction with persistent wheeze for weeks at a time. However, in these children its intensity will fluctuate considerably from time to time, and the fact that there is chronic obstruction can easily be missed. In very severe obstruction wheeze may not occur owing to the very small tidal volume. Some infants under the age of 12 months also develop a persistent wheeze. Asthma is discussed in detail in Chapter 26.

Hypersensitivity Pneumonitis. There are a host of conditions which fall into this category, including pigeon breeder's lung, farmer's lung, and humidifier disease. Exposure to doves, gerbils and parakeets can also bring about this syndrome.

Aspiration Bronchitis. The inhalation of oral or gastric contents, especially milk, can result in a chemical bronchitis with the production of wheeze. If recurrent, an allergic component develops that is probably due to the milk protein. Poor palatal-pharyngeal swallowing coordination, and gastroesophageal reflux are often involved.

"H-Type" Tracheoesophageal Fistula. This lesion, which may be very subtle, can contribute to recurrent wheezing because of the spillover of esophageal contents into the trachea. Cough is also a prominent symptom.

Cystic Fibrosis. Many infants with cystic fibrosis have a continuous bronchiolitis-like condition which may last for several weeks. Wheezing is a major component of the pulmonary symptoms, at times presenting more of a problem than the chronic cough. As the patient with cystic fibrosis reaches late adolescence, a low-grade bronchospasm becomes commonplace.

Immune-Deficiency Disorders. These conditions often have a suppurative bronchiectasis resulting from the inability to properly contain infection. Cough, often producing sputum, and low-grade bronchospasm poorly responsive to bronchodilators are features of this group.

Non-specific Infective Bronchitis. Although poorly classified and documented, there is a group of children whose symptoms resemble the chronic bronchitis of adulthood. Usually there is a history of exposure to tobacco smoke in the home. No consistent organism is isolated from these patients, who are often said to have "wheezing bronchitis" or "asthmatic bronchitis." Yet they do not have atopic disease.

Alpha-1-antitrypsin Deficiency. Although the symptoms of dyspnea and wheezing coupled with lower lobe emphysema, as seen on radiographs, usually do not develop until the third decade of life, certain younger patients with this disorder have the persistent wheezing that is poorly responsive to treatment and characteristic of this disorder.

Obliterative Bronchiolitis. This is an end-stage result of certain distal airway infections, notably influenza virus and adenoviral infections. Patchy areas of hyperinflation adjacent to areas of atelectasis result in a very uneven ventilation.

Congenital Heart Disease with Pulmonary Hyperperfusion. In congenital cardiac conditions with large left to right shunts, i.e., VSD and PDA, the increased pulmonary arterial flow causes congestion of the capillary bed. Interstitial fluid collects in the peribronchial space, compressing the small distal airways, leading to wheezing, hyperaeration and migratory areas of atelectasis.

Foreign Body. A foreign body is the most common cause of wheezing from large airways obstruction. Impacted esophageal foreign bodies may cause wheezing by tracheal compression.

Vascular Rings. Those anomalies of the vessels originating from the aortic arch may develop true encircling rings of the trachea and cause wheezing by direct tracheal compression. Often, after the surgical repair of the obstructing vessel, a defect in the tracheal cartilage may remain, resulting in continued wheezing and interference with normal cough mechanics by allowing almost complete tracheal closure to occur at the point of the cartilaginous defect.

Mediastinal Lymphadenopathy, Cysts and Tumors. Depending on the location of these masses, tracheal or bronchial compression may result, producing a persistent wheeze. Associated findings such as an irritative cough, lobar atelectasis, or swallowing difficulties may be present.

Tracheal and Bronchial Webs and Stenosis. Usually both an inspiratory and expiratory wheeze is produced by these lesions. While resting, the wheeze may be minimal or absent, but become obvious with activity, excitement or a respiratory infection.

Conclusion

Although "all that wheezes is not asthma," asthma is by far the most common cause of wheezing in childhood; the diagnosis must be considered in every child presenting with recurrent or persistent wheezing. A chest radiograph is indicated for all children with persistent wheezing to try to exclude local bronchial compression as the cause. Further investigations, which may include radiological screening, bronchography, endoscopic examination and pulmonary function tests, are indicated if the clinical pattern of the wheezing is not typical of asthma.

COUGH

"The cough-reflex is the watchdog of the lung"
.... Chevalier Jackson

Cough is perhaps the most common symptom of acute and chronic respiratory disease in children. Because of its audible nature, it attracts considerable attention. An extravagant amount of time and money is spent on treating this symptom, one of the most important vital protective mechanisms of the body.

Purpose and Function

Cough serves to clear foreign matter and excess secretions from the air passages of the lung. This mechanism of clearance is a protective mechanism of a primitive nature used when inhaled foreign particles, noxious gases, chemical irritants, etc., reach the tracheobronchial tree. One major function of cough is to protect the respiratory tract from inhalation of food or fluids, especially during swallowing.

Usually, the quantity of mucus secreted by the membranes lining the airway is small, and no cough is present. The action of the cilia covering those membranes is all that is needed to sweep the mucus, with any entrapped particles, up the airways into the pharynx. This mucociliary escalator extends from the terminal bronchioles of the lung; beyond that, other clearance mechanisms exist.

The fact that we normally cough little, and that persons unable to cough because of polio or spinal cord injuries may get along well for long periods of time, indicate that the normal mechanisms provide adequate clearance when they are operating properly. However, if the cilia are injured or destroyed, as frequently occurs in acute and chronic infections of the airways, or if there are excess secretions because of inflammation, cough then becomes a powerful and necessary supplementary clearance method.

Mechanism of Cough

Cough Reflex. A cough is induced by an irritation of the afferent fibers of the pharyngeal branches of the glossopharyngeal nerve, as well as the sensory endings of the vagus nerve in the larynx, trachea, and mucous membranes of the pharynx and larger bronchi. The impulses are transmitted to the cough center in the medulla and pons. Impulses from the cough center are then relayed via the vagus and spinal nerves from C_3 to S_2 to the muscles of the chest and the larynx. A considerable amount of air is inspired; the glottis closes, the vocal cords shut tightly to trap the air in the lungs; the muscles of the chest wall, abdominal wall, diaphragm and pelvic floor contract, pushing the diaphragm up while other expiratory muscles also contract forcefully. Pleural, alveolar and subglottic pressures rise to as much as 200 cm. H_2O, and the glottis suddenly opens. The combined effect of high intrapleural and intraabdominal pressures on expiratory volume flow rate creates a high linear velocity air stream with a high kinetic energy, which, upon opening of the glottis, makes possible the acceleration and displacement of any foreign material in the bronchi or the trachea.

It has been estimated that the linear velocities of air flow achieved in the trachea during a cough may well be as follows: in an uncompressed tracheal lumen with a diameter of 1.5 cm. and a normal expiratory flow rate of 1 liter/sec., it would be approximately 15 miles per hour; at a flow rate of 7 liters/sec. it could reach a hurricane velocity up to 100 miles per hour; if, in addition, the cross-section of the trachea is compressed to one-sixteenth of its normal area, the linear velocity can reach a speed of 600 miles per hour or 85 per cent the speed of sound.

It is important to appreciate that the cough reflex is under voluntary control and may be either inhibited or initiated at will. Voluntary inhibition because of pain prevents effective clearing of the bronchial tree of excess secretion, and central stimulation may be responsible for nervous coughing.

Not all patients nor all portions of the respiratory tree have the same stimulus threshold. Cough may be absent, at times, in a small infant with severe pneumonia or even though a foreign body is present in the tracheobronchial tree. Tolerance or decreased reflex excitability may also develop as in some patients with bronchiectasis or atelectasis where coughing is not continuous.

Clearing the Airways. The two main mechanisms by which coughing clears the airway are the "tussive squeeze" and the "bechic blast," both terms coined by the Jacksons.

Tussive Squeeze. The lung and smaller peripheral airways are compressed due to the high positive pleural pressure. Secretions and exudate are squeezed into the larger bronchi from which they can be expelled by blasts of high velocity air. The velocity of gas flowing in the alveoli and small airways is so low that little energy can be transferred to any retained secretions. During vigorous coughing, dynamic collapse of the peripheral airways due to the high intrathoracic pressure, especially at low lung volumes, may involve a large part of the bronchial tree, and the volume of air in the airways may be reduced to one-seventh the normal value. Cartilage rings in the large airways prevent complete collapse, but their lumina are considerably narrowed.

Bechic Blast. When high velocity expiratory air flows are produced in the upper airways, some of this momentum is transferred to the foreign matter, secretions or exudate, resulting in expectoration.

Peak velocity of gas in the trachea or larynx during a forcible cough may reach the astounding level of well over half the speed of sound or 180–300 m./sec. The rate of expiratory gas flow depends on two factors: the alveolar-to-mouth pressure gradient, and the volume of gas in the alveoli at the beginning of coughing. The greater the lung volume the greater the flow rate, hence the marked inspiratory effort which normally precedes coughing. In healthy young males an air flow volume of 12 liters/sec. can be achieved easily. Deep inspiration also enables the expiratory muscles to act with greater force. At lung volumes of less than 50 percent of normal the maximum flow rate is halved.

The velocity of gas flow at any point in the airways depends on the instantaneous flow divided by the total cross section of all airways of that generation. As the total cross section in area of all the small airways is over one hundred times that of the trachea or larger airways, the velocity of expelled air reaches a very high level in the large airways. This velocity is further increased as the diameter of the trachea and larger bronchi is narrowed by dynamic compression due to the high positive intrapleural pressure.

Etiologic Classification of Cough

The conditions which can lead to coughing are too numerous to list in detail. Some broad areas are listed as follows:

Infections

> Upper Respiratory. Acute rhinitis and/or sinusitis with post-nasal drip and irritation; acute tonsillo-pharyngitis; epiglottitis.
>
> Lower Respiratory. Acute spasmodic laryngitis ("spasmodic croup"); laryngotracheobronchitis; measles; pertussis and parapertussis; cystic fibrosis; bronchiolitis; bronchopneumonia; tuberculosis; bronchiectasis; atelectasis.

Parasitic infections. Ascariasis; visceral larva migrans.

Congenital anomalies. Pulmonary sequestration; diaphragmatic hernia; tracheoesophageal fistula of the "H" type; vascular rings; anomalous major vessels.

Allergy. Allergic rhinitis; asthma; hypersensitivity pneumonitis (pigeonbreeder's lung, parakeets, gerbils, etc.); allergic broncho-pulmonary aspergillosis.

Irritants. Tobacco smoke; fumes; perfumes; sprays.

Pulmonary edema. Congestive heart failure; hyperperfused lungs due to large left to right intracardiac shunts.

Acute aspirations. Hydrocarbons; talc; water; vomitus

Recurrent Aspirations. Palato-pharyngeal incoordination; gastroesophageal reflux; mongolism; familial dysautonomia.

Foreign bodies

Extrinsic irritation. Retropharyngeal abscess; mediastinal cysts or tumors; enlarged mediastinal or hilar lymphnodes; pleurisy; pleural effusion; emphysema.

Miscellaneous: Idiopathic pulmonary hemosiderosis; chlamydial infection.

Extrarespiratory: Impacted cerumen in the ear; foreign body in ear; external otitis; esophageal duplication.

Psychogenic or habit spasm

Special Kinds of Cough

Certain conditions, in their classic form, have characteristic coughing patterns which may be of help in diagnosis. Some examples are:

Sinusitis. Particularly bothersome at night after going to bed and in the morning upon arising.

Acute Spasmodic Laryngitis. Rather sudden onset of a tight, harsh, barking cough, often associated with inspiratory stridor which occurs during the night and disappears the next day.

Bronchitis. A deep and productive cough, especially of viral origin, which may persist 4–6 weeks after the associated signs of upper respiratory infection have gone.

Pertussis. Paroxysms of harsh, hacking cough, followed by a sudden, deep, tight, crowing inspiration or whoop.

Chlamydia. Occurs in infants, predominantly black, with an onset between 2 and 6 weeks of age of tachypnea and a distinctive cough. This cough is a series of harsh, staccato coughs, each separated by a brief inspiration and with no post-tussic inspiratory whoop. There are no systemic signs of illness and no fever and the course is protracted for several weeks. A history of inclusion conjunctivitis is only present in about half the cases.

Cystic Fibrosis. This should be a diagnostic consideration in infants and children who have a persistent cough and frequent respiratory infections. In infants, the cough may be paroxysmal and resemble that of bronchiolitis and not become productive until progression of the disease occurs.

Bronchiectasis. Paroxysms of cough productive of purulent sputum, particularly upon arising or with changes in posture.

Nocturnal Cough. This may be a sign of bronchial asthma not associated with wheezing detectable by auscultation. The cough may awaken the child early in the morning.

Chronic Aspiration and "H-Type" T-E Fistula. These infants may cough, choke and become cyanotic when feeding, especially with milk.

Postoperative Repair of T-E Fistulae or Vascular Rings. It is not unusual for a harsh, brassy, irritative cough to persist for several months after surgery because of the residual area of tracheomalacia.

Mediastinal and Hilar Lymphnodes. A harsh, repetitive brassy cough due to compression and/or infiltration of the bronchial wall.

Associated Stridor. Cough with stridor should always suggest laryngeal or tracheal pathology.

Foreign Body. The sudden onset of violent paroxysms of coughing and choking, especially in a toddler, should be investigated. This may be followed by a symptom-free period that can delay the actual diagnosis.

Adolescent Cough. The adolescent who develops a recurrent or chronic cough should be suspected of smoking.

Habit Spasm. This is a short, slight, dry cough which becomes worse when attention is directed to the cough and disappears during sleep. It frequently develops after a previous lower respiratory infection, yet persists long after any evidence of inflammation has disappeared. The cough is reinforced by the parents' concern, constant attention to and commenting about the cough and a general level of increased anxiety in the environment.

Psychogenic Cough. This occurs in older children and adolescents and has a non-productive, barking, foghorn nature which the patient delights in demonstrating, much to the irritation of his teachers, parents and physician. Its loudness and deep resonating nature are additional features. As in the habit spasm cough, no evidence of any underlying respiratory disease can be detected.

Hazards of Cough

Some hazards may arise in coughing. If severe enough, rib fractures may result. Tears at the gastroesophageal junction may produce some bleeding which can be difficult to tell from hemoptysis. Intrathoracic pressure may remain so high for a prolonged period of time with a severe paroxysm of coughing, that venous return to the heart is impeded, cardiac output falls and unconsciousness results—"cough syncope." Persistent coughing may interrupt sleep and this, together with the significant energy expenditure of cough, produces fatigue. In some patients, the force of the cough may precipitate vomiting, particularly when large amounts of mucus have been swallowed. Young infants may find it difficult to feed and fluid intake may suffer. Finally, the appearance of cyanosis in patients during prolonged coughing spells is evidence of hypoxia, and is a warning to use caution and oxygen if airway manipulation is being considered.

Sneeze

The sneeze reflex is very much like the cough reflex except that it is initiated by irritation to the epithelium of the nasal passages. Afferent impulses pass via the trigeminal nerve to the medulla where the reflex is integrated. A series of reactions similar to those which mediate the cough reflex take place. In a sneeze, however, the initial air block takes place mainly at the soft palate and uvula. The uvula is suddenly depressed and a large volume of air passes rapidly through the nose, helping to clear the nasal passages of foreign matter.

Thus, the respiratory system is equipped with a series of coordinated defense mechanisms that strive to keep the tracheobronchial airways open at all times.

BIBLIOGRAPHY

Kendig, E. L., Jr., and Chernick, V.: Disorders of the Respiratory Tract in Children. 3rd Edition. Philadelphia, W. B. Saunders, 1977.

> This is the most comprehensive of texts dealing with the entire spectrum of clinical conditions encountered in pediatric pulmonary disease. Some 68 separate chapters by 52 recognized experts provide a most authoritative coverage of the material.

Murray, J. F.: The Normal Lung. Philadelphia, W. B. Saunders, 1976.

> A current, comprehensive, readable and well-illustrated summary of the structure and function of the lung. Has good sections on growth and development of the lung and on defense mechanisms of the respiratory tract.

West, J. B.: Respiratory Physiology—The Essentials. Baltimore, Williams and Wilkins, 1974.

> This is a jewel of a book which was written as a core course for medical students. The emphasis is on gas exchange as the chief function of the lung.

Williams, H. E., and Phelan, P. D.: Respiratory Illness in Children. London, Blackwell Scientific Publications, 1975.

> Written by two well-regarded Australian pediatric pulmonary physicians, this text focuses more on the clinical pathophysiology and symptoms associated with the major areas of pediatric pulmonary disease. Very little of the text deals with neonatal pulmonary problems; its major focus is on the practitioner faced with the interpretation of symptoms characteristic of the more common pulmonary conditions.

24

Evaluation of the Cardiovascular System

Sidney Friedman, M.D.

Although the format of the procedure is basically the same as in the adult, evaluation of the cardiovascular system in infancy and childhood requires unique knowledge and skills. Evaluation should begin with a pertinent history, the questioning based upon an understanding of cardiovascular symptomatology in pediatric patients. A careful physical examination should follow, in which cardiac auscultation plays a major role. An electrocardiogram, chest radiograph, and blood count should be carried out routinely in all cardiac suspects. For the solution of more complex problems, special techniques, first of the non-invasive type and finally of the invasive variety, may be required.

HISTORY

The medical history in pediatric cardiac suspects may be shorter but is no less important than in adult patients. A clear stating of the circumstances and reasons that bring the patient to cardiac review is helpful not only to the physician but also in orienting parents to the goals of the examination. The chief complaint in over 90 per cent of patients who appear for cardiac evaluation in childhood is the recent discovery of a cardiac murmur. This is not surprising since congenital heart disease and rheumatic heart disease are the two major etiologic varieties of heart disease in the pediatric age group. Both are characterized by the presence of cardiac murmurs. The high frequency of functional or innocent cardiac murmurs in childhood also contributes toward the common appearance of this chief complaint. Other less frequent presenting complaints are cyanosis, congestive heart failure (often precipitated by a respiratory tract infection), failure to thrive, chest pain, exercise intolerance, and occasionally the discovery of an abnormal cardiac silhouette in a chest roentgenogram.

Although congenital heart disease does not usually follow a simple hereditary pattern, the family history should be discussed. There are rare families in which congenital heart disease is found in more than one member, the same lesion reappearing in two or three siblings (e.g., aortic stenosis, patent ductus arteriosus, atrial septal defect, tetralogy of Fallot, and pulmonary stenosis). In evaluating the possibility of rheumatic fever, it is important to establish a family history, since a familial pattern of incidence occurs in this disease. When questioning in relation to this illness, it should also be determined if there is a history of streptococcal infection prior to a suspected rheumatic episode.

The time of initial discovery of a cardiac murmur is of some diagnostic assistance and should always be established. Murmurs related to obstructive lesions are usually present at the first examination following birth. Murmurs dependent upon pressure differences between the right and left sides of the heart may not appear for several weeks or months after birth. Murmurs whose intensity is related to large stroke volumes may not be appreciated to be significant ones for a number of years.

Evaluation of the symptoms of cardiovascular disease should include questions about cyanosis, exercise intolerance, and shortness of breath. Cyanosis related to breath holding or exposure to cold, as with bathing, can be ignored safely. Parents are consistently poor observers of cyanosis, particularly of the milder varieties. In individuals with normal hemoglobin levels, Comroe demonstrated that only at arterial oxygen saturations below 75 per cent is clinical cyanosis apparent consistently to all observers in all subjects. Easy fatigability is best evaluated in the small infant by questions related to feeding patterns; this symptom may be interpreted erroneously by parents as a special need for sleep rather than intolerance to exertion. Respiratory distress is best assayed historically by questions related to the rate and regularity of respirations and the presence of retractions of the chest wall. Sighing type respirations are not cardiac in origin.

A complete history should include some evaluation of the patient's rate of physical growth. This is easily observed and appreciated by use of one of the standard growth charts, plotting weight or height against age. A graphic expression of this relationship in terms of a percentile of a standard growth pattern is helpful for rapid appreciation of gross deviations. A review of past medical illnesses, particularly with regard to the frequency of respiratory tract infections, is usually helpful since lingering, complicated respiratory tract infections are often associated with large arteriovenous shunts due to congenital heart disease. A list of the hospitalizations and their precipitating illnesses will quickly provide information regarding serious disease.

PHYSICAL EXAMINATION

One of the chief roles of the cardiac examiner is to arrange and produce the circumstances so that the patient is comfortable and in a favorable state of cooperation during the physical examination. Observations made with the patient struggling and crying, or even in a very fearful state, are of little value and may indeed be misleading. Infants up to the age of 6 months are readily placated with a few pleasant sounds or a bottle; between the ages of 6 months and 2–2½ years, a considerable effort must go into preparing a peaceful, productive examination. First, discard the white coat. Examination on the mother's lap rather than on the examining table is very helpful. Distractions with toys, pictures, and office artifacts are sometimes successful. Children beyond the age of 3 are almost uniformly won over by remarks showing interest in them as individuals, including overt flattery. Asking a preschool 3- or 4-year-old his grade in school almost always provides a cooperative subject. Another effective question is "How come you're so good?" Adolescents, particularly girls, are likely to become very apprehensive about a physical examination, especially when asked to disrobe. Provision of a private dressing room and appropriate gowns to minimize exposure are helpful measures as are a variety of verbal reassurances.

The findings of the physical examination are also profoundly influenced by the presence of fever or anemia. Both of these conditions produce high stroke volume and high cardiac output and thereby may alter the cardiac findings. Final interpretations of the cardiac examination should be deferred until anemia and fever are not present.

Vital Signs

The recorded physical examination should include *without fail* three vital measures of cardiovascular function: (1) the blood pressure, (2) the cardiac rate as well as the peripheral arterial pulse rate and character and (3) the respiratory rate and pattern. Too often these vital measurements are left for the end of the examination and then omitted entirely in the recorded examination.

Blood Pressure. Despite the increased difficulty in obtaining accurate determinations in small and uncooperative individuals, measurement of the blood pressure is an essential part of every pediatric examination. This particular determination is valid only if the infant is quiet and calm; crying, apprehension, and physical activity will markedly elevate the blood pressure. Apprehension in older children can be averted by a brief period of explanation and diversion, followed by a series of measurements, with greater credence being attributed to later determinations.

Aside from the need for a basal state, there are a number of details of technique which are important in accurately determining the blood pressure in smaller individuals. The proper width of the blood pressure cuff is critical for an accurate result; the proper size is one which covers approximately two-thirds of the upper arm or thigh. A cuff that is too narrow provides falsely elevated blood pressure values that are sometimes as much as twice the normal level. A cuff that is too broad produces smaller errors, but in the direction of falsely low values. Cuffs of several sizes should be available; veterinary medical supply sources are valuable in this effort. A nomogram for proper selection of cuff size, based on arm circumference and the child's height, is available.

The blood pressure should be measured in both arms and in at least one of the lower extremities. Occasional variations occur in the blood pressure level in the two upper extremities, e.g. supravalvular aortic stenosis, or absence or compression of one of the subclavian arteries (post-Blalock-Taussig operation). Comparison of the upper and lower extremity blood pressure may give information leading to the diagnosis of coarctation of the aorta.

The brachial artery is used for determination of pressure in the upper extremity. The cuff should be applied snugly and without bulges to the bare arm. It should be inflated rapidly to avoid venous congestion and deflated at a rate of approximately 5 mm. Hg/second. If the cuff is released too rapidly, the readings will be falsely low. If a second determination is made, the cuff should be deflated completely before restarting the second measurement.

Measurements in the lower extremities are made using the popliteal artery with the cuff applied around the thigh. After the age of 9 months, the systolic blood pressure in the lower extremities is normally higher than in the arms by about 10–20 mm. Hg. This is due to the fact that the arterial pulse wave is augmented by the rebound wave, an effect that increases with the distance from the heart. Prior to the age of 6 or 9 months, the flush pressure in the upper extremity is higher than in the lower, usually by 5 or 10 mm. Hg, due to the normal narrowing at the isthmus of the aorta. Diastolic pressures are usually equal in the upper and lower extremities.

Palpation. There are several techniques available for determining the arterial blood pressure in infants and children. The method of palpation permits a rough estimate of systolic pressure. In this technique, the cuff is inflated to a pressure well above that which will cause the peripheral arterial pulse to disappear on palpation and then the cuff is slowly deflated. The pressure level at which the palpable pulse reappears corresponds to a level approximately 10 mm. Hg below the systolic blood pressure.

Auscultation. The method of auscultation can be used for all ages, but is more difficult to apply in early infancy when vascular sounds are weak and difficult to hear. The pressure at which the first sound appears following deflation of the cuff corresponds accurately with systolic blood pressure measured intraluminally. There is less agreement concerning the indicator level which corresponds to the diastolic blood pressure. The point at which the Korotkoff sounds are first muffled or at which they disappear completely is variably taken as the level of diastolic blood pressure. It is wise to record both figures if there is more than a 5 mm. difference between the two.

The flush technique may be used in infants when auscultation is difficult. In the flush method, a cuff is placed on the thigh or forearm and an elastic bandage is wrapped snugly around the distal extremity which is then massaged to drain the superficial blood. The cuff is inflated to a pressure above the anticipated systolic level and the bandage is removed. The skin of the hand or foot appears pale and bloodless. The pressure at which the first flush of pink color appears in the skin of the blanched distal extremity is taken as the mean arterial blood pressure. The Doppler technique and a variety of electronic methods can also be used in problem situations.

The blood pressure of a child varies directly with age. Standard normal values are available. Neonatal pressures are most variable. There is a steady increase in blood pressure thoughout infancy and childhood, before stabilization at adult levels. The pulse pressure varies normally from 20 to 50 mm. Hg throughout childhood.

Cardiac Rate. Observation of the cardiac rate is also of fundamental value in evaluating the cardiovascular system. The cardiac rate can be determined prior to birth either by direct auscultation or by intrauterine electrocardiographic monitoring. This type of monitoring is commonly employed during labor, particularly in high risk pregnancies. The cardiac rate is used in determining the Apgar scoring after birth as a gauge of neonatal well-being. The normal fetal rate varies between 120 and 160/minute. Excessive slowing of the fetal heart is taken as a measure of fetal distress during labor. A slow fetal heart rate may also signal the presence of congenital heart block.

The cardiac rate in a newborn is rapid and subject to wide variations. In small infants, the apical rate should be counted for an entire minute, rather than placing reliance on the peripheral arterial pulse. For the first 15 or 30 minutes of life, the heart rate may commonly reach a level of 180/minute. Average values for a full term infant during the first week of life are 120 to 140/minute. The rate increases quickly with crying or feeding. A rate above 200/minute that persists when the infant is quiet should raise the possibility of a tachyarrhythmia, e.g. paroxysmal supraventricular tachycardia.

Respiratory variation of the heart rate is observed in many full-term newborn infants and often in premature infants. During sleep there may be periods of apnea and decreased heart rate; when respiratory movements are resumed, the rate again quickens. Cardiac arrhythmias of many types are encountered often during the neonatal period. When monitored continuously, approximately 10 per cent of full term newborn infants will show infrequent ectopic beats, primarily premature ventricular contractions. Forty per cent of premature infants studied in this way show periods of sinus bradycardia with or without nodal escape. These findings are not abnormal unless they persist.

As the infant ages, the heart rate tends to decrease. By the age of 2 years, a resting cardiac rate of 110/minute is normal. At the age of 6 years, the rate of 100/minute is normal. By the age of 10 years, the normal rate has decreased to 90 beats/minute, and in the adolescent period, values of 60 to 80 are common. Rates for males are generally below those of females.

During childhood the cardiac rate is very labile; it increases rapidly in response to muscular activity and emotional stimulation, and is often found to be higher after meals and in the afternoon. Persistent sinus tachycardia is often seen in the pediatrician's office because of fear or excitement. Parents should be asked to check the cardiac rate during sleep if there is any concern about this point since tachycardia from organic illnesses persists during sleep.

Rapid heart rates may be observed secondary to anemia, shock, or fever. The heart rate usually increases 8 to 10 beats/minute/F° temperature elevation. In the presence of rheumatic carditis, a tachycardia is present which exceeds the level to be expected from temperature elevation alone, and persists during sleep. Thyrotoxicosis is a rare cause of tachycardia during childhood. An increase in heart rate is present almost uniformly with congestive heart failure.

Adolescence. Sinus bradycardia is usually defined as a cardiac rate less than 100 beats/minute to infants, and less than 60 beats/minute in older children. Slow rates may be normal in athletes in high states of physical training and occasionally in newborns and premature infants. Other causes of slow cardiac rates in pediatric patients include increased intracranial pressure, hypothyroidism, and increased serum potassium levels.

Sinus arrhythmia is observed most frequently in adolescence, particularly in males. It is a phasic heart rate that is often but not necessarily associated with respiration; frequently the rate speeds with inspiration and slows with expiration. Sinus arrhythmia is often seen with a slow overall heart rate, but is usually abolished by exercise. It is an early evidence of cardiotoxicity due to digitalis.

Respiration. The respiratory pattern of the newborn infant may be very irregular and variable. In premature infants respiration may be characterized by periods of deep respiratory excursions which alternate with apnea or slow and shallow respirations. This type of irregularity of breathing usually disappears by the fourth week of life. Its persistence may indicate central nervous system disease or metabolic abnormalities which depress the central respiratory control center.

The normal range of rate of respiration varies from 30 to 50/minute at birth, to 16 to 20 at the age of 6 years, and 14 to 16 at puberty. The respiratory rate is markedly influenced by excitement or apprehension in young infants and for this reason is best determined during sleep or in a basal period. Rapid respiratory rates are observed in many pulmonary disorders and with infections, fever, poisonings (particulary salicylism), or in congestive heart failure, acidosis, or shock. Slow respiratory rates may be indicative of increased intracranial pressure, suppression of the respiratory center by sedatives, alkalosis, or poisons. The depth of respiration may be indicative of anoxia, the state of activity of the respiratory center, or the presence of acidosis or alkalosis.

The use of accessory muscles of respiration should be consciously observed and is the objective counterpart of the subjective complaint of dyspnea in adults. Flaring of the alae nasi, retraction of the intercostal spaces, other areas of retraction above and below the costal cage, and grunting with respiration represent use of accessory muscles of respiration. Respiratory distress may occur with exercise, pain, fright, anemia, cardiovascular disorders, hypothyroidism, and in many other conditions. Inspiratory distress occurs more frequently with high airway obstructions and expiratory distress with low obstructions.

INSPECTION

Important information related to the cardiovascular system can be gained by simple inspection. Ease and accuracy of an examination will be abetted if pertinent clothing, necklaces, bracelets, and nail polish are removed beforehand. First, a crude estimate should be made of the size and physical development of the patient in relationship to age. The weight and height can be expressed in terms of percentile values compared to a normal group of children of similar age. Whether or not the patient seems content, uncomfortable or interested in his environment should be included in the record of general inspection. The respiratory rate and effort can be noted by simple observation.

Identification of a variety of somatic syndromes, some representing chromosomal aberrations, can contribute toward the cardiac evaluation. The stigmata of mongolism should alert the observer to the possibility of an atrial or a ventricular septal defect, perhaps associated with an endocardial cushion defect and early pulmonary hypertension. The phenotype of Turner's syndrome should raise suspicion of coarctation of the aorta; this is found in 30 to 40 percent of such patients. The features of Noonan's syndrome should suggest the possibility of pulmonary stenosis associated with pulmonary valvular dysplasia syndrome. Marfan's syndrome should lead to a careful search for evidence of aortic and mitral valve dysfunction. Patients with stigmata of neonatal rubella should be observed for combinations of patent ductus arteriosus, pulmonary artery stenosis, pulmonary and aortic valvular stenosis, and coarctation of the aorta. Other less common congenital somatic syndromes also have characteristic cardiac manifestations.

Cyanosis is best observed in daylight or under incandescent lighting. Exposure to fluorescent light or low intensity light, particularly with exposure to cold, will spuriously enhance the apparent degree of cyanosis. Cyanosis may be generalized or regional. A comparison of the discoloration of the nail beds of the fingers and the toes should be made by placing them side by side. The presence of a preductal coarctation of the aorta is likely to produce only detectable cyanosis of the lower extremities. A variety of other complex congenital lesions may produce regional cyanosis.

Clubbing of the fingers and toes will occur in patients with large venous-arterial shunts associated with cyanotic congenital heart disease. Clubbing is rarely present in the absence of obvious cyanosis, nor does it often become apparent before the age of 6 months. A generalized redness of the fingertips may be evidence of mild arterial unsaturation, as is present with a large atrial septal defect. In the presence of more severe hypoxia, the angle between the base of the nail and the skin proximal to it may disappear and, still later, longitudinal curving of the nails with widening of the terminal phalanges develops. Polycythemia is almost uniformly associated with hypoxia sufficiently severe to cause clubbing. Clubbing will disappear in the course of 2 to 4 months following surgical relief of arterial unsaturation.

Inspection of the cervical veins may provide useful information concerning venous pressure. In the erect position, the external jugular vein should not be distended visibly. In the recumbent position, distention of the external jugular vein may be normal. This vein should collapse normally as the level of the patient is raised to approximately 45° from the horizontal table, if the muscles of the neck are relaxed.

With each heart beat two small venous pulse waves can be noted: the "a-wave" coinciding with right atrial contraction and the "v-wave" coinciding with right ventricular contraction. These waves, at times difficult to discern, alternate with more apparent phases of venous collapse. The collapse following the a-wave occurs as the right atrium becomes less distended following presystolic contraction, whereas the collapse after the v-wave occurs as the tricuspid valve opens. The a-wave, which occurs in presystole, can be timed with the apical impulse. A prominent a-wave in presystole can be noted in patients with tricuspid stenosis or tricuspid atresia, severe pulmonary stenosis, primary pulmonary hypertension, and cor pulmonale. It may be absent with right-sided heart failure, or in the presence of auricular fibrillation and other arrhythmias. The v-wave may become very prominent in patients with tricuspid regurgitation, and can be demonstrated by compressing the vein with the finger. The portion of the vein above the finger becomes distended from above while the portion below shows the systolic v-wave as blood from the right ventricle is regurgitated into the right atrium and then refluxed into the cervical veins.

Prominent arterial pulsations can also be observed in the neck in the presence of wide pulse pressures as seen with aortic regurgitation, coarctation of the aorta, patent ductus arteriosus, and large systemic arteriovenous fistulae. A variety of congenital deformities of the chest wall can be observed in children with cardiac abnormalities. A precordial bulge may provide information concerning the size and laterality of the heart.

Edema in small infants is usually initially observed as facial and periorbital swelling. This swelling results from the loose connection between the skin and subcutaneous tissues in these areas and the head-down position of the infant. Edema rarely occurs prior to hepatomegaly in right heart failure. In longstanding right heart failure, edema of the lower extremities and ascites may occur.

Pallor and jaundice of the skin may also be observed in certain cardiac conditions. Jaundice can be the result of prolonged right heart failure and chronic congestion of the liver. Pallor may be related to severe anemia and is prominent in proportion to the hemoglobin level in patients with rheumatic fever during the active stage of the disease.

Inspection of the teeth often provides general information concerning the standard of health care provided the patient. Dental health is related as well to prophylaxis against subacute bacterial endocarditis. Large tonsils and upper airway obstruction may be the visible causes for chronic hypoxia leading to pulmonary hypertension and cor pulmonale.

PALPATION AND PERCUSSION

Considerable information can be gained by palpation of the arterial pulses, usually at the site of the brachial and femoral arteries. A discrepancy in the volume of the pulses between the upper and lower extremities should raise the suspicion of a coarctation of the aorta. A strong, bounding pulse with a rapid collapse (water-hammer pulse) occurs in lesions associated with a wide pulse pressure. The latter include a large patent ductus arteriosus, aortic regurgitation, systemic arteriovenous fistulae, complete heart block, or certain high cardiac output states. In contrast, a weak pulse is palpated with severe aortic stenosis, pericardial tamponade, congestive heart failure, or in cardiovascular shock. The term paradoxical pulse is applied to variations in the amplitude of the arterial pulse observed by palpation during inspiration and expiration. In pulses paradoxicus, the pulse becomes weak or disappears during inspiration and reappears during expiration. This is observed with pericardial effusion or constrictive pericarditis, in severe primary myocardial diseases, and in frank congestive heart failure. Pulsus alternans is characterized by alternating strong and weak arterial pulses on palpation and is observed in advanced left heart failure. Pulsus bigeminus consists of a prominent pulse alternating with a prematurely occurring weaker one; this may be observed with digitalis intoxication and occasionally with no other evidence of heart disease.

Location of the apex beat is helpful in determining the spacial orientation of the heart as well as its size. In the usual levocardia with situs solitus, the apex beat is at the point furthest to the left and downward where the impact of the heart is palpable, and indicates a leftward orientation of the heart. In dextrocardia, the apical impulse is in the fourth or fifth interspace in the right midclavicular line. Displacement of the apex beat accompanies cardiac enlargement.

Palpation permits the recognition of a cardiac thrill which is the tactile appreciation of the vibrations observed as a cardiac murmur on auscultation. The location of the thrill may direct attention to a specific lesion. A thrill palpable in the second right interspace is usually associated with aortic stenosis. A thrill found to the left of the lower sternum and in the xiphoid region usually signals the presence of a ventricular septal defect. In valvular pulmonic stenosis, the thrill is often found to the left of the upper sternum. A palpable thrill in the suprasternal notch and over the vessels of the neck is often associated with aortic stenosis but may also be present with valvular pulmonic stenosis or other causes of turbulence in the great arteries such as a surgical systemic artery to pulmonary artery anastomosis.

The third major observation that can be made by palpation is the presence of an abnormal ventricular impulse. A sustained lift to the left of the lower sternum and in the xiphoid region indicates right ventricular overwork. In contrast, a sustained lift at the cardiac apex signifies left ventricular hypertrophy. The tactile character of the impulse varies in the right as compared with the left ventricular impulse.

Varying degrees of hepatomegaly can be appreciated by palpation and percussion. In small infants hepatomegaly is a sensitive and useful index of congestive heart failure. Massive hepatic enlargement may occasionally be observed by inspection. When the liver enlarges in a small infant, the liver edge and the anterior surface of the liver become more superficial and are palpable just beneath the anterior abdominal wall. Upon percussion, the dull note over the liver surface is also an accurate indicator of liver size.

Cardiac enlargement can at times be appreciated by palpation and percussion, particularly if the enlargement is more than slight. A roentgenogram of the chest is more valuable than physical examination in detecting slight changes in heart size. Detection of the left heart border by percussion or by identification of the apex beat is useful to this end.

AUSCULTATION

Successful cardiac auscultation requires favorable environmental circumstances. It is essential that the patient be relaxed and quiet. Next, the examiner must be in a comfortable position that can be maintained without fatigue or distraction for several minutes. He must have a free state of mind and the time to concentrate completely upon the task at hand. His stethoscope must be familiar to him and well-fitting, particularly with regard to the ear pieces and the length of the rubber tubing. While short tubing is of theoretical benefit with regard to acoustic principles, it will produce poor results if it forces an uncomfortable examining position. Finally, and most important, auscultation has to be done systematically with premeditation and conscious direction. Each auscultatory possibility has to be sought consciously and then noted as either present or absent. A large number of observations must be made concerning each cardiac sound or murmur. In order to make these observations accurately, the examiner must know all the acoustic possibilities beforehand, and process them through a mental checklist.

Heart Sounds

The identification of the first and second heart sounds should be the first goal of auscultation, thereby determining the two phases of the cardiac cycle, systole and diastole. The first heart sound is the louder of the two sounds at the cardiac apex and is synchronous with the apex beat. It is usually nearer to the second heart sound than the distance in time from the second sound to the first, since systole is usually shorter than diastole. The second heart sound is the louder of the two sounds at the base of the heart and two components are often heard intermittently.

The first heart sound results from vibrations associated with closure of the mitral and tricuspid valves. Mitral valve closure usually precedes tricuspid valve closure; asynchrony results in some splitting of the first heart sound, usually with an interval of less than 0.02 seconds. This interval is difficult to appreciate. The second heart sound is due chiefly to events associated with closure of the semilunar valves. Aortic valve closure usually precedes pulmonary valve closure; this results in an easily detectable duplication best heard in the second left interspace. The degree of splitting is variable (0.04–0.06 seconds), being wider during inspiration and in the recumbent position.

Evaluation of the second heart sound at the base of the heart with regard to intensity and splitting of components is one of the most rewarding efforts of cardiac auscultation in childhood. Observation of the two components of the second heart sound usually provides an accurate clue to the level of pulmonary artery pressure. The louder the second component of the second sound, the higher the pulmonary artery pressure. A reduction in the intensity of the second component in the pulmonary area suggests low pulmonary artery diastolic closing pressure, as with severe pulmonary stenosis. Accentuation of the second heart sound, especially with little or no audible duplication, usually indicates pulmonary hypertension.

A single second heart sound at the base of the heart may indicate either synchronous closure of the two semilunar valves or an inaudible pulmonary component. Wide splitting of the second heart sound is encountered with an atrial septal defect, moderate isolated valvular pulmonic stenosis, and with right bundle branch block.

A third heart sound can be heard in approximately 25 percent of pediatric patients between the ages of 2 and 12 years. This third sound is found in early diastole and is coincident with the phase of rapid filling of the ventricles from the atria. It is usually heard best at or just to the right of the cardiac apex in the recumbent position. Maneuvers to increase systemic venous return accentuate the third heart sound.

A fourth heart sound is not heard normally. When present, it is due to atrial contraction and is most often heard with right atrial hypertension. Accentuation by inspiration suggests the right-sided origin of this sound.

Clicking Sounds

Clicking sounds of diagnostic significance can be heard in early systole or in mid-systole. The early systolic ejection click is usually present to the left of the upper sternum and is observed in conditions associated with dilatation of the main pulmonary artery, ascending aorta or semilunar valve abnormality. Prominent ejection clicks are heard with aortic and pulmonic valvular stenosis. Similar sounds can be heard with coarctation of the aorta, truncus arteriosus, severe pulmonary hypertension, and idiopathic dilatation of the pulmonary artery.

Clicking sounds that occur in the middle of systole are due to dysfunction of the mitral valve. They are found often in connection with and introducing the late systolic apical murmur of mitral insufficiency associated with papillary muscle dysfunction syndrome. The click is coincident with the maximal excursion of the mitral valve leaflet connected to the abnormal papillary muscle. Redundant mitral valve tissue with or without mitral insufficiency, often found with atrial septal defects, may also be associated with midsystolic clicking sounds.

Murmurs

The analysis of each cardiac murmur should include an evaluation of the following six features: (1) timing, (2) acoustic quality, (3) intensity, (4) duration, (5) location and (6) transmission.

The timing of murmurs is facilitated by the proper identification of the first and second heart sounds. Systolic murmurs occurring between the first and second heart sound should be described with regard to the portion or portions of systole occupied. Similarly, the diastolic murmurs may be present in one or more of the three standard subdivisions of diastole (protodiastole, mid-diastole, or presystole). The continuous murmur overrides the second heart sounds and spills from systole into diastole.

The quality or acoustic characteristics of murmurs are described usually in a local jargon which may or may not be accurate with regard to the physical characteristics of the murmur, but which provides a group of individuals a method of communicating among themselves the acoustic characteristics of cardiac murmurs. Terms such as blowing, buzzing, musical, vibratory, harsh, rough, rumbling, expulsive, crescendo, and decrescendo fall into this category as do pitch (high, medium, and low) and the presence of peculiar overtones.

Grading the intensity of cardiac murmurs is valuable, especially for systematic comparison of murmurs in serial observations of a single patient. Levine's system, in which murmurs are graded from 1 to 6 for systolic murmurs and 1 to 4 for diastolic murmurs, was originated for use in adults. In the pediatric age group, the intensity of murmurs is not as accurately correlated with signficance of murmurs as in the adult age group. Many of the functional or innocent murmurs may be louder than the apical holosystolic blowing murmur of mild mitral insufficiency.

The duration of cardiac murmurs is usually expressed in the terms suggested by Leatham. An ejection murmur is compared to a pansystolic or holosystolic murmur. The ejection murmur is the murmur that does not extend throughout all of systole but occupies a variable portion of systole starting from the first heart sound. On graphic recordings, this murmur often has a diamond-shaped or crescendo-descresendo appearance. In contrast, the holosystolic murmur occupies all of systole from the first to the second heart sound and usually has a plateau of intensity; it is characteristic of the murmurs observed with a ventricular septal defect or mitral insufficiency. There are rare situations in which a long ejection murmur may be indistinguishable in duration from a holosystolic murmur. Occasionally, murmurs may be heard exclusively during late systole, as with the mitral insufficiency associated with posterior papillary muscle dysfunction syndrome.

Determining the point of maximal intensity of a murmur is very helpful in evaluation. Murmurs derived from events occurring at the mitral valve are apical in location. Sounds created at the pulmonary valve are heard in the second left interspace; at the aortic valve, sounds are heard in the second right interspace. The exception is the diastolic murmur of aortic insufficiency which is heard best to the left of the mid-sternum. Tricuspid valve deformities are reflected by sounds to the left of the lower sternum.

The degree and direction of transmission of a cardiac murmur is a useful diagnostic observation. Functional or innocent murmurs should not be audible over the posterior chest wall. The murmur of mitral insufficiency is transmitted to the left axilla; the degree of transmission correlates well with the severity of the valvular insufficiency. Pulmonic stenosis produces a murmur that is transmitted well to the posterior chest wall above the left scapula; aortic stenosis produces a murmur that is transmitted above the right scapula and is also carried over to the neck vessels. The murmurs generated by patent ductus arteriosus, coarctation of the aorta, and pulmonary artery stenosis are particularly heard well over the posterior chest wall; in contrast, the murmur of a ventricular septal defect is poorly transmitted to the posterior chest wall.

The following classification of murmurs has been modified from Leatham and provides a useful mechanism for categorizing both systolic and diastolic murmurs:

I.   Systolic Murmurs
    A. Ejection systolic murmurs
        1. Innocent, insignificant murmurs
        2. Systolic murmurs due to pulmonary or aortic valvular, infundibular or supravalvular stenoses
        3. Pulmonary or aortic systolic murmurs due to increased flow across these normal valves, as in atrial septal defect, ventricular septal defect, aortic or pulmonic regurgitation
        4. Systolic murmurs due to relative stenosis of the pulmonary or the aortic orifices, as in idiopathic dilatation of the pulmonary artery, dilatation of the ascending aorta or primary pulmonary hypertension.
    B. Regurgitant systolic murmurs
        1. Systolic murmur due to mitral or tricuspid regurgitation
        2. Systolic murmur due to ventricular septal defect
II.   Diastolic Murmurs
    A. Regurgitant diastolic murmurs (early diastolic murmurs)
        1. Diastolic murmur in aortic regurgitation
        2. Diastolic murmur in pulmonary regurgitation
    B. Ventricular filling murmurs (mid-diastolic murmurs)
        1. Diastolic murmur in atrioventricular valve stenosis, such as in:
           Mitral stenosis
           Tricuspid stenosis
        2. Diastolic murmur in relative atrioventricular valve stenosis due to increased flow and/or dilated ventricles, such as in:
           Atrial septal defect
           Ventricular septal defect
           Anomalous entrance of pulmonary veins
           Patent ductus arteriosus
           Mitral regurgitation
           Complete A-V block

Primary myocardial disease
Severe anemia
3. Diastolic murmur in the presence of obstruction at the mitral or the tricuspid orifices
Tumor; ball-valve thrombi
C. Atrial presystolic murmurs (late diastolic murmurs), such as in:
Mitral stenosis
Tricuspid stenosis
III. Continuous Murmurs, such as in:
Patent ductus arteriosus
Aortocardiac fistula
Coronary arteriovenous fistulae

Pericardiac Friction Rub

A striking extracardiac sound is the pericardial friction rub. It is usually present in both systole and diastole with variable relative intensity in the two portions of the cardiac cycle. This sound may be discovered in any location over the precordium, but is heard most frequently to the left of the lower sternum. Occasionally, it is very difficult to differentiate a pericardial friction rub from a combination of a systolic and diastolic murmur to the left of the sternum. The coarse, scratchy acoustic quality of the pericardial friction rub is the best clue. Bacterial or viral infection is the most common cause of acute pericarditis and a pericardial friction rub.

Innocent Adventitious Sounds

A large number of innocent adventitious heart sounds are encountered in the pediatric age group. A variety of functional or innocent heart murmurs, the venous hum, and the physiologic third heart sound are the most common sounds in this category.

Functional or innocent cardiac murmurs are found in approximately 50 percent of healthy children, especially between the ages of 4 and 8 years. The differentiation of innocent murmurs from those derived from serious varieties of heart disease can be accomplished in the vast majority of instances by auscultation alone. Considerable clinical experience indicates that properly identified innocent murmurs are indeed benign. The 20-year follow-up study of Marienfeld and associates demonstrated that no difference in the incidence of heart disease was found among a group of adult patients who as children had innocent cardiac murmurs compared with a similar group who had not shown such murmurs in childhood. Most functional murmurs disappear in later childhood; an estimated 90 percent are gone by the age of 14 years. The other 10 percent remain for varying periods of time, but the cardiac prognosis in a child is the same whether or not the murmur persists. Two principle categories of benign murmurs are recognized: (1) the mid-precordial musical murmur or the "twanging-string" murmur of Still, and (2) the basal ejection-type systolic murmur sometimes referred to as a "pulmonic-systolic" murmur.

Still's "twanging-string" murmur is the most common and easily identified of the innocent murmurs. Its musical quality has been described variously as buzzing or vibratory; it occupies the first one-third or one-half of systole and in graphic recordings has a crescendo-descrescendo (diamond-shaped) configuration. It is heard best over the midprecordium with the patient in the recumbent position, and often disappears or is not as loud in the erect position. The intensity is remarkably variable and is increased by exercise or other conditions associated with increased stroke volume. Intensity alone is not a useful criterion for the identification of this murmur; more important differential features are (1) the location of the point of maximum intensity over the midprecordium, i.e. to the right of the apex and to the left of the lower sternum, and (2) the characteristic musical acoustic quality. Approximately 60 percent of innocent murmurs are of the Still's variety (Fig. 24-1).

The next most frequent of the non-pathologic murmurs of childhood is the "pulmonic-systolic" or basal ejection-type murmur. This murmur is best heard in the second left interspace. It too is usually confined to the first one-third or one-half of systole. The acoustic quality is less characteristic and less easily identified than the Still's murmur. Its quality is relatively harsh or blowing, rather than musical or vibratory, and the pitch is usually low. Because the pulmonic-systolic murmur is usually of low intensity, it is not transmitted to the posterior chest wall. A palpable thrill is never associated with this murmur. As compared to the Still's murmur, it is less influenced by change in position, but is similarly accentuated by exercise. A much wider area of indecision exists with this murmur than with the Still's murmur in its differentiation from significant murmurs indicating the presence of heart disease. The basal innocent systolic murmurs are at times difficult to differentiate by auscultation from the murmurs of a small atrial septal defect, mild pulmonic or aortic stenosis, pulmonary artery coarctation, or aortic coarctation. A useful distinction is that these organic murmurs tend to be transmitted to the posterior chest wall in a high percentage of cases. The presence of an associated thrill is also an indicator of a significant murmur. Additional evidence of organic heart disease may also help to identify the significance of the murmur.

The venous hum is a continuous whirring sound occupying portions of both systole and diastole, heard best beneath the right clavicle when the patient is in the erect position. This sound can be attributed to the rapid passage of blood through the cervical veins. Although there are occasional exceptions, the venous hum usually disappears in the recumbent position. Compression of the cervical veins will cause the sound to

INNOCENT MURMUR   ORGANIC MURMUR

PHONOCARDIOGRAM

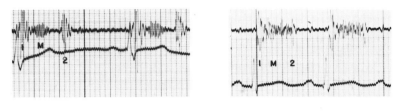

OSCILLOGRAM

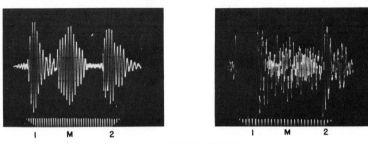

SPECTROGRAM

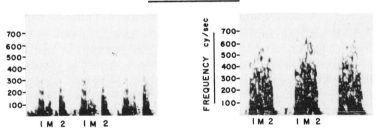

Fig. 24-1. Comparison of the phonocardiographic tracings, oscillo-scopic traces and sound spectrograms of patients with innocent (functional) and organic (mitral insufficiency) murmurs. The wave form of the innocent murmur is regular and of low frequency, similar to that of a musical tone. In contrast, the murmur of mitral insufficiency has a much higher frequency of vibration and a chaotic wave form, the acoustic properties of "noise."

disappear abruptly while extension of the neck will accentuate the intensity of the venous hum.

A positive correlation exists in the coincidence of a functional heart murmur, a venous hum, and a physiologic third heart sound. These three auscultatory findings tend to occur in the same patient, suggesting a common etiology. An increased velocity of blood flow and a high stroke volume are probably the underlying bases for all three of these non-pathologic adventitious sounds.

ROUTINE STUDIES

Three simple laboratory studies should be carried out routinely on all children undergoing formal cardiac evaluation: an electrocardiogram, chest roentgenogram, and a blood count.

Electrocardiogram

The electrocardiogram provides a wide range of valuable information. Cardiac rhythm can be established and abnormalities of rhythm or ectopic pacemakers identified. Quantitative indication of right or left atrial enlargement is provided by the electrocardiogram as is the presence and severity of right, left, or combined ventricular hypertrophy. The hemodynamic mechanism of ventricular hypertrophy, differentiating pressure overwork from volume overload, may also be ascertained. The severity of such lesions as isolated pulmonary stenosis or aortic stenosis can be judged by estimating the degree of right or left ventricular hypertrophy and the presence or absence of "strain" pattern. An excellent correlation exists between the height of the R wave in lead V_1 and the intracavitary right ventricular pressure in the presence of isolated valvular pulmonic stenosis. Left ventricular "strain" pattern is associated almost uniformly with severe aortic stenosis.

A number of specific electrocardiographic patterns related to individual congenital heart lesions are recognized. These include the picture of mirror image dextrocardia, the pattern of an endocardial cushion defect or a double outlet right ventricle, and the pattern of ventricular inversion.

The electrocardiogram can provide evidence of myocardial changes as seen in the presence of myocarditis, digitalis toxicity, or ventricular "strain." These non-specific alterations include prolongation of the P-R interval, T wave and S-T segment changes, and a variety of ectopic beats or arrhythmias.

Chest Radiograph

Cardiac size is the most useful information provided by the chest radiograph, but it is less valuable than the electrocardiogram in predicting right as opposed to left ventricular enlargement. Right atrial and left atrial enlargement are predicted more reliably by chest radiograph than ventricular enlargement. The chest radiograph permits an evaluation of the pulmonary vasculature, both arterial and venous. The side and size of the aortic arch may be valuable information in certain diagnostic and therapeutic situations. The large globular cardiac silhouette of pericardial effusion may also be suspected from the chest roentgenogram.

The chest radiograph is particularly valuable as a diagnostic aid in the cyanotic subject with tetralogy of Fallot, transposition of the great arteries, tricuspid atresia, and persistent truncus arteriosus. A small number of specific contours may be diagnostic, e.g. total anomalous pulmonary venous return of the supracardiac type (figure of eight) and total anomalous pulmonary venous drainage below the diaphragm. Corrected transposition of the great arteries and coarctation of the aorta each provide a number of valuable diagnostic signs in the plain films.

Blood Count

The routine blood count will give information concerning anemia (associated with a high cardiac output state) and polycythemia. The hematologic indices provide information concerning iron deficiency. Polycythemia is a reliable measure of chronic hypoxia due to cyanotic congenital heart disease. Relative anemia in polycythemic patients is of particular importance since its treatment with iron may improve exercise tolerance and avoid the complication of intravascular thrombosis.

NON-INVASIVE CARDIAC STUDIES

Phonocardiogram

The study first available historically in this category is the phonocardiogram, a graphic recording of the heart sounds and murmurs. Questions concerning the duration and timing within the cardiac cycle of murmurs, clicks and heart sounds can be readily resolved by this method. In a few instances, the quality characteristics of the wave form of the phonocardiogram may be useful, particularly in the identification of functional or innocent murmurs. A regular wave form at a low frequency (80–120 cycles/second) is seen regularly with functional murmurs and is presumed to be due to the vibration of solid structures as compared to the chaotic pattern of vibrations resulting from abnormal blood flow.

Vectorcardiogram

Vectorcardiography has relatively few special applications in pediatric cardiology as a supplement to the routine scalar electrocardiogram. There are certain lesions in which the estimate of intraventricular pressure can be derived more accurately from the vectorcardiogram as compared with the regular electrocardiogram. The degree of right ventricular hypertrophy in the pulmonary valvular dysplasia seen in Noonan's syndrome is an example; the level of left ventricular pressure in aortic stenosis is reflected more accurately in the vectorcardiogram than in the electrocardiogram, according to some observers. The direction of the vector loop (counterclockwise) can be helpful in identifying the presence of an endocardial cushion defect.

Echocardiogram

A more recently devised non-invasive technique is the echocardiogram. This is being tested widely now to determine its applications in pediatric cardiology. Movement characteristics of the mitral and other valves are visualized in the echocardiogram. Absence of the normal continuity of the aortic and mitral valve rings can be demonstrated in the echocardiogram in supporting the diagnosis of double outlet right ventricle. Abnormalities of the interventricular septum may be established by echocardiography leading to such diagnoses as asymmetrical septal hypertrophy or idiopathic hypertrophic subaortic stenosis. Pericardial effusion can also be detected in the echocardiogram. Future improvements in the technical aspects of scanning and recording capabilities of this non-invasive technique may indeed yield a very accurate picture of the structure and function of the intracardiac anatomy.

INVASIVE CARDIAC STUDIES

The most widely employed invasive technique is cardiac catheterization. This provides information concerning intracavitary and intravascular pressure, values of the oxygen content in blood specimens obtained from the various chambers and great vessels, the opportunity for selective angiocardiography and finally the detection of abnormal diagnostic pathways taken by the cardiac catheter tip. The balloon catheter used in the creation of an atrial septal defect may also be employed for the purpose of carrying out a trial banding of the pulmonary artery or trial occlusion of a patent ductus arteriosus. The response of the blood pressure, particularly in the pulmonary artery, to a variety of drugs and the administration of 100 percent oxygen inhalation is another diagnostic method in this category. Other invasive techniques include intracavitary electrocardiography and electrophysiologic investigations via a probing catheter, including His bundle recordings. The recording of selective dye dilution curves has been used effectively as a diagnostic tool in a number of laboratories.

BIBLIOGRAPHY

Comroe, J. H., Forster, R. E., Dubois, A. B., Briscoe, W. A., and Carlsen, E.: The Lung. Clinical Physiology and Pulmonary Function Tests. Chicago, The Year Book Publishers, 1955.

    A handbook that delineates concisely the principles of pulmonary physiology and pulmonary function testing.

Friedman, S.: The innocent (functional) cardiac murmurs of childhood. Clin. Pediatr. *4*:77, 1965.

Contains a description of the common innocent cardiac murmurs of childhood by clinical and laboratory means.

Leatham, A.: Auscultation of the heart. Lancet, *2*:703,757, 1958.

Provides a very useful classification of cardiac murmurs based primarily on timing and duration.

Levine, S. A.: Systolic murmur: Its clinical significance. JAMA, *101*:436, 1933.

An early reference to the use of a grading system for uniformity in expressing the intensity of cardiac murmurs.

Marienfield, D. J., Telles, N., Silvera, J., and Nordsieck, J.: A 20-year follow-up study of "innocent" murmurs. Pediatrics. *30*:42, 1962.

Confirms the benign nature of functional heart murmurs by means of a long-term follow-up study.

Moss, A. J., and Adams, F. H.: Problems of Blood Pressure in Childhood. Springfield, Illinois, Charles C Thomas, 1962.

25

Cardiac Disease

Sidney Friedman, M.D.

ETIOLOGY

Two major etiologic varieties of heart disease are encountered in childhood. These are congenital heart disease and rheumatic heart disease. Approximately 5–7 per one thousand newborn infants have a cardiovascular anomaly. Among school-age children, there is the same prevalence of heart disease, but increasing numbers of rheumatic subjects enter the group, reaching about 30–40 per cent of the total at high school levels. The implication is that congenital heart disease is a highly lethal variety of heart disease leading to death in early childhood in almost half the cases. This fact justifies the complicated diagnostic procedures and heroic surgical measures employed. In contrast, some 40–50 per cent of children, particularly those between the ages of 4 and 12 years, have innocent or functional murmurs. Although these murmurs are unrelated to the presence of heart disease, they require accurate recognition and differentiation from the pathologic sounds.

In contrast to the relatively low incidence of heart disease among pediatric patients (.5–1%), degenerative heart disease occurs in almost all adults as part of the normal aging process. Clinically manifest degenerative heart disease is almost an epidemic in the adult male population of the developed countries of the world; in the United States it accounts for approximately 50 per cent of total annual deaths. These differences in incidence lead to a fundamental difference in attitude between pediatric and adult cardiologists. The high incidence of functional or innocent murmurs and the low incidence of actual heart disease, prompts most pediatric cardiologists to question the presence of heart disease in presenting children. Among adult cardiologists, a very high index of suspicion of heart disease exists since almost all individuals beyond middle age have some degenerative changes.

Symptomatic Presentation

The symptomatic presentation of heart disease in childhood is quite different from that encountered among adults; chest pain is rarely evidence of heart disease. The vast majority (95%) of cardiac suspects in childhood are so designated because of the detection of a cardiac murmur. Cyanosis and symptoms of hypoxia are initial manifestations in many infants. Occasionally congestive heart failure will be the initial presenting manifestation, often precipitated by an intercurrent respiratory tract infection. Failure to thrive and easy fatigability are occasionally the chief complaint. Finally, the discovery of an abnormal appearance of the cardiac silhouette is not an infrequent mechanism for the suspicion of heart disease in pediatric patients.

FETAL CIRCULATION AND ITS CONVERSION TO THE POSTNATAL CIRCULATION

In the intrauterine circulation the oxygen supply of the fetus is obtained from the placenta, rather than the lungs. The oxygenated blood enters the right atrium, having arrived there via the umbilical vein, ductus venosus and inferior vena cava. This blood is immediately transferred to the left atrium by means of preferential streaming across the foramen ovale. The ductus arteriosus is patent and carries blood from the pulmonary artery into the descending aorta. This shunting of blood away from the pulmonary vascular bed is dependent upon the high pulmonary vascular resistance in the blood vessels of the lungs in the fetal state. The lungs receive approximately 10 per cent of the ventricular output.

The blood in the right atrium represents a mixture of input from the superior vena cava at about 30 per cent oxygen saturation and the blood coming in from the inferior vena cava which has an oxygen saturation of about 65 per cent. The latter represents a mixture of fresh placental blood obtained through the ductus venosus and reduced systemic venous blood from the lower part of the body. The mixing in the right atrium is not complete. Most of the more highly oxygenated blood from the inferior vena cava enters the left atrium through the foramen ovale. Most of that from the superior vena cava enters the right ventricle through the tricuspid valve; this blood enters the pulmonary artery and more than half of it passes into the descending aorta through the patent ductus arteriosus. The remainder circulates through the lungs and eventually enters the left atrium.

Left atrial blood is a mixture of pulmonary arterial blood which enters through the pulmonary veins and the blood arriving through the foramen ovale. The oxygen saturation of the mixture in the left ventricle supplying the head and the right arm is about 60 per cent. In contrast, the left arm and the lower part of the body are supplied by a mixture of left ventricular and patent ductus arteriosus blood with a less than 60 per cent oxygen saturation.

At birth, a sudden decrease in the pulmonary vascular resistance occurs due to expansion of the lungs associated with the onset of breathing. There is also an increase in systemic resistance due to the collapse and cutting of the umbilical cord. As the pulmonary resistance drops, the blood is diverted from the ductus arteriosus into the lungs via the pulmonary arteries; this supply eventually arrives in the left atrium. The sudden increase in the pulmonary venous blood entering the left atrium raises the left atrial pressure and results in closure of the flap of the foramen ovale. In this way the two circuits are separated; that is, the foramen ovale is closed by the increased left atrial pressure and the patent ductus arteriosus is bypassed by virtue of the sudden fall in pulmonary vascular resistance.

Although these dramatic changes occur within a few minutes or hours, they are not completed for days or weeks. The pulmonary artery pressure drops significantly in the first day of life but a further gradual fall occurs over the next 3 or 4 weeks. The ductus arteriosus constricts rapidly within minutes after the establishment of respiration but is not anatomically closed for 1 or 2 days.

CONGENITAL HEART DISEASE

Approximately 60 or 70 different structural abnormalities of the heart and great vessels may occur as congenital cardiac malformations. These lesions are compatible with fetal life but probably represent a small segment of all the potential cardiac malformations which may occur *in utero*. Many others, incompatible with fetal life, result in the death of the fetus. A number of malformations are not recognized at birth because their presenting manifestations depend upon the changes that occur normally in the conversion of the fetal circulation to the postnatal circulation.

Etiology

The etiology of congenital heart disease is largely unknown. Certain drugs such as thalidomide and LSD have been implicated following maternal ingestion in early pregnancy; intrauterine viral infection with the rubella virus is another established etiologic mechanism. Heredity seems to play a relatively minor role in the etiology of congenital heart disease in humans. However, with inbreeding in animals such as the dog, a very strong hereditary influence is demonstrable. When multiple instances of congenital heart disease occur in a single family, the specific lesions are frequently repeated.

In giving genetic counseling concerning congenital heart disease, an optimistic picture can be painted. Congenital cardiovascular anomalies appear in one of 200 pregnancies, in the absence of any previous family history. In a family that already includes one member with congenital heart disease, the risk is increased only to a level of one in 150. A family desiring more children should be encouraged to take this small risk. If two individuals in a family have the same lesion, subsequent pregnancies carry a considerably higher risk to future offspring, in the range of one in 20.

Incidence

Congenital heart disease is the most common etiologic form of heart disease in the pediatric age group. The acquired heart disease of childhood, rheumatic heart disease, is found only rarely under the age of 4 years. The majority of those who die with congenital heart disease do so in the first weeks and months of life. In considering all of the lesions of congenital heart disease, there is no predilection for males or females; in specific lesions, a sex predilection may exist. The frequency of the individual lesions is difficult to determine accurately and is dependent upon the method of data accumulation. Ventricular septal defect is the most common defect; patent ductus arteriosus is second and tetralogy of Fallot is third in frequency. Atrial septal defect, coarctation of the aorta, aortic stenosis, isolated pulmonary stenosis and transposition of the great vessels occur with almost equal frequency behind the first three. All other lesions are distinctly less common.

Classification of Congenital Heart Disease

The simplest and perhaps most useful classification of congenital cardiac anomalies was proposed by Dr. Maude Abbott of McGill University in 1936 in her historic atlas reviewing 1,000 autopsy specimens of congenital heart disease. She suggested three categories of lesions: (1) those without shunting of blood from one side of the heart to the other, (2) those with shunting of blood from the left side of the heart to the right, (3) those with shunting from the right side of the heart to the left.

The lesions that occur in the absence of shunting are primarily mechanical obstructions and the anomalies of position. Coarctation of the aorta, aortic stenosis, and mitral stenosis are a few examples of obstructive lesions; dextrocardia, single coronary artery, a constricting vascular ring and a right aortic arch are examples of the latter group. The name acyanotic group was used by Dr. Abbott for this category.

The cardiac anomalies with left to right or arterio-venous shunts are common since they are associated with prolonged survival and successful surgical treatment. The three common lesions in this category are atrial septal defect, ventricular septal defect and patent ductus arteriosus. A common feature in these lesions is the accentuation of the pulmonary vascular markings in the chest radiograph. Cyanosis is absent with exclusive left to right shunting. Less common examples of left to right shunting are partial anomalous pulmonary venous return, aortico-pulmonary window, and systemic arterio-venous fistula.

While the arterio-venous shunts are not associated ordinarily with cyanosis, Dr. Abbott offered the designation of cyanosis tardive for this category. This name is the result of her observation that late in the clinical course of children with large left to right shunts, cyanosis did sometimes appear. She was referring to the development of pulmonary vascular occlusive disease that results in high pulmonary vascular resistance and pulmonary hypertension (Eisenmenger complex). Under these circumstances, the pressure in the pulmonary circuit can exceed the systemic arterial blood pressure and reverse the direction of the shunt through the defect. This sequence does not occur frequently and is observed rarely in the first decade of life. Nevertheless, the consequences of such pulmonary vascular disease are devastating, since they preclude successful surgical closure of the defect.

The third category, the cyanotic group consists of those lesions with persistent right to left or venous-arterial shunting. The most blatant right to left shunt occurs in transposition of the great arteries since the entire systemic venous return enters the aorta from the right ventricle. Other common lesions of right to left shunting are: the tetralogy of Fallot, a combination of severe pulmonary stenosis and a large ventricular septal defect; severe valvular pulmonic stenosis with an interatrial right to left shunt; tricuspid atresia with hypoplasia of the right ventricle; persistent truncus arteriosus, single ventricle or single atrium; and a variety of lesions associated with pulmonary atresia.

A useful subdivision of the lesions with right to left shunting can be made, from a therapeutic standpoint, by use of the chest roentgenogram. One category includes the lesions with obstruction of pulmonary blood flow and, therefore, a paucity of pulmonary vascular markings; the heart is usually not enlarged. This group includes tetralogy of Fallot, tricuspid atresia with hypoplasia of the right ventricle, pulmonary atresia with or without a ventricular septal defect. If total correction is not feasible, improvement of hypoxia can be obtained by surgical measures for increasing pulmonary blood flow. The second category includes the cyanotic lesions associated with abundant pulmonary blood flow. In these lesions, cyanosis is not as severe, but the heart is enlarged and congestive heart failure may be a presenting manifestation. Examples of this subgroup are transposition of the great arteries, persistent truncus arteriosus, and single ventricle. Finally, another very useful diagnostic finding in cyanotic infants is an extreme left-sided picture in the electrocardiogram; this is strongly suggestive of tricuspid atresia with hypoplasia of the right ventricle.

Clinical Consequences of Congenital Heart Disease

Pediatric cardiac supervision and treatment is focused around several unfavorable clinical sequelae which occur frequently in patients with congenital heart disease. These include: (1) congestive heart failure, (2) hypoxia and its complications, (3) the prevention and management of pulmonary hypertension, (4) the bacterial complications of subacute bacterial endocarditis and brain abscess, and (5) syncope and sudden death.

Congestive Heart Failure. The wide variety of lesions of congenital heart disease produces a number of mechanical problems which may lead to congestive heart failure. In patients with severe obstructive lesions such as aortic stenosis or pulmonic stenosis, systolic overloading of the ventricles occurs. Severe degrees of systolic overloading are best reflected in the electrocardiogram in the form of right or left ventricular hypertrophy and "strain" patterns. Coarctation of the aorta and pulmonary vascular obstructive disease are other common causes for systolic overloading leading to congestive heart failure.

Diastolic overloading of the ventricle may occur in congenital heart disease as a result of the need for the right or left ventricle to handle increased volumes of blood presented during diastole. Left ventricular diastolic overloading may be associated with such lesions as patent ductus arteriosus or aortic insufficiency. Diastolic overloading of the right ventricle occurs commonly with atrial septal defect or anomalous pulmonary venous drainage. With diastolic overloading, the chest roentgenogram is most helpful in judging the specific chamber of increased volume and also the prominence of the pulmonary vasculature. A consistently accurate guide to the size of a left to right shunt related to diastolic overloading is the presence or absence of a mid-diastolic flow murmur, indicating augmented flow through either the tricuspid or mitral valves. In the presence of such a filling sound, a pulmonary to systemic flow ratio greater than 2 to 1 can be predicted accurately.

Hypoxia. In the absence of congestive heart failure and pulmonary disease, cyanosis in congenital heart disease is related to right to left shunting. The peripheral cyanosis of congestive heart failure usually is recognized by the evidences of a low cardiac output. The favorable response in skin color to inhalation of 100 per cent oxygen in patients with pulmonary disease usually differentiates this cause of cyanosis from that associated with central mixing of arterial and venous blood.

Cyanosis due to right to left shunting is dependent on a communication between the two circuits with a resistance to flow of blood on the right side greater than the resistance to the flow on the left side. The presence of inadequate pulmonary blood flow contributes quantitatively to the severity of cyanosis. Cyanosis is not due to diminished pulmonary blood flow per se. The expansion of the volume of pulmonary blood flow can favorably reduce the level of arterial unsaturation by exposing a larger volume of unsaturated blood to inspired air.

The clinical manifestations of hypoxia are clubbing of the fingers and toes, the development of polycythemia, shortness of breath on exertion, squatting and anoxic attacks. The latter two are found almost invariably in patients with cyanotic lesions associated with inadequate pulmonary blood flow. Anoxic attacks are paroxysms of cerebral hypoxia resulting from a temporary increase in right to left shunting. The attacks usually occur in infancy, beyond the age of 3 months, often in the morning following breakfast. Occasionally they are associated with bowel movements or feeding. The attack is marked by increased cyanosis, increased respiratory rate and effort, and a variety of subtle or obvious changes in the state of consciousness. The latter can vary from a staring spell to rolling back of the eyes, limpness, a convulsive seizure, or death.

Pulmonary Hypertension. In patients with large communications between the pulmonary and systemic circuits, a single mean pressure must be present in the two ventricles. A systemic blood pressure level is thus established in the pulmonary circuit. Patients with this hemodynamic arrangement have a tendency to develop histopathologic changes in the pulmonary arterioles consisting initially of medial muscular hypertrophy and later of intimal proliferation. The picture of medial hypertrophy is reactive and reversible following closure of the communication; the intimal proliferation is fixed and irreversible. Wide variation exists among different subjects and lesions in the duration of pulmonary hypertension necessary for the development of irreversible pulmonary vascular changes. The factors involved in the establishment of these changes in a given patient are poorly understood. Fixed pulmonary hypertension and pulmonary vascular occlusive disease are much more likely to occur in childhood in the presence of a ventricular septal defect or a patent ductus arteriosus than in atrial septal defect. Fixed pulmonary vascular resistance below the age of 2 years is unknown in acyanotic patients. In patients with or without congenital heart disease the persistence of the fetal pattern of pulmonary vascular resistance may contribute to the presence of pulmonary arterial hypertension. Lesions associated with left atrial hypertension due to mitral valve disease may predispose to the development of pulmonary vascular disease by elevating pulmonary venous pressure. Exposure to low partial pressures of oxygen as occur at high altitudes may be another provoking factor. An idiopathic variety of primary pulmonary hypertension is also known to occur in which the findings of cor pulmonale follow isolated pulmonary vascular obstructive changes.

In the clinical observation of patients with pulmonary arterial hypertension, two causative possibilities must be considered: augmented pulmonary blood flow and elevated pulmonary vascular resistance. When high pulmonary blood flow produces elevated pulmonary artery pressure, successful surgical closure of the underlying communication between pulmonary and systemic circuits results in a prompt fall in pulmonary artery pressure. By contrast, in patients with elevated pulmonary artery pressure due to high pulmonary vascular resistance (intimal proliferation) closure of the defect will not result in a fall of pulmonary artery pressure and may indeed be harmful if the defect has been acting as a site of right to left shunting and thereby as a safety valve for the right ventricle.

Bacterial Complications. Two major bacterial complications threaten patients with congenital heart disease: subacute bacterial endocarditis and brain abscess. Both are related to transient venous bacteremia, usually involving organisms of low virulence.

Subacute bacterial endocarditis occurs less frequently in infants and children than in adults. This inverse relationship to age is related to the duration of time necessary for the development of areas of endocardial or endothelial injury. The repeated impingement of a jet of blood against a localized area of endocardium can result in the formation of jet lesions or plaques at the site of endocardial injury. The wall of the pulmonary artery opposite the site of entry of the shunt of a patent ductus arteriosus or the right ventricular wall opposite a ventricular septal defect are common jet lesion locations. The deposition of fibrin on the surface of injured endocardium permits the embedding of passing bacteria and fosters their growth and proliferation, eventually with the formation of macroscopic vegetations. Cardiac anomalies associated with turbulence and high pressure are the ones most likely to be complicated by subacute bacterial endocarditis (e.g., aortic stenosis, coarctation of the aorta, ventricular septal defect, patent ductus arteriosus, mitral valve deformity and occasionally pulmonary stenosis).

When structures on the left side of the heart are the sites of subacute bacterial endocarditis, the signs and symptoms are not unlike those observed in adults with this complication superimposed upon rheumatic valvular deformity. These include high fever, weight loss, anorexia, splenomegaly, and evidence of systemic bacterial embolization such as petechiae. In children with congenital heart disease, the concept of right-sided bacterial endocarditis must also be appreciated. When the jet lesion is situated in the lesser circulation, the symptoms of embolization are related to pulmonary infarction. This may be recognized from changes in the chest roentgenogram and is manifest by chest pain and respiratory distress.

Subacute bacterial endocarditis may remain undiagnosed for several weeks. The initial fever and malaise often lead to no specific diagnosis and the administration of non-specific antibiotic treatment. The infectious process may be temporarily aborted only to recur after the cessation of antibiotic therapy. This sequence may be repeated several times before the underlying cause of the fever is established. The differentiation of a series of coincidental, self-limited infections of viral origin from subacute bacterial endocarditis is a frequent problem in patients with congenital heart disease. Withdrawal of antibiotic therapy for a number of days in order to obtain a series of blood cultures usually resolves the problem.

The organism most commonly involved in subacute bacterial endocarditis in childhood is the alpha hemolytic streptococcus. Most but not all of these organisms are sensitive to penicillin. Acute bacterial endocarditis associated with virulent hemolytic staphylococci may occur in association with septicemia. Finally, bacterial endocarditis with organisms of low virulence may complicate cardiac surgery due to contamination from monitoring devices, intravenous tubing, and other instrumentation.

Treatment depends upon the organism involved and its sensitivity. In instances of alpha hemolytic streptococcal endocarditis, a 4-week course of intravenous penicillin at a level of 10 to 15 million units/day is usually advised. Individualization of treatment based upon *in vitro* sensitivity studies is essential in dealing with the less common organisms.

Brain abscess in the pediatric age group is associated frequently with cyanotic congenital heart disease. The basis for this relationship is the diversion of peripheral venous blood into the systemic circulation, away from its usual pathway through the lungs. This route bypasses the filtering action of the pulmonary capillary bed, permitting the organisms of a casual venous bacteremia to find access to the arterial circulation. The poor local resistance of neural tissue to bacterial infection accounts for the predilection of the brain as the site of seeding of these organisms. The vital nature of the brain tissue and its enclosure in the inflexible calvarium accounts for the serious consequences of this complication.

The early diagnosis and successful treatment of brain abscess require a high index of suspicion of this complication in patients with cyanotic congenital heart disease. Unexplained headache, particularly if severe and unrelieved by symptomatic measures, should raise serious suspicions; fever, vomiting and changes in the state of consciousness are also common symptoms, and occasionally seizures and focal neurological signs may be observed. Evidence of increased intracranial pressure results from the expansion of this space-occupying lesion. Once suspected, brain abscess can be sought by brain scanning techniques, including the use of the computed tomography. Antibiotic therapy occasionally can be successful in the treatment of a small subarachnoid abscess which drains spontaneously into the subarachnoid space. However, most confined abscesses require surgical drainage or removal in toto for cure.

Syncope and Sudden Death. A number of congenital cardiac anomalies is known to be associated with syncope and sudden death. The mechanism is the presence of a low cardiac output resulting from such causes as a slow cardiac rate, a serious cardiac arrhythmia, severe obstruction to left ventricular outflow or inadequate pulmonary venous return to the left heart.

The lesion most frequently mentioned in association with syncope and sudden death is severe congenital aortic stenosis. Syncope in such patients should be taken as an indication of severe left ventricular outflow tract obstruction and should be an indication for prompt hemodynamic study and surgical treatment. In such patients, the electrocardiographic pattern of left ventricular hypertrophy and left ventricular strain is usually, but not invariably, present. In borderline instances, the T wave and ST segment abnormalities in the electrocardiogram may be provoked by exercise testing, indicating the need for measurement of the aortic valve gradient somewhat earlier.

Systolic gradients in pressure at the level of the aortic valve in excess of 70 to 80 mm. Hg are sufficient to warrant surgical relief of aortic stenosis. In childhood, this is usually carried out as a palliative procedure, by aortic valvulotomy, in preference to aortic valve replacement. The opportunity for effective relief of aortic stenosis is largely dependent upon the anatomic features of the deformed aortic valve. In the case of a unicommissural aortic valve, it is particularly difficult to obtain benefit from the method of commissurotomy. Sudden death may occur postoperatively in those patients who have had inadequate relief of aortic stenosis because of unfavorable anatomic features.

Dramatic episodes of syncope and sudden death may occur with extreme degrees of slowing of the cardiac rate. Congenital and acquired heart block may produce Stokes-Adams syncopal attacks. The cardiac rate is usually below 30/minute in patients suffering such episodes. The electrocardiogram usually shows complete atrioventricular dissociation with no relationship between the atrial and ventricular contractions. Treatment consists of the introduction of an electronic pacemaker.

The presence of severe pulmonary vascular disease may occasionally be associated with syncope and sudden death. The pulmonary venous return may be so limited by the pulmonary arteriolar occlusion that the left ventricular output is inadequate to perfuse the brain and myocardium. Syncope and sudden death may be manifestations of a variety of coordinated and uncoordinated tachyarrhythmias associated or unassociated with congenital heart disease. The ventricular tachycardias are more likely to produce serious symptoms and results than are the tachycardias of supraventricular origin.

Treatment of Congenital Heart Disease

Definitive treatment of congenital heart disease is primarily surgical. Since 1940 an increasing number of cardiac anomalies have become amenable to successful surgical treatment; at present, almost 85 per cent of all congenital cardiac lesions can be corrected or improved by surgical techniques.

All patients with patent ductus arteriosus or significant coarctation of the aorta should have surgical correction. Isolated atrial septal defect and ventricular septal defect should be corrected with the use of cardio-pulmonary bypass, if the left to right shunt is significant, that is producing a pulmonary to systemic flow ratio greater than two to one. Isolated valvular pulmonic stenosis requires surgical relief if the absolute right ventricular pressure is 80–90 mm. Hg in systole. The indication for surgical relief of aortic stenosis is a gradient in excess of 80 mm. Hg at the specific site of narrowing.

Patients with cyanotic congenital heart disease and inadequate pulmonary blood flow may require palliation by creation of a systemic artery to pulmonary artery shunt. The Blalock-Taussig anastomosis is preferred, but in very small infants it may be necessary to carry out an ascending aorta to right pulmonary artery (Waterston) anastomosis because of the small size of the blood vessels involved. Patients who reach the age of 5 to 10 years with tetralogy of Fallot, with or without earlier palliation, should have a total correction of the intracardiac defects. Only by eliminating the right to left shunting will the complication of brain abscess be avoided. The transatrial approach to the correction of the pulmonary stenosis and closure of the ventricular septal defect has reduced postoperative morbidity.

Complete transposition of the great arteries is treated initially by creation of an interatrial communication either by balloon-atrioseptostomy or by surgical means. After the age of 6 to 12 months, definitive treatment can be achieved by the technique of Mustard which transposes the systemic and pulmonary venous return by reorientation of the atrial septum. Combinations of lesions require individual methods of management and timing of application.

The medical management of patients with congenital heart disease consists largely in diagnostic evaluation of the anatomy and severity of the defect, the timing of surgical management, providing advice concerning physical activity, the handling of intercurrent infections and allied medical and surgical problems. Infants with large left to right shunts and pulmonary hypertension are particularly prone to atelectasis and pneumonitis, and often require repeated hospitalizations for treatment of these complications. Many patients with congenital heart disease require treatment of congestive heart failure by symptomatic measures. Most infants with congestive heart failure due to isolated coarctation of the aorta can be controlled by medical means alone. Similarly, most patients with ventricular septal defect can be successfully managed through infancy with the hope that favorable changes may occur spontaneously, either in the form of a reduction in the relative size of the defect or development of right ventricular outflow tract obstruction (self-banding). Spontaneous closure of a persistently patent ductus arteriosus may be awaited for approximately six months, but thereafter surgical closure is indicated.

Surgical banding of the pulmonary artery is carried out in the palliative management of patients with severe pulmonary artery hypertension. It is applicable only in patients with a large interventricular communication or a single ventricle who have a reactive pulmonary vascular bed. Reduction of the pulmonary artery pressure beyond the site of application of the band prevents the development of irreversible pulmonary vascular occlusive changes at the pulmonary arteriolar level. The introduction of an obstruction to right ventricular outflow is beneficial in the treatment of congestive heart failure by reducing the volume of left to right shunting through the interventricular communication and thereby diminishing the volume load of the left ventricle. The trend toward definitive correction of intracardiac defects in infancy will reduce the need for the use of the pulmonary artery banding procedure.

The use of prosthetic valves should be avoided assiduously in childhood. Nevertheless, occasionally no other solution exists for the management of a valvular abnormality. Currently, operations designed to restore continuity between the right ventricle and pulmonary arteries in patients with truncus arteriosus or pulmonary atresia are being developed, according to the method suggested by Rastelli. The anatomic features that make for success and failure are still being studied and eventually will become well established. The duration of effectiveness of the "conduit" procedures has yet to be determined. In considering the elective application of surgical treatment, an optimistic expectation that improved methods will be available in 5 or 10 years is not unrealistic when dealing with any problems for which no established procedure is now available. This has certainly been the case over the past 3 decades.

The medical management of anoxic attacks may present as an emergency situation. Use of the knee-chest position and the administration of oxygen aborts or terminates most mild attacks. In more severe instances, the use of parenteral morphine sulfate or propranolol, in that order, is effective. Oxygen and morphine should be given as promptly as possible and thereafter the patient should be left alone to rest without further handling for 30 minutes to permit these measures to become effective.

Dramatic improvements in hypoxia can be obtained sometimes in patients by the oral administration of iron, especially if a relative anemia exists as in patients with polycythemia. The elimination of this type of anemia will also reduce the risk of intravascular clotting that results in cerebral vascular thrombosis.

Systematic cardiac supervision in patients with mild congenital heart lesions at 6- or 12-month intervals permits (1) regulation of medications such as digitalis, (2) reinforcement of the need for prophylactic measures against subacute bacterial endocarditis and brain abscess, (3) evaluation of the degree of hypoxia by clinical and laboratory means (hemoglobin and hematocrit), and (4) the opportunity to provide advice about general health measures and activity restrictions. Finally, an annual or semi-annual discussion of the patient's cardiac problem, particularly with regard to the long range plans, the availability or lack of availability of surgical treatment, some of its details, risks, and results, make the actual encounter with these problems more readily bearable by parents when the hour of surgical action finally arrives.

RHEUMATIC FEVER

Rheumatic fever is a generalized inflammatory disease of unknown etiology that involves many organs of the body, but primarily the connective tissue system. The organs most commonly involved in the inflammatory process are the heart, joints, skin and the brain. Rheumatic fever is primarily a pediatric disease; its etiology is related to streptococcal infection which occurs more commonly in childhood than in adult life.

Despite a decline in incidence and severity over the past 50 years, rheumatic heart disease remains the second most common etiologic variety of heart disease in childhood. Among children of school age in Philadelphia, one half of the six cases per 1000 with heart disease are rheumatic. During the first 3 decades of this century, rheumatic heart disease was the leading medical cause of death among school-age children. The reduction in incidence and severity of rheumatic fever over the past several decades has occurred only in the developed countries of the world; the disease continues to be rampant in the underdeveloped areas.

A vast literature based upon epidemiologic, bacteriologic and serologic data has developed in the past 3 decades relating the beta-hemolytic streptococcus of Lancefield Group A to rheumatic fever. There is considerable evidence that the streptococcus is almost uniformly related in an undetermined way to the pathogenesis of rheumatic fever. The streptococcus is not directly invasive in its action in the disease. In current concepts, the streptococcus is related to rheumatic fever by an immunologic mechanism, either by a reaction of hypersensitivity or by the formation and reaction of autoimmune antibodies.

Clinical Characteristics

A very high percentage of rheumatic attacks are preceded by overt or subclinical streptococcal infection. The time interval between the preceding streptococcal infection and the onset of symptoms of rheumatic fever varies between 1 and 3 weeks in the majority of cases. Most patients with rheumatic fever fall into one of three categories with regard to the persistence of their rheumatic activity: (1) in a small number of patients, an acute or fulminating course terminates in death within a few days or weeks; (2) in a slightly larger group, a chronic course of low grade activity takes place, rheumatic activity persists over a period of months or years and never subsides completely, and eventually death occurs from profound cardiac involvement; (3) the majority of rheumatic subjects experience a recurrent form of rheumatic fever in which individual, identifiable, self-limited episodes of active rheumatic inflammation are followed by periods of complete quiescence or inactivity of the disease. In the absence of prophylactic measures, a high percentage of such patients experiences one or more recurrences of rheumatic activity with the hazard of cardiac involvement with each episode. Within a given period of rheumatic activity, readily recognizable variations in intensity occur commonly and may produce a polycyclic course. The age range in which initial attacks of rheumatic fever occur most often is 6 to 8 years. One per cent of all cases occur below the age of 4 years. Both initial attacks and recurrences occur less frequently beyond the age of puberty. Considerable variation occurs in the duration of rheumatic episodes; a range of from 2 weeks to 12 months is recognized. The majority of cases have an attack duration of 1 to 4 months. A trend exists among rheumatic subjects for the occurrence of the same individual manifestations of the disease in each recurrent episode. Thus, subjects with abdominal pain in an initial attack frequently manifest abdominal pain with a recurrent attack. Although this is a useful clinical characteristic of rheumatic fever from the diagnostic standpoint, exceptions to this trend occur. Of patients experiencing no evidence of carditis in the initial attack, approximately 14 per cent manifest definite cardiac involvement in a subsequent attack.

Diagnosis

An accurate decision concerning the presence or absence of rheumatic fever is of great importance to the individual patient. Since no specific diagnostic test is available, the diagnosis rests in each instance on clinical judgment. Errors in the direction of over-diagnosis or under-diagnosis are equally unfortunate. Failure to recognize rheumatic carditis promptly may result in delayed onset of treatment and increased residual cardiac damage. A false diagnosis of rheumatic fever may result in prolonged, unnecessary confinement.

During the mobilization of young adults for service in World War II, the problems related to the diagnosis of rheumatic fever were magnified suddenly. An arbitrary set of diagnostic criteria was proposed at this time by Dr. T. Duckett Jones for the purpose of minimizing errors. These criteria subsequently have been modified and are widely accepted. They separate the manifestations into two categories, major and minor manifestations of rheumatic fever. The major criteria consist of those manifestations that occur almost exclusively in rheumatic fever, although none is pathognomonic. The minor criteria are less specific and occur in a wide variety of inflammatory diseases. In order to fulfill the criteria of Jones for the diagnosis of rheumatic fever, at least one major and two minor manifestations, or two major and one minor manifestation must be present. In evaluation of an individual patient, the arbitrary nature of the system of Jones must be appreciated. It is designed to provide accuracy in diagnosis among large numbers of suspected subjects. An individual patient may have rheumatic fever with a clinical picture which does not fulfill these criteria.

The major criteria of Jones include migrating polyarthritis, chorea, subcutaneous nodules, erythema marginatum, and carditis. The presence of objective evidence of joint inflammation involving multiple joints in a migratory fashion is highly suggestive of rheumatic fever. The syndrome of chorea described by Sydenham in 1686 (St. Vitus dance) represents the central nervous system involvement in rheumatic fever and has four basic features: (1) muscular weakness, (2) muscular incoordination, (3) involuntary, purposeless movements which disappear during sleep, and (4) emotional lability. The average duration of an episode of chorea is 10 weeks, although extreme variability exists. Intensification of symptoms occurs for approximately 3 weeks, followed by gradual improvement. Unilateral or hemichorea occurs in about 10 per cent of the cases; in the remainder, involvement is grossly symmetrical. Chorea is more common in females than in males and rarely occurs beyond the age of puberty, except during pregnancy. Subcutaneous nodules are firm, round, non-tender nodules which vary from 0.5 to 2 cm. in diameter and are attached beneath the skin to tendon sheaths and fascia; the skin moves freely over them. Subcutaneous nodules occur in crops and are found over the extensor surfaces of the elbows, knees and wrists, in the occipital region, and over the spinous processes of the thoracic and lumbar vertebrae. They appear most commonly at least 3 to 5 weeks after the onset of clinical manifestations, often in association with carditis. Erythema marginatum is an erythematous nonpruritic skin rash. It is the least specific of the major manifestations of rheumatic fever. The rash has a pink color which fades away from its sharp scalloped edges and is found mainly over the trunk, occasionally on the extremities and rarely on the feet. The rash is recurrent and may migrate from one portion of the body to another. It is difficult to differentiate with certainty erythema marginatum from skin rashes due to hypersensitivity to drugs.

The cardiac involvement in rheumatic fever is the most important consequence of the disease because permanent damage to cardiac tissues may occur. All three tissue layers of the heart (the endocardium, myocardium and pericardium) may be involved in the inflammatory process producing the picture of pancarditis. Irreversible changes in the structure and function of the cardiac valves may result from endocardial involvement. Post-inflammatory scarring of the myocardium may lead to serious impairment of myocardial function especially in the presence of superimposed degenerative (aging) changes.

The pathophysiology of rheumatic heart disease in childhood is quite different from that in adults. In the pediatric age group, it is the active inflammatory processes involving the myocardium which produce the cardiac dysfunction (heart failure). In adult patients with rheumatic heart disease, cardiac failure is the result of the mechanical handicapping of valvular deformity and of impaired ventricular function due to earlier scarring of the myocardium. Rheumatic heart disease in the pediatric age group is a dynamic, active inflammatory process; in comparison, the process is mechanical and static in adult subjects.

The following clinical evidences of carditis are considered to be major manifestations, according to the criteria of Jones: (1) significant new or changing cardiac murmurs, (2) cardiac enlargement, (3) pericarditis and (4) congestive heart failure. Evidence of cardiac involvement such as electrocardiographic abnormalities, arrhythmias, inappropriate tachycardia, and changes in the quality of heart sounds are non-specific indications of myocardial disease and are not accepted as major criteria.

Murmurs. In childhood, endocarditis involves the mitral and aortic valves almost exclusively and the mitral valve in approximately 90 per cent of patients with overt carditis. In approximately half of the patients with mitral lesions, the aortic valve is also involved. Isolated involvement of the aortic valve occurs in only 10 per cent of cases.

The murmur of mitral insufficiency is the most commonly heard murmur of rheumatic heart disease in childhood. It is loudest at the site of the apex beat and is transmitted in the direction of the left axilla as well as to the back on the left side where it is usually best heard beneath the left scapula. Transmission to the vessels of the neck is poor. This murmur is holosystolic in duration and high pitched and blowing in quality. Its intensity is variable; occasionally it may be of only grade I or II intensity. It is heard better in the recumbent than in the erect position, sometimes only with the patient in the left lateral recumbent position. Occasionally, in a localized area at the apex, this murmur may acquire a very high pitched squeaking or screeching quality. This peculiar high pitched character is referred to as a "sea-gull screech" and is almost always present in a patient with active carditis. A good correlation exists between the severity of isolated mitral insufficiency and the distance of transmission of the murmur into the left axilla.

In the presence of mitral insufficiency, a mid-diastolic murmur may be heard at the cardiac apex with active rheumatic carditis. It is usually preceded by the appearance of a protodiastolic gallop sound. Differentiation of this sound from the physiologic third heart sound of childhood

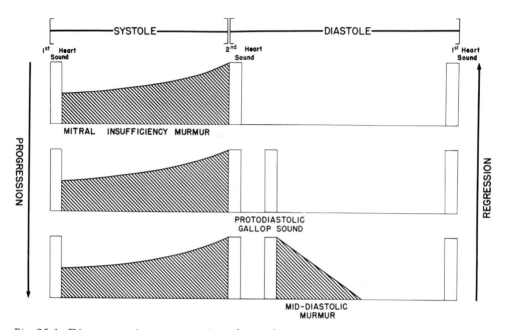

SYSTOLE   DIASTOLE

1st Heart Sound   2nd Heart Sound   1st Heart Sound

MITRAL INSUFFICIENCY MURMUR

PROGRESSION   REGRESSION

PROTODIASTOLIC GALLOP SOUND

MID-DIASTOLIC MURMUR

Fig. 25-1. Diagrammatic representation of auscultatory events resulting from mitral valve involvement during acute rheumatic carditis in childhood. Diagrams indicate initial appearance of holosystolic murmur of mitral insufficiency, followed by the appearance of a protodiastolic gallop sound, and of a mid-diastolic murmur. Arrows indicate the direction taken by the auscultatory events during progression and regression of cardiac involvement. (From Conn, H. L. and Horwitz, O.: Cardiac and Cardiovascular Diseases. Philadelphia, Lea and Febiger, 1971; p. 773.)

may be impossible. With progressive cardiac involvement, the proto-diastolic gallop sound becomes longer and takes on the duration and character of a cardiac murmur (Fig. 25-1). This mid-diastolic murmur is of medium or low pitch, vibratory in character, and usually does not extend to the first heart sound. It is heard best with the patient in the recumbent position. The murmur is attributed to "relative" mitral stenosis. It is not heard in the absence of mitral insufficiency and requires for its production the accelerated flow of an increased volume of blood through the mitral valve during the period of rapid filling of the left ventricle from the left atrium. The mid-diastolic murmur of active rheumatic carditis is often heard intermittently. The characteristic presystolic rumbling murmur of organic mitral stenosis is a rare finding in rheumatic heart disease of childhood. It is frequently heard together with the murmur of mitral insufficiency, but may occasionally occur alone.

Rheumatic involvement of the aortic valve results in the murmur of aortic regurgitation; the murmur of aortic stenosis due to rheumatic heart disease is almost never heard below the age of puberty. The murmur of aortic regurgitation is early diastolic in time, following immediately after the second heart sound. It has a high pitched decrescendo blowing character and is best heard in the third left interspace at the anatomic position of the aortic valve. It is transmitted toward the cardiac apex and is rarely heard over the posterior chestwall. This murmur may also be of very low intensity and is easily overlooked. Once associated with the peripheral evidences of aortic insufficiency, it rarely disappears.

Despite the fact that the auscultatory findings in rheumatic carditis do not accurately reflect the extent of myocardial involvement, the cardiac murmurs provide a valuable method of following the clinical course of the disease process. Changes in the intensity, quality and degree of transmission of murmurs reflect progression and regression of the rheumatic process. At the mitral valve the sequence of sounds and murmurs is orderly and repetitive during both progression and regression of the disease.

Cardiac Enlargement. Evidence of increasing heart size is another firm indication of active rheumatic carditis, usually indicating severe myocardial involvement. Chamber enlargement depends in part on specific valvular deformities; but, in the presence of diffuse myocardial involvement, a generalized form of enlargement results. Cardiac enlargement associated with rheumatic carditis is almost invariably associated with the characteristic murmurs of this disease; cardiac enlargement in the absence of characteristic murmurs is not rheumatic in origin. The prognosis in rheumatic fever is related more to cardiac size than to the presence of the various cardiac murmurs.

Pericarditis. Auscultatory evidence of inflammation of the visceral pericardium is another indication of the presence of rheumatic carditis. A friction rub may appear in any location over the precordium but is usually found in the left parasternal region. Frequently this adventitious sound is transient or heard intermittently. Electrocardiographic confirmation of pericardial involvement is usually available, especially in the acute stages. As in the case of cardiomegaly, a pericardial friction rub of rheumatic origin is almost always associated with the characteristic murmurs of rheumatic heart disease. Pericardial effusion may occur in association with acute rheumatic pericarditis, but the volume of such an effusion is usually small and cardiac tamponade rarely results. The problem that arises occasionally is the need to differentiate pericarditis with effusion from the large dilated flabby heart associated with congestive heart failure. The echocardiogram may be useful in separating these two entities.

Congestive Heart Failure. Congestive heart failure resulting from rheumatic heart disease in childhood is an indication of extensive myocardial involvement. Mechanical handicapping of the heart as a result of valvular deformity is rarely of sufficient severity in childhood to account for cardiac failure. Nevertheless, as in the case of cardiac enlargement and pericarditis, this manifestation of rheumatic carditis also does not occur in the absence of one or more of the characteristic cardiac murmurs of rheumatic carditis. The manifestations of congestive heart failure in rheumatic heart disease of childhood are not grossly different from those observed in adults, but the onset may be more abrupt and the progression more rapid. Evidence of left ventricular failure is frequently observed initially, but signs of right heart failure follow shortly thereafter. Tachycardia, tachypnea, dyspnea and orthopnea are often the first changes noted; hepatomegaly may occur early and is a valuable index of the severity of right heart failure in childhood. It is common for peripheral edema to appear later; pulmonary edema with basilar rales appears as a very late manifestation of congestive heart failure in childhood.

The minor manifestations of Jones are non-specific and occur in many inflammatory diseases. They provide only supporting evidence for the diagnosis and must be accompanied by at least one of the major manifestations in order to fulfill the criteria of Jones for the diagnosis of rheumatic fever. Minor criteria include fever, arthralgia, prolonged P-R interval in the electrocardiogram, increased erythrocyte sedimentation rate or other acute phase reactants, evidence of recent beta-hemolytic streptococcal infection, previous history of rheumatic fever or the presence of inactive rheumatic heart disease. Epistaxis, pallor, anemia, abdominal pain, pneumonitis, weight loss, easy fatiguability, headache and vomiting may also be considered minor manifestations of rheumatic fever.

Laboratory Aids in Rheumatic Fever

Because of the absence of any known pathogenetic agent of rheumatic fever, no specific tests for the detection or measurement of activity are available. As a result, a number of non-specific tests have been employed for these purposes. These tests fall into two categories which differ in their purpose and in their relationship to rheumatic fever: (1) the acute phase tests and (2) the antistreptococcal antibody determinations.

The acute phase tests are entirely non-specific in character and reflect quantitatively the destruction of tissue due to such diverse causes as inflammation, infarction or malignancy. The most widely used, oldest and simplest to perform of these tests is the erythrocyte sedimentation rate. Another acute phase test recently popularized is the determination of C-reactive protein, a substance that is not normally a component of serum but is found in many states involving tissue destruction. These determinations are useful primarily in following the activity of the rheumatic process after the diagnosis has been determined from other information. Certain special situations have been recognized in which the erythrocyte sedimentation rate gives results that cannot be reconciled with clinical evidence of rheumatic inflammation. In the presence of cardiac failure associated with rheumatic carditis, the erythrocyte sedimentation rate may be paradoxically decreased, often to a level that is within normal limits. In sicklemia, the erythrocyte sedimentation rate is known to be unreliable since the departure of erythrocytes from the normal shape of a biconcave disc results in failure of these cells to form rouleaux as large as would be formed by normally shaped erythrocytes under the same circumstances.

The second major type of laboratory determination which is useful in the evaluation of patients suspected of having rheumatic fever is the antistreptococcal antibody titer. Antibodies developed to a variety of antigenic components and products of the streptococcus may be measured and reflect recent immunologic experience with this organism. The antigen used for the longest time in this application is the streptococcal hemolysin; the determination is referred to by the contracted term antistreptolysin-0 titer. Titers of 200 or less are commonly found in a healthy population. Values in excess of 200 may be interpreted as an indication of recent streptococcal infection. Elevated titers are encountered in patients convalescing from acute streptococcal infections as well as in patients with acute rheumatic fever. Among rheumatic suspects the finding of very low titers or very high titers is a more significant indication of the absence or presence of the disease than titers in the middle range.

Various other antigens have been employed to measure antistreptococcal antibodies in patients with rheumatic fever. High levels of antibodies that have developed in response to hyaluronidase, an enzyme product of the streptococcus, have been found to correlate well with the presence of acute rheumatic fever. Other streptococcal antigens used for this purpose are streptokinase and desoxyribonuclease. The titer of antibodies in each of these may increase independently of the other, depending in part on relative amounts of antigen released by the infecting strain of streptococcus. Hence, conclusions derived from three antibody titer determinations are more reliable than from two, and two estimates are more reliable than one titer in identifying patients with recent streptococcal infection. A poor correlation exists between the clinical course of rheumatic fever and the antibody titer determinations. Once elevated, titers tend to remain at high levels for 3 to 6 months regardless of the duration of rheumatic activity. Antibody titers are usually increased significantly at the time of onset of symptoms of rheumatic fever.

Treatment of Rheumatic Fever

Therapy in rheumatic fever is non-specific, supportive and symptomatic. Since only the cardiac involvement leads to permanent residua, all major therapeutic efforts should be directed toward minimizing the damage resulting from carditis. For this reason, a period of complete bed rest is essential in patients with and without obvious cardiac involvement. Effective bedrest is difficult for children and requires determined and coordinated efforts from many paramedical sources. The arthritis

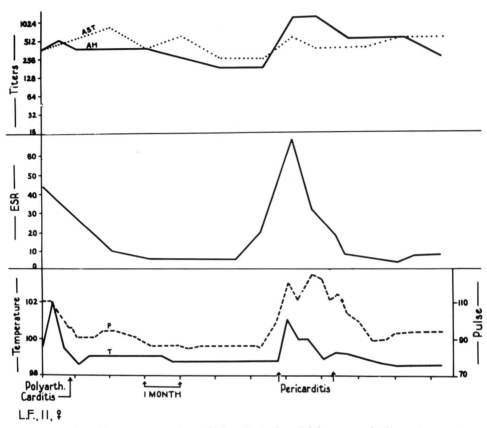

Fig. 25-2. Graphic representation of the clinical and laboratory findings in a patient with a polycyclic course of acute rheumatic fever. Lower panel depicts clinical findings. Middle panel demonstrates concurrent changes in erythrocyte sedimentation rate. Upper panel indicates antistreptococcal antibody titers which remain stable throughout fluctuating clinical course. (From Harris, T. N., Harris, S., and Nagle, R. L.: Studies in the relation of the hemolytic streptococcus to rheumatic fever. Pediatrics, 3:482, 1949. Copyright American Academy of Pediatrics, 1949).

and fever of rheumatic fever respond dramatically to salicylate therapy in large doses. The response of arthritis and fever to salicylates is so dramatic that it represents a valuable diagnostic aid. Severe nosebleeds requiring more than local pressure may occur during acute rheumatic fever. Cauterization of a bleeding point or the use of local hemostatic agents is often necessary. The use of a posterior nasal pack or replacement of blood lost during epistaxis is occasionally necessary. The treatment of chorea consists of minimizing physical and emotional stimulation to the child. Sedatives and tranquilizing drugs may be of some help in the management of choreic patients but do not alter the natural course significantly. Except for the component that results from iron loss due to severe epistaxis, the anemia of acute rheumatic fever does not respond to iron therapy.

Aside from restrictions of physical activity other symptomatic measures in patients with severe carditis and congestive heart failure include oxygen administration, diuretics and digitalis. Salt and water restriction may also be useful in the management of heart failure due to rheumatic carditis. Patients who show progressive cardiac involvement while under observation and maximal medical support should be considered for treatment with adrenal steroids. The efficacy of such treatment is unproven in controlled studies, but temporary suppression of the inflammatory process within the myocardium usually results in a suppression of the symptoms. Anecdotal reports of dramatic, life-saving reversal of congestive heart failure by adrenal steroid therapy have appeared on numerous occasions.

The majority of rheumatic attacks end spontaneously in 1–4 months. The identification of the time of cessation of the rheumatic activity is sometimes difficult and is a decision based on arbitrary clinical judgment. In general, the rheumatic episode may be considered terminated when all of the clinical and laboratory evidence of the disease has disappeared, or has reached a stable or plateau level. Further useful indications of inactivity of the rheumatic process are: (1) spontaneous rise of hemoglobin, (2) spontaneous weight gain, (3) disappearance of rheumatic pallor, (4) favorable changes in the patient's personality response, (5) disappearance of wide diurnal variations in body temperature, (6) non-occurrence of tachycardia following minor trials of physical exertion, (7) disappearance of minor variations in regularity of cardiac rhythm and (8) slow sleeping pulse rate. As a general guide, patients with no overt evidence of carditis are kept at bedrest for a minimum of 6 weeks, those with overt carditis for a minimum of 3 months.

Prevention of Rheumatic Fever

There are two aspects to the prevention of rheumatic fever: (1) secondary prevention, the prevention of recurrences of rheumatic fever in known rheumatic subjects by the daily oral administration of antistreptococcal agents; and (2) primary prevention, the prevention of either initial or recurrent attacks of rheumatic fever by the prompt and vigorous treatment of streptococcal infection. The basis for prevention is the interruption of the relationship between infection with beta-hemolytic streptococcus and the etiologic mechanism of rheumatic fever.

All individuals with a history of rheumatic fever or chorea, especially those who show evidence of rheumatic heart disease, should be placed on long-term antistreptococcal prophylaxis. The prophylaxis should be continued throughout the life of the patient or until new information demonstrates that such prolonged administration is unnecessary. Prophylaxis should be continuous throughout all seasons of the year rather than intermittent. For the prevention of streptococcal infection in known rheumatic subjects, the current recommended dosage of sulfonamides is 0.5 g. daily for individuals under 60 lbs. in body weight, and 1 g. daily for individuals over 60 lbs. For penicillin the recommended oral dosage is 400,000 units of penicillin G given daily on a fasting stomach. The newer forms of oral penicillin such as penicillin V or penicillin V potassium are equally effective, but are considerably more expensive. A single intramuscular injection of a slow-releasing preparation of penicillin such as Benzathine penicillin given at 4-week intervals has been demonstrated to be equally effective for antistreptococcal prophylaxis.

Penicillin is the drug of choice for primary prevention of rheumatic fever and should be continued for a period of 10 days. Effectiveness is based upon the bactericidal quality of penicillin against beta-hemolytic streptococci and is dependent upon the total eradication of streptococci from the throat. Penicillin may be administered either intramuscularly or orally. A single intramuscular injection of long-acting repository Benzathine penicillin is effective; a dose of 900,000 to 1,200,000 units is recommended. Using the oral route, a dose of 400,000 units (250 mg.) of penicillin V four times a day for a full 10 days is recommended. Therapy must not be discontinued despite the prompt favorable disappearance of the fever and other signs of infection.

Occasionally the failure of such treatment to prevent rheumatic sequelae has been reported. In most instances, failure of the antistreptococcal treatment to completely eradicate the organism has been responsible. The following principles must be applied if this method of prevention is to be successful: (1) the streptococcus itself must be eradicated—clinical cure alone is inadequate; (2) to achieve such eradication the bactericidal property of penicillin should be used—sulfonamides are ineffective for this purpose, and tetracycline compounds are effective, but not to the same extent as penicillin; (3) penicillin must be provided in adequate amounts for at least 10 days to insure complete eradication of the organisms. Treatment should be started as soon as possible, but a delay of up to 7 to 9 days may still prevent the onset of rheumatic fever.

CARDIAC ARRHYTHMIAS

The frequency of cardiac arrhythmias in the pediatric age group is far lower than among adult cardiac patients, in whom degenerative heart disease is the predominant pathologic process. The cardiac arrhythmias of rheumatic heart disease are benign and relatively uncommon. Temporary first degree heart block, occasional premature supraventricular or ventricular contractions, and rare instances of complete heart block occur during acute rheumatic carditis. In rare instances in childhood, auricular fibrillation and auricular flutter may occur in the chronic active form of rheumatic heart involvement. Myocardial disease (e.g. diphtheritic myocarditis) of any form may be an etiologic focus of arrhythmias. The cardiac arrhythmias observed with congenital heart disease are also rare and usually indicate a deteriorating state of myocardial function due to hypoxia or other deleterious causes. Arrhythmias are not uncommonly encountered in postoperative patients following surgery for congenital heart disease and they may pose a serious threat at this precarious time. A congenital anomaly of conduction manifest by a short PR interval and a prolonged QRS duration was described by Wolff, Parkinson and White in 1930 and is known to predispose to tachyarrhythmias. Occasional instances of isolated sinus node or atrioventricular node dysfunction occur.

Benign Arrhythmias

The most common arrhythmia of childhood encountered is sinus arrhythmia. This represents a phasic variation in the cardiac rate usually associated with respiration. It is per se a benign arrhythmia and indeed a normal variation. Occasionally it may occur as an early manifestation of digitalis toxicity. Sinus arrest is another benign cardiac arrhythmia of childhood. Another common arrhythmia is the sporadic appearance of premature contractions originating from atrial, nodal, or ventricular foci of origin. These occur rarely in the course of myocarditis or myocardial dysfunction and are occasionally a result of digitalis intoxication. More commonly, premature contractions from any focus occur without any other evidence of heart disease. Under these circumstances, the condition is benign and it is safe to attempt no specific treatment and urge no restriction of physical activity. Premature contractions create no important hemodynamic handicap in the absence of other evidence of heart disease and can safely by ignored. Occasionally premature contractions are first discovered following an illness, anesthesia, or chest trauma, but even this antecedent history does not necessarily establish the etiology. In most instances no etiology is evident. In approximately half of the cases, isolated premature contractions will disappear spontaneously without treatment.

Paroxysmal Supraventricular Tachycardia

Two serious cardiac arrhythmias are encountered in the pediatric age group, paroxysmal supraventricular tachycardia and congenital heart block. Paroxysmal supraventricular tachycardia is of special importance in young infants because it can precipitate a true medical emergency requiring prompt and precise treatment for survival. During such a tachyarrhythmia, cardiac rates between 200 and 400 beats/minute are common; congestive heart failure may develop within a few hours because of poor coronary artery perfusion and poor ventricular filling associated with extreme shortening of the diastolic interval of the cardiac cycle. Many patients are not brought to medical attention until after the onset of congestive heart failure, especially the young infant who cannot transmit any feeling of discomfort. Patients first encountered at this phase of the disease may die within minutes or hours unless the tachyarrhythmia can be converted.

Many patients with paroxysmal supraventricular tachycardia are male newborn infants in whom no other evidence of heart disease can be found. The diagnosis is made by the detection of a very rapid cardiac rate and the presence of signs and symptoms of congestive heart failure, if the tachycardia has persisted for more than 12 to 24 hours. Confirmation of the diagnosis requires an electrocardiogram; the tracing shows a very regular and rapid rate varying between 200 and 400 beats/minute. The QRS complexes are of normal duration and the P waves are usually not visible. The recording is also useful in ruling out the possibility of ventricular tachycardia which requires drug treatment quite different from supraventricular tachycardia.

The idiopathic variety of supraventricular tachycardia occurs predominantly in males, with its onset in the newborn period. The prognosis for these infants is excellent in the absence of any other evidence of heart disease. Recurrences are observed during the first year or two of life and rarely thereafter. Only in a minority of patients with paroxysmal supraventricular tachycardia is a detectable etiology manifest. The usual causative factors are intercurrent infection, organic heart disease, and the abnormal conduction mechanism described by Wolff, Parkinson and White.

The great majority of patients with supraventricular tachycardia will respond promptly to digitalization. A few require other medications such as propanolol or quinidine. In situations of severe congestive heart failure and impending demise, direct current cardioversion may save the patient's life. Following restoration of normal sinus rhythm, transient electrocardiographic changes may be present for several days, consisting primarily of T wave inversion. In small infants it is wise to maintain digoxin medication for 6 to 12 months following an episode of paroxysmal tachycardia in order to defer the possibility of a recurrence until the child is older and more tolerant of the insult of an extremely rapid heart rate. Eventually the digoxin medication must be discontinued on a trial-and-error basis and recurrences beyond the age of 1 year are rare.

Congenital Heart Block

Congenital heart block is a rare but important cardiac arrhythmia of infancy and childhood. Its earliest detection may occur *in utero*; it may be mistaken as a sign of fetal distress and therefore as an indication for caesarean section. Approximately half of the infants with congenital heart block have additional congenital intracardiac anomalies; in the other half the arrhythmia is the only abnormality.

Symptoms usually are not produced by complete heart block unless the cardiac rate becomes excessively slow; this rarely occurs in infancy and early childhood. Extreme slowing of the cardiac rate may occur in the second decade of life. Cardiac rates below 40 beats/minute may lead to dizziness and syncope. Major episodes of syncope with loss of consciousness or death (Stokes-Adams attacks) may be observed with congenital heart block. With technical improvements in the construction and longevity of pacemakers, the occurence of even a single Stokes-Adams attack should be considered an indication for artificial pacing.

The diagnosis of complete heart block can be made from the electrocardiogram. The tracing will show a lack of relationship between the atrial activity (P waves) and the QRS complexes representing ventricular activity. In the absence of intracardiac anomalies, the prognosis varies with the duration of the QRS complexes. The prognosis is best with a short QRS duration and least favorable in those patients with prolonged QRS duration. The QRS complexes of short duration indicate a pacemaker close to the AV node while those of prolonged duration having a bizarre contour result from a ventricular pacemaker well below the AV node. In the latter group, extremely slow cardiac rates and syncope are encountered more frequently.

HIGH CARDIAC OUTPUT STATES

A number of pathologic conditions may produce severe states of high cardiac output in the pediatric age group. Profound disturbances in cardiac function may result from the high stroke volume, increased circulating blood volume and accelerated velocity of blood flow in these clinical conditions. Congestive heart failure, reponsive only to the elimination of the cause of the high cardiac output state, may ensue.

The most common clinical state producing a high cardiac output is chronic anemia. To produce congestive heart failure, anemia must be of long-standing duration with a level of hemoglobin below 5 g./dl. In patients with intrinsic heart disease in addition to severe anemia, congestive heart failure may appear at higher hemoglobin levels.

Another common variety of high cardiac output state in childhood is that produced by the presence of a systemic arteriovenous fistula. An abnormal connection between a systemic artery and a systemic vein may occur in the cerebral circulation (vein of Galen aneurysm), in the coronary circuit, at the site of vascular tumors such as in hemangiomata of the liver or in peripheral arteriovenous connections, either congenital or acquired (Fig. 25-3). Acquired arteriovenous connections may result from

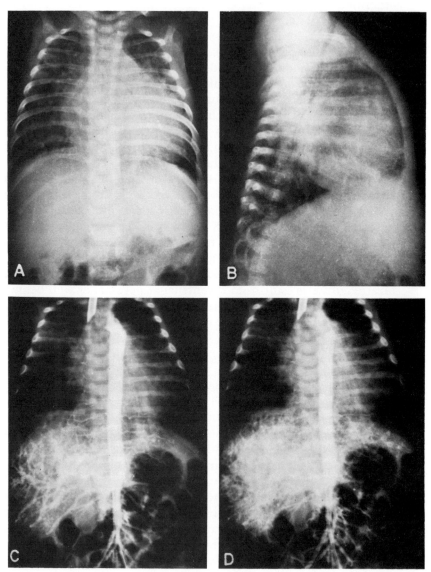

Fig. 25-3. Chest radiographs in the anterior-posterior (A) and lateral (B) views in infant with congestive heart failure resulting from multiple hemangiomata of liver acting as an arteriovenous fistula. Note cardiomegaly and prominent pulmonary vascular markings, similar to those seen with congenital heart disease. Abdominal aortogram (C and D) demonstrates multiple arteriovenous communications within the liver.

trauma, especially following arterial punctures either planned or inadvertent, as in a renal biopsy. A very rare cause of high cardiac output state in pediatrics is hyperthyroidism.

The physical findings in the high output states include a wide pulse pressure, with a slightly elevated systolic blood pressure and a distinctly lowered diastolic pressure. The arterial pulses are bounding in quality. A low pitched systolic murmur of the ejection type is present over the midprecordium. A variety of graphic studies have demonstrated the physical similarity between this type of murmur and a functional or innocent murmur of childhood. Transmission of the systolic murmur to the posterior chestwall is common in the high cardiac output states. Occasionally a mid-diastolic apical murmur of relative mitral stenosis will be heard due to the accelerated velocity of blood flow at the mitral valve during the period of diastolic filling of the left ventricle from the left atrium. Cardiomegaly and evidence of left ventricular hypertrophy in the electrocardiogram complete the picture.

There may be particular difficulty in differentiating the cardiac findings in a patient with a high output cardiac state due to a hidden arteriovenous fistula from the manifestations of congenital heart disease. This problem is accentuated in early infancy and in the presence of congestive heart failure. Occasionally the diagnosis of systemic arteriovenous fistula can be suspected from auscultation if a continuous murmur is discovered that indicates a flow of blood through the fistula during both systole and diastole. Auscultation should be carried out over the cranium, liver, or in other suspected areas for the presence of a continuous murmur. Visible vascular tumors involving the skin or mucous membranes should arouse suspicion of the possibility of a generalized distribution of such tumors including hidden sites. Hypertrophy of individual extremities or portions thereof may result from vascular anomalies of this type. Variations in surface temperature or discoloration of extremities may provide a clue to the presence of a vascular abnormality. Prominent pulsating jugular veins may be observed in the presence of a cerebral arteriovenous fistula; a loud cervical venous hum may be heard. During cardiac catheterization, the presence of highly oxygenated blood specimens from the jugular vein, superior vena cava and right atrium as compared to the inferior vena cava may result from the arteriovenous shunting within the cerebral circulation.

In radiographs of the chest obtained from patients with large systemic arteriovenous fistulas, the pulmonary vascular markings may be accentuated and mimic the plethora of pulmomary blood flow observed with intracardiac arteriovenous shunting. This radiographic feature results from an increase in circulating blood volume and the associated increase in pulmonary blood flow; mild pulmonary hypertension may also result from the overdistention of the pulmonary vascular bed.

Cyanosis may accompany the altered hemodynamics associated with congestive heart failure from this or any cause. The presence of cyanosis is not exclusively due to venous-arterial shunting via a cardiac anomaly.

While temporary benefit may be obtained from the symptomatic measures used in the treatment of congestive heart failure, the cardiopathy of high cardiac output states responds dramatically to the elimination of the cause. Transfusion of whole blood or packed red blood cells usually relieves the cardiac problem in chronic anemia; the surgical division of an arterio-venous fistula similarly produces a striking improvement in the cardiac difficulties in the presence of a large arterio-venous fistula. Hyperthyroidism can be treated medically, surgically or by radiotherapy.

PRIMARY MYOCARDIAL DISEASES OF INFANCY

The term *primary myocardial diseases of infancy* describes an artificial but useful category of cardiac lesions observed in small infants. In this grouping belong those infants with cardiomegaly and congestive heart failure who have no significant cardiac murmurs and hence are unlikely to have congenital heart disease. Anemia and hypertension are absent. All of these infants have in common evidence of left ventricular hypertrophy and left ventricular myocardial changes in the electrocardiogram.

The etiology of the lesions included in this category are not uniform: (1) interstitial myocarditis, probably of infectious (viral) origin with multiple offending agents, (2) endocardial fibroelastosis, a disease of unknown etiology which probably represents a non-specific tissue response to injury, (3) glycogen storage disease, type II, a hereditary metabolic disorder, and (4) a congenital cardiovascular anomaly, namely aberrant origin of the left coronary artery from the pulmonary artery. Each of these conditions of diverse etiology produces the same set of clinical and electrocardiographic manifestations, thereby constituting a useful diagnostic category. Several other very rare conditions such as medial necrosis of the coronary arteries, the involvement of the coronary arteries with the process of polyarteritis nodosa, and amyloid invasion of the myocardium can also produce a similar picture in infancy.

Interstitial Myocarditis

Myocarditis in infancy, especially in the newborn period, is not uncommon, and is usually of viral origin. Epidemics of myocarditis resulting from infection with Coxsackie B virus have been reported from a number of newborn nurseries. The viruses of mumps, chickenpox, rubella and the protozoan parasite of toxoplasmosis have been implicated, but in many instances the specific agent is undetermined.

The manifestations of myocarditis include tachycardia, cardiac enlargement, and congestive heart failure in the absence of significant cardiac murmurs. The electrocardiogram often shows non-specific myocardial changes including T-wave inversion, P-R interval prolongation, S-T segment depression and a variety of cardiac arrhythmias. Left ventricular hypertrophy is usually seen in the electrocardiogram, but a diffuse and balanced involvement of both ventricles may also be present.

The treatment of myocarditis in infancy is symptomatic and includes supportive measures such as digitalis, diuretics, oxygen, and salt and fluid restriction. Occasionally adrenal hormone therapy has been useful in temporarily suppressing the inflammation and edema of the myocardium. The adrenal steroids are helpful only if the pathology is self limited. In many instances, the eventual withdrawal of the adrenal steroids is accompanied by a return of the evidence of myocardial inflammation.

Approximately 50 per cent of patients with myocarditis recover and show no evidence of residual heart disease. It is the lesion with the best prognosis in the category of primary myocardial disease of infancy.

Endocardial Fibroelastosis

In this entity the endocardium of the heart develops a pathologic process resulting in thickening and rigidity of its inner lining; this thick, cast-like structure replaces the endocardial layer of the heart and interferes with ventricular filling as well as ventricular contractility. The left-sided chambers are involved most often although instances of four-chamber involvement have been reported.

Congestive heart failure is often the initial manifestation of endocardial fibroelastosis, usually precipitated by a respiratory tract infection during the third to sixth month of life. Physical examination reveals only cardiomegaly in the absence of a cardiac murmur. Occasionally involvement of the papillary muscles attached to the mitral valve leaflets produce mitral insufficiency. The chest roentgenogram shows cardiomegaly, primarily left atrial and left ventricular. The electrocardiogram provides evidence of left ventricular hypertrophy with T-wave abnormalities in the leads reflecting left ventricular activity, leads I and V 5–7.

There is usually a favorable initial response to digitalization and other symptomatic measures. However, subsequent episodes of congestive heart failure, often precipitated by intercurrent infection, are less responsive. Death often occurs around the age of 2 years, usually with the appearance of serious cardiac arrhythmias. In some instances, the process may become arrested and the child may survive for a decade or more.

In the primary form of endocardial fibroelastosis, no other evidence of heart disease is present. Secondary forms of endocardial fibroelastosis occur in the presence of congenital cardiac anomalies, usually left-sided obstructive lesions. Histopathologic examination of the endocardium permits identification of the primary and secondary forms.

Glycogen Storage Disease of the Heart and Skeletal Muscles

This form (type II) of glycogen storage disease is often referred to as Pompe's disease or cardiac glycogenosis. It is now known to be caused by the absence of a specific enzyme, acid maltase, essential for the breakdown of glycogen in striated muscle cells. When the enzyme is congenitally absent, glycogen is stored excessively in the cells of voluntary muscles and the syncitium of the myocardium. The presence of the glycogen eventually interferes with the contracting function of the involved muscles. Generalized skeletal muscle weakness and myocardial failure results.

Pompe's disease follows a Mendelian genetic pattern of transmission and multiple cases may occur in a single family. Clinical manifestations include the discovery of cardiomegaly in the absence of cardiac murmurs. The electrocardiogram is striking in its demonstration of a short P-R interval (less than 0.07 seconds), very high amplitude QRS complexes and marked S-T segment and T-wave changes. Left lower lobe atelectasis is very common in this disease because the enlarged heart compresses the left lower lobe bronchus. Death usually occurs in early infancy because of respiratory muscle weakness, aspiration, atelectasis and pneumonitis. Congestive heart failure rarely is the cause of death, but marked cardiac enlargement is the rule.

Aberrant Origin of the Left Coronary Artery from the Pulmonary Artery

In this congenital cardiovascular anomaly the left ventricular myocardium is perfused at low pressure with venous blood from the pulmonary artery via the left coronary which arises from the main pulmonary artery. This results in infarct-like changes in the left ventricular myocardium, often involving some of the papillary muscles attached to the mitral valve leaflets. As a result, cardiomegaly and congestive heart failure appear in the first month or two of life. Occasionally it is observed that infants with this anomaly have clinical episodes suggesting angina.

The physical findings include cardiomegaly, a prominent left ventricular impulse on palpation, the murmur of mitral insufficiency in 20 per cent of the cases and eventually the evidences of congestive heart failure. In rare instances, rupture of the left ventricular myocardium may occur with the complication of hemopericardium and cardiac tamponade.

Because of the potential for surgical treatment in this congenital anomaly, all patients with primary myocardial disease of infancy should be studied by cardiac catheterization technique with the possible exception of those with the obvious changes of glycogen storage disease. The presence of the aberrant origin of the left coronary artery should be established and the direction of blood flow in the left coronary artery specifically determined by cineangiography and oximetry. If the left coronary artery is acting as a venous conduit in an arterio-venous connection, with the right coronary artery as the arterial source, ligation of the left coronary artery improves myocardial perfusion as does the introduction of a graft from the aorta to the anomalous left coronary artery. If the direction of blood flow in the aberrant left coronary artery is from the pulmonary artery into the myocardium, ligation is harmful. Intractable congestive heart failure is an indication for surgical treatment. Dramatic improvement with long-term survival has been observed after ligation of the left coronary artery in a few instances.

MISCELLANEOUS CARDIAC DISEASES OF CHILDHOOD

Some of the common varieties of cardiac disease encountered in infancy and childhood have been reviewed briefly; a large number of less common examples of cardiac involvement is recognized. Among these are the cardiac components of systemic diseases, such as the cardiac involvement in collagen diseases and in rheumatoid arthritis. A serious aspect of acute glomerulonephritis is acute hypertensive cardiovascular disease. Cor pulmonale occurs in childhood; the most common causes are the chronic lung diseases of cystic fibrosis and upper airway obstruction. Cardiac manifestations are sometimes evident with hyper- and hypothyroidism. Neuromuscular dystrophies frequently include cardiac involvement. In somatic syndromes such as mongolism, Noonan's syndrome, arachnodactyly and gargoylism, a specific cardiopathy exists. Finally, the early origins of arteriosclerosis and the prevention of this common variety of adult heart disease by measures applied in the pediatric age group are currently under intensive study.

BIBLIOGRAPHY

Abbott, M. E.: Atlas of Congenital Cardiac Disease. New York, American Heart Association, 1936.

> Primarily of historical interest. The first organized treatise on congenital heart disease.

Conn, H. L., and Horwitz, O.: Acute rheumatic fever. *In* Cardiac and Vascular Disease. Philadelphia, Lea and Febiger, 1971; pp. 757–783.

> A complete treatment of rheumatic fever and rheumatic heart disease as they occur among pediatric patients.

Lambert, E. C., Israel, R., and Hohn, A.: *In* Cassels, D. E., and Ziegler, R. F.: Cardiac Arrhythmias of Infancy and Childhood: A Clinical Approach in Electrocardiography in Infants and Children. New York, Grune and Stratton, 1966.

> A brief review of cardiac arrhythmias as they present in the pediatric age group.

Markowitz, M., and Kuttner, A. G.: Rheumatic Fever: Diagnosis, Management and Prevention. Philadelphia, W. B. Saunders Company, 1965.

An excellent review of all current considerations concerning rheumatic fever in the form of a small volume [185 pages]; includes a section on community health services.

Nadas, A. S., and Fyler, D. C.: Pediatric Cardiology. Philadelphia, W. B. Saunders Company, 1972.

A clinically oriented reference book on entire subject of cardiac disease in infancy and childhood.

Perloff, J. K.: The Clinical Recognition of Congenital Heart Disease. Philadelphia, W. B. Saunders Company, 1970.

A complete and excellent review of the lesions of congenital heart disease with special emphasis on application of physical findings, particularly auscultation in diagnosis.

Ziegler, R. F.: Electrocardiographic Studies in Normal Infants and Children. Springfield, Illinois, Charles C Thomas, 1951.

A basic reference for electrocardiographic standard in pediatrics, including a careful statistical evaluation of all standard EKG values.

26

Bronchial Asthma

Eliot Dunsky, M.D.

Bronchial asthma is a major cause of chronic disease among children. It can be defined as an obstructive airway disease characterized by recurrent episodes of bronchospasm with a significant degree of reversibility. The main pathological features include: bronchial smooth muscle spasm, mucosal edema, and the accumulation of thick tenacious mucus within the bronchial lumen. All contribute toward the obstruction of the airway. The obstructive interference with ventilation produces the clinical picture characterized by coughing, shortness of breath, and wheezing. Asthmatic children typically have an increased responsiveness of their bronchi to various stimuli resulting in a narrowing of the airway. The key points that differentiate bronchial asthma from other obstructive lung diseases are its "twitchy" bronchi which tend to narrow upon minimal stimulation, and the characteristic reversible nature of the obstruction.

ETIOLOGY

The bronchospasm is episodic in nature, followed by asymptomatic periods of varying length. A smaller number of more severely affected patients may have continuous symptoms with marked exacerbations of bronchospasm occurring intermittently. Clinically, these children may present with a history of recurrent paroxysms of coughing, dyspnea, and/or wheezing. Some authors refer to asthma as a symptom complex rather than a disease because of the diverse etiologic factors that may produce the disorder.

In recognition of the heterogeneity of bronchial asthma, attempts at classification have been undertaken. Initially asthma was separated into two major subgroups. In the first group, extrinsic asthma or allergic asthma, symptoms are caused by the inhalation of a specific allergen (e.g., pollens, etc.). This reaction is known to be immunologically induced and associated with mast cell release of mediators that can produce bronchospasm. The second major group is intrinsic bronchial asthma or non-allergic asthma, in which no immunologic mechanism has been identified. These patients appear to have hyperirritable or "twitchy" airways. Thus, significant airway obstruction may be induced by the inhalation of non-specific air pollutants or by respiratory tract infections. Additional types of bronchial asthma that do not fit within either one of these two categories include exercise-induced and aspirin-induced asthma.

In order to explain the diverse etiologies producing what superficially appears to be a single clinical disorder, it has been proposed that asthmatics may have a common underlying defect. The theory postulates that asthmatics have a defect in or partial blockade of their beta adrenergic receptors. Stimulation of the beta receptors produces relaxation of the smooth muscle (i.e., bronchodilation).

The bronchial tree contains beta receptors which promote bronchodilation. Stimulation of these pulmonary B_2 receptors by catecholamines (e.g., epinephrine, isoproterenol, etc.) activates the target organ membrane enzyme, adenyl cyclase, converting adenosine triphosphate (ATP) to 3', 5'-cyclic adenosine monophosphate (cyclic AMP or C-AMP). An increase in C-AMP results in bronchodilation as well as the suppression of certain allergic reactions. It would follow, therefore, that a defect in the beta adrenergic receptor would ultimately predispose toward the development of bronchospasm even upon modest stimulation of the tracheobronchial tree.

In addition to this postulated biochemical defect it has long been recognized that bronchial asthma and allergy tend to occur with greater frequency in the offspring of asthmatic families. Some authors have suggested that asthma may be due to an autosomal dominant gene with incomplete penetrance. Up to one-half of the asthmatic patients have a positive family history, while the incidence of asthma in a control population appears to be less than 10 per cent.

PREVALENCE

Asthma in children most frequently has its onset during the first 5 years of life. A recent United States National Health Survey reports that the overall prevalence of allergy is 32.8 per cent in children under 17. One-third of these children suffer from bronchial asthma. Among the younger children, asthma occurs about twice as frequently in males as it does in females. In the older children, the proportion of males to females is approximately equal. The most severe forms of asthma appear to begin very early in life and affect more males than females.

MORBIDITY AND MORTALITY

The magnitude of asthma morbidity was documented in the U.S. National Health Survey; 22.9 per cent of all school days lost due to chronic disease was attributed to asthma. These statistics reflect only a part of the disability caused by asthma. The inability to compete effectively in sports, poor performance in school, and a general lack of energy are a few of the many sequelae of incompletely controlled bronchial asthma.

Approximately 200 childhood deaths due to bronchial asthma occur each year, yielding a mortality rate about 2 per 100,000. A much higher rate prevails in adults.

Autopsies performed on children who died of asthma reveal airway obstruction due to a narrowed bronchial lumen filled with inspissated mucus and epithelial debris. The lining of the respiratory mucosa is swollen and infiltrated with inflammatory cells including large numbers of eosinophils. Bronchial basement membrane thickening, hypertrophy of the bronchial smooth muscle and mucous gland hyperplasia and hypertrophy are frequent findings.

Asthmatic deaths have been attributed to: asphyxia due to respiratory failure, the use of sedatives or tranquilizers that may suppress the respiratory drive, the abuse of sympathomimetic inhalers, aminophylline toxicity, and the inadequate use of corticosteroid supplement in steroid-dependent asthmatics.

THE BETA-ADRENERGIC BLOCKADE
AND CYCLIC NUCLEOTIDES

It has been known for some time that both alpha and beta receptors exist in the lungs. Pharmacological stimulation of the alpha receptor tends to increase bronchomotor tone, while pulmonary beta receptor stimulation produces smooth bronchial muscle relaxation. Normally, a balance exists between relaxation and contraction. It has been postulated that patients with bronchial asthma have a partial blockade of their pulmonary beta receptors. The resulting imbalance tends to produce bronchospasm.

On a biochemical level this phenomenon can be explained by the alpha and beta receptor control of cyclic nucleotide concentrations.

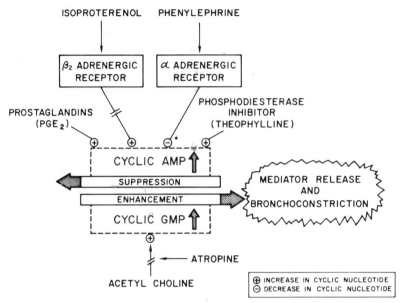

Fig. 26-1. Cyclic nucleotide control of mediator release and broncho-constriction.

The two cyclic nucleotides, cyclic 3'5' adenosine monophosphate (cyclic AMP) and cyclic 3'5' guanosine monophosphate (cyclic GMP) are important in asthma since they appear to play a regulatory role in both bronchial smooth muscle relaxation and immediate hypersensitivity reactions through opposing actions (Fig. 26-1).

An increase in intracellular cyclic AMP suppresses the release of mast cell mediators and promotes bronchodilation. Conversely, an increase in the opposing nucleotide, cyclic GMP, promotes both the release of mediators and bronchospasm. The level of cyclic AMP is increased by stimulation of the beta-adrenergic receptor by catecholamines (e.g., isoproterenol and epinephrine), while alpha-adrenergic agents (phenylephrine) suppress the level of cyclic AMP. On the other hand, the level of cyclic GMP may be raised by stimulation of the cholinergic receptors (by acetylcholine) and suppressed by cholinergic blockade (e.g., atropine). It should be noted that cyclic nucleotides are being broken down constantly by the enzyme phosphodiesterase. The inhibition of this enzyme appears to be the mechanism of action of the important anti-asthmatic drug (theophylline) by indirectly raising the intra-cellular cyclic AMP.

In addition, corticosteroids as well as prostaglandins of the E series produce increases in intracellular cyclic AMP. Corticosteroids appear to enhance the catecholamine effects on asthmatic beta receptors while prostaglandins seem to function via other independent receptors.

Considering the above factors, one can begin to comprehend why an asthmatic patient with sensitive cholinergic receptors and/or having a partial blockade of beta receptors might have a tendency to develop bronchospasm.

PATHOPHYSIOLOGY OF ASTHMA

Smooth muscle bronchospasm, mucosal edema, and the accumulation of large amounts of thick tenacious mucous diminishing the internal diameter of the bronchial lumen are the bases for the airway obstruction in bronchial asthma. Even a small change in the diameter of the lumen will produce a relatively large increase in airway resistance since the latter varies inversely to the fourth power of the radius of the lumen

$$\left(R \cong \frac{1}{r^4} \right).$$

Although most of the airway may eventually be involved in severe bronchospasm, it is the small airways (less than 2 mm. in diameter) that are usually affected. Since these small airways constitute only 20 per cent of the total airway resistance, it is not surprising that they may be obstructed partially; yet few if any symptoms may be clinically manifested. As the medium-sized and large airways become involved, airway resistance quickly and significantly increases, as do symptoms.

During normal inspiration the bronchi tend to dilate due to a transient negative intrapleural pressure (relative to intraluminal pressure) (Fig. 26-2). This is an active process secondary to muscular effort. On the other

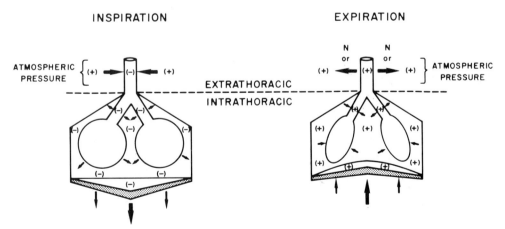

Fig. 26-2. Mechanics of obstructive airway disease.

hand, during the expiratory phase the elastic tissue of the lungs and thorax tends to passively return to its original position and thus act as the driving force that expels the inhaled air. If bronchial airway obstruction exists, expiration needs to be assisted by muscular compression of the pleural cavity; this assistance should include forceful elevation of the diaphragm and the use of the accessory muscles of respiration. The compression of the pleural space produces an increased positive pleural pressure. When this transmitted pressure exceeds the intraluminal bronchial pressure the bronchi tend to narrow and/or collapse. This is seen dramatically in acute asthma as the patient uses his accessory muscles to force air out of the lungs during a markedly prolonged expiratory phase. As a consequence of the turbulent air flow through narrowed and partially obstructed airways, wheezing may be heard on auscultation. As the airway obstruction proceeds, some airways collapse while others continue to function normally. In order to compensate for the hypoventilated area (distal to the obstructed airways) the patient increases his respiratory rate (tachypnea) and depth of respiration (hyperpnea). In attempting to produce the necessary driving pressure to overcome the increased airway resistance, the accessory muscles of respiration are recruited, resulting in an increase in the work of breathing. Even with prolonged expirations, not all the previously inspired air can be expelled, and a portion of the gas remains trapped.

As the quantity of air accumulates the thorax becomes hyperinflated. Pulmonary function studies of these patients reveal an increase in the residual capacity (air remaining in the lung after forced expiration); such patients ultimately will have both clinical and radiologic signs of pulmonary hyperinflation. In addition to increased airway resistance, the asthmatic lung has a decreased compliance and is a stiffer lung. Both of these changes cause an increase in the work of breathing, which in itself markedly increases oxygen consumption in the already hypoxemic patient. These disturbances of respiratory mechanics are further complicated by a deranged gas exchange. Normally, each terminal respiratory unit (alveolus) is both well-ventilated and well-perfused. Alveolar oxygen fully saturates perfusing hemoglobin. One of the pathophysiologic characteristics of asthma is the uneven match of ventilation to perfusion. Some alveolae are well-ventilated and well-perfused. Others are poorly ventilated with normal perfusion, while another group may be well-ventilated and poorly perfused due to pulmonary vascular constriction. In hypoventilated well-perfused respiratory units, hemoglobin can only be saturated partially with oxygen. This mismatch of ventilation to perfusion (V/Q) results in partially unsaturated hemoglobin. On the other hand, the remaining normal units which may be hyperventilated (due to tachypnea and hypernea) cannot saturate hemoglobin beyond its maximum carrying capacity (100%).

Partially unsaturated hemoglobin (returning from hypoventilated areas) is mixed with completely saturated hemoglobin (returning from well ventilated areas) resulting in less than 100 per cent saturation. The greater the mismatch between ventilation and perfusion the greater the resulting hypoxemia. This situation is analogous to a right-to-left cardiac shunt, as a certain amount of blood bypasses the functioning respiratory units of the lung. The exchange of carbon dioxide under identical circumstances in asthma is very different from that of oxygen. Carbon dioxide is 20 times more diffusible across the respiratory membrane than oxygen. Well-perfused hypoventilating respiratory units may not permit adequate local exchange of any gas including CO_2. During the mild asthma attack, in contrast to oxygen gas exchange, the remaining hyperventilating respiratory units may exchange ("blow off") large amounts of CO_2, more than compensating for those respiratory units that are failing. Arterial blood gasses clinically confirm this phenomenon during an acute mild attack of asthma, as patients are usually hypocarbic ($PaCO_2 \downarrow$) in the face of hypoxemia. As the asthmatic attack becomes more severe due to increased airway obstruction, the minute volume (the amount of air exchanged/minute) decreases. A point is reached when the patient's remaining functioning respiratory units begin to hypoventilate and the $PaCO_2$ begins to rise. If the trend persists and medication fails to reverse the respiratory obstruction, the patient may eventually enter into respiratory failure.

CLINICAL ASPECTS OF ASTHMA

Bronchial asthma may be classified into five separate groups, although it should be recognized that a single patient may have characteristics of more than one group.

Extrinsic Bronchial Asthma

This is allergic asthma and it is due to an IgE-mediated mechanism associated with the release of mast cell mediators. It is induced by an inhaled allergen and frequently there is a good correlation between the onset of symptoms and allergen exposure. For example, the symptoms may occur each year during the months of August and September at the time of ragweed pollination. In some patients symptoms may follow exposure to dust, molds, feather pillows, or animal dander. Antigen exposure may also produce the signs and symptoms of allergic rhinitis and conjunctivitis. Allergic asthmatic patients usually have positive skin tests to the appropriate antigen as well as a positive family history for allergy. In general, many allergic patients with asthma respond to avoidance and specific therapy. Their prognosis is generally better than those patients with non-allergic (intrinsic) asthma.

Intrinsic Bronchial Asthma

This group is characterized by highly irritable bronchi that easily develop bronchospasm upon exposure to non-specific stimuli. No immunologic mechanism has been implicated. Patients develop asthmatic symptoms following exposure to various stimuli including air pollutants, respiratory tract infections, weather changes, hyperventilation, exposure to cold air, emotional stress. Allergy skin tests are usually negative. Symptoms tend to be perennial or occur mainly during the winter months when respiratory infections are frequently encountered.

Mixed Type Asthma

Patients in this category have characteristics of intrinsic as well as extrinsic asthma.

Exercise-Induced Asthma or Exercise-Induced Bronchospasm

Exercise-induced bronchospasm (E.I.B.) can be defined as acute bronchospasm following strenuous exercise. Prior to exercise, patients may be asymptomatic and have normal polmonary functions. Five to 10 minutes after strenuous exercise patients may become dyspneic, tachypneic, develop coughing, or begin wheezing. Pulmonary functions indicate sudden onset of significant airway obstruction. These symptoms can be reversed quickly by beta-adrenergic stimulants or the asthma subsides spontaneously, usually within a period of less than 1–2 hours following onset.

Aspirin-Sensitive Asthma

The incidence of aspirin-induced asthma is probably less than 4 per cent among asthmatics. These patients may have a history of a triad of profuse rhinorrhea, hyperplastic sinusitis associated with nasal polyps, and marked bronchospasm following the ingestion of aspirin. The mechanism for this reaction is unknown but does not appear to be immunologic in nature. Because both aspirin and indomethicin are prostaglandin inhibitors, this may be the mechanism that underlies this type of asthma.

CLINICAL SIGNS AND SYMPTOMS

The presentation and course of bronchial asthma in children is highly variable. Symptoms may occur as acute recurrent episodes separated by asymptomatic periods. Other children have continuous symptoms with intermittent exacerbations of severe wheezing. The intensity of the symptoms can vary from mild or even unnoticed to severe, potentially fatal attacks necessitating immediate hospitalization. The presentation of asthma often mimics other respiratory diseases, but because its obstructive component is reversible, asthma differs from other obstructive airway disease.

The Asymptomatic Interval in Asthma

The majority of children with asthma have periods in which the patient looks and feels well. The physical examination may be completely within normal limits and pulmonary function studies within the range of normal values. Other asymptomatic asthmatic children demonstrate obstructive changes in pulmonary functions suggesting persistent small airway disease. Still others claim that they are asymptomatic and yet when asked to perform a forced expiration maneuver, numerous wheezes at the end of expiration are audible. These subtle changes are an indication that at least a number of apparently asymptomatic patients have a continuing obstructive airway disease and may require further therapy.

The Mild Asthmatic Episode

Patients with mild episodes of asthma may develop a dry, hacking cough, mild dyspnea, and a feeling of tightness in the chest. Many will have an elevated respiratory rate (tachypnea). Auscultation of the chest reveals good air entry into both lungs and diffuse wheezing associated with a prolonged expiratory phase.

The Moderate Asthmatic Episode

As the severity of the attack proceeds the signs and symptoms of the mild attack intensify. Wheezing becomes louder and expiration more prolonged and forceful. Air entry into both lungs may be unequal or its intensity may be diminished. The respiratory rate increases and hyperpnea developes. There may be a need for use of accessory muscles of respiration which include; flaring of the alae nasi, retraction of the intercostal and subcostal muscles, and prominent excursions of the abdominal musculature.

The Severe Episode of Asthma

When tachypnea and hyperpnea become maximal, the patient is in acute respiratory distress. The child may assume a sitting position, grasping the edge of the bed with his hands, fostering maximal utilization of the accessory muscles. Vomiting as well as complaints of chest and abdominal pain are frequently encountered. If airway obstruction progresses, breath sounds diminish, often to the extent of being inaudible, and as little or no air is being ventilated wheezing may cease entirely. Under such conditions a "silent chest" is often associated with either respiratory arrest or acute respiratory failure. In the moderate to severe attack of asthma the physical exam may reveal an increase in the AP diameter of the chest. The shoulders are raised high and remain in a fixed position, and the chest is hyperresonant to percussion. The development of hypoxia may present clinically as pallor or cyanosis. The lack of oxygen may produce anxiety, irritability, restlessness, or confusion. Signs of hypercarbia include headache, muscle twitching, confusion, somnolence, and finally coma. A technique often used for assessing the severity of an acute attack of asthma is the measurement of the pulsus paradoxus. The systolic blood pressure measured during both inspiration and expiration is recorded. The greater the difference between the inspiratory and expiratory systolic blood pressures the more severe the respiratory obstruction.

LABORATORY STUDIES

Sputum

Many asthmatic children swallow their sputum. For those who can expectorate, examination of the sputum offers useful diagnostic information. Eosinophils are often present in large numbers. Charcot-Leyden crystals, thought to be the breakdown product of eosinophils, are frequently associated with Curshmann's spirals (mucoid casts of the bronchioles). Secondary bacterial infections may be identified when the sputum contains large numbers of neutrophils and bacteria.

Blood Studies

Asthmatic children usually have a normal hemoglobin while children with other chronic pulmonary disease may have secondary polycythemia. The total white count is frequently elevated above 12,000 cells/mm³ during the acute attacks of asthma, but is normal when the patient is asymptomatic. Peripheral eosinophilia is observed frequently in both intrinsic and extrinsic asthma. Suppression of the eosinophil count may be used as a guide to the success of drug management (e.g., steroids). Asthmatics usually have normal serum electrolytes, although the use of steroids may induce hypokalemia.

Radiographic Findings

Asymptomatic patients and those with mild asthma frequently have normal chest radiographs. In more severely affected subjects radiographic changes include: pulmonary hyperinflation, depressed or flattened diaphragms, increase in the AP diameter of the chest, and prominent hilar bronchovascular markings. Following resolution of an acute attack of asthma many of these findings disappear. Persistence of hyperinflation may be a sign of moderate to severe chronic disease. Some of the pul-

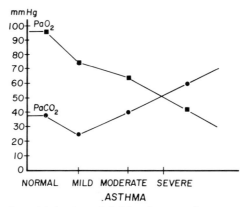

Fig. 26-3. Arterial blood gases in acute bronchial asthma.

monary complications seen on radiograph in asthmatic patients are: atelectasis, pneumomediastinum, pneumothorax, pneumopericardium and pneumonia.

Arterial Blood Gases and Asthma

Arterial blood gasses are probably the best available means for assessment of respiratory function in acute asthma. Between asthmatic episodes blood gases are often normal (PaO_2 = 90 ± 5mm.Hg, $PaCO_2$ = 40 ± 4mm.Hg and pH=7.4 ± 0.05). However, a small group of asymptomatic patients have a diminished PaO_2.

Hypoxemia of varying degrees if often noted in patients recovering from an acute attack of status asthmaticus for periods up to 6 weeks. During the mild paroxysm of asthma the child hyperventilates. Arterial blood gases at that time reveal a decrease in the $PaCO_2$ (hypocarbia) and a decrease in the PaO_2 (hypoxemia) (Fig. 26-3). As the attack progresses to moderate obstruction, the child can no longer hyperventilate and his minute volume decreases. Therefore, the $PaCO_2$ rises, often to a level that appears to be normal (40 ± 5 mm.). Although the $PaCO_2$, in this instance, appears to be normal, it represents a decompensatory phase and actually may herald subsequent respiratory failure. Finally, as bronchial obstruction becomes maximal, the muscles of respiration become fatigued, minute volume decreases further, and $PaCO_2$ continues to rise. When the $PaCO_2$ reaches 55 mm. the situation can be defined as impending respiratory failure, and at 65 mm. the patient is considered in frank respiratory failure.

Pulmonary function studies frequently used in the assessment and management of asthma include: the peak expiratory flow rates (PEFR); the vital capacity (VC); the forced expiratory volume in one second (FEV_1)

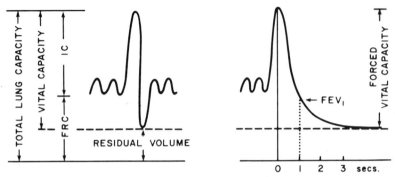

Fig. 26-4. Pulmonary spirometry and lung volumes. IC = Inspiratory capacity; FRC = Functional residual capacity; FEV_1 = Forced expiratory volume in one second.

and the maximal mid-expiratory flow rate (MMEFR) (Fig. 26-4). The peak expiratory flow rate is both quick and easy to perform, especially if serial measurements are required; PEFR reflects conductance in the larger upper airways. FEV_1, the amount of air that can be forcibly expelled in one second, for the most part measures larger but also some small airway resistance; it is effort dependent. Normally, the FEV_1 represents about 86 ± 7 per cent of the vital capacity of the normal child, while lower values indicate obstructive airway disease. Asymptomatic asthmatic children may have normal pulmonary function; however, a number of these children may have small airway obstructive disease that may not be picked up in study of the FEV_1 or the peak expiratory flow rate. Therefore, an earlier objective sign of obstructive airway disease may be reflected in an abnormal measurement of small airway resistance such as the maximal mid-expiratory flow rate (MMEFR). This value represents the mean flow rate in the middle portion of the forced expiratory volume. The MMEFR is often the earliest spirographic sign of active airway obstruction and is frequently the last to return to normal following cessation of an acute attack. In addition to evaluating the degree of obstructive disease at any one time, an inhaled bronchodilator will reveal the degree of reversibility of the airway obstruction. Pulmonary functions are taken before and after the administration of isoproterenol. Most asthmatics with bronchospasm have an increase of more than 15–20 per cent in their peak expiratory flow rates or their FEV_1. Patients with chronic bronchitis, emphysema and other obstructive diseases have less than a 15 per cent element of reversible obstructive airway disease. Significant reversibility of airway obstruction is the basis of the diagnosis of asthma.

Total and Specific IgE Levels

Many childhood asthmatics have an elevated total IgE. An elevated IgE suggests the presence of allergy. Children with either historical evidence or signs of respiratory allergy require skin testing or RAST (radioallergo-sorbent tests, Fig. 26-5) to identify the specific allergic etiology of this disease.

Allergy Skin Testing

Scratch, prick (puncture), and intradermal allergy skin testing tradi-tionally are used in a evaluation of specific allergy. A sensitive individual responds by developing an immediate hypersensitive reaction at the punctured site. This is interpreted as evidence of the presence of specific IgE class antibodies directed against the tested allergen. Within 15 min-utes a hive (wheal and flare) will develop. The size of the reaction is related to the degree of sensitivity.

DIFFERENTIAL DIAGNOSIS

The signs and symptoms of asthma can simulate a large variety of disease states. Fortunately, in the majority of instances the diagnosis of asthma is readily established. However, an initial diagnosis of bronchial asthma (especially in the young child) may be erroneous and some other underlying disease proved to be the etiologic agent at a later date.

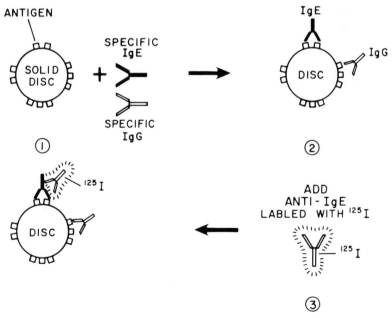

Fig. 26-5. Radioallergosorbent test (RAST).

Differential Diagnosis of Childhood Asthma

Upper Airway
  Foreign bodies
  Croup
  Laryngo- and tracheomalacia
  Retropharyngeal and peritonsilar abscess
  Aspiration syndromes

Lower Airway
  Foreign body aspiration
  Aspiration syndromes
  Vascular ring compression
  Compression of airways due to: lymphnode
    enlargement (T.B., etc.), neoplasm, congenital
    abnormalities (lobar emphysema, etc.).
  Bronchiolitis, bronchitis, bronchiectasis
  Pneumonia, primary (viral, bacterial, fungal) or
    secondary to underlying disease
  Immunodeficiency
  Cystic fibrosis
  Hypersensitivity pneumonitis
  Allergic bronchopulmonary aspergillosis
  Alpha-1-antitrypsin deficiency
  Persistent atelectasis
  Loeffler's syndrome
  Congestive heart failure

Foreign Bodies

Foreign bodies may be lodged anywhere along the airway. A history of sudden onset of coughing, stridor, and respiratory distress are frequently encountered. However, the symptoms may develop more gradually. Foreign objects in the esophagus can cause obstruction through pressure on the trachea. Clinically, this may be accompanied by difficulty in swallowing. Foreign body obstruction in the upper airway may be diagnosed with the aid of a lateral neck radiograph or may necessitate endoscopy.

Croup, Bronchiolitis and Cystic Fibrosis

Laryngotracheobronchitis, epiglotitis and bronchiolitis are discussed in Chapter 31. Cystic fibrosis is considered and discussed in Chapter 23.

Immunodeficiency

Patients with hypogammaglobulinemia may have a history of recurrent respiratory tract infections characerized by pneumonia, coughing, and wheezing. They often have poor lymphnode, tonsillar, and adenoidal development. Quantitative immunoglobin determinations diagnose the deficiency in most cases. Patients with defects in their cellular immune system or those with severe combined immunodeficiency are frequently so ill during the first 6 months of life, they are rarely confused with a typical case of bronchial asthma.

Hypersensitivity Pneumonitides

This group of pulmonary disorders is caused by the inhalation of organic dusts and proteins and characterized by recurrent episodes of coughing, fever, and respiratory distress. A few hours after exposure, fever, respiratory distress, leukocytosis and coarse rales appear, but the symptoms usually subside within 12 to 24 hours. The common bronchodilators are not effective. In contrast, corticosteroids do suppress symptoms.

Allergic Bronchopulmonary Aspergillosis

This disease may be mistaken initially for bronchial asthma. Clinical presentation usually includes recurrent episodes of coughing and wheezing, poor control of symptoms with antiasthmatic medications, fleeting pulmonary infiltrates, and the production of sputum, often brown in color and sometimes containing aspergillus hyphae. Blood studies may reveal peripheral eosinophilia and marked elevation of the total IgE. Skin testing with aspergillis extract produces both an immediate (20 min.) and a delayed reaction (4–8 hrs.). In addition, patients usually have precipitating antibodies directed against aspergillis.

Alpha-1-Antitrypsin Deficiency

This is an autosomal recessive disorder due to a deficiency of alpha-1-antitrypsin in the serum. Such children may present with the symptoms of lung disease including coughing, dyspnea, and wheezing. This is an obstructive lung disease characterized by air trapping and poor reversibility of airway obstruction. A family history of chronic lung disease or emphysema should alert the clinician to obtain a quantitative alpha-1-antitrypsin level.

COMPLICATIONS OF ASTHMA

Status Asthmaticus

Status asthmaticus may be defined as a persistent, acute attack of asthma which does not adequately respond to treatment either with sympathomimetics (epinephrine) or other commonly used bronchodilators (e.g., aminophylline). This complication can quickly result in asphyxia and therefore constitutes a medical emergency. Patients require constant monitoring and frequent reevaluation for possible modification of treatment. Predisposing factors to the development of status asthmaticus include; poorly controlled asthma, abuse of sympathomimetic nebulizers, respiratory tract infections. Patients may become dehydrated because of diminished fluid intake and concomitant increases in both sensible and insensible fluid loss (hyperventilation, vomiting, etc.). Those not responding to oxygen, fluid and electrolyte therapy, and intravenous aminophylline will require corticosteroid administration. The initial clinical assessment should include information about the presence of cyanosis, the quality of breath sounds on inspiration in both lungs, the use of accessory muscles of respiration, the intensity of wheezing, cerebral function, the state of hydration, and the possible presence of underlying disease. Etiological factors exacerbating or complicating asthma should be sorted out (e.g., infection, atelectasis, etc). Clinically, one can estimate the severity of status asthmaticus by using either a clinical scoring system and/or by measuring the pulsus paradoxus. Either of these techniques afford a non-invasive method of assessment and may be used serially to judge the patient's course and response to medication. The following studies are recommended: chest radiograph (PA and lateral), CBC and differential, total eosinophil count, NP and throat culture, sputum cytology, and serum electrolytes. Arterial blood gases are drawn if clinical judgement indicates that an accurate assessment of gas exchange is required. Arterial blood gasses can be interpreted as presented in Figure 26-3.

Atelectasis

In asthma, atelectasis occurs with greater frequency in the right middle lobe, possibly because the right middle lobe bronchus comes off at a sharp angle from the right main stem bronchus as well as being long and narrow. In many cases, atelectasis causes no obvious symptoms, or a mucous plug blocking the main stem bronchus may produce massive atelectasis of an entire lung with immediate symptoms of respiratory distress constituting an acute medical emergency.

Pneumomediastinum

Free air within the mediastinum is thought to be the result of air escaping from the ruptured asthmatic aveolae and dissecting its way along the bronchovascular tree to the hilum. Many patients are asymptomatic and the presence of a pneumomediastinum is made by the radiographic finding of retrosternal free air. Signs and symptoms of pneumomediastinum include chest pain, tachypnea and dyspnea. This complication is frequently seen in the younger asthmatic.

Pneumothorax

Fortunately, this complication occurs less frequently than does pneumomediastinum. However, the symptoms of pneumothorax are usually more prominent and potentially serious. They include sudden clinical deterioration, dyspnea, cough, air hunger, marked tachypnea, and frank cyanosis. Non-tension pneumothoraces with free air occupying less than 20 per cent of the hemithoracic volume are handled conservatively, while those exceeding 20 per cent often require insertion of a chest tube and suction.

Other complications encountered include pneumonia, bronchiectasis, and, rarely, cor pulmonale. Some of the more severely affected children may show signs of inhibition of linear growth, and/or deformity of their chest.

An important and often overlooked complication of asthma is the physical disability resulting from chronic lung disease. Frequent absences from school may interfere seriously with academic development. Poorly controlled asthmatics may be unable to participate in sports. Also, a number of children and their families may develop significant psycho-pathology as a result of the problems related to asthma or their existing psychopathology may exacerbate the asthma.

TREATMENT OF BRONCHIAL ASTHMA

The successful management of childhood bronchial asthma requires a careful assessment and identification of the type of asthma involved (in-trinsic, extrinsic, etc), its duration and severity, environmental and other provoking stimuli, and a history of response and side effects to medica-tions. In dealing with extrinsic bronchial asthma, environmental control as well as hyposensitization should be considered.

Environmental Control

Specific allergens identified as causative factors either by history or allergy testing and interpreted as being significant etiologically should initially be avoided and/or eliminated from the immediate environment. Common allergens known to produce asthma in sensitive individuals include: house dust, dog and cat dander, feathers, mold (damp base-ments), and bedding material (kapok and cotton fibers). Certain allergens such as dust may be partially eliminated through a concerted effort to lower its concentrations within the immediate enviroment.

Hyposensitization or "Allergy Injections"

Hyposensitization to various allergens may be accomplished by means of subcutaneous injections of the offending allergen administered in in-creasing amounts. Although the mechanism underlying successful hy-posensitization is not completely clear, it appears that these injections result in increasing IgG blocking antibodies, decreased cellular sensitiv-ity (histamine release), decreased specific IgE, and diminished allergen-

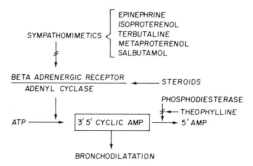

Fig. 26-6. Site of drug action in bronchial asthma.

induced symptoms. Indications for hyposensitization include correlation of symptoms following exposure (i.e., seasonal correlation), plus positive allergy tests (skin testing or RAST). If avoidance is unsuccessful and symptoms are not easily controlled with medication, hyposensitization is considered. The following allergens are frequently used for hyposensitization in asthma; pollens, dust, and molds. The use of bacterial vaccines to treat asthma is controversial. The traditional method of selection of the appropriate antigen (i.e., skin testing) has not proven to be of value in the case of bacterial vaccines.

Ingestants in Asthma

The ingestion of certain foods has been associated with asthma in childhood. Contrary to popular opinion, foods have not been shown as a major etiologic factor in asthma. Of those foods that do cause respiratory symptoms, milk and eggs are among the most common offenders. In addition to their respiratory symptoms, many children have concomitant dermal (urticaria-eczema) or gastrointestinal manifestations (diarrhea or colic). Allergy skin testing for foods is far less reliable than testing with other allergens. A more accurate technique for diagnosing food allergies is an elimination diet followed by a provocation test with the suspected food. We prefer to repeat this maneuver at least three times to clearly reproduce the respiratory symptoms before incriminating a specific food. Certain drugs, including aspirin, and tartrazine dyes (yellow dye #5) should be eliminated if they are suspected of inducing asthma.

Medical Treatment

Theophylline, a member of the methylxanthine group, has become a drug of choice in the management of childhood asthma today. Theophylline's action is accomplished through suppression of the enzyme phosphosdiesterase (preventing the degradation of cyclic AMP) with a resultant increase in cyclic AMP and bronchodilation (Fig. 26-6). This drug can be used concomitantly with beta-adrenergic sympathomimetics in a synergistic manner. The metabolism of theophylline in children may vary considerably among individuals. Therapeutic blood levels usually lie between 10 and 20 μg./ml. These levels are generally achieved by administering orally 5 mg./kg. of anhydrous theophylline three to four times per day. For children not responding adequately or experiencing side effects, a theophylline blood level may be determined and the drug dosage adjusted appropriately. Most oral theophylline preparations produce adequate blood levels within 15 to 60 minutes following ingestion. Rectal preparations are less useful because of their erratic absorption and possible prolonged duration of action. The intravenous use of aminophylline is limited generally to acute asthma in an emergency room or hospital setting. The toxic side effects of theophylline overdose include nausea, vomiting, hypotension, arrythmias, hematemesis, and convulsions. Toxicity is commonly encountered when the blood level exceeds 20 μg./ml.

Sympathomimetics

Sympathomimetics act through stiumlation of the beta adrenergic receptors producing an elevation in intracellular cyclic AMP and subsequent bronchodilatation (Fig. 26-6). Sympathomimetics used in the treatment of asthma are related to the parent compound phenylethylamine. Substitution in this compound can increase beta$_2$ activity as seen with terbutaline and metaproterenol. Certain adrenergic drugs are inactivated in the GI tract by a mucosal enzyme, catechol-o-methyltransferase. Therefore, drugs destroyed by these enzymes (epinephrine, isoproterenol, etc.) are only effective when injected or inhaled. Moreover, the latter two drugs also have a short half-life. Certain sympathomimetics may be administered orally, subcutaneoisly, by inhalation, and very rarely intravenously. Beta$_1$ drugs produce cardiac acceleration and beta$_2$, smooth bronchial muscle relaxation effects. The better known side effects include cardiac stimulation and skeletal muscle tremor.

Ephedrine

The main advantage of ephedrine is that it is inexpensive, can be administered orally, and has a duration of 4–6 hours. Unfortunately, children do suffer from annoying side effects such as insomnia, headache, and other signs of central nervous system stimulation. Addiction does not seem to be a problem.

Epinephrine

The medication is not effective orally; however, it can produce dramatic relief of bronchospasm within a few minutes following subcutaneous injection. It may also be inhaled as an aerosol. Epinephrine's main disadvantages are a very short duration of action and central nervous system stimulation. It is the drug of choice in acute asthma that does not respond to conservative treatment.

Isoproterenol (Isuprel)

Isuprel, a frequently inhaled anti-asthmatic agent, has both beta$_1$ and beta$_2$-stimulating capacities. It acts rapidly (within a few minutes) and has a relatively short duration of action. One of its breakdown products, 1-3 methoxyisoproterenol, is known to be a weak beta blocker. Therefore, it is conceivable that nebulized isoproterenol, especially when over-used, may act in a paradoxical manner and produce bronchospasm. Recent developments have made available new beta$_2$ preferential stimulators including terbutaline, metaproterenol, and isoetharine. Metaproterenol (Alupent) produces prolonged bronchodilatation associated with few of the beta$_1$ side effects. It is available in both oral and inhalation forms. Terbutaline and salbutamol are both more potent beta$_2$ stimulators than metaproterenol and may be administered by the oral, subcutaneous, and inhalation routes. One common side effect is muscle tremor which subsides following continuous treatment.

Expectorants

Expectorants are thought to increase the flow and clearance, of the respiratory tract mucous, as well as decrease its viscosity. Acute asthma results in the production of thick, tenacious mucous that often plays an important role in the pathophysiology of the disease. Oral or intravenous fluids increase the clearance of respiratory mucous and are considered by many to be the best expectorants. Both iodides and glyceryl guaiacolate have become the primary expectorants used in the treatment of asthma either alone or in combination with other anti-asthmatic drugs. There is evidence that glyceryl guaiacolate is not an effective expectorant in the normal dosage range. Iodides also do not seem to be effective expectorants.

Cromolyn Sodium

Cromolyn sodium (Intal, Aarane) unlike the preceding medications, does not appear to affect the level of cyclic AMP or directly cause bronchodilatation, rather it appears to prevent mast cell release of mediators through stabilization of the cellular membrane. Cromolyn sodium is inhaled as a powder which coats the respiratory mucosa. It is generally not effective when administered to patients having signs of acute asthma. When given prior to the onset of wheezing it may have a preventive action. The drug is expensive and usually requires long-term use. Efficacy may be delayed for 2–3 weeks after treatment has been initiated. In addition, the child must be able to inhale the drug properly. Side effects are limited to coughing, sore throat, skin rashes; pulmonary infiltrates have been reported rarely.

Corticosteroids

The mechanism by which corticosteroids produce striking relief of asthmatic symptoms is not well understood. Steroids appear to function in several ways including: stabilization of cell membranes, prevention of lysozomal enzyme release, potentiation of sympathomimetics on the B_2 receptor in asthmatics with an increase in cyclic AMP, and suppression of the cellular inflammatory response. Corticosteroids do not block antigen-induced immediate type allergic asthma but can prevent the late response that is often seen 4–6 hours after antigen inhalation. The suppression of late asthmatic responses may be due, in part, to corticosteroid suppression of the responding inflammatory cell accumulation at the reaction site.

Certain synthetic corticosteroids have a prolonged duration of action (e.g., dexamethasone) as a result of both long plasma and biological half-lives. Steroid preparation such as prednisone and prednisolone have shorter half-lives and may be administered as a single dose every other morning in an attempt to avoid hypothalmic-pituitary-adrenal (HPA) axis suppression. In contrast, daily treatment with doses as low as 2.5 mg. given on a daily basis has been shown to suppress the HPA-axis in children. Recently, an inhaled steroid, beclomethasone has been introduced for the treatment of bronchial asthma. Because of its high topical activity, a local therapeutic benefit can be derived at a dose small enough to avoid HPA-axis suppression or suppression of linear growth.

THERAPEUTIC APPROACH IN THE MANAGEMENT OF BRONCHIAL ASTHMA

The Acute Attack of Asthma

The presentation of a dyspneic wheezing asthmatic child is a commonly encountered clinical situation facing physicians who treat children. The following medical regimen is used in many pediatric centers:

Moist oxygen is administered by mask or nasal cannula. Subcutaneous injections of epinephrine are given every 15–20 minutes (usually two injections suffice, but 15 per cent of asthmatics who do not respond to two respond to three). Most patients respond and are sent home with a long-acting injection of epinephrine (Sus-phrine) as well as oral theophylline. Non-responders are hydrated and administered intravenous theophylline. Patients not responding to the foregoing treatment are considered to be in status asthmaticus and are admitted to the hospital. Radiographs are taken to rule out complications of asthma. Imbalance of fluids, electrolytes and/or pH are corrected. Patients not responding at this stage require intravenous corticosteroids. Children in status asthmaticus are continuously monitored utilizing clinical scoring, arterial blood gasses, and/or pulsus paradoxus. Asthmatic children entering respiratory failure will require further therapy with either intravenous isoproterenol or artificial mechanical ventilation. As the acute attack subsides, percussion and postural drainage, expectorants, and IPPB±Isuprel may be employed.

Subacute and Chronic Asthma

Therapy is initiated with a single oral theophylline preparation at a dose of 5 mg./kg. given 4 times a day. Clinical response with or without serum theophylline levels indicates the need for dosage adjustment. It should be noted that the metabolism of theophylline may vary greatly from one child to another, therefore individualization of dosage may be required.

Sympathomimetic agents are added to the regimen of non-responders. Oral preparations such as ephedrine, metaproterenol, terbutaline, etc., offer an oral, and in the case of metaproterenol and isoproterenol, an inhaled delivery system. Inhaled sympathomimetics often can reverse dramatically acute asthma early in the episode. The inhaler is preferably kept under parental control because of the propensity for abuse.

Children with continuing signs of asthma should receive a course of cromolyn sodium therapy. It is administered as an inhaled powder four times a day for at least a 1-month trial period. It is used solely as a preventative medication and not during a wheezing episode. Children not controlled by cromolyn inhalation may be considered candidates for steroid therapy.

Corticosteroids may be given as short-term treatment for unresponsive exacerbations of bronchospasm or as part of a long-term program to control severe chronic asthma. In either case, information on the potential side effects of this potent medication should be supplied to parents.

Short-Term Steroid Treatment. At one time or another, a number of asthmatic children develop marked obstructive respiratory symptoms either as an intermittent paroxysm of bronchospasm or as an exacerbation of chronic asthma despite the use of conservative treatment. Under these circumstances a short term (3–5 day) course for a short-acting steroid preparation (prednisone) may be administered at a dose of 2 mg./kg./day in divided doses.

Long-Term Steroid Therapy. Less frequently, asthmatic children will have recurrent acute attacks and/or chronic disability despite the proper use of all the previous mentioned medications. Under such circumstances long-term steroid therapy in addition to conservative therapy (i.e., theophylline, sympathomimetics) may be necessary to control symptoms.

Beclomethasone, a highly active steroid, can be used in an inhaled form that suppresses asthmatic symptoms while minimizing systemic side effects. Beclomethasone (Vanceril) is inhaled in very small amounts (100–400 μg./dose) up to four times per day. Of course, if the recommended dosage is exceeded, systemic side effects may occur.

Long-term oral steroid treatment should be considered either as continuous or alternate day therapy for those failing to respond to inhaled beclomethasone. The preferred alternate day course may be instituted by administering double the daily dosage as a single dose every other morning. And finally, the remaining individuals with persistent symptoms require daily steroid therapy with all its possible side effects.

A Partial List of Corticosteroid Complications

Cushingoid features including:
    acne, moonface, facial plethora, central obesity, striae, etc.
Suppression of linear growth and osteoporosis
Suppression of the HPA-axis
Muscle weakness and cramps
Subcapsular cataracts and glaucoma
Psychotic reactions
Pseudotumor cerebri
Hypertension
Peptic ulceration
Pancreatitis

It should be remembered that steroid dependent asthmatics require additional steroid during stressful periods (surgery, status asthmaticus, etc.) if a medical catastrophe is to be avoided. The state of steroid dependence may persist 1 year beyond the cessation of daily steroid therapy.

General Supportive Therapy

Hydration, expectorants, and percussion and postural drainage can significantly aid in the mobilization of tenacious bronchial secretions. Exercise-induced bronchospasm may be prevented with the pre-exercise use of theophylline, inhaled sympathomimetics, or Cromolyn. In general, the patient should receive enough therapy to permit him to function in a normal manner. Asthmatic children should be encouraged to participate in sports and other physical activities as long as their asthma is under control.

PROGNOSIS

As bronchial asthma is a highly variable disease, it is impossible to predict accurately its course in any individual child. Between one-half to two-thirds of affected children will be free of bronchospastic symptoms as adults.

Those children who develop severe chronic asthma often have a history of an early onset of their disease (usually before the age of 3 years) and have persistent abnormal pulmonary functions. Children who "outgrow" their asthma frequently suffer persistent allergic rhinitis and conjunctivitis. Another group of individuals with a history of resolved childhood asthma experience the onset of intrinsic asthma as adults.

BIBLIOGRAPHY

Pride, N. B.: Physiology. *In* Clark, T. J. H. and Godrey, S. (eds.): Asthma. Philadelphia, W. B. Saunders, 1977.

> An excellent review of pulmonary function tests and their use in the identification and interpretation of asthma.

Szentnanyi, A., and Fischel, C.: The Beta adrenergic theory and cyclic AMP-mediated control mechanism in human asthma. *In* Weiss, E. B., and Segal, M. S. (eds.): Bronchial Asthma, Mechanisms and Therapeutics. Boston, Little, Brown, 1976.

> A scholarly review of the Beta adrenergic blockage theory in asthma as well as a discussion of drug treatment and its effect on cyclic AMP.

Pediatric Allergy. Pediatr. Clin. North Am., *22*:1, 1975.

> This edition contains review articles on B-adrenergic bronchodilators, cromolyn sodium, Beclomethasone, and the treatment of status asthmaticus.

Lichtenstein, L. M., Ishizaka, K. Norman, P. S., Scbodka, A. K., and Hill, B. M.: IgE antibody measurements in ragweed hayfever. Relationship to clinical severity and the results of immunotherapy. J. Clin. Invest., *52*:472, 1973.

> A careful study of the effects of "allergy shots" in relation to suppression of symptoms and immunologic changes.

27

Common Allergic Disorders

Eliot Dunsky, M.D.

The term allergy or hypersensitivity disease includes a large and heterogenous group of immunologically mediated adverse reactions induced by either antigens or haptens. Antigens are high molecular weight complexes, usually containing protein, that elicit a specific immune response involving antibodies or immune lymphocytes. Haptens are low molecular weight substances that become antigens only when they combine with larger "carrier" molecules. Not all antigens cause allergic reactions. Those that do are referred to as allergens.

Many diseases can mimic closely the symptoms of allergy, just as allergy can simulate a disease of non-immunologic origin. In order to correctly label a child's malady as allergic in origin, an attempt to define the immunologic basis of the disease or reaction must be made. Within this context, symptoms alone may be misleading as to the origin of the disease. For example, gastrointestinal symptoms immediately following the ingestion of a specific food may be due to an enzyme deficiency rather than allergy (e.g., dissacharidase deficiency and milk ingestion) or "pneumonia" may be the result of allergic asthma rather than an infectious etiology.

THE IMMUNOPATHOLOGY OF ALLERGY

The main function of the immune system appears to be one of protection. However, under certain circumstances the immune response works to the detriment of the host. In allergic disease the host suffers an adverse reaction due to an altered or hyperresponsive immune response. In the case of autoimmunity an immune response is directed, at least in part, against the host's own tissue which has been perceived as foreign antigen.

In man, the components of an immunologic response may be divided into two basic groups: the humoral (antibody) and the cellular (lymphocyte) systems. Characteristically, the response of either or both systems is directed against the stimulating antigen with great specificity. This highly specialized defense mechanism begins with the differentiations of a primordial stem cell in the bone marrow. The totipotential stem cell undergoes differentiation into either B-cells (under the influence of the bursal equivalent) or T-cells (under influence of the thymus) (Fig. 27-1). B-cells further differentiate into plasma cells, which upon appropriate antigenic stimulation produce a specific antibody against a stimulating antigen. The immunoglobulins (antibodies) are plasma protein molecules composed of four pairs of polypeptide chains, two identical heavy chains and two identical light chains. When intact, the antibody configuration appears to be similar to the letter "Y" (Fig. 27-2).

The heavy chains may have a molecular weight of approximately 53,000 and the light chain a molecular weight of 22,000 (i.e., IgG). The linked heavy chain forms the entire length of the molecule, while the light chains parallel the heavy chains for only a section of their length, forming part of the two arm's of the "Y". These two arms of the "Y" are known as the Fab fragments and act as receptor sites for antigenic determinants. The foot of the "Y" or the Fc portion is adapted to attach to a cell surface.

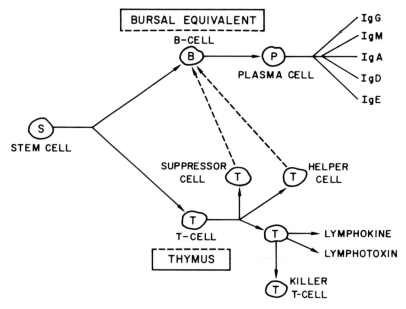

Fig. 27-1. The immune system, humoral and cellular aspects.

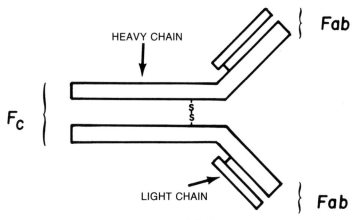

HEAVY CHAIN

Fab

F_c

LIGHT CHAIN

Fab

Fig. 27-2. Immunoglobulin structure.

Immunoglobulins

Depending on the characterization of their heavy chain, immunoglob-ulins can be divided into five classes (IgM, IgG, IgA, IgD, and IgE). IgM plays an important role in the primary immune response and usually is present in the form of a pentamer (five units joined together). Although this antibody is not as selective as IgG, it is more rapidly synthesized during the initial contact with the antigenic stimulus. IgG is the major immunoglobulin of the intravascular system. It plays its most significant role during the secondary or anamnestic immune response. IgG's speci-ficity and avidity for a given antigen is much greater than that of IgM. IgA is the major secretory immunoglobulin. Two units of IgA and their secretory piece are found in mucosal secretions and saliva; it is thought to play an important role in protecting the mucosal portals of entry. The role of IgD remains obscure. Immunoglobulin E plays a central role in immediate type allergic reactions. Even though it is present in extremely small amounts in the blood, it has the ability to attach selectively and remain fixed to mast cells and basophils for prolonged periods. The res-piratory mucosa is richly endowed with mast cells, and as might be expected, it is one of the most common sites for allergic reactions. Chil-dren with defective antibody production, particularly with diminished IgG, suffer from recurrent bacterial infections.

Delayed Response Mechanism

The other half of the dual system of immunity is the delayed or cell-mediated response mechanism that is mediated by specifically sensitized lymphocytes without the aid of immunoglobulins. Totipotential stem-cells in the bone marrow circulate through the thymus, and under influ-ence of the thymic hormone thymosin, evolve into T-lymphocytes (T-cells, Fig. 27-1). In man, these cells may be characterized *in vitro* by their ability to spontaneously form rosettes with sheep erythrocytes (E-rosettes) and undergo lymphoblastic transformation following concavalin A (con A) or phytohemagglutinin (PHA) stimulation. T-lymphocytes are resposible for rejection of foreign tissue grafts, contact dermatitis, reaction to invasion by certain bacteria (e.g., tuberculosis), viruses (e.g., measles), fungi (e.g., candida), and play an important role in the suppression of tumor growth.

In addition, T-cells indirectly regulate immunoglobulin synthesis by enhancing or suppressing the B-cell/plasma cell system production of antibodies (by means of T-helper or T-suppressor cells). Certain small T-lymphocytes are thought to be long-lived memory cells, which could explain the phenomenon of life long immunity (e.g., measles). When appropriately stimulated, T-lymphocytes can release soluble mediators that participate in the cellular defense mechanism in a number of ways. For example, migration inhibition factor (MIF) inhibits the migration of macrophages and therefore induces their accumulation at the site of inflammation. The T-cell may destroy the foreign cell (killer T-cell), "arm" macrophages by committing them to destroy another specific cell, or by secretion of a lymphotoxin directly kill the target cell (Fig. 27-1).

Circulating Serum Proteins

Aside from the specific sensitized responses of the immune system, there are a number of circulating serum proteins that may participate in and amplify immune reactions. A good example of this is the complement system which consists of 11 fluid phase proteins that upon activation bind to an antigen-antibody complex. Complement activation can take place by at least two pathways. The first or classical pathway necessitates the initial attachment of a subunit of the first component of complement (C_{1q}) to the Fc portion of the immunoglobin (IgG or IgM) in the antigen-antibody complex. The ensuing structural changes cause C_{1r} to enzymatically activate C_{1s} and the cascade begins. Activated C_{1qrs} initiates a cascade of the remaining complement components in the following order: C_4, C_2, C_3, C_5, C_6, C_7, C_8 and C_9.

The alternate pathway bypasses the classical initiation of the complement cascade via C_1. Instead, with the aid of the properdin system (that can be activated by aggregated IgA, bacterial polysaccharide and endotoxin lipopolysaccharides) C_3 is directly activated (bypassing C_1, C_4 and C_2) and from this point the cascade continues exactly as in the classical pathway.

Certain complement cascade products have specific biologic activities that play an important role in certain immunologic reactions in man. Soluble products of C_3 (C_{3a}) and C_5 (C_{5a}) are anaphylatoxins that cause mast cells to release histamine and can therefore simulate anaphylaxis and other immediate type allergic reactions. C_{3a} and C_{5a} are also chemotactic for inflammatory cells as is the C_{567} complex. Other functions of complement include viral neutralization and enhanced immune adherence (C_{3b}). The final attack sequence, including the activation of the terminal components C_8 and C_9, culminates in damage or lysis to the cellular membrane.

Classification of Allergic Response

To better conceptualize the various kinds of immune reactions, Gell and Coombs classified hypersensitivity responses into four basic categories (Fig. 27-3).

Type I or Immediate Hypersensitivity. Immediate hypersensitivity represents the immunologic basis of extrinsic (allergic) asthma, hayfever,

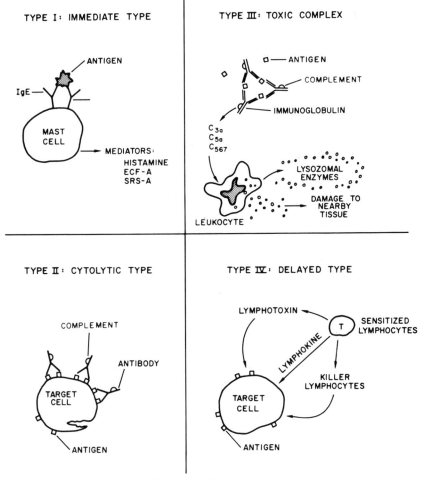

Fig. 27-3. Classification of hypersensitivity reactions.

anaphylactic reactions, and urticaria. Individuals suffering from these diseases apparently have the genetic potential, upon exposure to the appropriate antigen, to produce a specific antibody of the immunoglobulin E class (IgE). IgE has a number of special characteristics that include: (1) the ability to passively transfer hypersensitivity for up to 6 weeks in a normal individual; (2) its biologic activity is lost upon heating for 1–4 hours at 56°C; and (3) it does not fix complement.

IgE fixes firmly to the surface of mast cells and basophils by its Fc receptor. Mast cells are found in abundance in the respiratory mucosa, the gastrointestinal tract and the skin. When the specific antigen binds to IgE molecules on the surface of the mast cell, a number of biochemical events occur that ultimately cause the release of biologic mediators. These events and their clinical sequelae occur within a matter of minutes and hence the term immediate hypersensitivity. Although the antigen-IgE complex initiates the mechanism of mediator release, their final release is modulated by the cell's cyclic nucleotide concentrations (e.g., cyclic adenosine monophophate) (see Chapter 26). Among the mediators released are:

1. *Histamine*—a vasoactive amine which causes increased capillary permeability, edema, increased secretions of bronchial mucosa, and smooth muscle contraction. Its action on the target organ is blocked by antihistamines.

2. *Slow reactive substance of anaphylaxis* (SRS-A)—An acidic lipid of low molecular weight, is considered to be an important mediator producing prolonged smooth muscle contractions that are not blocked by antihistamines.

3. *Eosinophilic chemotactic factor of anaphylaxis* (ECF-A)—A polypeptide (molecular weight of about 500) that preferentially attracts eosinophils to the site of its release. The presence of ECF-A could explain the large number of eosinophils found at the site of an immediate hypersensitivity reaction.

Histamine and ECF-A are preformed and stored as granules within basophils and mast cells, while SRS-A is synthesized upon stimulation. The release of these mediators as a group can produce prolonged bronchospasm, swelling of the bronchial mucosa, hypersecretion of mucous within the bronchial lumen, and an influx of inflammatory cells—in short, the pathology of asthma. Mediator release in the skin can cause hives, while systemic release can result in anaphylaxis.

Type II or the Cytotoxic Reaction. This second type of reaction is due to antibodies, usually of the IgG or IgM class, directed against antigens or haptens on the cell membrane. These antigenic determinants may be absorbed onto the cell surface or be an intrinsic part of the cell membrane. In type II reactions the Fab portion of the molecule binds to the cell surface. Complement may then fix to the Fc portion of the bound antibody, and its activation under these conditions can result in damage or lysis to the cell membrane. Other cellular circulating elements so coated with antibody and fixed complement may be made more susceptible to phagocytosis and removal by the reticuloendothelial system rather than undergo lysis.

Clinical examples of the cytotoxic reactions include the hemolytic anemias of the newborn (Rh and ABO incompatibility) where maternal antibody (IgG) is directed against the newborn's RBC, transfusion reactions, Penicillin-induced hemolytic anemia, and Goodpasture's Syndrome. In the last example antibodies are produced against antigenic determinants on the pulmonary and glomerular basement membranes.

Type III or Toxic-Complex Reations. The type III reactions occur when circulating soluble antigen-antibody complexes are deposited in tissues.

If the amount of soluble circulating antigen is in slight excess to the amount of available antibody (IgG or IgM), soluble microcomplexes may be formed. Although they are small enough to avoid removal from the circulation by the reticuloendothelial system, they eventually settle in small blood vessels or the glomeruli of the kidney. Following tissue deposition, complement may bind to the Fc portion of the antibody within the complex. The ensuing complement cascade causes the release of chemotactic factors (C_{3a} and C_{5a}) that attract polymorphonuclear leukocytes. The lysosomal enzymes released by these leukocytes cause the actual damage to nearby cells and tissues. In addition, anaphylatoxins, also by-products of the complement cascade, cause local vasodilation and increased vascular permeability, thus permitting further immune complex deposition and continuing local inflammation.

Type IV Reaction, Delayed or Cellular Hypersensitivity. This fourth type of reaction is referred to as delayed hypersensitivity since the peak of the reaction usually occurs 24–72 hours following antigen exposure. Specifically sensitized T-lymphocytes, without the aid of immunoglobulin or complement, recognize antigens that have been processed by macrophages and react by either destroying the cell bearing these antigenic determinants or by secreting lymphokines.

Appropriately stimulated sensitized lymphocytes undergo lymphoblastic transformation and secrete soluble mediators called lymphokines (e.g., migration inhibition factor or MIF). Lymphokines may recruit macrophages and non-sensitized lymphocytes to the reaction site. Other lymphokines activate macrophages or lymphocytes against the foreign antigen. Still other lymphoblasts secrete lymphotoxin that directly damages the target cell.

Examples of delayed hypersensitivity include: contact dermatitis, tuberculin reaction, and foreign skin graft rejection.

Atopic Disease. The term atopy is used to describe a group of allergic disorders in which the affected children have a predisposition to developing immediate-type hypersensitivity to various environmental antigens. Atopic diseases include asthma, hayfever, urticaria (hives), and atopic dermatitis (infantile eczema). Although there appears to be a genetic basis for the development of atopy (many patients have some similarly affected relatives), the exact mode of inheritance is not clear. Atopic disorders are usually associated with the increased production of IgE against various antigens and the development of immediate hypersensitivity reactions. Atopy to both ingested and inhaled allergens tends to begin early in childhood. About 10–15 per cent of the population suffer from atopy. Allergic rhinitis and conjunctivitis are among the most common forms of atopy. Food allergy tends to occur early in infancy, while inhalent allergy tends to occur more frequently following infancy. Atopic disease, such as atopic dermatitis, is associated with a high incidence of allergic disease in the affected patient; nevertheless atopic dermatitis does not appear to be caused by an IgE mediated or any known allergic mechanism. Therefore in this latter case, "atopy" is used to refer to the high incidence of allergy in these patients rather than the etiology of the disease.

ALLERGIC RHINITIS AND CONJUNCTIVITIS

About 10 per cent of the population is affected at some time by the symptoms of allergic rhinitis or conjunctivitis. Symptoms may be present throughout the year (perennial allergic rhinitis, conjunctivitis) or they may have a seasonal periodicity (seasonal allergic rhinitis, conjunctivitis).

Seasonal symptoms are most often related to the release of pollen into the atmosphere during the spring and summer. The release of spores from molds growing on decaying vegetations during the summer may also produce a seasonal pattern. On the other hand, perennial symptoms may be related to allergens in the home, namely: house dust, mold spores (released from damp basements), or animal danders.

Common Inhaled Allergens

Pollen. Only pollen that is relatively small (10–40 μm) and light in weight can become airborn and be dispersed widely. Certain trees, grasses and weeds release such pollen, while pollen from flowers are so heavy as not to play much of a role in inhalant allergy. Depending on geography and climatic conditions, trees pollinate in the spring, grasses in the summer, and weeds in the summer and fall.

Molds. Fungal spores are present in the atmosphere throughout most of the year except when the ground is covered with snow. They reach their peak concentration during the late summer months when dead vegetation and a warm humid climate produce optimal growth conditions. Molds may also be found year round in the home. They tend to proliferate in damp areas (e.g., wet basement, bath area). Mold-sensitive patients have either a seasonal or perennial pattern depending on their sensitivity to specific molds and their exposure pattern.

Dust. House dust is a common indoor allergen. It is a product of partially decomposed epidermoid tissue, hair, bacteria, insects (mites) and other organic material (cotton linters from bedding, etc).

Animal Dander. Shedded epithelium from dog, cats, and other domestic animals can be potent allergens. Sensitive children have symptoms when exposed to the animal or the room in which the animal had been present. Even animal products such as horse hair in stuffed furniture or cattle hair in rug padding may induce symptoms.

Foods are not a common cause of respiratory allergy. In general, the few patients who have respiratory symptoms as a result of food allergy also have gastrointestinal, dermal, or anaphylactic symptoms. Food allergy will be discussed in greater detail later in this chapter.

Allergic Rhinitis

Symptoms may vary from occasional mild nasal stuffiness to an incapacitating chronic nasal obstruction and its associated complications (e.g., serous otitis media). Affected children may have a history of multiple paroxysms of sneezing, nasal congestion, nasal pruritis, and anterior and/or posterior nasal discharge. It is typical for these children to chronically rub their noses with an upward and outward movement of the palm of the hand. In so doing, the soft anterior third of the nose bends back forming a transverse nasal crease between the rigid upper two-thirds and the soft lower third of the nose. The nose rubbing maneuver is known as the "allergic salute" and the resulting nasal crease helps identify these allergic children. Patients may also complain of pruritis of the throat and ears. Many of these symptoms may be erroneously attributed to recurrent colds. When the obstruction is severe, the child becomes an obligate mouth breather. This may be associated with changes in phonation, postnasal drip, sore throat, hoarseness, and chronic cough. Allergic rhinitis may also be associated with recurrent serous otitis media and hearing loss. The physical examination reveals: (1) the presence of a transverse nasal crease, swollen and pale inferior nasal turbinates that may have a bluish discoloration; (2) clear mucoid discharge; (3) edema and bluish black discoloration of the skin just beneath the inferior border of both orbits ("allergic shiners"); and (4) mouth breathing and posterior pharyngeal lymphoid hypertrophy.

Allergic Conjunctivitis

This disorder may be associated with allergic rhinitis or occur independently. The symptoms are usually seasonal, but may be perennial. Affected children complain of pruritic conjunctivae, conjunctival discharge and in some cases photophobia. The child constantly rubs his eyes. The conjunctival blood vessels are injected and the inferior palpebral conjunctiva may demonstrate follicular lymphoid hyperplasia (which is often referred to as "cobblestoning"). Vernal conjunctivitis is a much more severe form of allergic conjunctivitis that appears each spring and summer. Patients characteristically have marked "cobblestoning" of the upper palpebral conjunctivae or develop an opacity at the corneal-scleral junction. Such lesions may damage the cornea and affect vision.

The diagnosis of allergic rhinitis and conjunctivitis may be confirmed with the aid of the following tests:

1. Nasal and conjunctival smear for eosinophils. Eosinophils are usually present in the secretions of the target organ. It should be remembered that eosinophils may be present in the secretions of normal infants up until the age of 6 months.

2. Allergy skin testing will help identify the specific offending allergen.

3. An elevated total IgE would be supportive of the diagnosis; however, many patients with allergic rhinitis and conjunctivitis have normal levels of this serum immunoglobulin.

The Differential Diagnosis of Allergic Rhinitis

Vasomotor rhinitis is a perennial rhinitis that does not have an underlying immunologic mechanism. Symptoms consist of chronic nasal congestion and rhinorrhea that is often provoked by nonspecific stimuli such as dust, chemicals, sudden temperature changes, etc.

Foreign bodies are occasionally placed in the nasal passage by a small child. It soon creates a local inflammatory reaction that produces a purulent, foul-smelling rhinorrhea.

Recurrent Colds. It is not uncommon for young children to have four to six colds per year. The symptoms of rhinorrhea may be associated with fever. Eosinophils are not abundant in the nasal mucosa nor is the typical history of pruritis noted.

Rhinitis Medicamentosa. Chronic use of sympathomimetic nasal drops has been associated with a syndrome of tachyphylaxis to the decongestant requiring frequent and increased dose administration as well as worsening nasal congestion. The rhinitis eventually subsides after the medication is discontinued.

Nasal polyps may occur spontaneously, or may be associated with chronic rhinitis of any etiology, aspirin intolerance, and cystic fibrosis.

A skull fracture involving the cribiform plate may cause persistent rhinorrhea as a consequence of cerebrospinal fluid (CSF) leakage; such cases are rare. These children may have a history of recurrent bacterial meningitis. Nasal mucous does not contain glucose, while CSF does. A dip stick indicating glucose in the nasal discharge confirms the diagnosis.

Treatment

Avoidance of contact with the allergen. Certain allergens can be completely avoided once identified. Foods can be eliminated from the diet, or a pet removed from the home. Dust control at home can significantly dimish the amount of allergen exposure. However, a number of allergens (e.g., pollen) cannot be effectively eliminated and therefore treatment will be required.

Antihistamines. Many medications have antihistaminic activity; they inhibit histamine's action of increasing capillary permeability, smooth muscle contraction, and induction of pruritis by competition for the H_1 receptor site on the target organ. Antihistamines do not effect H_2 receptor sites that can control gastric acid secretion. Since histamine is a major mediator of urticaria, allergic rhinitis, conjunctivitis, and pruritis in general, antihistamines have become the most popular therapeutic modality in the treatment of these diseases. The five groups of antihistamines include: (1) ethylenediamines—tripelennamine (Pyribenzamine), (2) alkylamines—chlorpheniramine (Chlor-trimeton), (3) *ethanolamines*—diphenhydramine (Benadryl), (4) *piperazine*—hydroxyzine (Atarax), and (5) *phenothiazides*—promethazine (Phenergan).

Antihistamine side effects include sedation, anticholinergic symptoms (dry mouth), gastrointestinal disturbances, central nervous system stimulation and drowsiness.

Sympathomimetics can be used both topically and orally. Topical therapy is generally avoided except for allergic conjunctivitis because of tachyphylaxis and rebound symptoms (rhinitis) associated with its prolonged usage. Oral sympathomimetics such as pseudoephedrine and Phenylephrine can be used alone or in combination with an antihistamine to reduce nasal and conjunctival congestion.

Cromolyn sodium, an inhibitor of mast cell degranulation, has been used with some success in the treatment of allergic rhinitis.

Corticosteroids. Topical steroids (dexamethasone or beclomethasone) are sprayed two–four times per day onto the nasal mucosa. This is an effective form of therapy for the more severe cases of allergic rhinitis, but may be associated with a number of side effects (e.g., septal perforation).

HMS Liquifilm (medrysone 1%) and similar steroids that do not have a tendency to raise intraoccular pressure are used in the topical treatment of severe allergic conjunctivitis and vernal conjunctivitis. Oral steroids are only used for short-term treatment of very severe cases. Injected long-acting depot steroids have no place in the treatment of this disease.

Hyposensitization. Allergy injection therapy is the only effective therapy that can actually cure allergic rhinitis and conjunctivitis. Indications include failure to suppress symptoms with conservative treatment (antihistamines/sympathomimetics) and intolerance or other adverse effects from these medications. This subject will be discussed in greater detail in the next section.

ALLERGY SKIN TESTING AND HYPOSENSITIZATION

Allergy Skin Testing

Allergy skin testing was developed empirically long before its immunologic basis was discovered. We now know that when an allergen comes in contact with sensitive individual's abraded skin a wheal and flare (hive) reaction occurs within 15 minutes. The immunologic basis of this phenomenon is an IgE-mediated immediate hypersensitivity reaction. A number of different methods for the introduction of the allergen are currently employed.

The scratch test involves a superficial scratching of the skin followed by a drop of a concentrated allergen placed on the abrasion. The more sensitive intradermal method necessitates the intradermal injection of a minute amount (0.02 ml.) of dilute antigen within the epidermis.

Both positive (histamine or histamine liberators) and negative controls are necessary for the proper interpretation of results. The more sensitive or allergic the individual, the larger the wheal and flare at a lower concentration of test allergen. However, a positive skin test only suggests the presence of specific IgE in the skin; only when positive skin tests correlate with the clinical history can the results afford the opportunity to identify allergen as an etiologic agent in the disease.

Common allergens used for testing include: trees, grasses, weeds, molds, dust, feathers, animal dander (dog, cat), foods, etc.

Hyposensitization

When allergen avoidance is impractical and conservative medical therapy unsuccessful in the suppression of the atopic symptoms of allergic asthma, allergic rhinitis, or allergic conjunctivitis, hyposensitization to the offending allergen should be considered.

Success in hyposensitization depends upon the correct selection of the offending allergen, the use of biologically potent allergen extracts, adequate dosage administration and appropriate frequency of injection.

Allergy injections are initiated at very dilute concentrations and the dosage increased on a weekly basis. The dose is increased until a maintenance level is reached. Improvement of symptoms with immunotherapy is slow and often not evident during the first 6 months. Side effects include both local and anaphylactic reactions.

Individuals with symptomatic improvement also undergo immunologic change including a rise in IgG blocking antibody, a loss of sensitivity to antigen-induced basophil histamine release, a decline in the level of specific IgE after a number of years of treatment, and a suppression of the rise of the level of specific IgE that normally occurs with each new seasonal exposure to the antigen.

URTICARIA AND ANGIOEDEMA

Urticaria (hives) can be defined as a disorder of the skin characterized by transient, erythematous, pruritic, superficial eruptions usually associated with an elevated central wheal. Angioedema is similar to urticaria; however, the deeper subcutaneous tissues are also involved.

Urticaria has two forms: acute and chronic. Acute urticaria is usually of short duration, often lasting less than a week. Urticaria persisting beyond 6 weeks is considered chronic. The hive itself is transient and often lasts less than 24 hours. It may be a discrete wheal and flare reaction taking a circular form, or the hives may coalesce to cover a large area of skin.

Angioedema usually involves swelling of the skin and subcutaneous tissues. The mucosal lining of the gastrointestinal tract as well as the upper airway may be affected similarly. In the latter case, death may occur due to asphyxia.

Immunologic Mechanism

An intradermal injection of histamine or a mast cell degranulator elicits the formation of a hive within 15 minutes. Histamine is an important vasoactive mediator stored in dermal mast cells that can be released during certain immunologic reactions. The IgE-mediated immediate hypersensitivity reaction (type I) has been implicated clearly in many cases of urticaria. Dermal biopsies often reveal an eosinophilic infiltration into the lesion. Histamine may also be released from mast cells during the complement cascade by the action of anaphylatoxin (C_{3a}, C_{5a}). Complement can be activated during type II and type III reaction or by the alternate pathway. However, many cases of urticaria have no clearly defined immunologic basis; therefore, urticaria appears to be heterogenic from a mechanistic point of view.

Etiological Factors

Allergens that are either ingested or injected are often the cause of urticaria while inhalant allergens are an uncommonly involved cause. Drugs are among the most frequently identified etiologic factors in urticaria. The lesions may appear within minutes following exposure or there may be a delay for days or weeks. Among the more frequently implicated drugs are: penicillin, sulfonamides and mast cell degranulators (e.g., codeine). The ingestion of certain foods can be associated with urticaria on an allergic basis. Foods commonly involved include: milk, egg, cola drinks, peanuts, citrus fruits, chocolate, fish, seafood, and strawberries. Food coloring (tartrazine yellow dye) and preservatives (benzoic acid) also have precipitated and prolonged urticarial reactions on a non-immunologic basis. Aspirin can also cause hives on a non-immunologic basis. Injectable drugs and vaccines as well as insect stings and bites may result in urticaria. Infections including viral (infectious hepatitis, infectious mononucleosis), bacterial (abscess, U.T.I.), and fungal (tinea pedis), as well as parasitic infestations are documented causes of hives.

Cholinergic urticaria is characterized by multiple tiny hives often provoked by exercise, over-heating, sweating, and emotional stress.

Physical urticarias are hives induced by cold, heat, pressure stroking (dermatographism), and light (actinic urticaria).

One should also bear in mind that urticaria may be the initial manifestation of an underlying disease state such as a malignancy (e.g., Hodgkin's) or a connective tissue disorder (e.g., systemic lupus erythematosis or periarteritis nodosa).

Differential Diagnosis

Urticaria Pigmentosa. These hives are associated with a local dermal accumulation of mast cells that present as slightly elevated brown pigmented macules or placques. When the lesion is stroked, hives appear locally.

Papular Urticaria. These are small pruritic papules that may present initially as a hive following an insect bite. Lesions usually last a number of days and have a tell-tale puncture in the center of the lesion.

Erythema Multiforme. Although hives may be present, other target lesions or iris lesions usually characterize this skin disorder.

Hereditary angioedema is an inherited disease characterized by recurrent episodes of angioedema. The swelling can involve the skin, the GI tract (abdominal cramps) or the respiratory mucosa (upper airway obstruction). There may be a family history of angioedema or a history of family members who died of asphyxia. Lesions are often precipitated by minor trauma. The disease is due to a deficiency of C_1-esterase inhibitor level.

Treatment of Urticaria

Obviously, identification and elimination of the etiologic antigen would be ideal. Unfortunately, no etiology is found in up to three-quarters of patients with chronic urticaria. Therefore, treatment is symptomatic. Antihistamines (hydroxyzine or chlorpheniramine) often provide some relief. Most cases of acute urticaria subside without an etiologic diagnosis.

Extensive urticarial lesions (giant urticaria) and angioedema may require treatment with epinephrine in acute situations. Steroids are indicated only under extraordinary circumstances.

ANAPHYLAXIS AND INSECT ALLERGY

Anaphylaxis is a systemic form of immediate hypersensitivity. Most of these reactions are believed to be an IgE-mediated (type I) reaction associated with the release of vasoactive substances. Other immunologic reactions (type II and type III) are capable of fixing complement and releasing anaphylatoxins (C_{3a}, and C_{5a}) as well as kinin-like substances (C_{2b}). The systemic release of vasoactive mediators can produce increased capillary permeability, peripheral vasodilation, bronchospasm, and severe hypotension.

Etiology

Almost any allergen can cause an anaphylactic reaction. The route of allergen administration plays an important role. Injection of allergens is more likely to cause anaphylaxis than oral or topical administration of the same allergen.

Drugs. Drugs are among the most common causes of anaphylaxis, Penicillin and its derivatives being prime offenders. Injected drugs such as foreign serums, hyposensitization serum, vaccines, enzymes as well as other proteins, are particularly potent inducers of anaphylaxis.

Intravenous radio contrast material can cause anaphylaxis or an anaphylactoid reaction. The latter has no immunologic basis and is thought to be related to the chemical liberation of histamine.

Chemical Histamine Releasers. Certain drugs such as codeine, morphine, d-tubocurarine are chemical histamine releasers that cause anaphylactoid reactions. Clinically, these reactions may be similar to anaphylaxis.

Foods can induce anaphylaxis in sensitive individuals. Among the common foods implicated are egg white, nuts, and seafoods.

Insects. Bees, wasps, yellow jackets and hornets (hymenoptera species) are common causes of insect sting anaphylaxis (see below).

Clinical Features

The systemic anaphylactic reaction often begins within a few minutes following exposure to an allergen. The earlier the onset the more severe the reaction. The patient suddenly feels weak and ill, is pale, diaphoretic, and suffers from vertigo. Cardiovascular symptoms result from a combination of systemic vascular dilation as well as fluid loss through transudation, resulting in intravascular hypovolemia and hypotension. Patients can develop the signs and symptoms of cardiovascular shock (pallor, diaphoresis, cold extremities, hypotension, weak thready pulse, etc). If not treated promptly such an anaphylactic response may terminate in fatal irreversible shock. Respiratory signs and symptoms of anaphylaxis include dyspnea, chest tightness, wheezing, and asphyxia due to edema of the mucosa in the upper airway. Some patients develop generalized urticaria and/or angioedema. Edema of the gastrointestinal mucosa presents clinically as abdominal cramps and nausea. Severely affected patients may loose consciousness and become incontinent.

Treatment of Anaphylaxis

The best treatment is prevention. Previous drug reactions as well as adverse reactions to environmental antigens should be assessed carefully and the appropriate avoidance measures recommended.

The treatment of choice for an acute reaction is subcutaneous epinephrine (0.01 ml./kg. of 1:1000 epinephrine). Patients in shock with poor peripheral tissue perfusion may require cautious intravenous administration of epinephrine (1:10,000).

Should the allergen be an injectant or insect sting in an extremity, a tourniquet should be placed proximal to the site of entry. Patients having signs and/or symptoms of shock require the administration of large volumes of intravenous fluids. Resistant hypotension requires intravenous vasopressor treatment: metaraminol (Aramine) or levarterenol (Levophed). Oxygen can be delivered via a face mask or nasal prongs. Following these urgent procedures antihistamine can be administered; however, its efficacy in anaphylaxis is not clear.

Patients with bronchospasm will need oxygen and intravenous aminophylline, as in the treatment of acute asthma. Those individuals with laryngeal edema that produces obstruction of the upper airway should undergo tracheostomy. Corticosteroids can be helpful in the treatment of anaphylaxis; because their biological action does not become prominent for a number of hours, these are not the first drugs administered.

Insect Sting Reactions

Over the past 10 years 300–400 deaths have occurred in the United States as a result of insect stings. Anaphylaxis is most often associated with the stings of hymenoptera species (bees, wasps, hornets, and yellow jackets) and the fire ant. Although atopic individuals have a greater tendency to develop anaphylactic reactions, they also occur in non-atopics. Most insect stings, including those of hymenoptera, result in a local reaction. In addition to bites and stings, the inhalation of insect products or parts (e.g., caddis fly and cockroach) has been associated with respiratory allergy in some patients. Clinically and immunologically insect sting anaphylaxis does not differ from other causes of anaphylaxis. Identification of the insect may not be possible. Allergy skin testing with various whole insect body extracts can identify the offending insect. More recently, skin testing with the insect venom alone seems more reliable in identifying the hypersensitive patient.

Treatment of Insect Stings

Anaphylaxis following insect stings is treated medically as in any case of anaphylaxis. In addition, patients with positive skin test correlating with an appropriate history are given hyposensitization beginning with a very low dose of insect extract. Allergy injections are usually carried out for a period greater than 10 years. This therapy appears to be satisfactory in the majority of cases. Patients are instructed to carry an insect sting kit containing epinephrine wherever they go. Avoidance methods include: no use of perfumes, scents, etc., wearing shoes outdoors, avoiding outdoor picnic and garbage areas, and not wearing brightly colored clothes.

ATOPIC DERMATITIS

Atopic dermatitis or infantile eczema is a common skin disease affecting between 1 to 3 per cent of all children. The skin lesions are highly pruritic, erythematous eruptions with a symmetrical distribution. Persistent scratching may induce exudative lesions in the acute stage or lichenification during the chronic stage. Often there is a positive family history for eczema. The lesions usually appear during the first 6 months of life and in most cases resolve between 2 and 4 years. However, some patients continue to have exacerbations or persistence of lesions throughout childhood and occasionally symptoms persist into adulthood.

Initially atopic dermatitis was thought to be an allergic disease because of its frequent association with other atopic disease (e.g., hayfever and asthma). But recent studies support the concept that the rash of atopic dermatitis is not caused by an IgE-mediated mechanism. Notwithstanding, these patients do have a number of immunologic abnormalities including a partial T-cell defect and a markedly increased level of IgE. How these findings relate to the etiology of the skin rash is unclear. An important characteristic of atopic dermatitis is the skin's low threshold for pruritis. Other characteristic dermal variations include abnormal blanching following stroking of the skin and an abnormal delayed blanching following intradermal injection of acetylcholine. The significance of these abnormal dermal vascular changes is not clear.

Clinical Course

During the first few months of life, symmetrical dermal lesions often present as fine pruritic papules over the cheeks and/or the extensor surfaces of the extremities. As the infant matures, the rash tends to localize over the flexural areas (anticubital fossa and popliteal fossa). Abrasion of lesions due to constant rubbing and scratching can produce a wet eczemoid lesion. When infected, such lesions are often covered with heaped up crusts filled with bacteria. At times, the exudative stage may become generalized involving most of the body, skin and scalp. In time, the chronic irritation of the skin produces a lichinified (thick, leather-like) skin lesion. Lesions often exacerbate during the dry winter months. The epidermis of these patients is delicate and has a marked tendency toward dryness and pruritis. The skin is easily irritated by soaps, detergents, rough or tight clothing (particularly wool). In the young child and infant certain foods may exacerbate lesions. The result may be a primary irritant effect in some cases. Elimination diets generally have not been successful in suppressing the lesions.

Treatment

Treatment is primarily aimed at suppression of the pruritis. Since the pruritis often occurs following drying and/or irritation of the skin, preventive therapy is a major goal. Dry skin can be hydrated with the use of moisture such as a hydrophilic ointment (e.g., Eucerin). Bathing is limited and a gentle soap (e.g., Dove) is used. Fingernails are cut short to minimize traumatic scratching. Clothing should be soft (cotton) and loose fitting. Rough sweaters and bedding are avoided. Persistent pruritis is treated with antihistamines (hydroxyzine) and topical steroids. Infected lesions are treated with frequent wet compresses and systemic antibiotics. The key to successful management is in-depth parental counseling in topical care of their child's skin.

Complications

Secondary bacterial infection of generalized eczema can lead to erythroderma. Patients exposed to herpes virus or smallpox vaccination may develop severe generalized viral lesions over their entire body known as Kaposi's varicelliform eruption. This latter complication has a 5 per cent mortality. Therefore, herpes lesions and smallpox vaccination contact must be avoided by patients with atopic dermatitis.

FOOD ALLERGY

The ingestion of a specific food can cause a variety of symptoms in the hypersensitive child, including anaphylaxis, urticaria, gastrointestinal disorders, wheezing, changes in personality, headaches, eczema, and enuresis. Other less documented disorders have also been reported as a result of food allergy.

Food allergy has a higher incidence in children than in adults. The foods commonly associated with allergic reactions include milk, egg, wheat, chocolate, corn, citrus fruits, nuts, legumes, berries, and seafood. The greater the cooking or processing of the food the less its allergenic capability. Allergic reactions to foods may be either immediate or delayed. The immediate type appears in many cases to be an IgE-mediated reaction. The mechanism for the delayed reactions are usually difficult or impossible to define immunologically. Unfortunately, the label of food allergy may be applied to young children and infants following a poorly defined reaction which may or may not be related to the food ingestion and which may or may not have an immunologic mechanism. The allergens in foods are usually proteins or polypeptides. When a certain food is suspected of being an allergen an attempt must be made to clearly document the mechanism. Allergy skin testing with food antigens is not always a reliable indication of allergy since food extracts may be poor allergens. In addition, one must consider that food additives, coloring, or contaminants may actually be causing the reaction, rather than the food itself.

Of all the foods thought to be allergenic in childhood, cow's milk is the one most frequently incriminated. The casein and lactoalbumin content of cow's milk has been shown to be the important allergens. A history of atopic reaction shortly after ingestion associated with positive skin tests confirms the diagnosis of immediate hypersensitivity. However, gastrointestinal complaints, colic, etc., may be related to a disaccharidase deficiency rather than milk allergy. Gastrointestinal allergy is often associated with peripheral eosinophilia as well as eosinophils in the feces. Milk ingestion can be associated with respiratory symptoms similar to asthma, pulmonary infiltrates, iron deficiency, anemia, and diarrhea. This phenomenon is known as Heiner's syndrome. The affected child has high titers of anti-milk precipitating antibodies. Symptoms subside when the patient is placed on a milk-free diet. Although food allergy often provokes cutaneous and gastrointestinal symptoms, respiratory symptoms are far less common; when foods provoke respiratory symptoms the patient frequently has dermal and/or gastrointestinal symptoms as well.

The final diagnosis of food allergy can be aided by repeated (3×) elimination and challenging diets. When a suspected food reproduces symptoms and its elimination causes a cessation of symptoms the diagnosis is confirmed. Of course, if the history suggests a violent reaction, this technique should be avoided.

Aspirin, food dyes and preservatives will be discussed in the drug allergy section.

DRUG ALLERGY

Almost any drug can cause an immunologically mediated adverse re-action in an appropriately sensitized individual. Certain drugs are fre-quent sensitizers (penicillins) while others are rarely allergenic (eryth-romycin).

Drug allergy or hypersensitivity reactions are one type of a variety of adverse reactions that may appear to be clinically similar. In order for a reaction to be classified as allergic some evidence suggesting its immu-nologic mechanism must be present.

Drug Reactions in Normal Individuals

Drug reactions can be divided into two major groups. The first group includes reactions that occur in many normal individuals; in this cate-gory are toxic drug effects, side effects, and secondary effects.

Toxic effects or overdosage is related to the drug's concentration in the body. This occurs when the drug is taken in amounts greater than nec-essary to achieve a pharmacological effect or may be related to a de-creased patient requirement because of drug clearance abnormalities (e.g., kidney or liver damage).

Side effects are certain undesirable pharmacological properties of the drug that can occur when the drug is administered at the recommended dosage. These adverse effects often are not related to the therapeutic function of the drug (e.g., drowsiness following antihistamine adminis-tration of tremor and excitement associated with sympathomimetics).

Secondary effects include reactions that are not directly caused by the drug's pharmacological action, but may result as a secondary conse-quence to the drug's action, as is seen with superinfections following antibiotic treatment (e.g., tetracycline).

Adverse Drug Reactions

A second category of drug reaction is related to an individual's special or unique sensitivity to the drug. This group of adverse reactions includes drug intolerance, idiosyncrasy, and allergy.

Drug intolerance is an adverse reaction related to the pharmacological action of the drug even when a very small amount of the drug is admin-istered. In other words, such individuals are exquisitly sensitive to the drug's pharmacological action (e.g., drowsiness from antihistamines when only a small fraction of the recommended dose is administered).

Idiosyncrasy is an adverse reaction due to an individual's biochemical abnormality. For example, a hemolytic anemia occurs in glucose 6-phos-phate dehydrogenase (G-6-PD) deficiency individuals when treated with nitrofurantoin.

Allergic reactions or hypersensitivity reactions occur in immunologi-cally sensitive individuals and are unrelated to the drug's pharacological action. Examples include penicillin causing anaphylaxis and neomycin-induced contact dermatitis. Most drugs are low molecular weight haptens that when combined with heavier carrier molecules in the body become allergens. Allergy to drugs occurs in only a small number of patients taking the medication. The reactions may occur 1–2 weeks following the initiation of therapy in a previously unsensitized child. Once the patient is sensitized, the allergic reaction may occur immediately following exposure to the drug again.

Mechanism

The mechanisms of drug allergy vary and can include any and all of the previously described four types of immunologic reactions. For example, type I reaction (e.g., anaphylaxis) can occur with penicillin therapy, as can type II (e.g., hemolytic anemia). Type III or toxic-complex reactions (serum sickness) can occur following foreign protein administration as with anti-snake venom treatment. Type IV or delayed hypersensitivity can present as cutaneous contact dermatitis following topical neomycin administration.

Allergic reactions to drugs include cutaneous reaction, anaphylaxis, serum sickness, pulmonary reactions, liver disease, renal disease, hematologic abnormalities, drug fever and allergic vasculitis.

Cutaneous Eruptions. Allergic dermal drug reactions include urticaria, angioedema, erythema multiforme, erythema nodosum, exfoliative dermatitis, etc. The term "fixed drug eruption" is used to describe the recurrence of a rash in the exact same anatomic site following subsequent exposure to the sensitizing drug (frequently barbiturates). Photoallergic reactions can occur in patients taking sulfonamides following activation of the drug by the sun's radiant energy; the rash appears on the exposed skin. Contact dermatitis occurs as a delayed reaction to topical medication, usually seen in the older child. It can result from sensitivity to a drug (e.g., neomycin) or a preservative in the medication (e.g., parabens).

Most allergic cutaneous lesions are highly pruritic, possibly their one clinical common denominator.

Anaphylaxis. Almost any drug can cause an anaphylactic reaction; however, penicillin and its derivatives are among the most commonly incriminated offenders during childhood (see section on anaphylaxis).

Serum sickness is an allergic reaction to injected foreign protein (e.g., equine-derived antisera). Symptoms include rash, fever, joint pain, lymphadenopathy, and nephritis. This is a type III (toxic-complex) reaction. Symptoms appear 7–10 days following administration of the medication. Today, equine-derived sera are rarely used, perhaps with the exception of anti-snake venom, but a similar clinical presentation has also been described following the use of other drugs (e.g., penicillin). When these symptoms are induced by a simple drug it is known as serum sickness-like disease.

Pulmonary Disease. Bronchospasm may occur as part of anaphylaxis or as a consequence of aerosolized antibiotics. The inhalation of pituitary snuff in the treatment of diabetes insipidus may cause asthma or a hypersensitivity pneumonitis. Nitrofurantoin, penicillin, and sulfonamides have been associated with pulmonary infiltrates, systemic illness, and eoinsophilia.

Liver disease can result from allergic reactions to salicylates, isoniazid, phenothiazines as well as repeated exposures to the anesthetic halothane.

Kidney Disease. The administration of methicillin has been associated with the development of antitubular antibodies and interstitial nephritis.

Drug Fever. Patients receiving drugs can develop a persistent high fever that may be associated with a leukocytosis. The symptoms usually appear about 1 week following the initiation of therapy with drugs like penicillin and sulfonamides.

Vasculitis. Some patients initially develop drug fever and/or erythema multiforme, and then go on to develop a generalized vasculitis as a result of drug treatment. Others will develop the vasculitis without fever or dermatological abnormalities.

Hematologic disorders caused by allergic drug reactions include hemolytic anemia (Coombs' positive anemia following penicillin therapy), thrombocytopenia and granulocytopenia.

Diagnosis

The patient's history is of primary importance in the diagnosis of drug allergy. In certain instances laboratory studies are very helpful (e.g., Coombs' positive hemolytic anemia, complement consumption in serum sickness). Immunopathologic studies may occasionally be of aid. Allergy skin testing has only been shown to be of value in penicillin allergy and only in the prediction of immediate type reactions.

In vitro tests for drug allergy have been disappointing with the exception of the radioallergosorbent test (RAST) for penicillin allergy testing. This is probably due to the fact that most drugs are haptens and/or metabolic products; therefore no antigen is readily available for laboratory use.

Treatment

The drug administration should be discontinued except when the treatment is required for a life-threatening illness in which no satisfactory alternative is available. Treatment following drug removal is symptomatic and includes the use of antihistamines, topical antipruritic, aspirin for systemic symptoms and occasionally steroids for severe reactions.

Desensitization consisting of injections of the offending drug beginning with minute amounts followed by frequent (every 15 min.) and cautious progressive increments has had some success in treating penicillin allergy.

This dangerous procedure is reserved for life-threatening illness when no alternative drug is available. Often a suitable drug with similar pharmacologic action and yet different chemical formulation may be used as a substitute.

BIBLIOGRAPHY

Fudenberg, H. H., Stites, D. P., Caldwell, J. L. and Weils, J. V. (eds): Basic and Clinical Immunology. Los Altos, Calif., Lange Medical Publications, 1976.

> Reviews clinical immunology including cellular and humoral mechanisms, immediate hypersensivity and complement.

Connel, J. T.: Allergic rhinitis. *In* Weiss, E. B., and Segal, M. S. (eds.): Bronchial Asthma, Mechanisms and Therapeutics. Boston, Little, Brown, 1976.

> The pathologic mechanisms, clinical evaluation, differential diagnosis and treatment of allergic rhinitis are discussed.

Norins, A. L.: Atopic dermatitis. Pediatr. Clin. North Am., *18*(3):801, 1971.

> A review of atopic dermatitis including etiologic, clinical and therapeutic considerations.

Sheffer, A.: Urticaria and angioedema. Pediatr. Clin. North Am., *22*(1):193, 1975.

> Immunologic and non-immunologic mechanisms in urticaria, hereditary angioedema, physical urticaria and aspirin intolerance are discussed.

28

Normal and Abnormal Emotional Development

Herman Belmont, M.D.

ASSESSMENT OF THE TOTAL CHILD

A thorough grounding in the fundamental aspects of child and adolescent mental health sciences is an integral part of the pediatric student's armamentarium. The more familiar the physician is with all areas of the child's development, the easier it is to treat the child patient as a total person. In fact, this orientation is a basic requirement in dealing with the rapidly and constantly changing child. There is a generally ordered sequence of progression in such comprehensive areas as the child's physical, cognitive, social, moral and emotional development, all proceeding concurrently, integrally related to and mutually influencing one another. Within each of these there are multiple lines of development.

Probably one of the most difficult questions the student must deal with concerns the boundaries of range of normal developmental manifestations for a particular child. A study of accumulatd knowledge about the various lines of development is helpful, but this is supplemented effectively by an extensive range of experience with large numbers of children whose developmental manifestations are carefully observed. From the beginning the pediatric student should make it a habit to carefully assess the child patient's developmental manifestations in all areas in relation to his chronological age. Gradually the student accumulates a useful reservoir of information about the expectations of a particular child's development. The student must ask not "What is normal?" but "What is normal for this or that chronological age and stage of development?"

As a child progresses through changing manifestations of development, the changes are sometimes referred to as "phases." The best aid in approaching the matter of phases is first a clear awareness of what takes place in the progressive normal development and what outer manifestations appear as a reflection of what is going on inside. The idea of "phases" has been exploited to cover many deviations and problems in the development of the personality that would hardly fall in the category of normal healthy development. Many parents have concluded a description of a chronically provocative and disobedient child with the question: "But don't you think it's only a phase, doctor?" or "He'll grow out of it, won't he?" Whether or not he'll grow out of it is, of course, an important part of the question.

A second consideration is whether or not a particular form of behavior at a particular time in the development is dynamic, flexible, changing or temporary—an expected behavioral response to what the child is normally struggling with within himself or in anticipation of problems he has to master. Or, is the behavior rigid and persistent, preventing him from moving on to the next stage of development and to further and better means of adaptation appropriate to his situation. A form of behavior is no longer a phase if it continues, no longer a dynamic surface manifestation of the child's current adjustment, but a fixed and lasting handicap preventing his growth and advancement to later stages of development and adaptation.

In differentiating what is a normal manifestation and what is pathological, the student has to consider also the nature of the eyes of the beholder and his experience. Who is looking at the child and observing? Sometimes a parent is either inexperienced or biased. This is why the mother of a first born child can be panicked by each developmental phasic manifestation as an abnormality, or the opposite—she misjudges abnormalities as "just a phase." With her second and third child she has learned what to expect, and when the child's development goes too far off course for too long, she sees a warning signal. On the other hand, the parent of a handicapped, retarded or psychotic child is often the last to recognize abnormal behavior for understandable reasons; sometimes one sees the opposite kind of bias. For example, the strait-laced and proper set of parents of an only adopted child had reason to believe that the child had been conceived illegitimately. Observing entirely normal phasic genital handling by the child at age 4 and 5, they were convinced that he was a potential sexual degenerate who had inherited the weakness of character and sins of his forebears. What they saw and interpreted was more a product of their worst fears than any objective view of what was happening.

Similar factors operate in the physician. Whether a child's particular manifestation is a matter for concern can only be learned through a thorough knowledge of all aspects of development and through observations of and familiarity with large numbers of developing children, comparing their characteristics.

Through understanding the parents and their position, it is possible to influence favorably their role in the child's development. For example, the parents' acceptance or rejection of pregnancy and their attitude prior to and during pregnancy may be determining factors in the subsequent parental input to the child's development. Reactions to a newborn child following a series of miscarriages or the loss of a child often results in parental protective overinvestment, and needs to be understood. In one instance, a mother may experience a letdown predisposing her to a subsequent postpartum depression, that is associated with cessation at the time of delivery of the previous intense investments and focus of the family on her welfare and well-being. A parent may have denied throughout a pregnancy the possibility of a child being born of other than the anticipated sex, resulting in serious interferences in parenting. While the possibilities are endless, the important thing is that the physician be sensitive and alert to the fact that parents demonstrate the same degree of variability in personality, attitudes and emotional responses as their children. With such an awareness the physician is immediately in a position to eliminate what is often a major void in the effective approach to the total child.

On the other hand, the pediatric student should not succumb to the common error of attributing to the parental role the sole responsibility for all that takes place within the child's development. It is a natural tendency for many parents to attribute such power and responsibility to themselves, and when their physician is equally inclined, they become burdened with feelings of guilt and self-criticism. Genetic and constitutional factors as well as a broader concept of environment go far beyond specific parental influences. The role of sociologic, cultural, economic and geographic factors, in addition to a host of potential acts of fate, must be considered. There is an interplay of nature and nurture (genetic and environmental factors) in development, in which it is believed there is an important genetic role in emotional disorders, though inheritance of human traits does not preclude environmental influences. They are not mutually exclusive but constantly interplay with one another. Identical twins may show a higher concordance rate than fraternal twins in such characteristics as independence, capacity for enthusiasm, guilt, introversion, and tendency to psychopathic disorders on a genetic basis. These factors, however, are subject to subsequent environmental influences. A healthy respect for the multiplicity of determinants in development and psychopathology enables the student to acquire a more mature and comprehensive approach to the specific problems of a specific child.

In considering the relationships of child psychiatry to pediatrics, it should be recognized that even today physicians tend to dichotomize the etiology of most illnesses. The tendency is to look at the etiology of an illness as either organic or psychologic. However, just as all development is multi-determined and physical development cannot be isolated from all other concurrent lines of development, similarly so-called physical pathology cannot be isolated from all of the other determinants of pathology. In terms of the relative role of strictly physical factors, as compared with psychological factors, there is a spectrum or complemental series ranging from those conditions which appear to have a predominant psychologic etiology, to those in which there is a balance of psychologic and physical factors, to those in which the organic etiology would appear predominant. Since developmental and pathological processes are never static and the effects of influencing factors are cumulative and epigenetic in any particular instance, it is difficult even to distinguish where the psychologic factors and physical factors begin. For example, mothering experiences in early infancy, the nature of stimulation and handling, the psychologic state of the mother, have been correlated with developmental manifestations ordinarily regarded as "organic." The establishment of respiratory equilibrium, vocalization, the extent of cerebral-neuronal dendrite development, susceptibility to infection, and cognitive development, are examples of areas that appear directly responsive to early environmental inputs.

STAGES OF EMOTIONAL DEVELOPMENT

Development differs from the concept of growth. Growth means an increase in physical size either of the total organism or its parts, involves relatively permanent tissue changes and is part of the child's progress toward physical maturity. Maturation, on the other hand, refers to those aspects of physical and psychological progression that relate to intrinsic sequential patterning of specific steps toward maturity, appearing on a built-in time-table based on largely biological or inborn sources. The concept of development encompasses the interaction of growth and maturational patterns on the one hand, and the total of past and present experience. Such interaction leads to the ultimate structure, function and behavior of the child.

The First Year

While development generally progresses through recognizable stages, the multivariant combinations of "nature" and "nurture" make each child different. Through genetic and constitutional endowment, some infants are extremely active and restless and respond vigorously to stimuli. Others are inactive and have to be prodded and urged to suck. Some children are born with a deficiency of phenylalanine hydroxylase and can become hopelessly retarded or relatively normal, depending upon how much phenylalanine is ingested during their earliest years. Some children, on the basis of genetic factors, are more susceptible to certain types of infection; for example, the concordance rate for infections with tuberculosis or scarlet fever is much greater in monozygotic than in dizygotic twins. But every child is born dependent and helpless, requiring supplies from the outside, usually at the mother's hands, for nutrition, sensory experience and care.

In the beginning, physiologic and psychic needs are not differentiated; the child has no real psychic structure, few memory traces and no concept of awareness of objects or of himself. It is only through his being repeatedly brought into contact with the outside world to fulfill basic needs that his primitive psychic functions, encompassed in the hypothetical term "ego," gradually develop. During feedings the child experiences sensations of taste, temperature, mother's warm arms and breasts, firmness, gentleness, or even her awkwardness. Continuous circular interactions between the child and the mother occur during the first months of life. With the routine pattern of hunger, discomfort, crying, and finally the appearance of mother to gratify him, the child gradually distinguishes parts of the outside world from himself. The hungry infant conjures up images of mother and sensations of being fed, and feels momentarily relieved. This form of imagery is a first step in mental functioning. Soon he cries, eventually realizing that only a real person gratifies him and he begins to differentiate reality from his own images of satisfaction. As his interactions with the outside world continue, action and trial action lead to the beginnings of thinking, memory traces are laid down, and he acquires knowledge. His perceptual-motor capacities grow and he begins to form concepts. He starts to possess a sense of identity, reality testing capacities, and relationships with objects. He learns to control and regulate the discharge of his drives, to postpone immediate satisfaction for future gain, to integrate and synthesize stimuli from all sources. He experiences anxiety and establishes psychic mechanisms for defending himself against anxiety. He adapts to and makes changes in the external world.

These are all functions in his developing ego and they continue throughout the years of his childhood. They evolve especially as a consequence of the repeated interactions between the child and the most important aspect of his environment, his mother, as she responds to his expressed needs.

The progress of development is irregular; there are forward spurts, there are regressions, and there are plateau periods where, presumably, consolidation of advances is taking place. Furthermore, developmental changes at any one time are irregularly distributed among the cognitive, social, emotional, and sensory motor areas.

Sometimes underlying developmental changes manifest themselves in behavior characteristic of the period, often identified as a "phase" or landmark in the course of development. The social smile, a highlight in the mother-child relationship and psychic development of the child, appears around the second or third month but may not come till as late as the sixth month. The child sees a face and smiles; we assume an association has been made between face and pleasurable gratification (by now he is capable of following a face with his eyes)—the child's beginning capacity to recognize and respond to a specific stimulus previously associated with pleasure. The response does not indicate a true object relationship but is a precursor to it. In blind children the smile response may be delayed until the fourth to sixth month (holding and talking to the child may also be associated stimuli involved in the smile response.). There is an important feedback factor here, for when the infant smiles the mother responds to him. Institutionalized children may have a delayed smile response. What is significant is that any face moving to and fro will elicit the same response. It is only through the child's repeated experience with the mother that over a further period of months her face (and their relationship) assumes a specificity.

At this time, the child's sensory and motor functions become more effective. Some surface manifestations of underlying development are so widely understood and accepted that they are taken for granted and not labeled as phases. The infant several months old tends to put everything he gets his hands on into his mouth,—food, an arm, a piece of clothing or a blanket. This is a reflection of the tremendous focus on the mouth during this period.

At around 5 to 7 months and for several months afterward however, we see a striking change in many children. The average child will now go through a period of fearing strangers. During the preceding months, as a result of his repeated feeding and child care experiences at his mother's hands, the child's powers of perception and recognition have developed. He recognizes his mother and sometimes his father, as differentiated from other people. We assume that he knows that when he is hungry, uncomfortable or has other needs, his mother alleviates them. As a concomitant of this degree of development, he is confronted also by his first great fear, namely, that these needs may not be fulfilled. Consequently, he cries when he is separated from his mother or doesn't see her. He also cries when a stranger tries to pick him up; this is not mother, thus he clings to her, denying the stranger's existence. This is evidence of healthy normal development in the child, who can now discriminate between mother and not-mother (object awareness). The potential for further development is established. An abnormal persistent fear which is no longer a phase, but intense, inflexible and exaggerated, indicates psychopathology.

Similarly, the child will cry when the mother disappears; this should not be regarded as evidence of his being "spoiled." His crying is a reflection of his fear of desertion and helplessness, in effect the fear that all his needs which have been fulfilled by the mother will go unnoticed if she is not there. In general, with every advance in development there is an associated threat or demand. The newborn has no threats; he has no object relationships, no perception of reality, and as yet no fears of desertion. The 5- to 7-month-old child can distinguish the mother from strangers, but he is not yet aware of her constant existence when she is not in view.

During this time the child continues to integrate his experiences into sets which hold together associatively—for example, pleasant, unpleasant, self, others, strange, familiar, real, imagined. He distinguishes emotions and uses them more appropriately, with greater specificity.

Throughout the child's development, particularly during the early months and years, we see how crucial the mother's role is and why we must constantly understand her needs and capacities for this role. While it is apt to be predominant, it need not be exclusive. Various members of the extended family, and particularly the father, also contribute to the "mothering" function.

During the child's initial stages of differentiation from his surroundings, beginning around 4 or 5 months of age, there is a progressive maturation of more complex locomotor functions, growing through circular reactions. There is also a development of sensory investigations, in which sensory experiences are associated with specific kinds of stimuli. After the first 6 months, the child may become attached to some inanimate object—for example, a diaper, a blanket, a stuffed fuzzy toy—which he seems to find a source of comfort. It is thought that such a "transitional object" serves as a bridge in the course of differentiation and separation of the child from his mother. The object simultaneously bears characteristics of both the mother (soft, warm and the odor of a piece of blanket) and the child himself. The transitional object may not be given up until grade school, though often earlier. Some children, such as recent generations of Japanese, who have had more continued closeness and body contact with the mother, seem to have less of a tendency to become involved with such transitional objects.

The Second Year

Toward the end of the first year, in a progressive movement toward separation and individuation as described by Margaret Mahler, there is a period of active practicing of motor skills and exploration of the environment. Words may begin to be used and identified with objects as well as in relation to needs. There are sharper sensory discriminations. The child practices moving away from the close tie to the mother; at times the child will crawl away from her and then return to "refuel." Other times the child seems temporarily almost oblivious to her. Many children around this time are weaned from the nipple, and the influence on the individual child of the wide variety of maternal practices in this area can be seen, ranging from sudden and abrupt interruptions of gratification to prolonged indulgence.

Earlier, objects were explored with the hands, mouth and teeth. Hands were brought to the mouth, at first accidentally and then intentionally, as certain actions became associated with particular effects. There was a constant striving toward mastery, such as climbing over objects, learning to back out, and standing up. The infant's sensory perceptions occurred at first in an all-or-none visceral type fashion, as, for example, with primitive sensations of equilibrium, tension, temperature, vibration, movement and the rhythm of rocking. At approximately 6 months, more discrete and specific sensations appeared with a gradual reduction of intuitive sensitivity in which the child became less alert to autonomic sensations.

By the second half of the second year, in a stage which Dr. Mahler refers to as a "rapproachement stage of the separation individuation progression," the child appears to become closer to the mother and wants to share experiences with her.

At about this time also, the child becomes more aware of himself and the things he can do, feel and perceive in the world around him. He is pleased with himself and in his newly acquired abilities, and he repeats them over and over, wanting to guard them jealously. When he is put to sleep, he is asked to relinquish his actions, perceptions and fresh conception of being a going concern. He fights it. He doesn't want to go to sleep but would rather stay up and play. He is not flexible about it, not having the wherewithal to reason and plan. He may need sleep badly and fight it, become cranky, insist on staying up, half asleep, and want to keep going. At about the same time the child may become negativistic, refusing to do as he is told and in fact doing just the opposite. He does this not because he is stubborn or mean, but because he wants to assure himself about something of which he is uncertain, that he is a capable individual with thoughts of his own. Without this progression and its necessary phasic consequences, he would never give up being a dependent non-entity. The sooner he develops this assurance that he can operate independently, the sooner he is able to abandon the earlier fear of being deserted in his helplessness. In a few months this phase subsides normally if he is helped to develop to the point where he has more and more assurance of his capabilities and independence and therefore has less need to prove them negativistically. If his behavior at this time is dealt with too punitively, the child may regard his independence as too dangerous and therefore not worthwhile. He may retreat to a continuing dependent kind of behavior.

As the child grows a little older, his education and social requirements, increasing expectations of him, and discipline continue. As a consequence of his normal development, more is required of the child and he finds himself in the midst of a struggle between his own strong wishes and the expectations of those around him, particularly his parents. Now it is no longer a matter of proving himself an entity in his own right but rather a contest between his own strong wishes and those of his demanding parents. He is torn between gratifying himself, for example, scribbling on a wall with a crayon, as opposed to losing his mother's approval and love; this is a difficult decision. Depriving himself of gratifications in order to retain her love and approval is crucial to the child's future evolution and socialization. This is a basic consideration throughout life and those children unable to work out these problems in relation to a loving, guiding, interested mother develop considerable potential impairment of this capacity.

The conflict over toilet training typifies this period. The child now shows more frequent temper tantrums as a surface reflection of his inner struggle. It is hoped that the child will resolve his second major fear, that of loss of his parents' love and approval, by taking over many of their expectations as his own. He masters his toileting functions, tantrums subside, and there is a greater degree of social compliance in the mastery of his impulses.

During this period, if the mother leaves the child who had been successfully trained, the child may regress and have to be retrained completely. This is because he has not yet internalized controls over these functions but carries them out to obtain the mother's approval and love. Eventually, when the child incorporates his mother's prohibitions and assumes her attitudes, he remains trained even if they are separated. In children taken into a foster home at this time, there may be a deficit or weakness in the new mother-child object relationship. The child is often so slow in toilet training that the foster mother becomes exasperated and has the child transferred to another foster home, even though he had just begun to approach achievement of training. Subsequently there is regression, infantile destructiveness, misbehavior, soiling, and poor control of impulses. This may lead to a vicious cycle in which each new foster parent reacts similarly and the child never has the opportunity to achieve a satisfactory object relationship. The same situation may arise when a mother has a career, has to work, and doesn't spend much time with the child, who is constantly shifted from one substitute caretaker to another. Without a satisfactory object relationship, the child may not be trained until later in childhood.

The Preschool Years

During the child's third year of life he gradually accepts separation from his mother and masters the concept of his mother's permanency even when she is out of his presence for increasingly longer periods of time. There is a greater interest in other adults and a sense of time, an increasing tolerance of small frustrations and a capacity to delay gratification for some future goals.

As the child moves through his preschool years, he achieves a greater mastery of his more impulsive desires, and his drives find expression in progressively more socially adaptive activities. He also moves more and more from a passive, helpless and dependent creature to one who participates actively in the mastery of his inner demands and his environmental expectations. The child between 3 and 6 generally shows forms of behavior that are a reflection of his further development. There is a beginning awareness of boy-girl differences, a greater familiarity with the various parts of his body and the pleasurable sensations derived from them, an activation of competitive and possessive drives and an expression of feelings of love and possessiveness, particularly for the parent of the opposite sex. The result of these developmental struggles is that the child appears concerned with another great fear, a fear of mutilation and injury. Very briefly, this threat may be understood as a symbol of the punishment the child fears for his emerging forbidden aggressive and rivalrous love feelings. He tries to cope with these, to him, dangerous impulses and the anticipated punishment in ways which give rise to certain behavioral manifestations of this period.

He may express his fear and anxiety by becoming babyish, whiny, peevish, and overly sensitive to the least hurt, thereby arming himself against a greater and more dangerous injury. Or he may assume the opposite attitude of extreme defiance and irritability. These are two principal methods that many children (and adults) use to cope with a great threat, such as serious illness or hospitalization—either they become overly fearful and helpless or they are uncooperative and rebellious in a denial of the situation.

In addition, the child may try to handle a danger he senses from those immediately around him in his family as punishment for his forbidden feelings and desires, by displacing the danger onto some distant and more easily avoided object, thereby developing a "phobia." It may then be some frightening picture in a book, a dog or some imaginary monster that is the "danger." These fears are common at this time and may be simply a surface reflection of the normal developmental struggle within the child. It is only when these fears become fixed, intense and prevent further progression in development that they are pathological.

Similarly, children now may develop a sleep disturbance. When the child gets into bed, he tries to stay awake and on guard against dangerous and frightening thoughts. He fights going to bed, fights going to sleep, and often sleeps fitfully and restlessly, awaking frequently. Night terrors and bad dreams are more common for the same reason. This is the time when a child is apt to be cowardly and overly sensitive to the slightest injury, crying and screaming over a tiny splinter. He is overly aware of defects and injuries in others. The child can ordinarily master this developmental hurdle with the help of understanding, kind and supportive parents until he re-establishes a more satisfactory equilibrium between the various forces within him, and gains satisfactory controls of his forbidden desires. He ordinarily accomplishes this by age 5 or 6.

The School-Age Child

When the child reaches school age, how he makes the transition for a large part of his waking day from the home and his parents to the school and a more intimate involvement with other adults and children, reflects the success of his developmental progress during the preceding years. With children of latency age, roughly 5 to 12, social, mental and emotional growth is favored, as with preschool children, by an opportunity to actively master and take over personal executive responsibility for what had previously been passively experienced (because the parent had assumed this function). Children need an opportunity for progressive and successive mastery and achievement of tasks which tax their capacity, but these tasks should neither frustrate them nor prove beyond their ability. They do better with gradual and modulated exposure to change, and subsequent development is best built upon previous favorable growth.

The child of 5 to 12 has a basic need for a continuing relationship with specific parent figures or their surrogates who provide some continuing point of reference in the process of personality growth and development. These parent figures offer the child as an individual a reasonable assurance of fulfillment of basic needs deriving from the reality of his dependence on outside supplies. This means "home," food, clothing, and affectional investment. The parents also serve as a model or standard of behavior with which to identify, by their function as individuals and in interrelations with spouse and children, as well as their mediation of stimulation and establishing limits for the child's behavior. The parents also need to give the child an opportunity for working out male or female sex role identifications and therefore both a male and female parent figure should be present during this time as in the preceding years. There is a continuing need for the parents to provide adequate support and understanding as the child moves through progressive developmental phases.

The crucial role of the continuing "parent" is supplemented by significant experiences with figures outside the home who serve as ego ideals for identification, sources and objects of affection, sources of stimulation and creativity, sources of patterns of limit and control, models for sex role identification and the means of acquisition and development of many ego skills. For these experiences outside the home to be meaningful and contribute effectively to development, they must in some way be sufficiently associated in nature to the child's prior experience in his home. Too abrupt a contrast renders the additional experience relatively less usable. To promote the most favorable significant experience with figures outside the home, the school seems to be the most fertile and most readily controlled answer for the greatest number of children.

Every child, especially during these years, needs continuing peer group relationships, not interrupted by forces outside his control, as an important factor in achieving ego growth. Peer relationships are important in terms of separation from parental dependency, firming up the child's own sense of identity and self-concept, and the development of a capacity for socially acceptable aggressiveness, group cooperation, and, in general, function within the more extensive social system. During this period we see an expansion in the child's intelligence, there is a broadening of his social understanding, his capacity for empathy and altruism; he displays a progressively better mastery of his environemnt, and we find him less readily regressing and disintegrating under the impact of crises. He shows progressively more effective synthesis and integration of external demands.

The school-age child notably develops a better capacity for coping with his earlier and more directly manifested drives and impulses. He does this in several ways. Through sublimation a child may express these drives with a changed aim. Thus a child who was sexually curious, a peeper with a desire to search and see, now diverts his expanded curiosity to many different areas. He also develops reaction formations, attitudes which are the antithesis of his earlier drives. The child who had little concern about nudity and was readily immodest, now seems to move rather automatically to a more modest orientation, becoming more self-conscious and not wanting to expose himself indiscriminately to others. A child who earlier expressed certain cruel and destructive drives now turns to kindness and a degree of social regard. The child who had been self-centered and personally oriented, now becomes not nearly as possessive and shows a relatively greater degree of generosity. There is also a marked increase in motoric discharge of the child's energies as a means of coping with forbidden drives. Play takes on a rapid pace and there is more involvement in games. When the child gets too tired, he uses his muscular system to discharge these strong drives and tensions, or else he becomes irritable, cranky and unhappy.

The Adolescent

Starting with the junior high school years, we come to a period in development about which a lot has been written, but this is still a difficult period to understand. This is especially true because of its manifest behavior—it seems to be changing constantly. The characteristics of adolescence have been described as rebelliousness, a search for independence, a period of volatile emotions, trouble in handling sexuality, questioning values and ideas, and searching for identity. These characteristics reflect underlying dynamic, complicated transitional changes from childhood to adulthood. These are important tasks which the adolescent has to achieve, and they are not simple. He must establish a considerable degree of detachment from parents, releasing himself from emotional dependence; as he gets older this can become confused with his continuing economic dependence. Often the parental ties are too threatening, too stimulating and too frightening, and when they are abruptly interrupted, the teenager may shift his feelings with the same intensity toward some other leader or peer group. He may deal with his feelings by turning them into their opposite. Thus one frequently sees an adolescent who is moving toward independence, who appears to have great love for his parents, but then in a reverse behavior pattern begins to demonstrate feelings of intense hate, contempt and revolt.

Another task of the adolescent is to find his personal identity, who he is. He literally goes around asking "Who am I?"—"What is the meaning of existence? of life?" He reads and engages in philosophical discussions, searching for knowledge. He has to come to terms with his drives, his feelings of inferiority and inadequacy. He has to master his relationships with his own and the opposite sex. He must be able to move from selfish, self-centered love to tender object love, to understanding and valuing the love object for the object itself. He has to achieve a sense of responsibility toward himself and other persons, to find a career and some direction.

It is impossible at this point to detail the fascinating vicissitudes of this period of the child's development. However, brief examples can be given of what is going on at this time. During the child's early adolescence the pediatrician particularly needs to be aware of the marked disparities between different parts of the child's physical development as well as disparities between his development and that of his peers. This plays an important role in the psychological development of the child. Size and relative development of arms, legs, breasts, secondary sex characteristics, are a great source of concern for young teenagers. They feel inferior and ashamed, and try to defend against the feelings of being clumsy, awkward and inadequate. They may withdraw or try to overcompensate to get the admiration of others, or they may express complete denial of their situation by exaggerating their defects and trying to make themselves look ugly and as clumsy as possible. At this time parents need help in knowing how to support the teenager's vulnerable ego; the pediatrician can assure the parents that patient understanding and time will accomplish more than long lectures and nagging.

Teenagers have a shaky self-esteem even though they may act unconcerned and indifferent. There is an ever-present fear of loss of ego control in the management of the drives which become intensified at this time, with an accompanying fear of not being able to control them. As part of this, there is at times a fear of losing one's mind as well as a fear of dying and a preoccupation with life, a questioning of whether they will ever reach adulthood. With the reactivation of forbidden drives and their intensification, there is a resulting fear of the possible consequences if the teenager fulfills these wishes. One way the teenager handles these earlier drives directed toward the parent, and is assisted in his struggle between his conflicting dependent and independent wishes in relation to his parents, is to put some distance between himself and his home. Often the adolescent looks to the peer group, or some adult whom he adopts as an ideal figure. These figures can be used to bolster the threatened ego controls as the young person has to move further from the parents.

During the ages of 14 to 16, it is not uncommon to see regressive manifestations, inasmuch as there is a tendency to turn to regression as a defense against the anxieties derived from the strongly emerging forbidden drives of childhood. A young man of 14 or 15, in his anxiety, can suddenly behave completely like a dependent baby in the classroom, at home or outside among his friends. He is sensitive, vulnerable, and given to crying easily. But paradoxically, when you try to help him and give him some advice, he is resentful and rejects it because this makes him feel too much like a baby. He struggles back and forth. He doesn't want to be a baby, he wants to grow up. At the same time, when you deal with him man to man as you would with an adult, he is unable to handle it and retreats. There may be regressions in eating habits during this time, and interestingly enough, even to transitory wetting, soiling and anal masturbatory activity. If the regression does not elicit an overreaction from those around him, the adolescent will generally swing back and forth, and gradually wind up ahead.

Girls, like boys, may show mixed reactions to cleanliness and dirtiness. They may be very clean during this period as reaction against their revulsion with menstruation; on the other hand they may be haphazard and negligent about their physical appearance. Physical examinations, relative to menstrual functions, are generally resented.

When acne appears, the teenager becomes sensitive. In his mind it definitely is connected with constipation and/or masturbation, and discussion is distasteful. Often he will not follow the recommendations of the dermatologist because "he knows what it is really all about." Also as a part of the reactivation of earlier drives in addition to regression, there is a good bit of exhibitionism, peeping, showing off, and exposure of parts of the body. There may be some normal fleeting transvestitism, perhaps as a regression to the period when there was a great emphasis on who had the penis and who did not. During this time also, the boy has a lot of trouble coping with his erections because they occur easily, usually at the wrong time and the wrong places. He becomes too excited too easily in response to slight stimuli.

Now one often sees regressions, not only in instinctual manifestations but also in the level of ego function. There may be regressions back to the period when there were no internalized prohibitions and all limits came from the outside. The teenager at this time often views the outside adult as potentially punitive and judgmental. He feels the doctor will be critical and therefore is apt to be guarded and secretive when they meet.

Object relationships during the pubertal period seem directed toward the opposite sex more for narcissistic gratification than for any interest in the object itself. There is a tendency to collect as many "scalps" as possible. The teenager also is busy sampling and exploring a wide variety of social interests; if the parents try to force the child into a particular niche, he may become fixated at a narrowly restricted orientation and lose his potential for development in different directions.

As we move into the post-pubertal period, around age 15 to 19 or 20, we see the adolescent searching for a greater degree of stabilization. This is when he has to solidify and synthesize his ideals and contradictions, his identifications with the peer group, his values, and precipitate out of that a composite that works for him. Also, he must discover a way of coping with the forbidden incestuous feelings directed toward his immediate family and find other outlets for his sexual drives and fantasies. He may once again find some kind of suitable working relationship with his family, not the earlier dependent and clinging tie, but now sufficiently secure and comfortable so that he can relate to them as one individual to another. He gradually comes to terms with his ideas about religion, his own personal philosophy, what his vocational strivings will be and where he is and where he's going.

Simultaneously, there is a progressive development of the child's identity. Starting with a negativisitic identity at the 18-month-old level, and succeeded by an identification with the characteristics of the parent of the same sex, now in puberty and in post-puberty additional identifications are made through ideal objects, through the peer group, and through parents. A healthy identity prevents the child from rejecting parental attitudes totally and yet allows him to be partly different from the parents and partly like them. The truly healthy and workable identity is an amalgam of all the different sources and not a drive in one direction. What started out as a helpless and dependent non-entity psychically has now emerged into a complex and independently functioning young adult.

WORRISOME DEVELOPMENTAL MANIFESTATIONS

Various developmental manifestations can present problems for those dealing with children. Here, the physician is of assistance to both the child and the parents through a greater developmental perspective and a multidimensional approach.

A parent's concern about a child's thumbsucking—an entirely normal manifestation of the child's early strong sucking needs—cannot be dealt with arbitrarily. A number of significant factors need to be taken into account. Some parents regard thumbsucking as an offensive and disgusting habit that will result in dental malformations. In other cases, the physician must evaluate the role of the parent in indirectly encouraging the child to use sucking satisfactions as a form of universal gratification whenever he has a need that is not gratified. Such a parent will put a nipple in the child's mouth each time he cries, for whatever reason. The physician must teach parents the role of constitutional variations in sucking needs of different children; e.g. an infant whose hunger needs are satisfied before his strong sucking needs are fulfilled during a feeding has to do some supplementary sucking.

Early in the child's development, when object relationships are not yet established, parents may observe occasional rhythmic genital stimulation concurrent with feeding. Such an entirely normal manifestation may become the focus of especially sensitive and overly watchful parents. Timely, supportive reassurance of the parents may forestall complicating over-reactions. Most children engage periodically in masturbatory activity, and unless this lasts as a fixed and all-encompassing activity, it may be regarded as a normal manifestation of development.

Children during the first year may show disturbances at bedtime, with restlessness and crying as soon as the mother leaves the child's bedroom. Such manifestations are understandable in terms of the child's normal development as helplessness in the absence of his newly recognized source of gratification. Some parents respond by holding the crying child and carrying him throughout a large part of the night, lest he be subjected in the parents' absence to undue anxiety. Others will try to "break the habit" by leaving the child to cry himself to sleep over long periods. In the first instance, aside from making the parents angry with the child, he becomes a participant in a ritual which can interfere, if continued long enough, with the entire process of separation-individuation. In the second instance, there is a potential interference with his basic trust in the newly emerging environment. The pediatrician may help the parents resolve the dilemma by the following program. The parent may allow the child to cry for 4 or 5 minutes, return to the room to comfort and quiet him, and leave again. If the crying is resumed, the entire procedure is repeated, and as many times as necessary. If the crying continues, in a few days the period is increased to 5 or 6 minutes and so on without permitting the crying period to last beyond a 10-minute period, which appears to be too anxiety producing. Through such an approach the parents can appreciate the young infant's need for gently titrated support, without interference with the gradual progression of growth and mastery. Sudden and excessive interruptions of the mother-child relationship may, on the other hand, result in prolonged complications with developmental regressions and even disturbances in feeding.

We have already discussed the meaning of transitional objects, negativism of the 18th-month period, and temper tantrums. With the patient understanding that these are temporary surface manifestations of underlying developmental changes, they soon pass. With overly severe responses, these manifestations may be compounded and persist in the form of real problems. Appropriate support by physicians helps to ameliorate such excessive responses.

We know that many transitory forms of behavior in the school-age child and adolescent reflect the ebb and flow of dynamic development. These do not constitute a problem unless they become marked and persistent, either because of constitutional variations in the child, developmental interferences from the environment, or some combination of these.

Sometimes there is a lag or a precocity or an unevenness in maturational steps. These can be a problem, particularly if the environmental responses and supports for them do not enable their satisfactory mastery. Children are born with variations in capacity for eating, for speech development, for development of control of bowel and bladder functions, and for sleeping. Some children show long continued hyperactivity or hypoactivity, some are significantly precocious or mildly retarded in cognitive development. There are variations in achieving autonomy from parents. Other children have significant delays in speech development and disorders in articulation and language comprehension. Such deviations in maturational patterns can complicate a child's development, adding a special quality and cast to what he brings into the child-environment interactions. What evolves in the subsequent development of these children also depends on the ability of the parents to cope with the deviations and to move them toward an adaptive integration with a child's other capacities.

DEVELOPMENTAL INTERFERENCES

Every child, in addition to showing behavioral manifestations of underlying developmental changes which are ordinarily transitory, also experiences conflicts inherent in the process of development, such as his need to adjust to the relinquishment of nipple feeding, or the struggles between indulgence of his wishes and a fear of losing his parents' love. What must be considered constantly is the extent to which external interferences disturb the "typical unfolding of development."[3] In other words, to what extent are unjustified demands being made of the child that do not take into account his capacity to cope with them?

Parental Interferences

These interferences include parental over-or under-reactions at specific developmental phases, inadequate supplementary or auxiliary supports of development by the environment (mother), qualitatively noxious attitudes and orientations on the part of significant persons in the child's environment, and any number of acts of fate. The young infant needs protection by a person who is capable of nurturing both the child's mind and body, which are at first inseparable. In the fulfillment of his bodily needs, feeding him, bathing him, changing him, the child's emotional needs are also being carried out, if the child-caring person deals with him in a warm and tender and feeling way, interacting and responding appropriately to his needs. Serious developmental interferences result from a lack or a deficiency of a need-satisfying adult, with whom the child can interact continuously, who responds to his signals of distress and calls for comfort and gratification, who establishes an emotional communication with him and eventually becomes someone he can love and trust.

Similarly, throughout the child's development he should have adult figures who can relate to him and provide him with appropriate developmental necessities. Unfortunately many children are unwanted and in homes where the adult responsible for their care sorely lacks the capacity to fulfill their needs. This is often the case of children who are born out of wedlock, children of young and immature mothers, or where mothers are badly handicapped by serious problems such as alcoholism, drug addiction, serious mental illness, or if the mother must work and no adequate mother substitute is provided for the child. Children experiencing severe forms of neglect exhibit a clinical failure to thrive without sufficient organic disease to account for it. This is characterized by failure to grow and gain weight, by developmental slowness, by occasional vomiting or diarrhea, by feeding difficulties and by weakness, fatigability and irritability. Lesser degrees of deficiency and deprivation in mothering are frequent developmental interferences.

Qualitative inadequacies in maternal attitudes act equally as interferences with child development; a mother's over-concern has been regarded as contributing to frequency of colic manifestations in children. Rene Spitz has related infantile neurodermatitis, fecal play, persistent hypermotility and rocking in children, to characteristic and specific maternal attitudes. Tens of thousands of children are victims of severe child abuse, occurring when a non-accidental physical attack or physical injury is inflicted by a person charged with the responsibility of caring for a child. The parents who abuse their children almost always have severe social problems, marital discord, as well as financial difficulties. Many of these parents appear to be in a state of continual anger and the only stimulation needed for direct and violent expression of this anger may be some normal difficulty of child rearing.

In addition to these examples of gross quantitative and qualitative developmental interferences, there are a number of so-called acts of fate that modify and interfere with development. Divorce and separation of parents disrupt the family structure, with emotional repercussions in the parents, varying degrees of object loss for the child, sometimes questions of placement, involvement of the child in extensive unpleasant legal contests, problems of divided loyalties, and many other associated difficulties. Similarly, we can list the death, serious illness, prolonged absences, and working habits of parents. Even the timing, spacing, number and sex distribution of the child's siblings, as well as the child's ordinal position in the family, will affect him directly, and indirectly through the parents. The nature of the extended family, their illnesses, deaths and demands on the parents, may be crucial interfering determinants in the child's development. This is to say nothing of an often neglected area, the impact of pets, their loss and illnesses. When a family moves frequently and the child's object ties with peers and his familiar environment are interrupted repeatedly, when he is subjected to sexual abuse or seduction, when he is regularly exposed to the authority of a humiliating and ridiculing or physically abusive adult, such as a parent, teacher or a sitter, the child's ego capacity may be unable to cope with such interferences.

The more thoroughly the pediatrician has mastered the developmental vicissitudes of children, the more effectively does he strive to soften the impact of such developmental interferences, to give the parent insight into the child's needs at these times, and to bolster a badly fractured or strained ego in the child.

The Hospitalized Child

For the physician, a most important interference with the child's development is his illness or hospitalization. Such experiences are often referred to as "traumatic," meaning that the child is subjected to stimuli that come in such abundance, intensity and unfamiliarity he cannot assimilate and master them. The age and stage of developmental progression of the child at the time of his illness or hospitalization is of fundamental significance in understanding the meaning of these experiences for him.

The Infant. Up to the age of 6 months, a hospitalized child tends to show varying degrees of agitation in response to changes in his customary environment and differences in patterns of handling him. After 6 months, having a degree of ego and object differentiation, the child shows manifestations of stranger and separation anxiety as a consequence of his removal from regular contact with the mother. In effect, the child's beginning basic trusting relationship with her has been jarred and disrupted.

Between the ages of 6 and 18 months, the child is working through his differentiation and practicing stages of separation individuation, described earlier. In the face of disruptions of the child's delicately established identity and object relationships that result from his abrupt separation from his mother, there may be degrees of regression and retreat to earlier levels of development accompanied by sleep and feeding disturbances.

Ages 2 to 6. In the period from 1½ to 2 years, the child is extremely sensitive to the threat of separation or desertion. He is now working through the rapprochement stage of the separation individuation process, where he has moved for a period into a closer interaction with his mother. This is also when the child is trying to develop a sense of autonomy that is threatened by the enforced separation and restrictions of movement often associated with hospitalization.

In the third year, hospitalization may be viewed as a punishment for forbidden activities or even wishes; this is understandable when we recall that the child is struggling between the gratification of his own wishes and the fear of loss of his parents' love and approval. Therefore, during hospitalization he may respond with a rigid reinforcement of control of all of his impulses or else turn in the other direction and yield to all the partially repressed and recently abandoned pleasures and forbidden activities, such as wetting and soiling and babyish demanding behavior. There may be a reactivation of whining and clinging, crying, temper tantrums and destructive behavior.

From ages 3 to 6, mutilation anxieties are high and although separation anxiety is diminished at this stage, there is a real threat of loss of physical integrity and a sense of initiative. The child is apt to interpret all forbidden actions and thoughts as punishable by physical mutilation, body damage and even castration, and so may react to the hospitalization and threatened medical and surgical procedures by denying his anxiety through acting completely contrary to what might be expected of someone who was ill. He may refuse to cooperate or accept any limitations. In fact, he may engage in overt misbehavior. Another form of response to the situation is to submit completely and become a perfect patient. This is in complete compliance with the dangerous and threatening environment. At times some children will retreat to earlier levels of functioning.

The School-Age Child. A child in the early school years, from 6 to 8, continues to have a high degree of mutilation anxiety and a fear of loss of control and mastery. Since his superego has by now been fairly well established and functions with some degree of severity, he may interpret the hospitalization experience as a punishing one, retaliative for all of his wrongdoings. As the child gets older, the effects of hospitalization continue to reflect his principal problems at those times. A young teenager may regard hospitalization as threatening to expose his hidden and embarrassing masturbatory activities. In the midst of a dependence-independence struggle, removal to a hospital bed in which he is bathed, nursed, and at times even fed, may be unbearable.

The Physician's Role

The physician can play an important role in ameliorating this developmental interference. He can strive to keep at a minimum all the changes in the child's daily living situation. For example, is the child treated at home wherever possible? If the child has to be removed to the hospital, are there arrangements available for the parents to be with the young child and to visit the older child frequently? Are medications being administered by the least traumatic route and frequency? Are medical and surgical procedures, laboratory studies, restrictions of diet and movement, length of hospitalization or restriction of activities kept at the minimum necessary for the best medical management of the problem? Finally and most important of all, where changes in the child's management or environment are unavoidable, does the physician make every effort to reduce the traumatic impact of these experiences?

The physician has the responsibility to communicate at the child's level of understanding and prepare him for each new experience to which he will be subjected. If he receives an explanation of a laboratory procedure, a restriction in activity and a separation from home in advance, the experience may still be unpleasant, but is less likely to be as upsetting. Unfamiliarity and unpreparedness for intense stimuli make it more difficult for the child's ego to assimilate and master the situation. When the child is unable to do this, he must resort to less satisfactory responses, to earlier seemingly less threatening levels of development, denial of painful aspects of reality, and arrests and fixations in development which may serve as foci for later neurotic development or character changes.

Just as there is an advantage in explanation and preparation in advance of procedures, there is also real value in simple clarification as procedures are being carried out, thereby reducing the completely helpless, dependent and passive aspects of these experiences. Finally, where it has been impossible to prepare a child in advance of or during his illness and hospitalization experiences, it is important that he be given an opportunity, after the fact, to discuss and understand fully all that has happened and its significance for him. He may have many questions, he may have considerable confusion about the meaning of his experiences, or he may have distorted the reality in terms of his own personal and age-appropriate fantasies. Ample opportunity for discussion of misconceptions can be invaluable in enabling a child to master the trauma inherent in most medical experiences.

DEVELOPMENTAL ARRESTS AND FIXATIONS

There are disorders in children that can derive from a lack of progress in the development of certain ego functions or in the advancement of the drive development, as opposed to manifestations of internal psychic conflict or a conflict with the environment. Here we see children who may retain feeding habits from early periods of development, restricting their diet to particular foods or to foods that do not require chewing. Some children show persistent enuresis, soiling, and characteristics of immaturity appropriate to a much younger age. Not all cases with these symptom manifestations are examples of developmental arrest, since these symptoms may also be expressions of other forms of psychopathology. However, a fair proportion of these children do show a prolonged continuation of characteristics ordinarily regarded as belonging to the early preschool years. These are children who also appear overly oriented in the direction of personal gratification without an appropriate balance in relation to the expectations and requirements of society, children who are more self-centered and less object oriented, who tend to readily deny the demands of reality. The capacity to postpone immediate gratification for future gain is not well developed. The result is that these children have not been able to relinquish gratifications associated with soiling, wetting and impulsive discharge. Instead, they have prolonged the direct or relatively direct discharge of early forms of satisfaction without the expected modification of these drives to social requirements. Similarly, some children continue in later years to express directly drives which were normal and expected at early periods in development, such as various exhibitionistic and voyeuristic (peeping) tendencies.

Developmental arrests and fixations can be serious handicaps to effective function and need to be watched carefully and studied in the perspective of a particular child's developmental circumstances. When it becomes evident that the behavior is fixed and unchanging despite early modifications in the child-rearing practices or other factors which appear to contribute to them, it is advisable to seek consultation and, if necessary, treatment, before these problems are further compounded. Simply eliminating the behavioral manifestation through threat or prohibition may lead to more serious problems. A child of latency age was found to be a severe stutterer. His mother related that he had been enuretic since infancy, and that she had "cured" this by placing a meat cleaver on his night-table one evening, threatening to chop off his penis if he wet again. He had stopped wetting that night but from that time on began to stutter.

PSYCHOPATHOLOGY DERIVING FROM INTRAPSYCHIC CONFLICT

The personality structure of the preschool child is fundamentally different from that of the school-age child. How the preschool child's needs and wishes are dealt with is to a greater degree determined by the expectations, prohibitions and threats of the world around him. And for the young child the parents constitute the principal representative of the external environment. During the preschool years of development, therefore, the child's behavior quickly and easily reflects change in the parental expectations. To some extent, even in these early years and especially when the child's development is precocious, his personality begins to take over some of the functions of regulating and controlling instinctual wishes, but even in those cases such controls continue to bear a close relationship with the external world. These controls are not firmly established, are readily influenced from the outside, and require continuing support from the parents in order to be maintained.

As a consequence of developmental changes during the latter part of the preschool period, the child in grade school adopts within his own psychic structure many of the prohibitions and controls previously applied from without by the parents. He has established identifications with important child-rearing figures and has internalized their prohibitions and controls. From this point on, the child's behavior will be responsive not only to continuing external threats and influences, but now in addition there is a continuing potential for conflict of an intrapsychic nature. This is a conflict between the child's wishes and his own prohibitions as embodied in his superego structure. The superego within his personality structure continues to retain the punitive qualities and characteristics it held at the time the superego was laid down around the age of 5 or 6. This is why the child can develop a conflict that is not understood rationally in terms of current environmental circumstances. Such a conflict is intrapsychic between several personality structures, and has a pathology that cannot be resolved by altering the current environment. This is evidenced by the continued existence, and even the development of the symptomatology, in the face of often optimal environmental circumstances. Such intrapsychic pathology often requires intensive psychotherapeutic intervention beyond the scope of the pediatrician.

On the other hand, children at any age can develop symptomatology when confronted with an overly stressful environment and show improvement when the environmental stress is alleviated. Here, the therapeutic approach is a relatively greater degree of environmental modification.

The school-age child continues to be dependent on his environment, so that there is an overlap and interplay between intrapsychic and environmental factors; both must be evaluated carefully in assessing psychopathology and determining the appropriate therapuetic approach. While the final eruption of psychoneurotic symptomatology may be precipitated by some environmental circumstance, the symptomatology is characteristically well-rooted in earlier predisposing developmental fixations and intrapsychic conflict. It is not likely to be very responsive to environmental changes. Specialized psychiatric intervention is necessary.

EGO DISTURBANCES

Certain children show significant disturbances in one or more of the principal functions of the ego, that hypothetical portion of the psychic "structure" which mediates and integrates internal drives and external reality. Some of the functions of the ego have already been indicated in the review of the young child's development. They consist of perceptual-motor functions, memory, thinking, object relations, reality testing and a sense of identity, defense, and integration and synthesis of stimuli from all sources.

Serious disturbances of one or more of these crucial functions markedly impair the child's developmental progress. Such impairments are seen in organic brain syndromes, childhood psychoses and in ego weaknesses of lesser degree. Mental retardation also constitutes a type of ego disturbance, namely, that of noticeable impairment of the ego's cognitive functions.

Children with minimal brain dysfunction, either of organic etiology or from severe developmental deprivation, may show, in addition to localized manifestations of a neurological nature, a wide constellation of characteristics. In addition to a persistent reluctance to let go of a situation once it has been structured, often there is increased irritability, excessive reactions of rage and despair, excessive crying, or withdrawal due to frustration. These children tend to be overly talkative and repetitive, somewhat awkward and deficient in perceptual-motor functions, clumsy, and therefore somewhat destructive; they over-react to frustration, to which they are easily susceptible. They are also somewhat guileless with a capacity to misjudge social situations; they miss the point, and therefore tend toward social immaturity. They are often not accepted by their peers, are excluded, and lack adequate social experiences. These characteristics further contribute to difficulties in school adjustment and performance.

A severe form of ego disturbance is the childhood psychosis. Here there is a marked impairment of the child's sense of identity, reality testing and object relationships, including interpersonal communication. One type of childhood psychosis, early infantile autism, first described by Leo Kanner, consists of a caricature of the earliest levels of psychic development that continue to manifest themselves. These children appear to be living in complete detachment from the world around them and the circular interactions between child and parent are broken down.

In another form of childhood psychosis the symbiotic psychosis described by Margaret Mahler, the child seems never to have mastered the separation-individuation process. He apparently relates in a seemingly satisfactory way with his mother until a point somewhere in the second or third year when special ego adaptations are required of him in response to special demands or stressful circumstances; he responds with a markedly disturbing reaction. The child either clings desperately to his mother searching for some kind of union with her, or easily slips back into a regressed level of isolated, detached and autistic function. It is as though in the face of some external demand, the resources of the ego are incapable of coping and resort to either progressively increased demands on his mother as an auxiliary ego, or to a severe regression. The child's capacity for functioning in any of the ego areas is thus seriously impaired.

There are also a number of children who from time to time show rather erratic pictures of development. On examination they evidence combinations and degrees of disturbance of one or more of the ego's functions, without necessarily demonstrating the global nature of the severe ego disturbances that have been previously described. These children remind one of the extreme examples of developmental deviations referred to earlier, with excesses and deficiencies in development of sensory function, motility, speech, or object relations. It is as though the governor or executive apparatus of the psychic structure were out of commission and the various functions of the ego were being expressed without appropriate modulation and integration.

These children are both distressing and markedly distressed. They exhibit degrees of disruption and disorganization of the core aspects of the entire psychic function; the roots of these difficulties are often inborn or the product of early environmental insults and as such require long, intensive and sometimes heroic interventive therapeutic efforts.

The subject of mental deficiency, a special type of ego disturbance of complex etiology, will be discussed elsewhere in this book.

While the above areas of pathology have featured predominant characteristics and etiological determination, there is a considerable overlapping of these categories, both in terms of characteristics and etiology. Many behavioral manifestations are determined in a composite fashion. In some instances the same symptomatology may individually have a variety of causes. Delinquent behavior in children, learning and reading disorders, and chronic hyperactivity are examples of conditions which may derive from multiple etiologies separately or in combination with one another. Any of these conditions could result from one or another developmental deviation, or from various developmental interferences which have been described as modifying the child's optimal development.

Similarly, arrests in instinctual and ego development, psychosis, organic brain syndrome, various ego weaknesses, mental retardation, psychoneuroses, may be the major causative factors in any of these pathological categories. For example, a delinquent child may be performing antisocial acts out of a sense of overwhelming guilt and a search for punishment, while on the other hand the same antisocial act might be a consequence of his limited cognitive development, psychosis, or a severe weakness in reality testing and internal controls, either organically or functionally determined. The same may be said for learning disorders and other symptom complexes.

REFERRAL

It is the primary care physician and not the child psychiatrist to whom parents and community turn for early guidance and understanding of healthy child development and rearing, as well as for a comprehensive approach to the ill, hospitalized or even dying child. He is the key mediator and purveyor of all we have learned about child and adolescent mental health. Only after the physician has thoroughly explored questions about the child's development or problems in his "total" development, may he turn to a child psychiatrist or other mental health specialist for consultation in certain cases where the problem exceeds the experience and realm of comprehensive pediatric practice.

REFERENCES

1. Kanner, L.: Autistic disturbances of affective contact. Nervous Child, 2:217, 1943.

   The classic first description of the syndrome of infantile autism of Leo Kanner.

2. Mahler, M. S.: Of Human Symbiosis and the Vicissitudes of Individuation. New York, International Universities Press, Inc., 1968.

   A detailed exposition of the principal stages of separation-individuation researched by the author.

3. ———On Child Psychosis and Schizophrenia: Autistic and Symbiotic Infantile Psychoses. The Psychoanalytic Study of the Child: 7:286-305, 1952.

   An early description of the syndrome of symbiotic psychosis as resulting from the child's lack of readiness for and failure in the process of separation and individuation.

4. Nagera, H.: Early Childhood Disturbances, the Infantile Neurosis, and the Adulthood Disturbances. Monograph Series of the Psychoanalytic Study of the Child, #2. New York, International Universities Press, 1966.

   A detailed dissection of the etiologic and dynamic nature of a hierarchy of early childhood disorders, delineating the relative roles and interplay of external and internal developmental interferences.

5. Spitz, R. A.: The psychogenic diseases in infancy: An attempt at their etiologic classification. The Psychoanalytic Study of the Child, 6:255-275, 1951.

   An etiologic classification of psychosomatic diseases in infancy constructed on six qualitative variations of inappropriate maternal attitudes and two quantitative variations in mother-child relations.

29

Mental Retardation

David Baker, M.D.

Mental retardation (or subnormality) is a major chronic handicap with profound implications for total life adjustment. The modern definition of mental retardation (significantly subaverage general intellectual functioning originating during the developmental period and associated with impairment of adaptive behavior, learning and social adjustment) views broadly not only cognitive ability (as measured by "intelligence tests") but the total resultant summation of a person's competency in social adaptation. The term "mentally retarded" is limited to those persons who have inherent mental deficiency as a result of anatomical, physiological, or biochemical impairment of central nervous system (CNS) function. Those who are unable to function intellectually or socially at the level expected by their chronological age as a result of non-CNS disability, sensory deprivation, social-cultural deprivation, or emotional disturbance, can best be described as having "pseudo-retardation."

As noted in Table 29-1, the majority of retarded people fall into the "mild" or "borderline" groups. Opinion is divided as to whether the persons who appear normal on physical and neurological examination are retarded because of polygenic inheritable factors (familial retardation) or socio-cultural determinants. Siblings of mildly retarded patients show a higher frequency of mild retardation when compared to the siblings of severely retarded patients, who are likely to be normal in intelligence. The mildly retarded are "educable," that is, capable of learning elementary reading, spelling, arithmetic; with modern educational and vocational training and community-based supportive programs, they are capable of being employed and becoming independent and self-sufficient.

The moderately retarded, in educational terms, are "trainable" and have potential for self-care and activities of daily living. These patients

Table 29-1. Characteristics of Varying Degrees of Mental Retardation

I.Q. = M.A./C.A.	S.D.	Function	Physical findings	Family history of mental retardation	Socio-cultural factors	Prevalence (%) M.R.	Total Pop.	Therapeutic goals
Borderline 70–84	−1.01 to −2.00	Basic academic skills "Slow learner"	Essentially normal	+	4+	67	13	Basic academic & social skills to be capable of self-support and independent living in community
Mild	55–69 −2.01 to −3.00	Educable (vocational training)	"	+	3+	22	2.7	"
Moderate	40–54 −3.01 to −4.00	Trainable	Increasing frequency of neurologic deficits Stigmata of dysmorphism	Only in cases due to genetic disorders	0	6	0.2	Self-care skills involving activities of daily living and sheltered workshop
Severe	25–39 −4.01 to −5.00	Dependent		"	0	3	0.1	Protective care at home or group home
Profound <25	−5.00	Totally dependent		"	0	2	0.05	Custodial care

need supervision. Employment in a sheltered workshop while maintaining residence at home or in a group home is a feasible goal.

The severely or profoundly retarded are unable to provide for their own needs and are dependent upon others for care. In this group are seen the various morphological stigmata of congenital malformation and genetic disorders, as well as the signs of severe neurological damage from pre- and perinatal insult to the CNS.

The prevalence of mental retardation (I.Q. less than 70) is estimated to be about 1 per cent of the adult population, but 3 per cent of newborns will be identified as retarded at some point in their lives. In children, mental retardation is second only to learning disabilities in frequency, and it is more often seen than cerebral palsy (0.5%) or epilepsy (0.5–1%). The prevalence of mental retardation increases during the school years as tests require greater comprehension for children of increasing age, and also because of ascertainment of intellectual subnormality as the child fails to cope with the demands of the school. The child who can learn by rote and can manage tasks requiring only concrete thinking may fail a test requiring abstract conceptualization, yet the "6-hour retarded child" (in school) may show good adaptive ability in a social setting other than school.

ETIOLOGY OF MENTAL RETARDATION

Infection

Prenatal infection includes the various intrauterine infections such as rubella, syphilis, cytomegalic inclusion body disease, toxoplasmosis, and infection due to herpes virus. Postnatal infections that cause mental retardation may be due to bacteria or viruses, including postinfectious encephalitis.

Toxic Agents

Mental retardation may be induced in the perinatal or neonatal period by maternal ingestion of intoxicants, toxemia of pregnancy, and kernicterus associated with hyperbilirubinemia related to blood group incompatibility and various other causes. In older infants and children, retardation can be a result of postimmunization toxicity after administration of pertussis and smallpox vaccines, and as a result of ingestion of lead and other toxic agents, causing encephalopathy.

Trauma or Physical Agents

These include interferences with fetal circulation, birth injury, anoxia at birth, and postnatal injury due to cranial trauma or battered child syndrome.

Disorders of Metabolism, Growth or Nutrition

Included here are the varied disorders of metabolism related to lipid, protein, and carbohydrate disorders. Among the various important causes are hypoglycemia, PKU, galactosemia, homocystinuria, and protein/calorie malnutrition. Endocrine disorders such as hypothyroidism are estimated to occur in one of 6,000 newborns; these too cause mental retardation.

Other Causes

Mental retardation may also be associated with gross postnatal brain disease, congenital defects, chromosomal abnormalities, prematurity, major psychiatric disorders, and psychosocial environment factors such as deprivation and cultural-familial retardation. Children suffering cultural-familial retardation usually suffer only mild impairment, while environmentally deprived children have more severe retardation. The relative incidence of genetic chromosomal disorders and inborn errors of metabolism as causes of mental retardation is 14 per cent; thus, various factors including social and economic factors cause the bulk of mental retardation (Table 29-2). Emphasis on good prenatal care and nutrition, prevention of accidents, abuse, neglect and poisoning are likely to result in decreased incidence of retardation. Advances in methods of immunizations and treatment of infectious diseases also contribute.

Table 29-2. Relative Frequency of Causes of Mental Retardation

Etiology	Percentage
Inborn errors and hereditary disorders	4
Early influences on embryonic development (Chromosomal changes 10%; multiple congenital anomalies 23%)	33
Maternal and perinatal causes (Fetal malnutrition 1%; prematurity with hyperbilirubinemia, hypoglycemia, trauma, hypoxia 11%)	12
Acquired childhood diseases	4
Environmental and social problems	19
Cause unknown	28

PREVENTIVE ASPECTS

Even before pregnancy occurs, prevention of mental retardation is possible. All women of childbearing age should be immunized with rubella vaccine. Family planning education can be helpful in avoiding high risk and unwanted pregnancies.

With pregnancy, efforts should turn toward preventing contamination of the fetal environment with bacteria, viruses, and teratogenic agents. Good prenatal care insures that the fetus is monitored for intrauterine growth impairment and for the ill-effects of maternal toxemia or diabetes. Close monitoring during labor and delivery allows early detection of fetal distress.

Recent advances in neonatology have resulted in improved care for high-risk newborns, including early detection of metabolic defects. Proper therapy of infantile diarrhea and avoidance of hypertonic dehydration can minimize mental impairment from those sources.

In older children, good nutrition and good medical care are of particular importance. A consistent immunization series should be given to each child. Parents should be educated on safety measures to prevent accidents, trauma, and poisonings. Medical practitioners should be alert for signs of child abuse and neglect.

EARLY IDENTIFICATION AND DIAGNOSIS

Regular developmental assessments should be performed, especially in infants and children at high risk. This includes regular measurement of growth parameters, including head circumference. Examinations should be performed to detect sensory handicaps as a part of the routine child care program.

Once suspicious signs are noted, a complete diagnostic work-up should be pursued with respect to determination of etiological factors (both primary and contributing factors) and a functional assessment of the degree of retardation in various aspects of development (Table 29-3). Appropriate referrals to sub-specialists should be considered if the physician wishes to coordinate the work-up himself or to a center which offers complete diagnosis and evaluation services by a team approach. In any event, the primary physician should take the responsibility for ensuring that the diagnostic services are completed satisfactorily, that the family is thoroughly informed, and that parents have adequate opportunity to ask questions, ventilate their concerns, and assume that there will be a planned comprehensive program for follow-up care and supervision.

The primary physician most likely makes the initial identification of the severely to moderately retarded child who presents with craniofacial abnormalities, microcephaly, neural tube defects, or other dysmorphic features at birth, or who shows rather clear cut developmental delays early in infancy and childhood. The mildly to borderline retarded group may not be recognized as early, especially when these children get poor or sporadic medical supervision. They may be referred from day care centers, preschool nursery programs, or, unfortunately, later in elementary schools.

Attention to developmental assessment (as outlined in the chapter on Child Development) should enable the physician to detect children with milder degrees of retardation prior to school entrance. These children usually exhibit delays in development, particularly in language, personal-social, and adaptive behavior, and may show unusual degrees of responsiveness in terms of being hypoactive or, on the other hand, may be hyperkinetic.

MANAGEMENT

The physician must face the problem of how to tell the parents that they have a retarded child, and how to help them provide for the needs of the child in order to stimulate maximum developmental potential while at the same time to rear their other children and deal with their own wounded feelings. He must recognize the parents' right to complete, accurate information and their responsibility to make major decisions affecting the child in the context of their own family situation. Physicians do not realize how vital a role they play with regard to their influence on the family and how influential their support can be in helping the family cope with these difficult situations.

Table 29-3. Checklist for Remediable Conditions

Condition	Procedure
Specific sensory deficit: Vision, Hearing	Careful examination; oto-audiologic and ophthalmic evaluation
Seizure phenomenon including "convulsive equivalent"	EEG
Metabolic and endocrine disorders	Metabolic screening tests, T_3, T_4, GTT*
Systemic disease including failure to thrive	Appropriate workup
Toxic (exogenous factors)	Pb and EPP† levels
Increased intracranial pressure	Funduscopic examination; skull film, brain scan
Ongoing active and progressive disease	Tests for metabolic disorders affecting CNS; CSF exam; brain scan, EEG
Other specific etiologic factors	Serology for rubella, herpes virus, cytomegalic inclusion disease, toxoplasmosis, STS
Genetic factors	Family history; buccal smear; karyotype; biochemical and enzyme studies; examine other family members; genetic counseling
Learning disability	Psycho-educational evaluation; educational programming
Speech and/or language disorder	Language/speech/hearing evaluation and appropriate therapy

*Glucose tolerance test
†Erythrocyte protoporphyrin

Parental reactions to the diagnosis of retardation initially involve shock, depression, and disbelief. It is extremely important to tell *both* parents the diagnosis at the same time and to plan several sessions after the initial statement so that they can air their feelings and questions. Often the parents do not hear the entire message the first time because they are emotionally upset and cannot focus on the issues. The diagnosis should be validated in a most authoritative fashion. One should anticipate that parents will have doubts and may want other professional opinions; indeed, the physician should encourage them to seek the opinions of a competent specialist rather than to let them "shop around" and perhaps fall into the hands of charlatans. One should not give false reassurance ("The child will grow out of it") in an effort to spare their feelings. Yet one should be extremely sympathetic and recognize that the parents experience a loss and while going through a period of grief and mourning may have difficulty relating to the physician who bears the bad news. The parents often view themselves as being damaged since they have given birth to a damaged child.

When the diagnosis is made in the postpartum period the problem can be especially distressing, as in the case of the newborn with Downs syndrome or other genetic or congenital defects, in the case of Downs syndrome with older parents, and especially in the case of the first baby. During the pregnancy the parents usually anticipate the possibility of the child being abnormal and the first question asked is in regard to that. One should not delay telling the parents that the child is abnormal if this is the case, and then help them make an identification and attachment with the baby to help them cope with the problem.

In the case of the child who has a gradually evolving picture of retarded development, the initial identification attachment of the child to the parents has been made; the problems of coping with the diagnosis will then include denial and ambivalence. After the initial shock phase, the parents often experience feelings of rejection, or they may compensate and overprotect the infant. Often excessive pressure of a coercive nature is placed on the child who is viewed as "lazy." In any event, parental attitudes of coercion, rejection or overprotection will compound and interfere with the further development of the child.

Therefore, close follow-up with anticipatory guidance and counseling should be planned. A long-term longitudinal "life-cycle" approach will deal with problems presented at each stage of development of the child. Also one must deal with the significance of mental retardation to the parents. They often view the child as having null potential and fail to recognize that the child will make developmental progress, although at a slower rate than normal children. Often young parents will not inform other family members or other children in the family; they should be encouraged to do so promptly because they will need the additional support of their extended family.

During early infancy problems center around basic home care such as feeding, sleeping, and other problems familiar to physicians who take care of infants. Later, concern will be focused on motility, toilet training, and still later on language development, socialization, and need for a preschool stimulation program.

It is important to convey the value of the child to the parents. The child should receive regular immunizations and care of intercurrent illnesses. It is important to let the parents know what to expect and to set up goals for the next epoch of development. Parents should be praised and reassured for doing a good job in taking care of their children; the positive aspects of the child should be stressed, but in a balanced, realistic fashion. The opportunity to talk with other parents who have had similar problems and who have learned methods of coping is a very therapeutic experience.

In the past, institutionalization had been recommended freely. It has been shown that a nurturing, stimulating home environment will provide the opportunity for maximal development and no effort should be spared to build into the program support for the family to rear the child at home. Indications for institutionalization are highly selective and should be reserved when other measures fail and the family cannot cope with the child. However, it must be recognized that the care of an extremely handicapped child can be a tremendous burden. Many programs are being offered for respite care or part-time placement; in this way the family can have a vacation knowing that the child will receive care. This may be necessary at times when there is a breakdown in the family's capacity to meet the child's needs and should be looked at as part of a positive therapeutic program rather than a negative event.

Community Mental Health and Mental Retardation Centers offer counseling including home visits by mental health workers and by parents who have retarded children. These services should be used freely.

Parents should be encouraged to join and participate in parents' organizations for the benefit of group therapy, to be involved actively and effect change in the local community to improve the care of the retarded. The history of mental retardation illustrates the relationship between society and an underprivileged minority. Indeed, the way in which a society deals with its handicapped is a measure of its state of civilization with respect to moral and ethical matters.

"Scientific" ideology and the eugenics movement were well-intended but misguided forces in segregating the retarded (including many individuals who now are viewed as socioculturally deprived) into institutions in the early part of the century where they languished. The efforts of organized parents groups (The National Association for Retarded Citizens) with the help of visionary humanistic professionals (such as Grover Powers, former professor of pediatrics at Yale University) were instrumental in changing this picture and are part of the story of a broad movement for human rights and the dignity of the individual.

One may view parental counseling in terms of epochal phases in which crucial decisions are made in the course of development. The major epochs include care during infancy, preschool programs, school age programs, problems related to pubertal and adolescent development, and vocational training. Adolescents with emerging sexual drives and poor self controls present many problems. Recreational and socialization programs are needed for the retarded who have problems being accepted by other children and being isolated from the community.

The physician must be familiar with resources within his community which offer services to the retarded. Furthermore, he should make efforts to improve the quality of these services by supporting parents groups, establish educational programs, and community mental health/mental retardation centers. His influence in the community is considerable, something which physicians often underestimate. His involvement in giving support to child abuse programs, immunization programs, and supportive services to the school will also be of importance with respect to the problems of mental retardation.

BIBLIOGRAPHY

Milunsky, A.: The Prevention of Genetic Disease and Mental Retardation. Philadelphia, W. B. Saunders, 1977.

> The author, a geneticist, writes knowingly of the recent advances in this rapidly growing area. The ratio of information acquired to time expended reading this work is very high. A wide range of topics is covered, including the causes and prevalence of mental retardation, principles of genetic counselling, prenatal diagnosis, prevention of prematurity and perinatal morbidity, lead intoxication, infectious diseases and early intervention. Legal, economic and eugenic issues are discussed.

Richmond, J. B., Tarjan, G., and Mendelsohn, R., (eds.): Mental Retardation: A Handbook for the Primary Physician. 2nd ed. Chicago, American Medical Association, 1974.

> This is a brief overview of the subject and is useful as a desk reference.

Smith, D. W., and Simons, F. E. R.: Rational diagnostic evaluation of the child with mental deficiency. Am. J. Dis. Child., *129*:1285-1290, 1975.

> This article clearly presents a practical approach for diagnostic procedures and data illustrating the relevance of various studies in relation to the history and physical examination.

30

Seizures and Other Paroxysmal Disorders

Michael H. Mitchell, M.D., and Peter H. Berman, M.D.

Paroxysmal disorders are recurrent, reversible alterations of brain function. Several occur frequently in children; particularly syncope, migraine, breath-holding and seizures. Although not subjects of this chapter, recurrent neurologic dysfunction also characterizes certain other diseases such as drug abuse and rare inborn errors of amino acid and urea metabolism.

Paroxysmal Disorders

Seizures	Paroxysmal vertigo
Migraine	Others
	Hypoglycemia
Syncope	Psychiatric disorders
	Drug abuse
Breath-holding spells	Certain in-born errors of metabolism

SEIZURE DISORDERS

Seizures are more frequent in children than in adults and are among the commonest neurologic disorders in pediatrics. It is stated that 4–8 per cent of *all* children experience one or more seizures between infancy and adolescence. This higher frequency of seizures in childhood reflects a greater seizure susceptibility in the immature brain which many children eventually outgrow, particularly when they are otherwise neurologically normal.

The stage of cerebral development strongly influences seizures. Examples discussed later in this chapter are neonatal seizures, infantile spasms and febrile convulsions where the onset, types and duration of seizures are remarkably age-dependent. Although the relevant processes are not well understood, cerebral maturation is a major factor determining whether seizures will be outgrown, change in type or persist to become epilepsy in adulthood.

EPILEPSY

Seizures often occur in non-epileptic children. Frequently seizures mark the onset of such serious acute brain diseases as intracranial infection, head injury and various toxic/metabolic disorders. Also, about five per cent of small children have seizures triggered by high fever (see Febrile Convulsions) as opposed to epilepsy which affects only 0.5 per cent of children in the same age group.

Epilepsy, a Greek word meaning "seizure," is a heterogenous group of disorders having in common a susceptibility to recurring seizures caused by intrinsic congenital or acquired brain abnormalities which in any particular patient may or may not be demonstrable by present-day diagnostic techniques. The types of seizures and the presence or absence of non-seizure abnormalities such as mental retardation or physical deformities greatly depends on what brain disease is present in each case. In fact, when seizures are completely or nearly completely controlled through good medical management, a large proportion of epileptic children live unhampered lives, do well in school, get a driver's license and pursue a satisfying adult career. Although we do not ignore the terms "epileptic" or "epilepsy," we prefer the official label "seizure disorder" which is more objective, more comprehensible to laymen and far less prejudicial when it appears in the child's school or medical records.

DESCRIPTION AND CLASSIFICATION OF SEIZURES

Hughlings Jackson's 1880 definition of seizure remains one of the best: "A seizure is an occasional, excessive and disorderly discharge of neurons resulting in an excess, distortion or deficit of central nervous system function. These disruptions of CNS function will vary according to the area of seizure onset and pathways of spread within the brain."

Our description of seizures (Table 30-1) is derived from the recently developed International Classification which is based on both clinical and electroencephalographic (EEG) abnormalities. This description successfully characterizes most childhood seizures.

Table 30-1. Seizure Classification with Examples of Clinical and EEG Findings

Seizure type	Examples of seizure activity	Typical EEG Findings
Partial seizures		
Motor (Focal motor)	Jacksonian march, adversive, speech arrest	
Sensory (Focal sensory)	Localized cutaneous, visual, auditory, smell, taste or vertiginous sensations	1. Focal abnormality* 2. Normal†
Complex (Psychomotor)	Impaired consciousness, visual or auditory misperceptions or hallucinations, anxiety, automatisms, déjà vu, visceral sensations. (Note: typical postictal lethargy and headache).	
Multifocal	Multiple partial seizures	Multifocal abnormalities
Generalized seizures		
Major motor ("convulsion" or grand mal)	Tonic-clonic. Sometimes purely tonic or clonic. "Secondary generalized major motor seizures" are very common—e.g., those with an aura, preceding partial seizure or localized EEG abnormality	1. Focal abnormality* 2. Normal† 3. Bilaterally synchronous discharges‡
Absence (Petit mal)	Brief loss of consciousness with or without eye blinking, automatism, clonic jerks or changes in tone. (Note: No postictal symptoms)	Bilaterally synchronous discharges especially 3/second spike-wave
Myoclonic	Massive or localized single jerks, often occurring in clusters. One characteristic type is infantile spasms	Various bilateral discharges‡ (Hypsarrhythmia in infantile spasms)
Atonic	Abrupt loss of tone, resultant fall frequently causing facial injury. Often associated with myoclonic seizures	
Akinetic	Inability to move (without loss of tone)	
Hemiconvulsions	Clonic or tonic-clonic activity in infants involving one entire side of the body	Contralateral discharges

*Focal paroxysmal discharges or disturbances of background rhythms (see Fig. 30-1).
†EEG may become positive with special techniques (e.g., sleep recording or nasopharyngeal leads).
‡Such as spike-wave, polyspike or paroxysmal slow waves (see Fig. 30-3).

PARTIAL SEIZURES

"Partial seizures" is a relatively new term used in the International Classification to encompass manifestations of localized seizure involvement of the brain (Fig. 30-1). The cerebral localization can be inferred by history or observations of the initial symptoms or motor phenomena. Often a description by the parent or other observer must be sought since the patient may have partial or complete amnesia for the attack. Sometimes the history will give a better localization for the origin of partial seizures than the EEG.

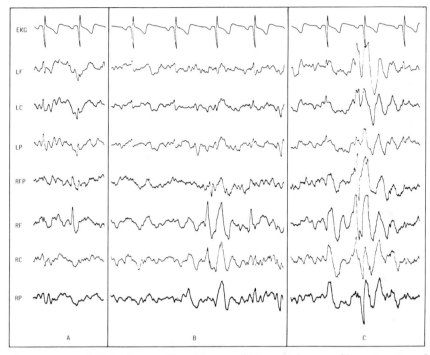

Fig. 30-1. Focal EEG abnormality: 13-year-old boy with neurofibromatosis and recent onset of partial and major motor seizures (also see Fig. 30-2, C). EEG shows focal right frontal spike (A), more extensive right hemisphere discharge (B) and discharge spreading to left hemisphere (C). (EKG = electrocardiogram, L = left, R = right, F = frontal, FP = frontopolar, C = central, P = parietal.)

Partial Motor Seizures

The most typical "focal" or partial motor seizure is tonic stiffening and/or clonic jerking of the face or extremity contralateral to the cerebral focus. Most often the initial involvement is rather diffuse, for example an entire extremity or the face and upper extremity. Relatively rare are *Jacksonian seizures* which begin in a highly localized part and then "march" in a way predictable from the functional anatomy of the motor strip: for example, an initial twitching of the thumb spreading to the fingers and then simultaneously to the face and lower extremity. These seizures, the Jacksonian especially, indicate a focus in or near the contralateral pre-central gyrus (motor strip).

Adversive seizures are also common. The head and eyes are turned contralaterally from the focus and the extremities on both sides may assume characteristic postures, particularly extension of the contralateral and flexion of the ipsilateral extremities in a manner similar to the infantile tonic neck reflex. Sometimes the contralateral rotation of the head and trunk is so strong that the patient actually turns in circles. Adversive seizures usually result from contralateral cerebral foci but they may be anywhere in the hemisphere, particularly in frontal, temporal or occipital areas.

Purely *inhibitory seizures* causing only temporary paralysis of the affected part are rare. When the hemisphere dominant for speech (usually the left) is involved, speech arrest or aphasia may accompany partial seizures. Postictal (Todd's) paralysis of the parts involved in a partial motor seizure frequently occurs and usually clears within several hours.

In children, partial motor seizures, focal or multifocal, often accompany acute, non-localized disturbances in brain function such as meningitis, hyponatremia or neonatal hypocalcemia. Although each case must be evaluated carefully, partial seizures in these situations very often do not indicate permanent localized brain damage. Epileptic children with stereotyped partial seizures and well-defined EEG foci (see Fig. 30-1) can be assumed to have a cortical lesion but it is remarkable how often one fails to demonstrate the lesion by sophisticated tests. When demonstrable, examples of lesions causing chronic partial seizures are cysts, vascular anomalies, other cerebral malformations and brain tumors. Figure 30-2 shows several examples demonstrated by computerized tomography.

Partial Sensory Seizures

Partial sensory seizures occur when irritative foci affect cerebral cortical sensory areas; thus, they can be categorized as somatic and special sensory seizures. *Somatic sensory seizures* arise from the contralateral post-central gyrus (sensory strip) and are most frequently described as a numbness or tingling, although pins and needles, movement, warmth and other sensations may be felt in the body part affeced by the seizure. The initially localized sensations may spread on the involved side as does a Jacksonian motor seizure. Due to the proximity and overlap of the Rolandic motor and sensory strips, motor seizure phenomena often occur concurrently.

Special sensory seizures arise from the occipital visual, temporal auditory-vestibular and olfactory, and Sylvian taste areas. Occipital visual seizures are usually elementary phenomena such as flashing lights and need to be differentiated from migraine attacks. More complex visual seizures, such as change in size or color of objects seen, usually arise from temporal lobe association areas. Seizures from the other sensory areas produce hallucinations of sound, motion, smell or taste which, because of their close proximity to other temporal lobe structures, are very frequently the aura to a complex seizure (see below).

Complex Partial Seizures

Complex partial seizures (also commonly called "psychomotor" or "temporal lobe" seizures) are fascinating, particularly because they affect

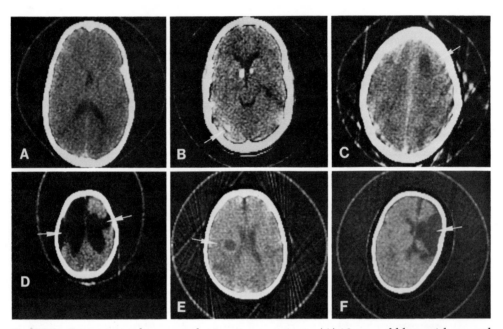

Fig. 30-2. Computerized tomography in seizure patients. (*A*) 10-year-old boy with mental retardation, seizures and large head. CT scan is normal. (*B*) Tuberous sclerosis: adolescent with typical skin manifestations, seizures and multifocal EEG discharges. CT scan shows the dense periventricular and cortical (arrow) hamartomas. (*C*) Cerebral tumor: Adolescent with neurofibromatosis, recent onset of partial and major motor seizures, and focal EEG. CT scan shows right frontal lesion (cystic astrocytoma). (*D*) Prenatal infection: Infant with developmental delay, chorioretinitis, myoclonic seizures and multifocal EEG. CT scan shows multiple cystic areas, (arrows) and ventricular enlargement presumably due to 3rd trimester *Herpes simplex* infection. (*E*) Cerebral abscess: Child with cyanotic congenital heart disease developed major motor seizures with focal EEG. CT scan shows left hemisphere lesion (arrow) which disappeared with antibiotic therapy. (*F*) Hemiplegic cerebral palsy: Child with hemiplegia, focal motor seizures and focal EEG attributed to birth anoxia. CT scan shows small right hemisphere with large cystic area (*arrow*).

areas of the cerebral cortex serving such complex functions as emotion, memory, other intellectual activities and the highest levels of autonomic system integration.

Although the pattern of seizure phenomena varies greatly from patient to patient, the attacks are usually clinically characteristic and indicative of origin in one or the other temporal lobes, especially the anterior and medial "limbic" portions. Adolescence and young adulthood are particularly important times for the development of complex partial seizures, most likely due to the combination of pre-existing lesions and maturational characteristics of the temporal lobe.

Complex partial seizures can be described as five general types: (1) arrest of activity with staring only, (2) arrest of activity with staring followed by automatisms, (3) psychic seizures, (4) seizures with visceral phenomena and (5) progression to secondary generalized seizures. These seizures are frequently considered in the differential diagnosis of childhood behavioral and psychiatric disorders.

Attacks causing *arrest of activity* with staring typically last 1–2 minutes, rarely more than 5 minutes. Consciousness is impaired and the patient usually cannot remember the attack. These "psychomotor lapses" are frequently misdiagnosed as simple absences (petit mal) but they are different due to their longer duration, postictal confusion and EEG findings. Arrest of activity with staring followed by simple or complex automatisms is similar with the additional phenomenon of *automatisms*, which are repetitive, automatic-looking movements. Simple automatisms include various oro-facial movements such as lip-smacking, chewing or mumbling, and movements of the hands like pulling at clothing, rubbing the face or fumbling with objects. Because simple automatisms also occur in absences, there is further potential confusion between these two very different seizure disorders (see also Generalized Seizures).

Complex automatisms encompass more integrated motor activity such as running in circles, removal of clothing or continuing in a rather aimless way some voluntary activity that was in progress before the seizure. Often the automatic behavior reflects a partial awareness of the environment.

Psychic seizures are consciously experienced by the patient. Affective components are common, usually fear or anxiety, and are generally recognized by the patients as not being real. Only a few patients describe the affective experiences as being pleasant. Memory phenomena include the famous déjà vu (a peculiar and inappropriate sense of familiarity), a sudden feeling of strangeness of the current environment, or a recollection from the past. Perceptual distortions of sight or sound can be striking such as the "zoom lens" phenomenon where objects in the environment seem to shrink or enlarge. Hallucinations, such as formed visual or auditory images or reliving a past experience, can be stereotyped or vary from attack to attack.

Visceral phenomena, both subjective and objective, frequently occur. The olfactory hallucinations, (usually distinctly unpleasant odors), are often associated with other phenomena such as déjà vu or may simply be the aura to a major motor seizure. Visceral sensations are quite common—frequently a peculiar abdominal distress which may become a "rising sensation" of abdominal discomfort moving upwards in the trunk to the throat or head. In children, "abdominal epilepsy" refers to paroxysmal abdominal pain as a seizure manifestation; it is a relatively rare cause of the syndrome of recurrent abdominal pain in children, however. Objective autonomic changes include pupillary dilatation, tachycardia, hypertension, changes in visceral motility and irregular respirations. The external autonomic changes may suggest rage or panic to an observer but usually the patient is immobile and unconscious.

Multifocal Seizures

Children with multifocal seizures fall into two large groups: First, are those with acute brain disturbances such as anoxia, bacterial meningitis, encephalitis, hypoglycemia, hyponatremia, hypocalcemia or lead intoxication. Clearly their prognosis depends on whether the acute cerebral insults are fully reversible or not. The second group is composed of epileptic children who usually have other signs of diffuse brain injury, particularly mental retardation. The seizures in such children are often difficult or impossible to fully control and consist of various partial motor types such as jerky eye movements, tonic adversive posturing, and localized clonus. The children may also suffer generalized attacks such as major motor, myoclonic, atypical absence and atonic seizures.

GENERALIZED SEIZURES

The several types of generalized seizures imply diffuse discharges that occur synchronously in both cerebral hemispheres. Apparently all of us have cerebral mechanisms for the most common type of generalized seizure, the major motor seizure, so it is not surprising that major motor seizures are common and occur in many different clinical settings. Probably most major motor seizures are secondary generalized seizures resulting when initially localized discharges rapidly become diffuse. On the other hand, certain epilepsies, particularly typical absences and a few patients with major motor seizures, are called primary generalized seizures because at present no localized "generator" has been found to explain the bilaterally synchronous EEG discharges in these cases.

Major Motor Seizures

After early infancy major motor seizures are by far the most common seizure type, occurring, for example, in about 80 per cent of epileptic children and most children with febrile convulsions. Among epileptic children with major motor seizures about half also have other seizure types. When parents say "convulsion" they usually mean a major motor seizure and, when asked, will usually recall their fear that their child was dying when the convulsion began.

The attack may occur abruptly or be preceded by an aura or by nonspecific prodromal behavioral changes such as irritability. When an *aura* is experienced beforehand, there definitely is a focal origin of the convulsion. Basically, auras are initial partial sensory seizures progressing immediately to a secondary generalized major motor seizure.

Next there is a sudden loss of consciousness, a fall if the child is not supported, and a generalized muscle contraction resulting in the *tonic phase* of diffuse rigidity, arrest of breathing, cyanosis and upward deviation of the eyes. Sometimes there is a piercing cry, biting of the tongue or cheek and loss of urine. The tonic phase is followed by a *clonic phase* of repeated flexor spasms of the entire body. Jerking respirations now resume and the intervals between clonic jerks lengthen until clonus ceases. Pooling of pharyngeal secretions is prominent. Autonomic phenomena also occur, including pupil dilatation, skin vasomotor changes, piloerection, sweating, tachycardia and hypertension.

The clonic jerks are followed by the *postictal phase* with unconsciousness, flaccid muscles, absent tendon reflexes and extensor plantar reflexes. As patients awaken, they are confused and frequently so irritable that they become combative if restrained. Often there is a postictal headache and desire to sleep. Unfortunate consequences can occur if the postictal state is mistaken for intoxication or some sort of antisocial behavior. The patient cannot remember the attack, but knows that it occurred because of postictal discomfort.

In children there is considerable variation in the severity and duration of the convulsive phase as well as the length of postictal CNS depression. Typically the tonic and clonic phases together last about 2 minutes, but often are shorter or longer, up to 5 minutes. Although most children suffer no discernible brain injury from occasional brief major motor seizures, there is always the risk of anoxia, especially if status epilepticus develops. *Major motor status epilepticus* refers to convulsions prolonged over 15 minutes or recurring so frequently that the patient does not recover consciousness in between; it is a true medical emergency.

Besides typical tonic-clonic major motor seizures, there are purely tonic or clonic variants. As a rule tonic seizures are brief and often occur during sleep. Purely clonic generalized seizures occur mostly in small children, especially in febrile convulsions.

The EEG during a major motor seizure reveals generalized high frequency discharges during the tonic phase and spike-wave discharges in the clonic phase. During the postictal phase brain waves are initially depressed in amplitude and then abnormally slow. This postictal slowing subsides gradually and will sometimes require 7–10 days to fully disappear.

Absence Seizures

Absence or petit mal seizures are in essence "blank stares" with sudden, brief interruption of consciousness.

Typical absences form a relatively distinctive, and well-known entity in epilepsy which is largely confined to children over 5 years of age and adolescents. However, it is found in only 5 per cent of all childhood epilepsy patients. The term *petit mal* should probably be avoided because many laymen and some physicians use it to describe any seizure other than a convulsion resulting in much unnecessary confusion.

Absences commonly last less than 10 seconds and infrequently more than 30 seconds. They are subdivided into simple and complex forms; both can occur in the same person. In a simple absence the patient suddenly stares blankly, stops verbal or motor activity and is unconscious but does not fall. The attack begins and ends abruptly with the patient fully alert afterward. Occasionally during the seizure, the patient continues some simple motor activity such as walking. Although the patient is typically unaware of the seizure itself, he or she frequently detects it from the interruption of ongoing events. Those attacks that last over 10 seconds tend to be complex with additional features such as eyelid fluttering, drooping of the head, myoclonic jerks or automatisms. Typical automatisms would be fumbling of the hands, lip-smacking or verbal stuttering.

In the untreated patient with typical absences, the attacks are extremely frequent and the EEG is virtually always abnormal. Twenty to 40 attacks per day are common, and there may be hundreds. The EEG displays sudden generalized bursts of 3 per second spike-wave complexes (see Fig. 30-3) during and between attacks. Clinical attacks and EEG discharges can often be induced by asking the patient to hyperventilate, stroboscopic light stimulation or emotional tension (e.g., the normal anxiety of being called upon in class). When the EEG discharges last 4 seconds or more, consciousness is transiently impaired even though a clinical attack may not be obvious. Since absences typically begin between age 5 and 10 years, teachers or parents frequently misinterpret them initially as daydreaming or peculiar mannerisms.

Another feature of children with typical absences is that they are usually neurologically normal otherwise. A few show learning disabilities, particularly when seizure control is difficult. Less than 5 per cent are

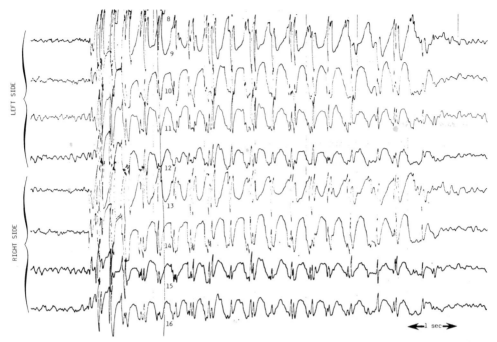

LEFT SIDE

RIGHT SIDE

←1 sec→

Fig. 30-3. Generalized EEG abnormality: 16-year-old girl has had absences since age 8 years. EEG shows bilaterally synchronous polyspike-wave discharges ("primary bilateral synchrony") at about 3/second. In early childhood she had several febrile and afebrile major motor seizures. In spite of continued daily absence seizures she is doing relatively well in tenth grade. Family history is positive for epilepsy.

retarded. In many patients a positive family history suggests an autosomal dominant genetic etiology.

Finally, it is important to differentiate absences from brief, complex partial (psychomotor) seizures because of the occurrence of staring and automatisms in both. As opposed to absences, brief psychomotor seizures generally last more than 30 seconds, are often preceded by an aura, may cause only partial alteration of consciousness, produce postictal confusion and often headache, and usually show localized EEG abnormalities. This differentiation is important because of significant differences in drug therapy. Usually the prognosis for seizure control and outgrowing the seizures in adolescence or young adulthood is good. However, about 50 per cent of patients have one or several major motor seizures during their course and a minority remain epileptics in adult life.

"Atypical" absence seizures do not differ much clinically from "typical" absences but are very different in the total clinical picture and EEG findings. Children in this category are heterogeneous but the majority is retarded or borderline. One large group, called "petit mal variant" or Lennox-Gasteaut syndrome, exhibits mental retardation, "slow" (2/second) spike-wave discharges and multiple types of seizures including absences, tonic seizures in sleep, and myoclonic/atonic seizures (see below).

Petit mal status or "spike-wave stupor" is a prolonged confusional state lasting hours or even days with associated continuous spike-wave discharges. This may occur in atypical or typical absence seizure states. The diagnosis is confirmed by obtaining an immediate EEG.

Myoclonic and Atonic Seizures

Myoclonic and atonic seizures are a difficult topic in childhood epilepsy because these children (1) are often hard to classify, (2) tend to vary greatly in the severity and type of seizure and causative factors, and (3) have a high incidence of other neurological problems, particularly mental retardation.

Myoclonus is a sudden involuntary jerk which may be generalized or localized to one body part. Patterns of seizure myoclonus vary; some forms of myoclonus are not seizures, such as the normal myoclonic jerks that occur when one is falling asleep.

Atonic seizures cause a sudden loss of tone of a few seconds duration. As "epileptic drop attacks," atonic seizures often result in serious facial injury because of their sudden, unpredictable onset. In all myoclonic/atonic seizure disorders most patients experience other seizures types as well, particularly atypical absences, multifocal motor, and generalized tonic or tonic-clonic seizures.

Infantile spasms are the most characteristic syndrome of myoclonic epilepsy in infancy. Infantile spasms are often the first recognized neurological symptoms in a baby who will later be retarded and are frequently responsive to a unique treatment, e.g., ACTH or corticosteroids. Infantile spasms characteristically begin around the sixth month and have usually ceased by the second birthday. The attacks are a 2- or 3-second generalized muscle contraction causing flexion of the trunk and extension of the arms—hence descriptive names like infantile spasm, "salaam attack" or "lightening spasm." Like other myoclonic seizures, infantile spasms tend to occur in clusters, particularly during drowsiness or arousal. Usually the EEG shows a continuously abnormal pattern called "hypsarrhythmia."

SPECIFIC CAUSES OF SEIZURES

Table 30-2 lists causes of seizures in three critical age groups. This diversity of causes emphasizes the importance of considering seizures as symptoms of CNS involvement and the need to treat the underlying cause if possible as well as the symptom.

Table 30-2. Causes of Seizures by Age Group*

Newborn period	Infancy-childhood	Adolescence
Anoxia or ischemia	Febrile convulsions	Unknown
intrapartum	Unknown	Trauma
postpartum	Perinatal insult (see Newborn	Anoxia or ischemia
Infection	Period)	Infection
meningitis	Cerebral malformation	Drug abuse
sepsis	Trauma	Perinatal insult
generalized *Herpes simplex*	accidents	Genetic
Metabolic derangement	child abuse	Brain tumor
(see Table 30-3)	Anoxia or ischemia	Vascular malformation
Prenatal abnormality	Infection	or disease
cerebral malformations	meningitis brain abscess	
intrauterine infections:	encephalitis Reye syndrome	
rubella, cytomegalo-	Genetic	
virus, toxoplasmosis,	non-degenerative, e.g., classic	
syphilis and others	absences	
neurocutaneous syndromes	neurocutaneous syndromes	
tuberous sclerosis	inborn errors: aminoacidurias,	
Birth injury	hypoglycemias, lipid storage	
Drug withdrawal	diseases, hemoglobinopathies,	
barbiturates	etc.	
narcotics	Metabolic derangement	
Unknown	hypocalcemia	
Inborn errors of metabolism	hypoglycemia	
(see Table 30-3)	hyper- and hyponatremia	
	uremia	
	Intoxication	
	drug ingestion	
	lead poisoning	
	Brain tumor	
	Vascular malformation or disease	

*Listed by approximate order of frequency

PATHOGENESIS OF SEIZURES

Metabolic Factors

Neurones function by conducting electrochemical impulses along their membranes and affecting other neurones through synaptic neurotransmitters. Derangement of these neuronal membrane functions is the physiological hallmark of seizure activity. Normally, the central nervous system depends on a continuous blood oxygen and glucose supply because CNS stores of glycogen and high energy compounds are very limited. During a major motor seizure cerebral energy metabolism increases while blood oxygen and glucose supplies tend to decrease due to impaired cardiorespiratory function from the convulsive activity. Cerebral anoxia, acidosis and circulatory disturbance pose serious threats for brain damage during prolonged major motor seizures.

Normal neuronal energy metabolism produces high energy compounds, particularly ATP which maintains the neuronal resting potential and repolarization through the Na^+-K^+ ATPase membrane "pump." During both normal and seizure-induced neuronal depolarization, Na^+ rushes into the neurone and then repolarization is rapidly accomplished by curtailment of the Na^+ influx and a transient K^+ outflow. The Na^+-K^+ ATPase pump then reestablishes the resting ion gradients (low intracellular Na^+, high intracellular K^+. Other factors influencing depolarization/repolarization include: (1) Ca^{++} and Mg^{++} which seem to modulate Na^+-K^+ permeabilities, (2) neurotransmitters, such as the excitatory transmitter acetylcholine which increases Na^+ permeability and the inhibitory transmitter gamma-aminobutyric acid (GABA) which appears to increase K^+ permeability, (3) Cl^- which affects membrane potentials, (4) glial cells which may stabilize neurons by taking up excess extracellular K^+, and (5) many other poorly elucidated factors including structural characteristics of the membrane macromolecules, actions of other neurotransmitters, and influences of trace metals such as zinc and manganese.

A number of systemic metabolic disturbances are routinely complicated by seizures. Anoxia and hypoglycemia, for example, destabilize neuronal membranes through impaired energy metabolism. Seizures typically accompany states of hyponatremia, hypocalcemia and hypomagnesemia. Striking seizures and EEG changes occur in infants who are vitamin B_6 deficient probably through insufficiency of GABA whose synthesis is B_6 dependent. Experimentally, poisoning of the Na^+ - K^+ ATPase pump produces seizures.

Epilepsy: Cellular and Physiological Factors

The intrinsic cerebral abnormalities underlying chronic seizure states appear variable, especially when the great diversity of epilepsy in childhood is considered. Many theories suggest defects in neurotransmitters and synapses, such as: (1) a genetic deficit of inhibitory neurotransmitters like GABA causing abnormal cortical excitability, (2) neuronal groups becoming hypersensitive as the result of loss of afferent connections, (3) abnormal post-synaptic receptors and (4) mechanical distortion of neuronal processes. Other theories attribute neuronal hyperirritability to disturbed membrane depolarization/repolarization from defects in cellular energy metabolism of Na^+ - K^+ ATPase pump function. Another theory suggests a glial cell abnormality such as defective glial K^+ uptake resulting in neuronal depolarization from excessive extracellular K^+.

In humans and in experimental animals much is known about the epileptic focus. Such foci commonly show glial cell proliferation, partial loss of neurons, and partial loss of synapses from the remaining neurons. In some patients the focus is a definite pathologic lesion (see Figure 30-2), examples of which are (1) localized malformation of cortical blood vessels, (2) scars from old injuries such as trauma, hemorrhage, anoxia or infection, (3) cysts, (4) foci of active infection, (5) the malformations of neurocutaneous diseases such as tuberous sclerosis, or (6) tumors. In humans, virtually all epileptogenic foci lie in the cerebral cortex, although foci in deep neuronal groups can occur.

Electrical recordings from cortical foci reveal characteristic autonomous, rhythmic, highly synchronized discharges which represent bursts of action potentials and activity of both inhibitory and excitatory synapses. If the firing of these cells becomes sufficiently synchronized, then the scalp EEG will show typical discharges such as spikes, as in Figure 30-1. However, the scalp EEG will fail to record some foci because of remote location or insufficient synchronization. Through their axonal processes, the neurons of the focus propagate their abnormal discharges to other areas of the brain (see Figure 30-1), and it is the balance of inhibitory versus facilitory responses of the neurons outside the focus that determines whether or not a clinical seizure results. Present evidence indicates that partial seizures and secondary generalized seizures occur when an excitatory feedback circuit is set up from the focus to other cortical neurons and deep neuronal masses such as the thalamus and basal ganglia.

The "primary generalized epilepsies" are less common and more poorly understood than focal epilepsy. The most characteristic generalized epilepsy in childhood is typical absences (petit mal) where genetic and maturational factors suggest a biochemical defect.

Genetic and Maturational Factors

The strong influence of cerebral development on seizures has already been mentioned and will be noted again in the subsequent sections on Neonatal Seizures and Febrile Convulsions. Adolescence is also a critical time where maturational influences have variable expression: a long-standing cerebral lesion may now first manifest itself with seizures or a pre-existing seizure disorder now may be "outgrown" or become worse.

Genetic influences can be principal or contributing causes for seizures and are of greater overall importance in children than adults. Autosomal dominant inheritance (with variable penetrance) is implicated in typical febrile convulsions and classic absences. In EEG studies of relatives of children with various seizure disorders, the 3-second EEG discharge (Figure 30-3) is frequently expressed as an autosomal dominant trait even in nonepileptic relatives. Genetic predisposition is also seen in post-traumatic epilepsy where the likelihood of a seizure disorder resulting from serious head injury is up to five times greater in those patients having a positive family history for epilepsy.

Cerebral Damage From Seizures

It has already been emphasized that anoxic brain damage may occur when ventilation is impaired, as in prolonged major motor seizures or newborn apneic seizures. Another concern is that the abnormal neuronal activity of seizures might injure brain cells, particularly in infancy where cell maturation and growth are very active. In neonatal rats, brief electroshock seizures (less than ½ second of convulsive activity once daily for 10 days) causes reduced brain size, cell number and rate of early motor-reflex development. In humans, infantile spasms may be an instance where frequent seizures and continuous cerebral discharges partially cause the associated mental retardation. In poorly controlled seizure patients the neuronal and glial abnormalities seen in epileptic foci may reflect a progressive deterioration. In animals normal neuronal groups can be induced to become "epileptic cells" by frequent low-intensity stimulation ("kindling") or by bombardment from a distant epileptic focus ("mirror focus"). Both the kindling and mirror focus phenomena can be prevented by phenobarbital treatment. One hopes that adequate anticonvulsant therapy will not only save children from anoxia but also help prevent other potentially adverse effects of seizures upon cerebral development and subsequent seizure susceptibility.

Factors "Triggering" Seizures

Although most epileptic seizures seem to happen spontaneously, there are many patients who are more apt to have attacks under certain conditions. Sometimes this is characteristic of the type of seizure disorder, as for example the induction of absences by hyperventilation, photic stimulation and anxiety. Many patients with various types of seizures are sensitive to one or more of the following: (1) diurnal cycle—sleep deprivation often induces seizures and some patients only have attacks, asleep, awake, drowsy, or on arousal; (2) emotional stress—in fact many completely controlled patients will start having seizures again when under stress; (3) menstrual cycle, particularly the several days before each period; (4) infections, even without fever, often exacerbate childhood seizure disorders (besides febrile convulsions which are discussed in a later section); (5) alcohol and illicit drugs—seizures may occur as the patient recovers from a "high" and there is often sleep deprivation and failure to take anticonvulsant medication as well; and (6) medications—occasionally an anticonvulsant paradoxically *worsens* a seizure disorder (e.g., phenytoin in absences) and convulsions can be induced by large intravenous doses of many drugs (penicillin, phenothiazines, antihistamines, local anesthetics, etc.) although this is rarely a problem when these drugs are given properly.

NEONATAL SEIZURES

Due to nervous system immaturity seizure manifestations in neonates are very different. They often are fragmentary and subtle, especially in prematures. Apneic spells can be caused by seizures. Sustained tonic seizures are relatively uncommon but can seriously impede ventilation. The EEG is helpful in confirming the presence of seizures and estimating prognosis.

The principal causes of neonatal seizures are summarized in Table 30-2. The major cause is hypoxia and/or ischemia occurring during labor or in the early newborn period from conditions such as premature placental separation, breech delivery, meconium aspiration or respiratory distress syndrome. In premature infants, severe hypoxia is often associated with intracranial hemorrhage and seizures.

Metabolic disturbances (Table 30-3) are frequently involved in neonatal seizures. Severe systemic neonatal diseases such as anoxia or sepsis are very often complicated by varying combinations of acidosis, hypoglycemia and hypocalcemia. Significantly less common are "pure" states of hypoglycemia, hypocalcemia or hypomagnesemia. Although rare, inborn metabolic errors must be considered since some are treatable (e.g., vitamin B_6 dependency and several of the amino acid disorders). Hyperbilirubinemia and intrapartum physical brain injuries are now less frequent due to improvements in obstetric and neonatal management. Since many congenital brain anomalies are not recognizable on physical examination, these are responsible for a significant group of otherwise unexplained neonatal seizures. Finally, when the mother is a drug addict or otherwise on large doses of medication, the infant may demonstrate withdrawal symptoms such as irritability and seizures.

As in other ages, seizures in the neonatal period must be considered symptoms of brain involvement; prognosis for the future brain development depends largely on the cause of the seizures. Overall, roughly 1 per cent of all newborns have seizures and of these, one-half to two-thirds will subsequently be normal. As examples of prognosis determined by cause, seizures from hypoxia-ischemia and intracranial infection carry a

Table 30-3.   Metabolic Causes of Neonatal Seizures

Anoxia

Acidosis, hypoglycemia and/or hypocalcemia complicating neonatal stresses such as anoxia, ischemia, sepsis or birth trauma

Primary hypoglycemia: Small-for-dates babies, infants of diabetic mothers

Primary tetany ("Benign neonatal tetany") due to hypocalcemia, hypomagnesemia and/or hyperphosphatemia, usually around the second week of life.

Hyponatremia: inappropriate ADH syndrome

Hypernatremia

Hyperbilirubinemia: hemolytic disease, liver dysfunction

Inborn errors of metabolism: Maple syrup urine disease and other amino- and organic acidopathies; B_6 dependency very high risk for subsequent brain impairment while those due to "benign neonatal tetany" (the primary or uncomplicated type of hypocalcemia, hypomagnesemia and/or hyperphosphatemia) generally have an excellent prognosis for subsequent normal brain development.

FEBRILE CONVULSIONS

"Febrile convulsions" is the term most widely used for seizures in small children triggered by fever. Febrile seizures affect about 5 per cent of children and are therefore about 10 times more frequent than is epilepsy in the same age group. Typically, the child is 1 or 2 years old and has a brief major motor seizure at the onset of a fever usually caused by an upper respiratory infection.

Although the pathophysiology is not well understood, it is clear that there is an age-dependent sensitivity of the nervous system to the triggering of seizures by fever. As seen in Figure 30-4 which graphs the age of occurrence of initial and recurrent febrile convulsions, the average age is 18 months, with most attacks occurring between age 6 months and 3 years. A genetic factor is also involved, since the family history is often positive for febrile convulsions in parents or siblings.

By definition, the diagnosis of febrile seizures excludes all other identifiable causes of seizures accompanying fever. An important differential diagnosis must always be considered including encephalitis, bac-

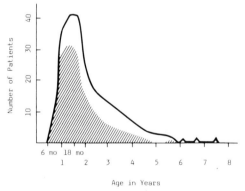

Fig. 30-4. Age when febrile convulsions occur. Upper curve: all attacks, initial and recurrent. Shaded area: initial attacks only. (Based on 200 children with initial and recurrent febrile convulsions reported by Frantzen, E., Lennox-Buchthal, M.A., and Nygaard, A.: Longitudinal EEG and clinical study of children with febrile convulsions. Electroencephalogr. Clin. Neurophysiol. *24*:197, 1968.)

terial meningitis, intracranial abscess, electrolyte disturbance, lead poisoning, trauma and many others.

Most often the convulsion is a single episode occurring within minutes or hours of the onset of a fever that is usually 102°F or higher. During high fever any child may exhibit periods of abnormal lethargy and minor twitching; these are often the prodrome to a seizure in the child susceptible to febrile convulsions. The seizures are most often generalized tonic-clonic and of less than 2 minutes' duration. However, about 8 per cent are akinetic and might easily go unnoticed if someone were not with the child at that moment. As with other convulsions, parents are usually extremely frightened, and often think the child may be dying. Although the interval may be only 15–20 minutes, the child is already recovering from postictal lethargy by the time he is seen by a physician whose examination usually reveals some common illness such as pharyngitis, otitis media, pulmonary infection, roseola or gastroenteritis.

Three fourths of attacks are of this uncomplicated or "simple" variety while one-fourth are considered "complicated" (see Table 30-4) because they are (1) prolonged, i.e., lasting more than 15 minutes; (2) multiple, i.e., more than one seizure per febrile illness; or (3) focal, i.e., a partial motor seizure which is often followed by a postictal hemiparesis. When the seizures are prolonged or multiple, they may become overt status epilepticus.

Sequelae of Febrile Convulsions

It is clear that the majority of children with febrile seizures will be normal. However, there is a risk, perhaps approaching 0.5 per cent of death or overt brain injury resulting from an unusually severe attack. Consequently, there is great concern about the 28 per cent incidence of potentially dangerous "complicated" attacks that may occur in any child and cannot be definitively predicted. It is known that the child is at greater risk for a subsequent complicated attack when (1) the seizure occurs in a child under 18 months of age, (2) there have been many febrile convulsions, (3) a previous complicated febrile convulsion has occurred, and (4) the child's previous neurodevelopmental status is not normal. These risk factors are discussed below in relation to indications for treatment.

The risk for subsequent epilepsy in the febrile convulsion group as a whole is 2 per cent or about four times greater than other children. However, as shown in Table 30-4, the epilepsy risk is lower in children with febrile convulsions who are neurologically normal and much higher in those who were not previously normal. At the present time it appears that most children with neurologic handicaps and a past history of febrile seizures were already neurodevelopmentally abnormal prior to the seizures.

Table 30-4. Febrile Convulsions: Risks for Immediate Complications, Subsequent Non-febrile Seizure and Subsequent Epilepsy

Sequelae	% of all children experiencing febrile convulsions
Immediate complications	
Immediate cerebral injury (e.g., death or hemiplegia)	0.5
"Complicated" attack (i.e., seizure > 15 minutes duration, focal or > 1 per day)	28
Subsequent single non-febrile seizure	1
Subsequent epilepsy	
All children with febrile seizures	2
Specific risk factors for epilepsy	
Prior neurologic status normal	
Uncomplicated first seizure	1.1
Complicated first seizure	1.7
Prior neurologic status not normal	
Uncomplicated first seizure	2.8
Complicated first seizure	9.2
Number of febrile seizures > 3	
Prior neurologic status normal	1.0
Prior neurologic status not normal	9.0
Age at first seizure	
0–6 months	5.7
> 12 months	2.0

From Millichap, J. G.: Febrile Convulsions. New York, Macmillan, 1968, and Nelson, K. B. and Ellenberg, J. H.: Predictors of epilepsy in children who have experienced febrile seizures. N. Engl. J. Med. *295*:1029, 1976.

Management

After an uncomplicated febrile seizure, the physician's principal concerns are differential diagnosis, treatment of the febrile illness and whether to give prophylactic therapy. Diagnosis requires careful clinical assessment to exclude intra- or extracranial disease capable of producing seizures with fever. Lumbar puncture should be performed whenever necessary to exclude meningitis and determination of glucose, electrolytes and calcium should be made. Fever is controlled by salicylates, tepid baths and treatment of infection. However, because so many febrile seizures occur at the onset of fever, it is impossible to prevent most attacks by antifever treatment or by phenobarbital given only at the time of fever.

There is no question that those children at greater risk for a subsequent complicated attack (see Sequelae above) should receive continuous phenobarbital prophylaxis (3 mg./kg./day in two divided doses). Whenever a high-risk child does not tolerate phenobarbital another anticonvulsant (such as primidone or phenytoin) should be used. There is much debate about whether a normal child over 18 months of age with an uncomplicated attack should receive continuous daily phenobarbital; one compromise in these children is to initiate treatment after a second attack and continue it until age 3 years.

DIAGNOSIS

Diagnosis requires that other paroxysmal disorders be excluded and the type of seizure(s) established by a good history and, when possible, observation of the attacks. Careful general physical, neurological and developmental examinations must be done, particularly to search for other evidence of neurologic dysfunction (e.g., signs of meningitis in a child with acute seizures and fever, or signs of cerebral palsy in an infant with seizure disorder and high-risk birth history).

The principal laboratory test is the EEG but since it can be normal or non-specifically abnormal in children with seizures, it cannot replace good clinical judgment in seizure diagnosis. In addition, an occasional child will have an "epileptiform" EEG without having epilepsy (e.g., siblings of children with absences). The yield of EEG abnormalities can be increased by "activating" techniques such as hyperventilation, flashing light (photic) stimulation, recording of drowsiness and sleep, and use of nasopharyngeal electrodes.

Other diagnostic tests are directed to the cause rather than the physiology of seizures. Computerized tomography (see Figure 30-2), is a revolutionary advance for the diagnosis of brain diseases. General indications for computerized tomography are: (1) all seizure disorders where partial seizures, EEG or clinical findings implicate a focus, (2) the presence of other findings suggesting potentially progressive cerebral disease, and (3) seizures refractory to therapy. Other tests which should be done in most patients are glucose, calcium, urine screening for inborn errors of metabolism, and skull radiographs. When acute seizures occur the following additonal tests must be considered: lumbar puncture for CSF examination and culture, blood electrolytes and gases, toxicological studies (lead, drugs, poisons) and other studies indicated by the individual clinical picture. In most instances when a child experiences seizures, a pediatrician or neurologist should be consulted for help with diagnosis and management.

TREATMENT

A comprehensive treatment plan for seizures should include the following measures:

Seizure Treatment

For convulsions: (1) maintain good airway and ventilation
during attack, and (2) instruct parents (sometimes teachers
and other laymen) to perform appropriate first aid and to
avoid harmful measures (e.g., abandoning the patient to
seek help, spoon in mouth, etc.)

Strive for optimal anticonvulsant medication therapy to
eliminate or minimize both seizures and medication side-
effects

Counsel patients and parents about medication effects and
therapy objectives

Maintenance Anticonvulsant Therapy

The current principal anticonvulsants are listed in Table 30-5 with oral
doses, therapeutic blood levels and general indications for use. The goal
of drug therapy is to approach as closely as possible complete suppression
of seizures with no significant side effects and can be attained in a majority of children. In a sizable minority one must compromise between
incomplete control of minor seizures and drug side effects; unfortunately,
in a few children seizures are inadequately controlled even at toxic doses.
In general, the least toxic drug likely to be effective should be started in
conventional doses and increased, or other drugs added depending on
response, side effects and blood levels. Often drug combinations are used
to get stronger anticonvulsant action with fewer side effects or to widen
the anticonvulsant spectrum.

Blood anticonvulsant levels have recently become widely available and
are now a cornerstone of good management. Levels should be checked
(1) about 6 weeks after initiation or significant modification of therapy,
(2) whenever side effects develop such as sedation or incoordination, (3)
whenever seizures relapse or fail to respond, and (4) at routine intervals.

Other laboratory tests should be done periodically to monitor for adverse effects of long-term anticonvulsant therapy such as bone marrow
depression, osteomalacia (presumably due to interference with vitamin
D metabolism) and liver toxicity. Such tests include complete blood
count, calcium, phosphorus, alkaline phosphatase and liver function
texts.

Anticonvulsant doses should usually be given twice daily (e.g., phenobarbital 30 mg. at breakfast and 60 mg. at dinner) which is compatible
with the 12- to 48-hour half-lives observed when the drugs of Table 30-
5 are given orally to children. Tablets or capsules favor more accurate
dosage than liquid preparations. Because a blood level plateau will not
be reached until a drug has been given orally for 1 to 3 weeks, it is
sometimes advisable to give an *oral loading dose* of twice the daily dose
for 2 days or a *parenteral loading dose* (see Treatment of Status Epilepticus, below, for doses).

Phenobarbital (see Table 30-5) deservedly remains the most widely used anticonvulsant in infants and children because of its very broad spectrum of anticonvulsant activity and greater safety. It is effective in major motor seizures, prevention of febrile convulsions, and many instances of partial seizures. Occasionally it is effective by itself in controlling absences and myoclonic seizures. It is used very often in combination with other drugs, especially phenytoin. It is absorbed well orally and intramuscularly and with caution can be given intravenously. Side effects include hyperactivity in small children and sedation; allergic rashes occur occasionally.

Primidone (Mysoline), another barbiturate, is unusual in that metabolites (principally phenobarbital and phenylethyl malonamide) as well as the parent molecule are all effective as anticonvulsants. Primidone is generally used as an adjunct drug, particularly when phenobarbital is ineffective, and for psychomotor seizures.

Phenytoin (Dilantin) is the second most widely used pediatric anticonvulsant. It is effective against major motor and most partial seizures but is generally ineffective in preventing febrile convulsions or absence seizures. It is much more variable than phenobarbital in its absorption and

Table 30-5. Drugs for Maintenance Anticonvulsant Therapy

Drug	Total Daily Dose		Therapeutic blood level (µg./ml.)	General therapeutic indications
	Infants & small children (mg./kg./day)	Older children mg./day		
Phenobarbital	3–6	60–120	10–40	All partial & generalized seizures. Febrile convulsions
Phenytoin (diphenylhydantoin, Dilantin)	5–7	100–400	10–20	Partial and major motor seizures.
Carbamazepine* (Tegretol)	10–20	200–1200	3–10	Partial, especially psychomotor, and major motor seizures.
Primidone* (Mysoline)	12–25	250–1500	(Use pheno-barbital level)	Partial, especially psychomotor, and major motor seizures.
Ethosuximide (Zarontin)	20–40	250–1250	40–100	Absence seizures with generalized spike/wave EEG.
Clonazepam* (Clonopin)	0.03–0.1	1–5		Refractory absence, myoclonic and major motor seizures.

*Initially use smaller doses to avoid excessive sedation

subsequent hepatic metabolism, so that much greater variation is encountered in the dose necessary to achieve the same blood level in different children. Some infants require very large doses (10 mg./kg./day or more) to reach therapeutic levels.

Cosmetic side effects occur to some degree in most children who take phenytoin over a long period even when blood levels are kept in the therapeutic range of 10–20 mcg./ml. These include hyperplasia of the gums, increased body hair and possibly coarse facial features. At toxic levels ataxia, sedation and even *increased* seizures may occur.

Phenytoin may be given orally or intravenously but not intramuscularly because of very poor absorption of the drug from muscle.

Carbamazepine (Tegretol) has emerged in the last decade as a highly effective anticonvulsant with a relatively broad spectrum including psychomotor seizures, other partial seizures and major motor seizures. In comparison with phenytoin, carbamazepine does not have cosmetic side effects and is roughly equivalent in the incidence of grave side effects, such as bone marrow depression and liver damage.

Ethosuximide (Zarontin) is one of a group of drugs including other succinimides and trimethadione whose use is largely restricted to absence seizures with generalized EEG discharges (classic petit mal). Because of lesser toxicity, ethosuximide is definitely the drug of choice for typical absences.

Patients with absence seizures should also receive phenobarbital to prevent the frequently associated major motor seizures. In a minority of children ethosuximide is ineffective because of gastric irritation or failure to control absences; in these instances valproate or clonazepam should be tried.

Clonazepam (Clonopin) is a benzodiazepine that has proved useful in maintenance anticonvulsant therapy. It is helpful in a number of refractory seizure states including infantile spasms and other myoclonic seizures, refractory absences and akinetic seizures.

Sodium valproate is a new, highly effective anticonvulsant which is expected to assume major importance particularly in treating absence, major motor, myoclonic/atonic and complex partial seizures. Valproate doses are 15-40 mg./kg./day.

Steroid therapy (ACTH 40-80 units/day or prednisone 2 mg./kg./day) is specifically used for infantile spasms, with seizure control in about 70 per cent and some improvement in 20 per cent of patients. Many other anticonvulsants are available but should generally be reserved for refractory seizure cases and used only by physicians thoroughly experienced with them because they either tend to be less effective or more toxic than the drugs listed in Table 30-5.

Other modes of therapy include surgical excision of epileptic foci. This method can be employed occasionally when a well-defined focus lies in a non-vital brain area and the patient has proved refractory to drug therapy adequately monitored by blood level measurements. Recently electrical stimulators have been implanted upon the cerebellum, presumably stimulating inhibitory cerebellar pathways to the cerebral cortex, but this remains an unproved mode of therapy. In children with refractory myoclonic seizures, it is sometimes helpful to induce a chronic state of acidosis through a ketogenic diet containing high fat intake or medium chain triglycerides.

Therapy of Status Epilepticus

Major motor status epilepticus is a medical emergency in which convulsions continue for more than 15 minutes or recur so quickly the patient does not recover consciousness in between. In this situation, patients become hypoxic and acidotic and small children also may become hypoglycemic. This occurs most commonly in an epileptic patient who suddenly discontinues medication or develops an infection, which may be as minor as a cold. When status epilepticus develops without a previous history of seizures, it usually implies a very serious illness, such as encephalitis, electrolyte disturbance, hypoglycemia, head trauma or extremely high fever. In any case, the first priority is to establish an airway and oxygenation by proper patient positioning, removal of secretions, administration of oxygen and when necessary, artificial ventilation. Next, an intravenous line should be established for administering medications and glucose and obtaining appropriate blood determinations such as glucose, electrolytes and blood gases.

The drug of choice is diazepam (Valium) given intravenously at 1 mg./minute until the seizure begins to stop. If diazepam is given more rapidly than this, depression of respirations is likely to occur. Intravenous diazepam will usually terminate the seizure within several minutes. However, the half life after intravenous administration is only about 15 minutes, so that a long-acting anticonvulsant such as intramuscular phenobarbital 6–10 mg./kg. or intravenous phenytoin 5–10 mg./kg. must be given to prevent seizure recurrence before the diazepam wears off. The total dose of diazepam required to stop an attack of status epilepticus varies greatly. Usually the maximum doses required are 0.3 mg./kg. in infants or 5–10 mg. in older children.

In infants or in dehydrated children, it may be very difficult and time consuming to achieve an intravenous injection. Here, intramuscular phenobarbital 8–10 mg./kg. often is effective within 15 minutes and allows the nurse or assistant to administer the medication while the physician concentrates on establishing good ventilation and other essential supportive measures.

A continuous partial motor seizure is called focal or partial status epilepticus and may result in depression of consciousness and respiration, particularly in infants and small children. It is treated in the same way as major motor status. Petit mal status epilepticus, discussed under Absences, usually responds well to intravenous diazepam (5-10 mg.).

MIGRAINE

Migraine in childhood begins typically between age 5 years and adolescence and is much more common than is generally realized. Furthermore, at least 10 per cent of cases begin before age 5. During childhood the sex incidence is equal, but females predominate by a ratio of 3 or 4 to 1 in adolescence and young adulthood. In older children and adolescents the headache usually identifies the condition and is the principal source of concern, but in small children headache may be minimal or absent so that the clinician must include the many other manifestations of migraine in the differential diagnosis of a wide variety of intermittent disorders of the nervous and autonomic systems.

CLASSIC AND COMMON MIGRAINE

These affect 2.5 per cent of all children at age 7 years and 5 per cent at age 15. The well-known classic form, which comprises only 10 per cent of cases, displays the characteristic "aura" of visual disturbances such as flashing lights, "colors" or blindness, followed by the intense throbbing unilateral pain of "hemicrania" in the eye, forehead and temple with associated photophobia, nausea, vomiting and abdominal distress. Sometimes the patient will experience the aura without proceeding to headache. Occasionally the aura will be other focal symptoms such as parasthesias or aphasia.

Common migraine is far more frequent but less characteristic, having diffuse rather than unilateral pain and frequently no visual aura. The prodrome of common migraine is more apt to consist of personality change, lightheadedness or nausea. Typically, attacks of both types of migraine will last several hours inducing the child to retire to a dark room to "sleep it off," but in some individuals attacks last only a few seconds while in others one attack may go on for several days. Syncope occurs fairly often in migraine children, sometimes leading to misinterpretation of migraine phenomena as seizures.

PATHOGENESIS

The pathogenesis of migraine is obscure although the occurrence of initial vasoconstriction of cranial vessels followed by headache-producing vasodilatation is well established. The aura is attributable to ischemia from vasoconstriction affecting retinal or occipital areas.

Precipitating factors should be carefully reviewed in each case. Emotional stress (such as school examinations or psychosocial problems) plays a major role but in most cases should be regarded as "triggers" rather than causes per se. Among the many non-emotional migraine triggers are fatigue, automobile riding, minor blows to the head and minor infections. Although frequently mentioned, allergy and specific dietary intolerances appear to be of little or no significance in most migraine patients.

MIGRAINE EQUIVALENTS

Migraine equivalents are frequently encountered among children with migraine although migraine is not the only cause for these symptom complexes. They are especially important in children under 5 years of age where motion sickness, syncope, cyclic nausea and vomiting, recurrent abdominal pain, paroxysmal dizziness, head banging or episodic behavioral changes may precede the onset of typical migraine headaches by a number of years. The cyclical vomiting syndrome is occasionally severe enough to cause secondary dehydration and acid-base disturbances. The benign paroxysmal vertigo syndrome (see Paroxysmal Vertigo) consists of attacks of dizziness which generally cease within a year; like other migraine equivalents, it may be recognized as part of the migraine complex only through a positive family history or by the onset of typical headaches several years later.

Complicated Migraine

Complicated migraines are rare forms in which hemiplegia, ophthalmoplegia or other focal deficits accompany the attack and clear only slowly over several days time. However, a permanent deficit attributable to vasospastic infarction sometimes occurs.

Cluster Headache

Cluster headache is seen in adolescence or adulthood, usually in males, and consists of very intense, transient unilateral pains around the eye which recur for an hour or so forming a "cluster" of attacks. Associated ipsilateral autonomic symptoms are very characteristic including nasal stuffiness, Horner's syndrome, tearing, facial erythema and sweating, and painfully dilated temporal artery. Cluster headache does not typically induce visual auras, nausea and vomiting. Cluster is a cyclical disorder and even though there is usually only a single cluster of attacks per day the pain can still be disabling, particularly when a given cycle is prolonged over many days or weeks.

DIAGNOSIS AND TREATMENT

Since there is no specific test, diagnosis must rest on a good description of the attacks, family history and a negative physical examination including blood pressure, optic fundi, ears and paranasal sinuses, cranial auscultation, general physical examination and, of course, neurological examination. In terms of laboratory tests plain skull films should be done in all cases. In selected cases it may be helpful to do EEG, computerized tomography (CT scan) or radioisotope scan.

Drug therapy for common and classic migraine is straightforward when salicylates provide adequate relief or when attacks are too short for any drug to be effective. In practice, ergot preparations are usually impractical for use in children. Other symptomatic medications for severe attacks are sedatives such a diazepam and mild analgesics such as codeine.

In some patients headaches can be prevented with the daily administration of certain non-analgesic medications such as phenytoin (Dilantin), phenobarbital, cyproheptadine (Periactin) and propanolol (Inderal). Because of the cyclical nature of migraine, prophylactic medications should be discontinued periodically to see whether they are still needed.

Therapy also requires ascertaining precipitating factors in each case since this may give an opportunity to avoid attacks (so long as overprotectiveness of the child is also avoided).

Frequently parents are more concerned than the child due to the widespread misbelief that a child cannot have headaches without serious cranial pathology. In this situation the physician's identification of migraine and reassurance are usually more therapeutic than any medication.

SYNCOPE

Syncope (fainting) is the most common paroxysmal disorder—so common that virtually everyone has fainted or at least felt faint. Many children are subject to frequent fainting, which is often misdiagnosed as seizures, even though a careful history usually indicates the correct diagnosis. On the other hand, unwitnessed seizures, brief major motor seizures or akinetic seizures may be erroneously attributed to fainting, especially when the full history is not available.

The usual vasovagal syncope is: (1) nearly always precipitated by stress or excitement, such as minor injury or an emotionally startling experience; (2) is found when the patient is upright and is aborted by lowering the head; (3) begins gradually with lightheadedness (the "I'm going to faint" sensation) and pallor; (4) results from temporary loss of vasomotor tone with bradycardia or even asystole; and (5) is typically associated with normal physical examination, ECG, and EEG. In a prolonged faint such as "pallid breath-holding" in young children, there can be brief tonic and clonic convulsive movements due to transient cerebral hypoxia which tends to cause further confusion with epileptic seizures. Important reasons to differentiate vasovagal syncope from epilepsy include the nonresponsiveness of syncope to anticonvulsants and the serious implications of a misdiagnosis of epilepsy. More serious types of syncope must be excluded such as cardiac arrhythmia, anemia, hypoglycemia, drug side effects, peripheral neuropathy and anomalies of the heart or great vessels.

In cases of straight-forward vasovagal syncope, there is virtually no likelihood of cerebral damage and the neurological prognosis is excellent. Therefore, therapy consists mainly of reassurance along these lines and advice to abort impending attacks by lowering the head.

BREATH-HOLDING SPELLS

Breath-holding is relatively common in infants and toddlers and can be very frightening to the inexperienced parent. All infants may hold their breath briefly during crying, but about 5 per cent of all children 6–24 months of age have *cyanotic breath-holding spells* in which they become blue and arrest breathing while crying and then lose consciousness for a few seconds. If the apnea persists for 30 seconds or more there will be tonic stiffening of the extremities and sometimes a few clonic jerks. The crying always has a precipitating event such as frustration, pain, anger or fear. The loss of consciousness and brief convulsive features result from hypoxia although the mechanisms causing the hypoxia and cyanosis are less well established; among those suggested are glottic closure, diminished cardiac output, increased oxygen utilization and right-to-left shunting.

In most instances the attacks begin between 6 and 18 months of age, occur at irregular intervals of days or weeks and are outgrown by 4 years of age. About 30 per cent have one to several attacks per day. In spite of this considerable frequency of cyanotic attacks the prognosis is excellent; these children are nearly always neurologically normal and do not suffer any secondary central nervous system damage. The diagnosis is based upon the characteristic history, especially the preceding precipitating event and the short period of crying just before apnea and loss of consciousness. The main differential diagnoses are epileptic seizures and congenital heart disease.

Pallid "breath-holding" spells occur in the same age group but less commonly than cyanotic breath-holding. The pallid variety are most often triggered by fright or minor injury resulting in pallor followed by loss of consciousness. They are actually vasovagal syncope of early childhood.

Treatment of breath-holding, especially of the cyanotic type, centers on explanation and reassurance for the parents. The attacks do not respond to anticonvulsants which are often prescribed for an erroneous diagnosis of seizure disorder. In the majority of cases the breath-holding becomes manageable as soon as the benign nature of the condition is explained to the parents and the child's subsequent emotional development is normal. However, in some particularly severe cases, the breath-holding is greatly aggravated by parental overindulgence occasioned by fear of triggering more attacks or by serious parental psychiatric problems resulting in anxiety or frustration in the child. In these cases a more detailed assessment of the family and consideration of psychotherapy will be necessary.

PAROXYSMAL VERTIGO

The benign paroxysmal vertigo syndrome of childhood consists of frequent brief attacks of dizziness and inability to stand during which the child becomes frightened and pale and attempts to lie or sit down before he falls. On examination during an attack the child is alert and is likely to exhibit nystagmus. It is usually self-limited and disappears within a few months to a year. The usual causes (ear disease or migraine) are benign, but similar vertiginous attacks can result from temporal lobe seizure foci or posterior fossa tumors. Clearly, children with attacks of vertigo should be carefully evaluated neurologically and otologically.

"Dizziness" is such a commonly used term by children and adults that some suggestions on how to evaluate this symptom are in order. Usually when patients say they are dizzy, they imply a lightheaded, pre-syncopal sensation; this should generally be evaluated as a syncope problem. Patients will also use "dizziness" to describe vertigo, that is, the illusion of movement of either the patient or the environment. Diagnostically it is important to try to establish whether the patient is describing lightheadedness as opposed to "true" vertigo. Although establishing the illusion of movement is very important, the nature of the sensation such as spinning, rocking or falling is of relatively small diagnostic value. Vertigo can be a component of syncope, but when it is the outstanding symptom the patient will usually require more extensive diagnostic investigation (e.g., ENT and neurologic consultations, skull radiographs, audiogram and electronystagmogram, EEG, CT scan, etc.).

Unfortunately, some children simply cannot describe what they mean by dizziness. In these instances the associated features may be of greater diagnostic value; for example, fright or pain inducing loss of consciousness in vasovagal syncope as opposed to sudden inability to stand with preservation of consciousness in typical attacks of benign paroxysmal vertigo.

BIBLIOGRAPHY

Seizures

Livingston, S.: Comprehensive Management of Epilepsy in Infancy, Childhood and Adolescence. Springfield, Ill, Charles C Thomas, 1972

Schmidt, R.P. and Wilder, B.J.: Epilepsy. Contemporary Neurology Series No. 2. Philadelphia, F. A. Davis, 1968.

Wright, F.S. *et al.*: Seizure disorders. *In* The Practice of Pediatric Neurology. St. Louis, C. V. Mosby, 1975.

> These three books provide extensive clinical and basic information on seizures and other paroxysmal disorders.

Gonzales, C., Grossman, C.B. and Palacios, E.: Computed Brain and Orbital Tomography. New York, Wiley, 1976.

Laffey, P., Mitchell, M., Teplick, G. and Haskins, M.: Computerized Tomography in Clinical Pediatrics. Philadelphia, Medical Directions, 1976.

> These two basic books cover computerized tomograpy which is an important new radiologic technique for diagnosis in seizures and other brain diseases.

Berman, P.: Management of seizure disorders with anticonvulsant drugs: Current concepts. Pediatr. Clin. North Am., *23*:443, 1976.

> A summary of newer information about the use of anticonvulsant drugs.

Jeavons, P.M., Clark, J.E. and Maheshwari, M.C.: Treatment of generalized epilepsies of childhood and adolescence with sodium valproate. Develop. Med. Child. Neurol. *19*:9, 1977.

> An excellent article on clinical use of the important new drug valproate.

Neonatal Seizures

Rose, A.L. and Lombroso, C.T.: Neonatal seizure states. Pediatrics *45*:404, 1970.

Volpe, J.J.: Neonatal seizures. Clin. Perinat. 4:43, 1977.

> These articles describe well the special characteristics of neonatal seizures.

Febrile Convulsions

Lennox-Buchthal, M.A.: Febrile convulsions: A reappraisal. Electro-encephalogr. Clin. Neurophysiol. 32 *(Suppl)*: 1973.

Millichap, J.G.: Febrile Convulsions. New York, Macmillan, 1968.

> These two texts are extensive reviews of the problem of febrile convulsions.

Nelson, K.B. and Ellenberg, J.H.: Predictors of epilepsy in children who have experienced febrile seizures. N. Engl. J. Med. *295*:1029, 1976.

> This is an important article regarding the prognosis of febrile convulsions.

Faerø, O. *et al.*: Successful prophylaxis of febrile convulsions with phenobarbital. Epilepsia, *13*:279, 1972.

Thorn, I.: A controlled study of prophylactic long-term treatment of febrile convulsions with phenobarbital. Acta Neurol. Scand., *60*: *(Suppl)* 67, 1975.

> These two articles describe phenobarbital efficacy and side-effects for preventing febrile convulsions.

Migraine and Other Paroxysmal Disorders

Friedman, A.P. and Harms, E.: Headaches in Children. Springfield, Ill., Charles C Thomas, 1967.

Lombroso, C.T. and Lerman, P.: Breatholding spells (cyanotic and pallid infantile syncope). Pediatrics, 39:567, 1967.

Prensky, A.L.: Migraine and migrainous variants in pediatric patients. Pediatr. Clin. North Am. 23:461, 1976.

These three sources provide more information on migraine, childhood headache and breatholding. (Additional information is also found in references 1 and 3 under Seizures.)

31

Serious Infections

Hugh L. Moffet, M.D.

The infections discussed in this chapter are especially important because they can kill or permanently damage normal children. Chapter 32 discusses other infections which are much less likely to cause death or permanent damage.

EPIGLOTTITIS

Epiglottitis is one of the most serious emergencies of the potentially fatal infections of children. It occurs most frequently in children 2 to 5 years of age, but has been reported in every age group, including newborn infants and adults. Typically, the epiglottis, along with the entire upper larynx, is very red and edematous.

Epiglottitis also has been called supraglottic laryngitis. Usually it can be distinguished on clinical grounds from subglottic laryngitis or "croup," which is discussed in the next chapter. Epiglottitis is usually caused by *Hemophilus influenzae*, type b.

Inspiratory stridor, a crowing-like sound, is the hallmark of high respiratory obstruction and is seen in epiglottitis, as well as in croup, foreign body, or other high respiratory obstructions. Because of the severity of the upper airway obstruction in epiglottitis, an emergency airway is often needed yet often attempted too late and under unfavorable conditions.

Typically, the child is previously normal and has not had past episodes of croup. The parent may telephone to report fever and cough, but it is the hoarseness, the muffled or guttural voice, and the unwillingness to speak that should be recognized by the physician or nurse as potentially serious symptoms. The course of the illness is marked by changes which occur in a matter of hours, rather than days. The parents should bring the child directly to the office or emergency room if they recognize anxiety (probably secondary to hypoxemia) or if the child appears seriously ill.

On physical examination, the child, usually of preschool age, often appears anxious and acutely ill. The sternum may sink in on inspiration. The child sits and barely moves, leaning forward with the chin up to allow a maximum airway. Auscultation shows decreased breath sounds. Drooling indicates difficulty with swallowing. Restlessness, like anxiety, suggests hypoxia and impending respiratory arrest. Direct visualization of the epiglottis by gagging the child with a tongue blade should not be attempted if the child appears seriously ill or requires restraint in the supine position, since this may produce aspiration of secretions and additional laryngospasm and edema. High fever is usually present, somewhere in the range of 104°F (40°C). Tachypnea is proportional to hypoxemia; cyanosis is a late sign.

Diagnosis and Treatment

The physician should try to distinguish epiglottitis from subglottic laryngitis (croup), although this is not always as easy as is sometimes implied. Unnecessary restraint and manipulation, such as might be necessary for laboratory tests, should be avoided if the child appears seriously ill. If the patient appears likely to need an airway soon, both an anesthesiologist and an otolaryngologist should be summoned immediately.

If the patient does not appear seriously ill, a white blood count and differential, and lateral neck radiograph should be obtained. Leukocytosis is typically present. The lateral radiograph of the soft tissues of the neck may reveal unsuspected supraglottic obstruction in early or doubtful cases, but is not necessary or advisable in seriously ill patients. A chest film can be obtained at the time of the lateral neck exam. It usually is normal, and is useful primarily to exclude a foreign body. After an airway is provided by intubation or tracheotomy, a chest film is useful to show the location of the tip of the tube.

A blood culture usually reveals bacteremia with *H. influenzae* after 24 hours. However, the seriously ill patient should not be restrained for a blood culture until an airway is assured. If epiglottitis is suspected, a physician always should accompany the patient and should be prepared to intubate or to ventilate the patient with a bag and mask if respiratory arrest suddenly occurs.

Plan

Often a patient with epiglottitis has endotracheal intubation or tracheotomy before a detailed note is written. However, a flow sheet should be begun as soon as the patient is seen. Respiratory rate and effort, pulse, and general appearance (anxious?, restless?, breathing carefully and deliberately?) should be recorded. Restraining the patient in the supine position for blood pressure or venipuncture (as for blood gases) usually aggravates the illness, and should not be done unless an adequate airway is present. If possible, a parent should be continuously present to comfort the child. Mist apparently has a soothing effect on the inflamed larynx. Oxygen should be used to lessen the hypoxemia. The patient should always be attended and accompanied by a person capable of providing intubation or assisted ventilation with a bag and mask.

In 1978, either nasotracheal intubation or tracheotomy are acceptable methods for providing an airway in epiglottitis. The method used depends on the availability of an anesthesiologist or otolaryngologist and medical and nursing personnel experienced and skillful in management of each method.

Antibiotics effective against *H. influenzae* should be given, although this has a lower priority than an emergency airway, if one is needed. A single intramuscular injection of a corticosteroid, such as dexamethasone, may sometimes lessen edema and "buy time" before an airway can be achieved, particularly en route to the hospital from the doctor's office or patient's home. However, routine use of corticosteroids has been shown to be of no statistical value in prospective, placebo-controlled studies of subglottic laryngitis.

ACUTE PNEUMONIA SYNDROMES

Classification

Pneumonias can be classified into syndromes using the variables of type of onset, course, severity, radiologic appearance and presence of underlying disease. The onset can be acute, subacute, or chronic; progressive or improving; recurrent or a first episode. It can also be classified as mild, moderate, or severe, as estimated by clinical observations, or by quantitation of respiratory acidosis and hypoxemia.

On the basis of the chest film, pneumonia can be classified as lobar, segmental, subsegmental, lobular, interstitial, perihilar, or miliary. Combinations of these forms may occur. Additional anatomical features may be present such as pleural thickening, effusion, cavitation, pneumatoceles, or pneumothorax.

Pneumonia can occur in normal individuals with no known underlying disease, it may be secondary to events such as aspiration or stasis, or it may be concurrent with underlying diseases such as cystic fibrosis of the pancreas or a malignancy.

Etiology

Most acute pneumonias are caused by infectious agents. These agents include viruses, bacteria, mycoplasmas, mycobacteria, or fungi. Unfortunately, etiologic diagnoses are not so easy to determine or so accurate as is sometimes implied, and conclusive evidence of the etiology is not obtained in most cases. The most frequent etiological diagnoses associated with various acute pneumonia syndromes are listed in Table 31-1.

It is useful to give a descriptive diagnosis for the primary diagnosis or statement of the problem, using above variables listed in Table 31-1. The etiologic diagnosis can then be expressed as a probability, along with a statement of other reasonable possibilities. Examples of such preliminary clinical and probable etiologic diagnoses include: acute lobar pneumonia—probably pneumococcal; severe bilateral interstitial pneumonia—probably due to influenza virus; recurrent right middle lobe pneumonia—probably pneumococcal or consider partial bronchial obstruction; right upper lobe pneumonia with cavitation—probably tuberculosis; bilateral interstitial pneumonia—complicating acute leukemia—probably *Pneumocystis carinii*.

Acute Lobar or Segmental Pneumonia

Acute lobar or segmental pneumonia sometimes has been called typical pneumonia, in contrast to atypical pneumonia, discussed later. The following characteristics can be considered typical. Significant fever of >102°F (39°C) is usually present. Chills often are noted in older children and adults. Often there is a toxic appearance, defined as appearing acutely ill, anxious and distressed. Definite chest signs are usually present and lateralized. These include consolidation as defined by dullness to percussion, decreased breath sounds, increased fremitus, and sometimes bronchophony. Fine end-inspiratory rales are often present.

Pleuritic pain or lateralizing differences in inspiratory expansion may be noted. Older children may fail to breathe deeply when asked to do so, or complain of pain and cough when they do. Shallow breathing (splinting) is sometimes the only sign suggesting that a child with high fever may have pneumonia. Grunting may be noted in infants or young children. Pleurisy is often used as a lay term or as an older medical term for pleuritis or pleural pain. Pleurodynia refers to pleuritic pain without pneumonia or pleural effusion and is characteristically caused by Coxsackie B virus.

In typical pneumonia, the chest radiograph shows a dense infiltration. It may appear segmental, lobar, or even spherical, but does not have multiple or diffuse "thin" infiltrates. Response to penicillin is often dramatic, with the temperature falling from the range of 104°F (40°C) to about 98°F (36.7°C) within 8 to 12 hours after the first dose of penicillin. The temperature often stays at a normal level.

Atypical Pneumonia Syndromes

Criteria for atypical pneumonia are the opposite of those for typical lobar pneumonia. The following features are usually regarded as "atypical."

Table 31-1. Acute Pneumonia Syndromes

Problem Pattern	Most Frequent Etiologies
Lobar, segmental, spherical pneumonias; or Pneumonia with effusion	*Strep. pneumoniae* *H. influenzae*, if preschool *Staph. aureus.* if less than 1 year old
Bilateral interstitial pneumonia; or Mild subacute pneumonia with minimal infiltrates	*Mycoplasma pneumoniae* or adenovirus, if school age Respiratory syncytial virus, if infant (2 years of age) *H. influenzae*, if preschool
Cold-agglutin positive pneumonia	*Mycoplasma pneumoniae* or adenovirus
Fulminating pneumonia	Influenza virus, if during outbreak *Mycoplasma pneumoniae*, if sporadic Chickenpox or measles, if immunosuppressed
Pneumonia complicating other diseases Cystic fibrosis	*Staph. aureus* *Pseudo. aeruginosa*
Immunosuppressed state or malignancy	*Staph. aureus* *Pseudo. aeruginosa* *Pneumocystis carinii* *Candida albicans*, tuberculosis, systemic mycoses
Pneumonary infiltrates with eosinophilia (PIE Syndrome)	Unknown Aspergillosis Ascariasis
Miliary pneumonias	Tuberculosis Unidentified causes, presumed to be viral
Nodular pneumonias	Disseminated bacteremias, usually *Staph. aureus* Disseminated fungemias, usually *Histo. capsulatum*

Subacute Onset. The onset is gradual, with cough for several days before the patient seeks medical attention. Chills, fever, and toxicity are minimal or absent.

Prominent Extrapulmonary Features. Headache, sore throat and pharyngeal exudate are often present and more prominent than the nonproductive cough or dyspnea.

Minimal or Disparate Chest Signs. Rales may be bilateral or localized, but there is often a disparity between auscultatory and radiologic findings. The chest radiograph often shows more extensive involvement than the clinican hears and in different locations than suspected. Sometimes the radiologic findings are minimal when the patient is cyanotic, with an alveolar-capillary diffusion block. Hypoxemia secondary to the diffusion block may produce a more rapid respiratory rate than might be expected from the minimal involvement by chest radiograph.

Chest Infiltrate Not Lobar or Segmental. The infiltrate is patchy, or mottled, with varying degrees of density, without a single dense area of consolidation. There may be a wedge-shaped or linear infiltrate, or a bilateral interstitial infiltrate.

No Clinical Response to Penicillin.

No Significant Leukocytosis.

Slow Course. The patient improves gradually and sometimes has a prolonged convalescence.

Exclusion. There are a number of other clinical patterns of pneumonias that are not typical of lobar pneumonia that can be excluded from the group of atypical pneumonia because of distinctive features. Most of these acute pneumonia syndromes are listed in Table 31-1: progressive or fulminating pneumonia, pulmonary infiltrates with eosinophilia, miliary or multiple nodular pneumonia, and bronchiolitis with minimal pneumonia (see p. 575).

Classification of Atypical Pneumonia Syndromes. Various classifications can be used to describe atypical pneumonias. "Non-bacterial pneumonia" is a term used sometimes. This has the disadvantage of implying that bacterial causes have been excluded, when this can rarely be done with certainty. "Non-bacterial" is a conclusion usually based on such observations as failure to respond to penicillin therapy, absence of leukocytosis, and sparse infiltrate.

"Cold agglutinin-positive pneumonia" is a diagnosis sometimes used, although many atypical pneumonias are not associated with cold agglutinins. Cold agglutinin-positive pneumonia should not be equated with mycoplasmal pneumonia. In children, many cold agglutinin-positive pneumonias are not associated with serologic evidence of *M. pneumoniae* infection, and some patients with mycoplasmal pneumonia do not have positive cold agglutinins, even when studied serially.

"Mycoplasmal pneumonia" should not be used as a syndrome diagnosis without laboratory proof of etiology, since many atypical pneumonias are not caused by *M. pneumoniae*. Furthermore, it is not possible to distinguish mycoplasmal pneumonia from other atypical pneumonias on clinical grounds.

In summary, it is useful to preserve the definition of atypical pneumonia as a clinical-radiologic one, recognizing that the syndrome can be caused by a number of specific agents. However, it is useful to specify the features of the pneumonia which are atypical (usually the subacute course) and to add an additional descriptive diagnosis, using available objective information. Examples of useful working diagnoses include: (1)

cold agglutinin-positive pneumonia, (2) subacute pneumonia with bilateral interstitial infiltrates, (3) subacute pneumonia with patchy pneumonitis of both lower lobes, (4) right upper lobe pneumonia, unresponsive to penicillin.

Pneumonia with Effusion

When a plural effusion is associated with an acute segmental or lobar pneumonia, pleural fluid should be obtained by thoracentesis. Gram stain and culture will usually reveal *Staph. aureus* in infants or children whose pneumonia has progressed while receiving parenteral penicillin. *Strep. pneumoniae* was formerly the most common cause, but is less common since penicillin has been used so widely. *H. influenzae* is an occasional cause of purulent pleural effusion (empyema) in preschool children.

When the pleural effusion is small, and is associated with a mild, subacute pneumonia, the cause is more likely to be *Mycoplasma pneumoniae*. A thoracentesis to obtain fluid may not be necessary if the illness is mild or if testing for cold agglutinins is positive.

Progressive or Fulminating Pneumonias

Progressive pneumonia can be defined as pneumonia that becomes worse radiologically and clinically, in spite of antibiotic therapy which should be effective against the presumed etiologic agent. In this situation the physician should consider penicillin-resistant staphylococci or gram-negative rods, including *Klebsiella* or *P. aeruginosa*, and change antibiotic therapy to treat these possibilities. However, progressive pneumonia can be caused by non-bacterial infections or even a malignancy.

Fulminating pneumonia can be defined as a severe bilateral pneumonia, with an unusually rapid progression, clinically or radiologically, over a period of 24 to 48 hours. Usually, fine moist inspiratory rales are heard in all lung fields, and the patient may be suspected of having acute pulmonary edema. Possible etiologies include influenza virus and *Mycoplasma pneumoniae* (Table 31-1). Oxygen is a very important part of therapy.

Pneumonia Complicating Other Diseases

In some acute or chronic diseases, particular etiological agents or anatomical types of pneumonia are found more frequently than in normal individuals. Cystic fibrosis and acute leukemia are examples of this situation (Table 31-1).

Cystic Fibrosis of the Pancreas. Chronic and recurrent bacterial pneumonias are a frequent complication of this disease. The usual etiologic agent is *Staph. aureus* or *Pseudo. aeruginosa*. Staphylococcal empyma is unusual in patients with cystic fibrosis, except in the first year of life.

Malignancy or Immunosuppressed State. Patients with malignancies such as leukemia, or patients receiving immunosuppressive therapy as after organ transplantation, have special risks for organisms rarely associated with pneumonia in normal individuals (Table 31-1). *Pneumocystis carinii* is a parasite that can cause pneumonia in this group of patients. Fever, marked tachypnea, cyanosis, and bilateral diffuse alveolar densities are found characteristically.

Pulmonary Infiltrates with Eosinophilia (PIE Syndrome)

This syndrome diagnosis is now used to include all of the variable clinical patterns with any type of pulmonary infiltrate and eosinophilia of the peripheral blood. Loeffler's pneumonia (Loeffler's syndrome) was the term formerly used for this pattern. Loeffler originally described transitory infiltrates with few symptoms and a benign course, but the syndrome has been expanded in common usage to include illnesses with severe symptoms and a prolonged course.

In some cases, the pulmonary infiltrates are caused by trapping of worm larvae in the smaller blood vessels of the lung. In other cases, both the pulmonary infiltrates and the blood eosinophilia appear to be a hypersensitivity phenomenon, (e.g., during desensitization to poison ivy).

Miliary and Nodular Pneumonias

Miliary refers to the size of a millet seed. Miliary or nodular pneumonia is an anatomic diagnosis based on a chest radiograph that shows multiple circular densities. In general, miliary refers to small densities (usually about 2 mm. in diameter) and nodular refers to larger densities (usually about 6 mm. or more in diameter). For convenience, the general term nodular is used to include finely nodular and coarsely nodular disseminated patterns.

In experimental miliary tuberculosis in rabbits, using bovine tubercule bacilli the miliary lesions become visible about 3 weeks after the intravenous injection. Relatively evenly distributed densities of the same size result from a gradual release into the blood of small particles of infectious agents. If dissemination of bacteria or emboli to the lung occur irregularly, it usually produces larger densities with more focal involvement of some parts of the lungs.

Acute Nodular Pneumonia. The possible etiologies include miliary tuberculosis, multiple septic emboli, and disseminated fungus diseases. Other infectious causes, such as a virus, or non-infectious causes, such as acute pulmonary edema, should be considered.

ACUTE NEUROLOGIC SYNDROMES

Acute infection of the central nervous system is the most likely cause of a febrile illness with manifestations of central nervous system involvement (Table 31-2). Bulging fontanel, headache, or vomiting suggest the

Table 31-2. Manifestations of CNS Infections

Sign or symptom	Suggests
Headache Vomiting Bulging fontanel	Increased CSF pressure
Stiff neck	Meningeal irritation
Crying when handled Disturbed consciousness (Lethargy, irritability)	Brain involvement
Fever	Infection

presence of increased intracranial pressure. Stiff neck, or crying when handled, suggests meningeal irritation. Papilledema is unusual in any of the acute neurologic infections, but should be excluded before doing a lumbar puncture. If marked papilledema is present, chronic increased intracranial pressure is likely to be present, and lumbar puncture should be avoided as it might result in downward movement of the brain stem into the spinal canal, with compression of the vital centers, and death.

A change in consciousness, such as confusion or disorientation, is an alarming sign that suggests a disturbance of cerebral cortical function, probably caused by cerebral hypoxia, inflammation, or edema.

These general signs of an acute CNS infection described in Table 31-2 should be regarded as indicating a medical emergency until proved otherwise; they should indicate to the physician the necessity of a lumbar puncture. The illness can then be classified as a particular anatomic syndrome on the basis of both the clinical and spinal fluid findings (Table 31-3).

Purulent Meningitis. This is best defined by a cerebrospinal fluid (CSF) that is cloudy and contains more than 1,000 neutrophils/mm.[3] Whether or not a bacterial etiology is proved by culture, purulent meningitis is almost always bacterial. When the term meningitis is not further modified, it usually means purulent or bacterial meningitis.

Nonpurulent Meningitis (Aseptic Meningitis Syndrome). This is best defined on the basis of a CSF cell count of about 10 to 500 leukocytes, usually predominantly lymphocytes. Patients with CSF cell counts in the intermediate range of 500 to 1,000 leukocytes can usually be classified tentatively as either presumed bacterial meningitis or aseptic meningitis syndrome on the basis of CSF cell count differential, glucose, protein, Gram stain, and state of consciousness.

Acute Encephalitis. This is best defined as an acute illness, with a severe and non-transient disturbance of consciousness and a CSF cell

Table 31-3. Classification of Acute Neurologic Syndromes (Usually Infectious)

	Spinal fluid findings			
	Leukocytes (per mm.[3])	*Protein (mg/dl.)*	*Glucose (mg/dl.)*	*State of consciousness*
Purulent meningitis	>1000 (Mostly polys)	>100 (high)	<30 (low)	Variable
Non-purulent meningitis (Aseptic meningitis syndrome)	10–500 (Mostly lymphs)	Variable	Variable	Usually normal
Encephalitis	10–1000 (Mostly lymphs)	Normal	Normal	Severely disturbed
Encephalopathy	Normal (<10)	Normal	Normal	Severely disturbed

count characteristic of non-purulent meningitis. Ordinarily, the number of cells is less than 500, and rarely exceeds 1,000/mm.[3]

A disturbance of consciousness should be considered non-transient if it persists for more than 8 hours and should be distinguished from febrile delirium, which occurs only at the time of a high fever.

Acute Encephalopathy. This is best defined as the acute onset of severe and non-transient disturbance of consciousness and a normal CSF cell count (<10 leukocytes/mm.[3]).

Other manifestations of brain disease, such as convulsions and abnormal focal neurologic signs, are variably present. Thus, encephalopathy has the same clinical pattern as encephalitis, but has a normal CSF cell count. This distinction between encephalitis and encephalopathy is a useful one, because the causes of encephalitis are usually infectious or postinfectious, whereas the causes of encephalopathy are usually toxic, metabolic, or vascular.

Meningismus. This term should not be used unless the spinal fluid is normal and the patient has a stiff neck due to local or reflex irritation. Streptococcal pharyngitis and pneumonia are frequent causes of meningismus. Acute juvenile rheumatoid arthritis and tetanus are uncommon causes.

Benign Intracranial Hypertension. This is defined by increased CSF pressure, as manifested by a bulging fontanel or papilledema, with infection, tumor, sinus thrombosis, and obstruction of the ventricular system specifically excluded. It can be produced by tetracycline therapy, early congestive heart failure, or hypervitaminosis A.

Meningoencephalitis. The term "meningoencephalitis" has the disadvantage of failing to identify patients who should be diagnosed as having "encephalitis," a disease distinguished by severe cerebral signs and high probability of brain damage. A severe and persistent disturbance of consciousness (at least 8 hours) is an early and relatively reliable indication of a poor prognosis. Non-purulent meningitis and acute encephalitis also differ in probable etiologies, another reason to try to avoid lumping them together as "meningoencephalitis."

Purulent Meningitis

Definitions. Purulent meningitis is a medical emergency. Early intensive therapy is essential to prevent brain damage or death. Typically, purulent meningitis is manifested by clinical signs of acute neurologic infection and cloudy spinal fluid. Usually, the CSF has more than 1,000 leukocytes/mm.³, with a predominance of neutrophils, a low CSF glucose (often 0 to 10 mg./dl.), and an elevated CSF protein (usually more than 100 mg./dl.). Some patients with early or partially-treated bacterial meningitis may have cell counts, glucose and protein which are in the same range as those found in non-purulent meningitis (aseptic meningitis syndrome). Therefore, it is more practical to use the term purulent or non-purulent meningitis as a preliminary diagnosis.

Ventriculitis may occur without meningitis, particularly if the CSF flow is obstructed. This is most likely to occur as a complication of neurosurgical shunting operations for hydrocephalus; ventriculitis is discussed on page 544.

Mechanisms. The lowered CSF glucose concentration is the result of defective glucose transport into the CSF and increased utilization of glucose in the brain. The CSF glucose also depends on the blood glucose concentration. Thus, a simultaneous blood glucose determination is usually obtained to help interpret the CSF glucose. A CSF glucose less than 40 per cent of the blood glucose is usually abnormally low.

The elevated CSF protein is due to increased permeability of the blood-CSF barrier, allowing plasma proteins to enter the CSF. An active exudation of serum protein into the CSF occurs and at autopsy a thick exudate can usually be seen covering the meninges.

Possible Etiologies. Most purulent meningitis is caused by *H. influenzae, Neisseria meningitidis,* or *Streptococcus (Diplococcus) pneumoniae.* The probability of these three agents depends on the age of the patient: between 1 month and 5 years of age, *H. influenzae* accounts for more than half; between 5 years and 30 years of age, the meningococcus accounts for more than half; and after 30 years of age, the pneumococcus accounts for more than half of the cases.

In the first 30 days of life, the most common causes of purulent meningitis are enteric bacteria (such as *E. coli*) and the Group B streptococcus. Other bacteria which rarely cause meningitis, except in the newborn period, include *Listeria monocytogenes* and *Staph. aureus.*

Early Clinical Diagnosis. In young infants, it is important to do a lumbar puncture and examine the spinal fluid whenever the neck is questionably stiff or the anterior fontanel is questionably bulging, even if the patient does not appear severely ill. Disturbed consciousness (lethargy, irritability) and crying when handled are especially important symptoms suggesting early meningitis, since a stiff neck may be absent or appear late in young infants. A convulsion which occurs in a child with fever should not be diagnosed as a simple febrile convulsion unless a lumbar puncture reveals a normal CSF.

Emergency Treatment (Before Lumbar Puncture). In rare cases, the illness is so severe that supportive therapy should be begun before the diagnostic studies. For example, in patients with meningococcemia, suspected because of hypotension and purpura, a good intravenous route should be obtained and treatment of shock begun before doing a lumbar puncture. Meningococcemia may occur without meningitis, and the early treatment of septic shock is more important than determining whether or not meningitis is present. Patients with evidence of life-threatening brain swelling should be treated with mannitol before a lumbar puncture is done.

Spinal Fluid Examination. Complete examination of the CSF should be done in order to detect any abnormality that may be helpful in the diagnosis. A Gram-stained smear should be examined even when few or no white blood cells are found. This policy can lead to error when a few organisms are found that may have originated on the slide or in the stain, but detects the rare instances in which many organisms are found in spinal fluids without many white blood cells, as may occur in pneumococcal meningitis. The meningococcus is the organism most frequently missed on smear but found on culture, and *H. influenzae* is often misinterpreted on the smear as another organism. Therefore, if the smear is not typical, and the child is less than 12 years old, ampicillin and chloramphenicol therapy are used for treatment of purulent meningitis until the culture results are available.

Glucose and protein should be determined and are especially valuable in non-purulent meningitis (see p. 541).

Therapy should not be delayed until the results of spinal fluid examinations are available, if the fluid appears cloudy. As soon as the CSF is recognized to be grossly purulent, (cloudy, like diluted milk), a bolus of intravenous ampicillin (one-fourth the total daily dose) should be given. If there is likely to be a delay in starting the infusion, the ampicillin should be injected into an antecubital vein, or intramuscularly if an intravenous route is not quickly obtained.

Non-Purulent Meningitis

Definitions. Non-purulent meningitis can be separated from the other syndromes of presumptive CNS infections by the absence of severe cerebral manifestations, such as a severe disturbance of consciousness, and by a spinal fluid cell count in the range of 10 to 500 leukocytes/mm.[3] (see Table 31-3). Aseptic meningitis syndrome, serous meningitis, benign lymphocytic meningitis, non-paralytic poliomyelitis, viral meningitis, and meningoencephalitis are terms with similar meanings. However, "non-purulent meningitis" or "aseptic meningitis syndrome" is the most useful preliminary diagnosis for this syndrome, since it emphasizes the possibility of a number of different causes.

Importance of CSF Glucose. A decreased CSF glucose concentration is usually present in purulent meningitis but often has little more than supportive diagnostic value since the purulent spinal fluid already indicates the presumptive diagnosis of bacterial meningitis. A lowered glucose suggests severe brain involvement, and in non-purulent meningitis, a low CSF glucose is correlated with a more chronic infection or more serious etiologic agents, such as tuberculosis. Therefore, in patients with non-purulent meningitis, a decreased CSF glucose has special diagnostic value. It is useful to divide non-purulent meningitis into two subgroups: non-purulent meningitis with a decreased CSF glucose and non-purulent meningitis without a decreased CSF glucose. A lowered CSF glucose can be conservatively defined as a CSF glucose less than 40 per cent of the blood glucose, or less than 40 mg./dl., if the blood glucose is not known. It is important to measure the blood glucose concentration as well as CSF glucose in order to interpret the CSF glucose as a percentage of the blood sugar.

An elevation of CSF protein concentration is often present when there is a decreased CSF glucose. However, a slightly elevated protein may be a result of laboratory variability or may come from slight bleeding during the procedure of lumbar puncture.

Non-Purulent Meningitis with Low Glucose

Tuberculous Meningitis. There are three factors that are especially important in evaluating suspected tuberculous meningitis: tuberculin test, chest roentgenogram, and exposure history. If the intermediate strength tuberculin test is negative, the chest roentgenogram is normal, and there is no history of exposure to tuberculosis, tuberculous meningitis is unlikely.

A second lumbar puncture and CSF examination should be done if the CSF glucose is borderline low on the first exam. This is very useful because during the course of untreated tuberculous meningitis there is almost always a progressive fall in the glucose, a rise in the protein, and a continuation of the CSF lymphocytosis.

Partially Treated Bacterial Meningitis. Decreased CSF glucose may be present if the patient has been receiving an antibiotic for several days and has an unrecognized bacterial meningitis. In this situation, the protein is often elevated. Since the prior antibiotic therapy often prevents recovery of the infecting organism on culture, the frequency of partially treated bacterial meningitis as a cause of this syndrome is unknown. However, this pattern of CSF findings is seen often enough on the 48- to 72-hour follow-up examination of a patient treated for a known bacterial meningitis that a partially treated unrecognized bacterial meningitis should always be considered.

The following are rare causes of this syndrome:

Meningeal Neoplasm. Low cerebrospinal fluid glucose may occur in neoplastic meningitis, but the cells are usually predominantly neutrophils in this exceedingly rare disease.

Cryptococcal Meningitis. Cryptococcal meningitis is a rare cause of non-purulent meningitis with a low glucose and a high protein, and typically occurs in a compromised host. The budding yeast forms can usually be seen in an India ink preparation of the CSF. It often grows out in a few days on most of the solid media usually used for the culture of *Mycobacterium tuberculosis*. A latex agglutination test, using CSF, may be of diagnostic value. Other fungal diseases, such as histoplasmosis or coccidiodomycosis, may resemble cryptococcal meningitis. It is important to detect fungal causes of non-purulent meningitis because therapy with amphotericin B is often lifesaving.

Mumps. Aseptic meningitis due to mumps virus has been shown to be associated occasionally with slightly decreased CSF glucose concentration.

Lymphocytic Choriomeningitis. CSF glucose may be slightly decreased in non-purulent meningitis caused by this virus.

Amebic Meningitis. Low glucose and high protein are produced by amebic meningitis, but the cells usually are predominantly neutrophils in this exceedingly rare disease.

Non-Purulent Meningitis with Normal Glucose

Viral Meningitis. Viruses are the most common cause of this syndrome, but are not the only cause. In three large series with viral cultures of patients with aseptic meningitis syndrome, the most common viral causes were Coxsackie virus, (about 20 to 50%); ECHO virus (about 10 to 15%); and mumps virus (about 5 to 15%).

In the United States, coxsackieviruses and echoviruses characteristically are found in the summer and fall, but echoviruses may be found all year. A history of exposure to mumps should be sought, and close examination for parotid enlargement should be done. The above viruses can often be recovered on culture in a virus diagnostic laboratory, so that viral cultures of throat, rectum, and CSF should be done, if facilities are available.

Serologic tests can be done for a number of viruses, including mumps, California encephalitis, lymphocytic choriomeningitis, Eastern equine encephalitis, Western equine encephalitis, and St. Louis encephalitis viruses. However, other than mumps, these viruses are relatively uncommon in the United States, except in occasional localized outbreaks. Pet hamsters or mice can be sources of lymphocytic choriomeningitis virus infection. These antibody studies require the study of two sera, the first obtained as soon as possible after the onset and the second obtained 3 to 6 weeks later.

Poliovirus infection is a rare cause of aseptic meningitis syndrome in the United States. However, poliovaccine virus can also be recovered as a coincidental finding unrelated to aseptic meningitis. Therefore, a history of past immunization or recent exposure to poliovaccine should always be sought in patients with aseptic meningitis syndrome. Arbovirus infection was demonstrated in about 1 per cent of patients studied with aseptic meningitis, in one study; but arboviruses are more likely to be associated with a clinical diagnosis of encephalitis. Herpes simplex virus is recovered from the throat in about 1 per cent of patients but this usually is coincidental.

Unknown Etiology. About 30 to 50 per cent of patients with non-purulent meningitis have negative cultures and negative serologic studies for viruses.

Partially treated bacterial meningitis can be a cause of non-purulent meningitis with a normal CSF glucose, but the frequency of this etiology is unknown. Observation of CSF cell count, glucose, and protein during antibiotic therapy of proven bacterial meningitis shows that the range of these values overlaps that of viral meningitis. However, the mean CSF glucose of many patients is often normal after a few days of appropriate antibiotic therapy. The mean CSF protein is usually still elevated at this time.

Conclusive evidence that the preceding antibiotic therapy can sometimes modify the CSF findings, resulting in a non-purulent meningitis with normal CSF glucose and protein can be seen in individual case histories. Occasionally, patients have been observed after some antibiotic therapy and have not had antibiotics continued. Relapse has then occurred within a day or two, with more typical findings of a bacterial meningitis with a positive culture. The recovery of the bacterial pathogen from spinal fluid or blood in patients with prior antibiotic therapy and spinal fluid findings of a non-purulent, lymphocytic meningitis with normal glucose and protein clearly establishes partially treated bacterial meningitis as one of the causes of the "aseptic meningitis syndrome." Part of the confusion can be explained by the variation in the definition of aseptic meningitis. Recently, the terms purulent and non-purulent appear to be used more frequently and have the advantage of avoiding the etiologic implications of the term "aseptic."

Leptospirosis. This was the cause of about 4 per cent of 430 cases of aseptic meningitis in one study. Clues to this diagnosis include the presence of conjunctival effusion, muscle pain, tenderness, and a rash. Jaundice, tender liver, microscopic hematuria, pyuria, and proteinuria may also be present.

Brain Abscess. The CSF protein may be elevated, but the CSF glucose is not lowered in a brain abscess. Increased intracranial pressure and lateralized neurologic signs suggest this diagnosis. Computerized brain scan techniques are useful in confirming and localizing a mass.

Acute Encephalitis

This syndrome is defined on page 537, and is characterized by a severe disturbance of consciousness and CSF lymphocytosis. Outbreaks of acute encephalitis are typically caused by an arbovirus, such as California encephalitis virus or St. Louis encephalitis virus. Often there is no etiology found for sporadic cases of encephalitis, although *Herpesvirus hominis* occasionally can be shown to be the cause.

No specific treatment is effective for any viral encephalitis, except that new antiviral agents are being investigated currently for treatment of herpesvirus encephalitis and may prove effective.

Acute Encephalopathy

The CSF is normal in acute encephalopathy, whereas there is a CSF lymphocytosis in acute encephalitis. Distinguishing between these two syndromes is clinically important, because specific therapy is often possible for an acute encephalopathy.

The possible etiologies of an acute encephalopathy include trauma (particularly head injury), poisoning (such as by lead, carbon monoxide, alcohol, or other drugs), metabolic disorders (such as diabetic acidosis, uremia, or hypoglycemia), and circulatory disorders (such as hypertension or water intoxication). Infectious causes (such as viral hepatitis or cerebral malaria) rarely are associated with the presence of CSF pleocytosis.

Infected Neurosurgical Shunts

In patients with hydrocephalus, a shunt (plastic tubing with a valve) is often placed between a lateral ventricle of the brain and the peritoneal cavity. These shunts may act as a foreign body and provide a place for bacteria to lodge during a transient bacteremia. Shunt infections typically occur months after the operation to insert the plastic tubing, but occasionally occur in the immediate postoperative period.

Shunt infections have many features in common with subacute bacterial endocarditis. The infection is often caused by a low virulence microorganism such as *Staph. epidermidis*. Fever is prominent, but systemic toxicity is uncommon. It is important to obtain proper specimens and obtain the organism for susceptibility testing. The infection may involve only the peritoneum, distal tubing, or valve; but if the ventricles are infected, the bacteria are transmitted through the tubing to the peritoneal cavity.

The infection should be treated with a bactericidal antibiotic, and concentrations adequate to kill the organism must be obtained in the CSF.

An antibiotic may be injected easily into the ventricle if a reservoir has been inserted with the tubing. Occasionally high doses of antibiotics given systemically and intraventricularly may cure an early infection, but usually the tubing must be removed.

MENINGOCOCCEMIA, HIGH FEVER AND SEPTIC SHOCK

Meningococcemia

Meningococcemia is a life-threatening emergency able to produce death a few hours after onset in a previously normal person. Meningococcal disease occurs most frequently in infants and small children, although a smaller peak in frequency occurs in young adults, primarily because of outbreaks in military bases among new recruits (Fig. 31-1).

Meningococcemia is typically manifested by high fever, septic shock, and disseminated intravascular coagulation. Each of these features will be discussed in the context of other possible causes, since a number of other diseases can resemble acute meningococcemia. Purulent meningitis is often present with meningococcemia, and is discussed in the preceding section (p. 539).

High Fever

This is a frequent problem in children. High fever is only rarely a manifestation of bacteremia, but should always be considered. The patterns and most frequent etiologies of acute fever syndromes are shown in Table 31-4.

Table 31-4. Acute Fever Syndromes

Problem Pattern	Most Frequent Etiologies
Fever without localizing signs (including normal urine microscopic)	
With hypotension, petechiae or seriously ill appearance	Septicemia, especially meningococcemia
With marked leukocytosis, in preschool child, not seriously ill	"Occult" bacteremia, especially pneumococcal or salmonella
Without marked leukocytosis, not seriously ill	Echovirus or Coxsackievirus Roseola syndrome, if infant Group A streptococcus Parainfluenza virus
Fever with upper respiratory symptoms and signs	(See Influenza-like illness and Table 32-6)

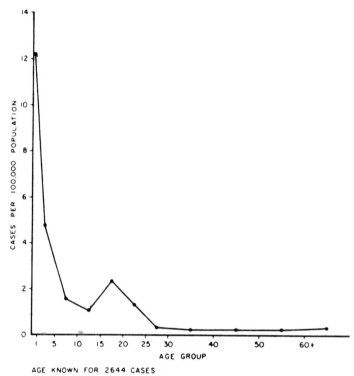

AGE KNOWN FOR 2644 CASES

Fig. 31-1. Meningococcal disease attack rates by age group USA–1969. (Moffet, H. L.: Clinical Microbiology. Philadelphia, J. B. Lippincott, 1975, p. 77.)

Symptoms. Children themselves rarely have complaints related only to fever, but headache or vomiting may occur concurrently. The parents may note hot skin or may have detected the fever by taking the child's temperature.

The state of consciousness is the most important symptom related to high fever. Decreased alertness, lethargy, or irritability should raise the question of a serious illness; whereas an active, alert, playing child is unlikely to have a serious cause of high fever. A petechial or purpuric rash (see p. 580) is not likely to be the presenting complaint in meningococcemia because it is typically preceded by other symptoms, particularly high fever. If a generalized petechial or purpuric rash is one of the presenting symptoms, the patient is either seriously and near fatally ill with bacteremia and disseminated intravascular coagulation, or else has a non-infectious cause of the rash, such as thrombocytopenic purpura or anaphylactoid purpura (see p. 580).

Objective Findings. The general appearance and the vital signs are the most important objective observations and should be evaluated immediately on examination of the child with high fever. The blood pressure may not be obviously low when the child is first seen, but the blood pressure cuff should be left in place for further determinations and to establish a trend for the blood pressure. The pulse should also be taken several times during the initial observation period to see if there is any trend.

The general appearance of the child is extremely important, but too often is described poorly. The observations useful in describing the general appearance of a febrile child need to be emphasized. Anxiety may be manifested by an anxious facial expression. Usually the skin is warm and flushed. Occasionally, the child appears pale because of cutaneous vasoconstriction. Lack of spontaneous activity and lack of interest in the surroundings, particularly the parents, indicates a decreased alertness. More severe depression of consciousness may be manifested by lethargy or staring. Irritability or persistent crying after minimal stimulation suggests cerebral involvement and possibly meningitis.

Assessment. Several major decisions need to be made in the assessment of the child with high fever. In general, the younger the child, the more cautious the physician must be. The first consideration is whether the child may have a bacteremic disease. If a child appears seriously ill or has a decreased state of consciousness or meningeal signs, a lumbar puncture is indicated, as discussed on p. 537. If a petechial or purpuric rash or hypotension is found along with the high fever, a blood culture should be obtained as an intravenous route is established, and intravenous antibiotics (usually including ampicillin) should be begun. The pulse, blood pressure, and general appearance should be closely monitored.

If the evaluation is negative for meningeal signs (see p. 537), petechial rash, hypotension, and focal areas of pain or tenderness, and the child's general appearance is good, bacteremia or meningitis is unlikely. If the physical examination and urinalysis are normal, the patient should be classified as having "undiagnosed fever" or "fever without localizing signs." The diagnostic plan can then be more deliberate and logical. In children who do not appear sick at all, and who have a negative physical examination, only observation may be indicated. A urinalysis should be done to look for pyuria or bacteriuria (see p. 581). A throat culture for Group A streptococci is usually indicated. In some patients, evaluation should include a white blood count with differential and a chest film.

The most common course of fever without localizing signs is either recovery without a specific etiologic diagnosis or development of specific localizing signs of an infection (such as pneumonia, otitis media, or a "viral rash"). Occult pneumococcal bacteremia is an uncommon cause of high fever. It typically occurs in preschool children, with high fever, marked leukocytosis (over 20,000 with a left shift), and only minimal upper respiratory symptoms.

Recently the use of blood cultures in young children with high fever and marked leukocytosis has been advocated to detect bacteremia, especially occult bacteremia. The disadvantages include the expense, the detection of skin contaminants such as *Staph. epidermidis*, and the absence of any clear evidence that this helps the clinician in the management of the child. In 1978, selective use of blood cultures in outpatients is still being investigated as a potentially helpful procedure. Currently it is advocated by some, but is done by very few clinicians in private practice.

Septic Shock

Parents report that the complaints which precede septic shock typically include high fever, a general appearance of being seriously ill, and later may include a petechial or purpuric rash.

The child who usually appears anxious with warm and flushed skin is in septic shock ("warm shock"). Later, the skin of the hands or feet may be cold. The entire skin should be examined for petechiae. The patient should be examined carefully for signs of meningeal irritation.

High fever and tachycardia (which usually accompanies fever) should stimulate the physician (or nurse or nurse's aide) to take the child's blood pressure. A low or falling blood pressure in this context should be presumed to indicate septic shock.

Treatment. Almost all authorities agree a rapid infusion of intravenous fluids is indicated to increase plasma volume. Beyond this, treatment is controversial. Most authorities recommend adrenal corticosteroids—not because of adrenal insufficiency (which is not present), but to counteract peripheral vascular disturbances and protect inadequately perfused cells. A recent prospective controlled study in adults indicated a corticosteroid was clearly more effective than a placebo in septic shock.

Disseminated Intravascular Coagulation (D.I.C.)

Disseminated Intravascular Coagulation (D.I.C.) is a serious and often terminal event in fulminating infections. Endotoxin release or tissue damage from the infection is the usual initial step that releases clotting factors which produce intravascular coagulation. The clotting factors become depleted so that D.I.C. is clinically manifested by signs related to bleeding, rather than clotting.

The petechial or purpuric rash of meningococcemia is a manifestation of D.I.C. In meningococcemia, purpura is associated with a higher mortality than petechiae.

Oozing after a venipuncture may be the first sign noted. In meningococcemia, petechiae may be the first indication of D.I.C. in a child with high fever. Sophisticated laboratory tests for D.I.C. are sometimes available, but the smear of peripheral blood is readily available and typically shows decreased platelets and deformed erythrocytes (including burr cells, helmet cells, and other fragmented erythrocytes).

Usually, the presumptive diagnosis of D.I.C. can be made by an experienced physician on the basis of fever, hypotenson, and a petechial rash. Laboratory confirmation can be obtained later from blood obtained just before the physician began emergency therapy.

Treatment. The use of heparin is controversial. It is not useful in some diseases with D.I.C., such as hemolytic uremic syndrome. In meningococcemia, the data are conflicting. Heparin therapy corrected the coagulation disorder, but did not reduce mortality in most prospective studies in meningococcemia. However, it is recommended by some experienced clinicians. Replacement of coagulation factors is contraindicated because this increases the intravascular coagulation.

ACUTE BONE AND JOINT INFECTIONS

Orthopaedic infections can be classified into syndromes according to the anatomical area involved (Table 31-5).

Definitions

Acute arthritis is defined as a warm, swollen, erythematous joint and can have causes other than infections. Purulent arthritis can be diagnosed when fluid containing many neutrophils is aspirated from a joint. In children, it is almost always caused by a bacterial infection, although the culture is not always positive. Septic arthritis implies bacterial arthritis, confirmed by culture. Synovitis can be defined as inflammation in a joint with sterile fluid and no preceding antibiotics. Usually the fluid is relatively clear and non-purulent.

Osteomyelitis can be defined as infection of a bone. Discitis is a term sometimes used to describe an inflammation of an intervertebral disc, often involving the adjacent vertebral bodies.

Cellulitis can be defined as inflammation (localized redness and

Table 31-5. Bone and Joint Syndromes

Problem pattern	Most likely etiologies
"Cellulitis" over an extremity or joint	Consider underlying arthritis or osteomyelitis
Osteomyelitis (diagnosed by tender bone)	*Staph. aureus* *Salmonella* if sickle cell disease
Septic arthritis (diagnosed by aspiration of joint)	*Staph. aureus* *H. influenzae,* if preschool child Gonococcus, if sexually active female Meningococcus, if signs of septicemia

warmth) of the skin and underlying soft tissue. Cellulitis over a bone or joint often is a manifestation of infection of the bone or joint.

Septic Arthritis

Septic arthritis is important because early diagnosis and proper treatment usually can prevent deformity or impaired function. A presumptive diagnosis of septic arthritis can often be made by immediate examination of the joint fluid, which is usually cloudy, with bacteria and segmented neutrophils seen on Gram stain and a decreased glucose concentration. Moderately high fever, erythema over the joint, and exquisite pain on motion of the joint are usually present. The joint is typically held in the position of least pain (usually flexion).

Classification of Acute Arthritis. *Acute monarticular arthritis* is characterized by rapid onset, usually with fever. When a child has fever with a single hot, tender, swollen joint, septic arthritis is the most likely diagnosis; joint aspiration is necessary. Cellulitis near a joint may resemble acute arthritis, but usually joint infection is not the cause of the cellulitis if the erythema is not distributed symmetrically around the joint. Diagnostic aspiration usually should be done if there is a reasonable suspicion of increased fluid in the joint. The risk of introducing bacteria from cellulitis into the joint is small compared to the risk of a delay in the diagnosis of septic arthritis.

Occasionally, a coagulation defect will be unrecognized until bleeding into a joint occurs after minor trauma and aspiration of the joint fluid reveals a hemarthrosis.

Acute Polyarticular Arthritis. Acute arthritis involving more than one joint in a child usually raises the question of acute rheumatic fever. However, septic arthritis can occasionally occur in more than one joint, particularly with staphylococcal bacteremia or during the newborn period.

Subacute Arthritis. This can be defined as arthritis with gradual onset over several days or a week, with little or no fever, and slow progression or recurrences of limitation of motion, tenderness, and swelling. The most likely infectious causes are partially treated septic arthritis or tuberculous arthritis. Rheumatoid arthritis, aseptic necrosis, or neoplasm should also be considered.

Importance. Subsequent growth of the child is likely to exaggerate any deformity caused by septic arthritis. Therefore, a suspected joint infection should be managed with diagnostic and therapeutic vigor. Diagnostic joint aspiration should be done promptly in acute monarticular arthritis when joint swelling or tenderness is recognized. Antibiotic treatment should be started after the joint fluid is aspirated, Gram-stained, and sent for culture. Septic arthritis of the hip is especially urgent because destruction of the epiphysis or epiphyseal growth plate can result in unequal leg length or fusion of the joint, with severe gait disturbances.

Mechanisms. The blood supply to the head of the femur (or the humerus) is by way of the proximal metaphyseal (retinacular) arteries, which lie within the joint cavity. These vessels can be compressed by increased intra-articular pressure, with ischemia and destructon of the epiphyseal growth plate the result. Therefore, most orthopaedic surgeons urge prompt open drainage followed by continuous irrigation for treatment of septic arthritis of the hip.

The action of proteolytic enzymes in pus—even when it is sterile—can destory joint cartilage, the result being joint deformity and crippling. Therefore, preservation of joint cartilage is another reason for vigorous and continuous removal of pus from joint spaces.

Etiologies. *Staph. aureus* is the most common cause of septic arthritis. In preschool children, *H. influenzae* is the next most frequent cause. Less common etiologies include the Group A streptococcus and pneumococcus. The gonococcus should be considered in sexually active females. Gram-negative enteric bacteria should be considered in the newborn period or in debilitated or compromised patients.

Treatment. A penicillinase-resistant penicillin should be given intravenously, unless a Gram stain clearly indicates gram-negative rods. If a joint or blood culture reveals *H. influenzae* or a penicillin-susceptible organism, therapy should be changed to the appropriate antibiotic.

Acute Osteomyelitis

Osteomyelitis can be defined as any infection of a bone. Osteomyelitis usually is an acute illness. However, it occasionally is subacute, chronic, or recurrent—particularly when treatment has been delayed or is inadequate.

Acute Hematogenous Osteomyelitis. In this pattern, the child typically has high fever and appears acutely ill. Young or newborn infants may be less febrile or less ill-appearing. There is marked redness, swelling, and tenderness over the involved bone, usually the tibia or femur. Marked leukocytosis with a neutrophilia is usually present, and the blood culture is usually positive for *Staph. aureus*.

Subacute Hematogenous Osteomyelitis. Brodie's abscess is a term sometimes used for a subacute pyogenic abscess of a bone, and typically occurs without fever or leukocytosis, even when the disease has not been modified by antibiotics. Subacute hematogenous osteomyelitis appears to have become more common in recent years, in part because of increased use of antibiotics. In one series, about one-third of children with osteomyelitis did not have fever over 100°F at the time of admission to the hospital. The fever and symptoms may also be modified by aspirin, and in some patients the infection becomes localized without antibiotic therapy. The organism is usually *Staph. aureus*. Treatment should be vigorous, just as for acute osteomyelitis.

Osteomyelitis can occur as an extension of an adjacent infection, such as overlying abscess, burns, and compound (open) fractures. Osteomyelitis can also occur after penetrating injuries. Puncture wounds of the foot may result in *Pseudomonas aeruginosa* infection of soft tissue, bone, and especially cartilage. Typically, the patient improves the first day or so after the injury, then develops increased swelling, pain, and tenderness. Local pain is often significant, but fever and leukocytosis are usually mild or absent. Radiologic evidence of bone destruction usually is not seen for several weeks. Damage to the metatarsal joint is common, so that antibiotic therapy with gentamicin and surgical drainage is indicated when *Pseudo. aeruginosa* is cultured from a puncture wound of the foot.

Osteomyelitis can occur after inoculation of bone following operations, such as open reduction of fractures, craniotomies, or other operations involving bone. Gram-negative enteric bacteria also should be considered as possible infecting agents in these forms of osteomyelitis.

Mechanisms. Acute hematogenous osteomyelitis can occur in any bone, but the usual sites are the long bones (femur, tibia, humerus), near one end (the metaphysis), where the blood supply of the bone is most dense. However, the blood supply differs with different age groups and inflences the clinical pattern, as described below, under age factors.

As pus forms and pressure increases within the metaphysis, the pus perforates the growth plate or the cortex, lifting up the periosteum. Periosteal elevation is not visible on radiograph until new bone is laid down and calcified, which takes at least 10 days.

Destruction of bone (lytic lesions) is usually not visible until about 1 to 3 weeks after the onset. Radiologic signs of soft tissue swelling, such as elimination of fascial planes, can be seen after a few days. However, this swelling also can be noted by examination of the patient. Thus, the diagnosis of acute hematogenous osteomyelitis *must be made on clinical grounds*, and antibiotic therapy must be begun before definitive bony changes can be seen by radiograph.

Age Factors. Over 85 per cent of acute hematogenous osteomyelitis occurs in children 16 years of age or younger. In general, three age-related patterns can be distinguished for long bones.

1. *Infantile form.* This form typically occurs in patients less than 1 year of age. The infection usually spreads from the metaphysis to the epiphysis and joint, because the blood vessels of the shaft penetrate to the epiphysis. The periosteum is usually quickly perforated, and pus can often be aspirated from just below the skin. Epiphyseal growth centers may be damaged, with shortening of a limb if a long bone is involved.

2. *Childhood form.* This form typically occurs in patients 1 to 15 years of age. The infection usually is localized to the metaphysis and does not penetrate to the epiphysis, because blood vessels do not penetrate the epiphyseal plate. Damage to the growth cartilage or joint is very rare.

3. *Adult form.* This form typically occurs after 16 years of age. The growth cartilage has been resorbed, and the metaphyseal infection can

penetrate to the epiphysis and joint. Chronic infection is more frequent in adults than in children.

Etiologies. *Staph. aureus* is the most common cause of osteomyelitis in children. *Salmonella* species are a frequent cause in children with sickle cell disease, but are not a consideration in sickle cell trait or normal individuals.

Treatment. After at least one blood culture has been obtained, treatment should be begun with a penicillinase-resistant penicillin, using the intravenous route. An operation to open the bone for drainage may be necessary in patients who are treated late or who do not respond well after 1 or 2 days of intravenous antibiotics.

Cellulitis

Cellulitis is defined as a localized inflammation of the skin, recognized by a localized area of redness and warmth. Fever may be present. Erysipelas is an older term for severe streptococcal cellulitis, with a sharply demarcated border. Lymphangitis is a thin line of redness, typically extending from an infected wound and following the lymphatic drainage up an arm or a leg.

The location of the cellulitis is very important. The descriptive diagnosis should always state the location, since there may be a serious infection underneath the cellulitis. The center point of the cellulitis may give a clue to the underlying disease (Table 31-6). The most important possible underlying diseases are osteomyelitis, septic arthritis, peritonitis, sinusitis, or deep wound infection.

Infectious Causes. Group A streptococcus is the most common cause of uncomplicated cellulitis in any location, including perianal cellulitis. The source of entrance of the organism may be a small wound that is not detectable. Severe necrotizing cellulitis or fasciitis is usually caused by beta-hemolytic streptococci, although other organisms may be found.

Hemophilus influenzae is the usual cause of facial cellulitis in infants under 2 years of age. Periorbital cellulitis is usually secondary to ethmoid

Table 31-6. Possible Causes of Cellulitis

Location	Consider
Periorbital	Ethmoid sinusitis
Abdomen	Peritonitis
Extremity	Osteomyelitis or septic arthritis
Around a wound	Wound infection
Over an enlarged node	Adenitis or abscess
Perianal	Group A streptococci
Face (over cheek)	*Hemophilus influenzae* (in infant)
	Staphylococcus aureus (in newborn)
Over both tibia	Erythema nodosum
Over sacrum	Pilonidal cyst infection

sinusitis and is also often caused by *H. influenzae*. It is rare for this organism to produce cellulitis of an extremity without involvement of an underlying joint, but underlying septic arthritis should always be considered. Typically, cellulitis due to *H. influenzae* has a purple-like color, and may be mistaken for a bruise.

Cellulitis related to *Staph. aureus* is usually caused by underlying osteomyelitis or a wound infection. Facial cellulitis in a newborn infant can be a manifestation of underlying staphylococcal maxillary osteomyelitis.

Laboratory Approach. White blood count and differential suggest infection in most patients with an infectious cellulitis. A blood culture should be obtained before starting therapy. Needle aspiration of an area of cellulitis for Gram stain and culture can be done. It is most likely to be useful if there is a bleb, or underlying abscess, elevated periosteum, or joint effusion.

Treatment. In most cases of simple cellulitis, Group A streptococcus is the suspected cause, and parenteral penicillin and close observation are indicated. However, a penicillinase-resistant penicillin should be used if septic arthritis or osteomyelitis is suspected as the possible underlying cause of the cellulitis. In facial or orbital cellulitis, ampicillin is the drug of choice.

BIBLIOGRAPHY

Moffet, H. L.: Pediatric Infectious Diseases: A Problem-Oriented Approach. Philadelphia, Lippincott, 1975.

A detailed discussion of serious infections

Epiglottitis

Battaglia, J. D., and Lockhart, D. H.: Management of acute epiglottitis by nasotracheal intubation. Am. J. Dis. Child., *129*:334–336, 1975.

A description of good success with intubation in one center.

Johnson, G. K., Sullivan, J. L., and Bishop, L. A.: Acute epiglottitis. Review of 55 cases and suggested protocol. Arch. Otolaryngol., *100*:333–337, 1974.

An excellent plan for management of epiglottitis.

Pneumonia

Dees, S. C., and Spock, A.: Right middle lobe syndrome in children. JAMA, *197*:78–84, 1966.

The importance of allergy in recurrent right middle lobe pneumonia.

Loda, F. A., Clyde, W. A., Jr., Glezen, W. P., Senior, R. J., Sheaffer, C. I., and Denny, F. W., Jr.: Studies on the role of viruses, bacteria, and *M. pneumoniae* as causes of lower respiratory tract infections in children. J. Pediatr., *72*:161–176, 1968.

The frequency of various causes of pneumonia in children.

CNS Infections

Adair, N. V., Gauld, R. L., and Smadel, J. E.: Aseptic meningitis, a disease of diverse etiology: Clinical and etiologic studies on 854 cases. Ann. Intern. Med., *39*:675–704, 1953.

The frequency of various causes of aseptic meningitis.

Converse, G. M., Gwaltney, J. M., Jr., Strassburg, D. A., and Hendley, J. O.: Alteration of cerebrospinal fluid findings by partial treatment of bacterial meningitis. J. Pediatr., *83*:220–225, 1973.

Partially-treated bacterial meningitis as a cause of "aseptic" meningitis.

Myers, M. G., and Schoenbaum, S. C.: Shunt fluid aspiration. An adjunct in the diagnosis of cerebrospinal fluid shunt infection. Am. J. Dis. Child., *129*:220–222, 1975.

A discussion of shunt infections.

Swartz, M. N., and Dodge, P. R.: Bacterial meningitis—a review of selected aspects. New Engl. J. Med., *272*:725–731, 779–787, 842, 847, 898–902, 954–960, 1003–1009, 1965.

A very comprehensive review.

Fever, Sepsis, Shock

Dechovitz, A. B., and Moffet, H. L.: Classification of acute febrile illnesses in childhood. Clin. Pediatr., 7:649–653, 1968.

A classification based on a study of cases.

Schumer, W.: Steroids in the treatment of clinical septic shock. Ann. Surg., *184*:333–341, 1976.

A discussion of the evidence favoring the use of steroids in shock.

Torphy, D. E., and Ray, C. G.: Occult pneumococcal bacteremia. Am. J. Dis. Child., *119*:336–338, 1970.

Fever and high white blood count can be due to this syndrome.

Bone and Joint Infections

Goetz, J. P., Tafari, N., and Boxerbaum, B.: Needle aspiration in *Hemophilus influenzae* type b cellulitis. Pediatrics, *54*:504–506, 1974.

A description of the usefulness of direct needle aspiration in cellulitis.

Nelson, J. D., and Koontz, W. C.: Septic arthritis in infants and children: A review of 117 cases. Pediatrics, *38*:966–971, 1966.

A good review of septic arthritis.

32

Common Infections

Hugh L. Moffet, M.D.

UPPER RESPIRATORY INFECTIONS

Upper Respiratory Infection (URI) is a vague diagnosis too often used by physicians who are capable of making a more precise diagnosis. Lay people are usually perfectly satisfied with the diagnosis of "URI," but the physician should be more specific. The more accurate descriptive diagnoses the physician should consider are shown in Table 32–1, and are discussed sequentially in this chapter.

Table 32–1. Alternatives to the Diagnosis of URI

Upper Respiratory Infections
  Common cold syndrome
  Purulent rhinitis
  Gingivostomatitis
  Pharyngitis (tonsillitis)

Pararespiratory Infections
  Acute otitis media
  Mastoiditis
  Sinusitis
  Cervical adenitis
  Parotitis

Influenza-like Illness or Bronchitis (see Table 32–6)

Acute Fever Syndromes (see Table 31–4)

Common Cold Syndrome

This syndrome is manifested by sneezing, a watery nasal discharge, nasal obstruction, and no significant fever. The illness usually lasts a few

556

days. Relief of symptoms can be obtained by a variety of over-the-counter or prescription medications, but a reasonable case can be made for simple therapy with rest, fluids, and appropriate doses of antipyretics as needed for discomfort.

Purulent Rhinitis

This syndrome is manifested by thick green or yellow-colored nasal discharge. It may be caused by sinusitis, a foreign body in the nose, or a self-limited infection of the nasopharynx. Excoriation around the nose suggests a Group A streptococcal etiology, especially in a preschool child. A culture for Group A streptococci is indicated if this organism is suspected. If found, it should be treated as described in the chapter on antibiotics.

Gingivostomatitis

Swollen red bleeding gums (gingivitis), ulcerations of the mucosa of the cheek (stomatitis), and ulcerations of the tongue (glossitis) are usually caused by *Herpesvirus hominis* (Herpes simplex virus). Vesicles, ulcers, and swelling of the lip (labiitis), or vesicles or ulcers on the face, near the mouth or nose (rarely near the eye), or, rarely, a pustule or ulcer of a sucked thumb or finger may also be seen.

There is no specific treatment for herpes stomatitis. The first infection in a young infant occasionally requires intravenous fluids because of fever, refusal to eat because of a painful mouth, and dehydration. Many local treatments have been recommended but none is truly needed. Many preventive measures, from vaccines to hypnosis, have been recommended; but all have been shown to be of no value when prospective controlled studies have been done.

Pharyngitis

All children with pharyngitis, defined as a red pharynx or tonsils, should have a throat culture done to detect Group A streptococci.

Streptococcal pharyngitis. This is defined as pharyngitis with a positive culture for beta-hemolytic streptococci. The positive culture could be a coincidental finding in a child with a viral pharyngitis, but for practical purposes, the physician acts on this definition. About 5 per cent of normal children have a positive throat culture. The physician should *not* obtain a throat culture unless there is sufficient suspicion of streptococcal disease so that the child would be treated if the culture is positive.

Small numbers of Group A streptococci in a child's throat may be due to a transient or convalescent carrier state; there is a rough correlation between number of streptococcal colonies and the severity and significance of the illness. Therefore, semiquantitative estimates of numbers of colonies on a sheep blood agar plate (this can be done in a doctor's office) are more useful clinically than methods that can detect small numbers of organisms after growth in broth, which is sometimes done in fluorescent antibody methods.

Children with streptococcal pharyngitis as defined above should be treated with penicillin (or erythromycin if there is a penicillin allergy) as described in Chapter 33.

Non-streptococcal Pharyngitis. This is defined as a red pharynx or tonsils with a negative culture for beta-hemolytic streptococci. The throat culture is especially useful in excluding Group A streptococci as a cause of pharyngitis, so the doctor can avoid unnecessary use of antibiotics.

The most common causes of non-streptococcal exudative pharyngitis are adenoviruses in young children and infections mononucleosis in older children (more than 10 years of age). If ulcerations are present in the posterior pharynx, infection with herpes simplex or coxsackievirus (herpangina) should be suspected. Other viruses, such as parainfluenza virus, can cause pharyngitis. However, pharyngitis should not be confused with tracheitis, defined by cough and the child's pointing to the trachea, rather than to the tonsillar nodes, as the area of maximum discomfort. In addition, "sore throat" caused by a virus is often associated with cough, hoarseness, or conjunctivitis, with minimal evidence of focal disease of the pharynx.

Diphtheria is practically the only non-streptococcal, bacterial cause of pharyngitis. It is very rare and usually has a membrane. Antitoxin therapy of diphtheria is more important than antibiotic therapy.

Gonorrhea is a rare cause of symptomatic pharyngitis in adolescents. The gonococcus can be detected in the pharynx only if a special medium is requested by the physician because of a clinical suspicion of the disease.

Infectious Mononucleosis. Severe non-streptococcal pharyngitis is the typical manifestation of clinically apparent infectious mononucleosis in adolescents and young adults. Anterior and posterior cervical lymphadenopathy, splenomegaly, and atypical lymphocytes in the peripheral smear are often present. If the heterophile antibody of infectious mononucleosis is present (most conveniently detected by the Mono-Spot test), the patient is said to have heterophile-positive infectious mononucleosis, which is caused by infection with EB virus. Reference laboratories can study acute and convalescent sera for EB virus antibodies, but this is not necessary if a Mono-Spot test on a second serum is positive.

Heterophile-Negative Infectious Mononucleosis-Like Illnesses. Children less than 10 years of age usually have mild or asymptomatic infections with EB virus. Even when young children have infectious mononucleosis-like illnesses, they rarely have a positive test for the heterophile antibody of infectious mononucleosis.

Heterophile-negative infectious mononucleosis-like syndrome is a useful problem-oriented diagnosis if a patient has clinical features resembling infectious mononucleosis, atypical lymphocytosis, but a negative heterophile test. The possible causes of this syndrome are shown in Table 32–2. Reference laboratories can test paired sera for antibodies to EB virus (the most common cause of this syndrome), cytomegalovirus, or *Toxoplasma gondii*.

No specific treatment is available for infectious mononucleosis. Rare complications include rupture of the enlarged spleen, fatal hepatitis, and pharyngeal airway obstruction. Therapy with corticosteriods is indicated when the patient appears to be in danger of these latter two complications. However, routine use of steroids for relief of symptoms in the uncomplicated patient is probably not justified.

PARARESPIRATORY INFECTIONS

Acute Otitis Media

The diagnosis and treatment of acute otitis media are controversial subjects for several reasons including the following:

1. Difficulties in visualization. Examination of the tympanic membranes often require adequate removal of ear wax. This is often difficult to do in young children, so that visualization of the tympanic membrane may be inadequate.

Table 32–2. Infectious Mononucleosis-Like Syndromes

Problem pattern	Most probable etiologies
Heterophile-positive illnesses Pharyngitis, generalized lymphadenopathy or splenomegaly, atypical lymphocytosis	Infectious mononucleosis (EB virus infection)
Asymptomatic child	EB virus infection, possibly convalescent from months earlier
Heterophile-negative illnesses Pharyngitis, generalized lymphadenopathy or splenomegaly, atypical lymphocytosis	EB virus Rarely cytomegalovirus, or adenovirus
Generalized lymphadenopathy or splenomegaly; atypical lymphocytosis	EB virus Cytomegalovirus, adenovirus, or toxoplasmosis
Fever; atypical lymphocytosis	Adenovirus Unidentified agents Cytomegalovirus Viral hepatitis

2. Difficulties in interpretation. Even when visualization of the tympanic membranes is adequate, interpretation may be difficult, especially for the physician without much experience with otitis media.

3. Differing definitions and terminology. In published studies, a variety of syndromes have been lumped into the category of acute otitis media, with few or no clinical subgroups.

4. Variable drainage. The drainage of the middle ear by the eustachian tube usually has not been considered in clinical studies. However, eustachian tube function is probably an important variable in the course of the illness. Relief of obstruction in an infected closed area has an important role in infections elsewhere and undoubtedly is important in otitis media.

5. Variable medical care. Social and economic differences appear to be involved in variations in results of studies of acute otitis media. Eskimos and native Americans have more severe and more frequent middle ear disease, presumably because they receive less adequate medical care. Studies based on children taken to an emergency room with fever and otalgia are not comparable to studies based on private practice in an office, in which asymptomatic middle ear effusions can be detected by a routine examination.

Controversy about otitis media will probably continue until these variables are clearly identified and controlled in prospective studies. Recognizing these difficulties is a first step in interpreting the literature about otitis media and should be remembered as one reads the rest of this section.

Clinical Diagnosis of Otitis Media

History. Middle ear effusions can be detected by pneumatic otoscopy in the routine examination of an asymptomatic child, but in many published series of acute otitis media, the child was brought to the physician because of ear pain (otalgia), nasal discharge, fever, or decreased hearing.

Otalgia. Ear pain can be a result of acute otitis media. Fluid in the middle ear may cause ear discomfort, with the infant "pulling at the ears." However, many patients with acute otitis media do not have ear pain, even before spontaneous perforation. Furthermore, ear pain in children has many causes other than otitis media—for example, otitis externa. Air pressure differences between the middle ear and the pharynx may be caused by temporary eustachian tube obstruction and can be associated with transient ear pain without otitis media.

Rhinitis. Nasal discharge, which is often purulent, is frequently found in association with otitis media.

Past Otitis Media. A history of previous otitis media often can be elicited in children with a current episode and is strong evidence for a recurrence. The history of a draining ear is also presumptive evidence of past otitis media in a patient who has not been seen before by the physician.

Fever. Acute otitis media often is associated with fever in the range of 101 to 102°F (about 38–39°C). Higher fever is unusual. Some children with acute otitis media have no fever. The true frequency of otitis media as a cause of fever has not been adequately studied. However, it is likely that many children with high fever and erythematous but mobile tympanic membranes are wrongly diagnosed as having acute otitis media.

Supine Swallowing. Feeding a supine infant by propping the bottle is a predisposing factor in acute otitis media. Nasopharyngeal secretions are pooled near the eustachian tube and are drawn into the middle ear by the negative pressure there, since swallowing opens the tube to equilibrate the pressure in the middle ear with the pressure of the nasopharynx, as can be demonstrated by the use of thin solutions of radiopaque media.

Hearing Loss. Sometimes hearing loss can be recognized by the parents of older infants and children. History of hearing loss is often more reliable than physical examination of a sick, irritable child. Decreased hearing is frequently associated with fluid in the middle ear.

Examination. The ear should be examined as thoroughly as possible before attempting to remove ear wax, since awkward attempts to remove wax sometimes make adequate removal and visualization more difficult. Suctioning is the most effective method of removing wax. A bent 14-gauge blunt needle attached by tubing to a trap and suction machine can be used and is especially useful for sticky wax.

Water irrigation may be useful if there is no perforation, and can be done by a nurse or aide using an ear syringe or a water-jet machine usually used for cleaning between teeth (Water Pik). The water-jet machine should be set at its lowest force, since perforation can occur at the highest force. Tools, such as a dull loop or a dewaxing speculum, can be used, but cotton swabs usually are not useful. Wax solvents followed by water irrigation or suction have been found useful by some physicians. However, severe local reactions to such solvents have been reported.

Appearance of the Tympanic Membrane. After the wax has been adequately removed, the tympanic membrane should be carefully examined. The color of the eardrum is normally gray or pink, but can be red, blue, or injected (prominent blood vessels). Tympanic membranes are often red in a crying infant. The drum normally appears thin and reflects the otoscope light. Diseased drums can appear dull or thick, with an absent light reflex. The drum can be bulging or retracted (atelectatic). Perforations, calcification, whitish exudate, or bullae may be noted on examination of the drum surface.

Mobility. The mobility of the drum should be tested as this is a very important guide to middle ear disease. The motion of the drum is observed while the examiner alternately puffs and sucks on a soft rubber tube attached to the otoscope head. The drum normally moves easily, but moves poorly or not at all when fluid is present in the middle ear. An immobile drum usually indicates middle ear fluid. Rarely is an immobile drum caused by a rigid or scarred membrane, or an undetected perforation. The redness of an ear drum may be only transient and not indicate an infection if it is freely mobile.

Impedance Testing. Recently, impedance testing has been used for the detection of middle ear fluid. The method is also useful for detection of perforations and for evaluation of hearing. Impedance testing has not yet been widely used in office practice, but eventually will have more frequent use.

Hearing Tests. In children with ear infections, hearing should be tested using methods appropriate for the age of the patient.

Ear Puncture. The procedure of ear puncture is not widely used in office practice. However, the clinicians who have used this procedure in their office have made important contributions to knowledge about the diagnosis and treatment of otitis. This procedure has been particularly useful in defining the frequency of various microorganisms recovered from the middle ear. This procedure can be dangerous in inexperienced hands and should not be attempted by untrained persons.

Characteristics of Middle Ear Fluid. This fluid can be defined in accurate terms only if examined directly, which is possible only if there is spontaneous perforation with drainage, or if ear puncture or myringotomy is done. The middle ear fluid may be purulent (cloudy, with many white blood cells), serous (clear, yellow, like serum), or mucoid (sticky, with threads of mucus). (See Table 32-3).

Definitions. Several definitions of acute otitis media have been used in published studies. Some studies have defined acute otitis media as an immobile, bulging, or dull drum, not necessarily abnormally red. Other studies have defined otitis media as an eardrum at least two-thirds of which is red, but do not mention mobility of the drum. Combinations of these definitions may have been used, without details to indicate different clinical subgroups. Thus, proper interpretation of published studies requires careful reading to determine the definitions used.

In order to obtain accurate data and clarify the efficacy of treatment in future studies, it will be important to identify clinical subgroups of acute otitis media, as can be done with problem-oriented diagnoses.

Treatment. In most children, otitis media of recent or unknown onset is treated with an antibiotic even though some patients may have a serous otitis media. Ampicillin is usually used for children less than about 6 years of age, in order to treat *H. influenzae* as well as *Strep. pneumoniae* and beta-hemolytic streptococci. Erythromycin and sulfa can be used if the child is allergic to penicillin. In older children, penicillin alone is usually used.

Oral decongestants, often combined with an antihistamine in commercial preparations, are usually used in an attempt to open up a possibly obstructed eustachian tube. However, the efficacy of oral decongestants in the treatment of otitis media has not been adequately studied.

Table 32-3. Acute Otitis Media and Draining Ears

Problem pattern	Most probable etiologies
Draining Ears	
Perforated otitis media	Strep. pneumoniae
	Group A streptococcus
Otitis externa ("swimmer's ear")	Pseudo. aeruginosa
	Other enteric bacteria
Acute Otitis Media	
If defined as "red ear drum"	Any febrile respiratory
	infection or crying
If defined as "immobile drum"	Eustachian tube dysfunction,
	possibly sterile,
	possibly bacterial
If defined as "red, bulging,	S. pneumoniae
dull, immobile drum"	H. influenzae
	Group A steptococcus

Acute Mastoiditis

Acute mastoiditis can be defined by clinical criteria without radiologic evidence of mastoid disease. Chronic mastoiditis can be defined by radiologic evidence of bony destruction, without any recent clinical findings.

The mastoid air cells communicate with the middle ear, so the mastoid bone is usually involved to some degree in all purulent middle ear infections. Acute mastoiditis typically occurs when the purulent infection spreads to the mastoid in the absence of drainage through the eustachian tube or through perforation of the eardrum. It can be considered an abscess in which antibiotic therapy can aid in localization but which often requires surgical drainage.

Clinical Diagnosis. Acute mastoiditis should be suspected when there is pain behind the ear and tenderness on pressing the mastoid bone. The tympanic membrane looks abnormal and is often distorted. Perforation of the tympanic membrane with ear drainage may be present. In some cases, the skin overlying the mastoid is red and edematous, and the ear may be pushed forward by the swelling behind it. The ear canal may be narrowed by swelling. Radiologic examination of the mastoid may show destruction of the air cells, although this is often not present early in the disease.

Culture of ear drainage and blood is indicated, and if positive may indicate a change from the initial therapy.

Treatment. Antibiotic therapy should be given by the intravenous route, to prevent spread to the central nervous system and to aid localization of the disease. If antibiotic therapy is begun early in the illness, ampicillin alone usually will produce improvement in about 1 day. Ampicillin is preferred for children because it is effective against *H. influenzae*, as well as the streptococcus and pneumococcus. In seriously ill patients or cases where the disease was recognized late, both methicillin and chloramphenicol may be indicated if there is a concern for possible ampicillin-resistant *H. influenzae* or penicillin-resistant *Staph. aureus*, and insufficient time to watch for a clinical response to ampicillin.

Operative drainage of the mastoid area may be necessary, although it is usually not more urgent than in any other abscess. The patient's general condition should be stabilized. Intravenous ampicillin should be given preoperatively to aid localization and to prevent dissemination during operation. Early or mild mastoiditis often can be successfully treated without surgery.

Complications. Acute mastoiditis has become very rare in recent years because of early antibiotic treatment of otitis media. However, it still occurs and if untreated can extend to produce brain abscess or meningitis. Facial palsy or lateral sinus thrombosis are very rare complications.

Sinusitis

Acute purulent sinusitis can be defined as pus in a sinus cavity, as when pus is seen to appear at a meatus immediately after wiping the area, or when pus is obtained on cannulation or puncture of a sinus. In many cases, acute sinusitis must be a presumptive diagnosis based on the clinical criteria described below. Chronic sinusitis is a presumptive diagnosis based on radiologic evidence of mucosal thickening. Purulent rhinitis can be a manifestation of acute purulent sinusitis.

Infection of a sinus cavity is usually secondary to obstruction of the meatus of the sinus, but the sinus must be developed enough to have a cavity to obstruct. Thus, the potential for sinus infection depends on the development and pneumatization of the various sinus cavities. The ethmoid sinuses are the first paranasal sinuses to develop. Ethmoid sinusitis may occur as early as 6 months of age, with most cases occurring between 1 and 3 years of age. Orbital cellulitis may occur as an extension of ethmoiditis and is discussed on page 566. Maxillary sinusitis is unlikely to occur before 5 years of age. Frontal sinusitis is uncommon before adolescence.

Predisposing Factors. Allergy is often a predisposing factor in sinusitis. Dental infections are a possible source of sinusitis in adults but are very rarely a source of sinusitis in young children. Massive contamination of the sinus by bacteria with resultant sinusitis can occur from swimming underwater, from a foreign body in the nose, or from trauma. Viral infections as a cause of obstruction predisposing to sinusitis have not been studied adequately.

Clinical Diagnosis. Acute purulent sinusitis should be suspected when there is a purulent nasal discharge from the anterior nares or the posterior nasopharynx. Tenderness to pressure over the sinus, decreased transillumination, and localized pain are strongly indicative of sinusitis. Fever to 101 or 102°F (38–39°C) may be present. Nasal obstruction secondary to edema or purulent secretions may be present.

Radiologic demonstration of an air-fluid level usually indicates purulent sinusitis. Radiologic evidence of "clouding" or opacification of a sinus has usually been interpreted as evidence of past or present sinus disease. However, a controlled study has indicated recently that radiographic signs of mucosal thickening, opacity, or polyps are found in many children without clinical evidence of acute sinusitis.

Possible Etiologies. The bacteria recovered from patients with acute purulent sinusitis are the "normal flora" of the nose, (*Neisseria* species, *Staph. epidermidis,* and *Staph. aureus*) and the common respiratory pathogens, (pneumococci, beta-stretococci and *H. influenzae*). More than one organism is often recovered. Enteric bacteria are less commonly recovered. Anaerobic bacteria, such as anaerobic streptococci, *Corynebacterium, Bacteroides,* and *Veillonella* are frequently recovered from sinuses of adults with chronic sinusitis, but they have not yet been shown to be important in sinusitis in children (See Table 32-4).

Diagnostic Approach. Radiographs of the sinuses should be done, but be interpreted with caution. Gram-stain and culture should be done if an adequate specimen can be obtained after wiping the meatal area. In

Table 32-4. Sinusitis, Orbital Cellulitis, Acute Conjunctivitis

Problem pattern	Most probable etiologies
Acute sinusitis	Undetermined etiology, probably those listed below
	S. pneumoniae, Beta hemolytic streptococci, H. influenzae in preschool children
Orbital cellulitis	Same as acute sinusitis
Acute conjunctivitis Purulent	S. aureus, if newborn
	H. influenzae, if preschool
	N. gonorrhea less common
	Chlamydiae
Non-purulent	Adenovirus
	Measles, if susceptible

one study, nasal cultures correlated with maxillary sinus puncture in about two-thirds of the patients.

Treatment. The most important part of therapy is to relieve the obstruction. This can be done by nasal vasoconstrictor drops or sprays for the first few days of acute sinusitis. Vasoconstrictors should not be used for prolonged periods. Antihistamines may be effective if allergy is a predisposing factor. Oral vasoconstrictors have not been studied in a controlled fashion.

Antibiotic therapy can be based on the Gram stain of pus obtained from near the meatus until culture results are available. In the absence of clear guidance from the Gram stain, ampicillin is a reasonable choice, particularly for preschool children, so that effectiveness against *H. influenzae* is included. Clindamycin appears to be a reasonable choice for adults with chronic sinusitis presumably caused by anaerobes, but it has not yet been adequately studied in children. Penetration of some antibiotics into the sinuses has been studied; however, the clinical efficacy of various antibiotics has not been investigated adequately in a controlled study.

Irrigation of the sinuses may be indicated for some patients. Operative cannulation or puncture is very rarely necessary in children. Aspirin or codeine may be indicated for relief of pain.

Complications. Brain abscess, meningitis, or thrombosis of a major intracranial vessel are very rare complications of sinusitis. Orbital cellulitis is discussed in the following section.

Association With Other Diseases. Purulent otitis media sometimes occurs with purulent sinusitis. Bronchiectasis is often secondary to or associated with sinusitis. Kartagener's syndrome is the triad of sinusitis, bronchiectasis, and situs inversus, and it is usually suspected if the chest radiograph is properly labeled as to right or left side.

Cystic fibrosis of the pancreas should be considered in patients with chronic sinusitis or nasal polyposis. Angiofibroma of the posterior nasopharynx occurs typically in adolescent boys and may produce refractory sinusitis because of obstruction.

Orbital Cellulitis

Orbital cellulitis (or periorbital cellulitis) is diagnosed by redness and edema of the eyelids and periorbital area of one or both eyes. Fever and leukocytosis are usually present. Cellulitis of other areas of the face, particularly the cheek area, should be referred to as facial cellulitis, often caused by *H. influenzae* in infants, but not secondary to sinusitis.

Mechanisms. Orbital cellulitis is usually an extension of an infection. In young children, ethmoid sinusitis is the usual source of the infection in orbital cellulitis. A traumatic wound near the eye is an occasional source of the infection. It is useful to distinguish these two sources, since penicillin-resistant staphylococcal infection is a significant hazard from traumatic cellulitis, whereas orbital cellulitis secondary to ethmoid sinusitis usually responds to intravenous ampicillin. Orbital cellulitis is rarely an extension of a sty or a pustule near the eye, or of a dental abscess.

Clinical Diagnosis. Fever, redness, and swelling of the periorbital area indicate a presumptive diagnosis of orbital cellulitis. Other common findings include eye pain, headache, and purulent nasal discharge. In severe cases, there may be proptosis, limitation of eye motion, and decreased vision. Loss of retinal vein pulsation indicates thrombosis, but often the fundus cannot be adequately examined. Bilateral proptosis indicates cavernous sinus thrombosis. The severity and toxicity of the illness may be modified by preceding oral antibiotics.

Differential Diagnosis. Purulent conjunctivitis can produce enough surrounding edema and erythema to resemble orbital cellulitis. Gonococcal conjunctivitis is particularly likely to be severe enough to resemble orbital cellulitis. Herpes simplex or vaccinia virus can produce cellulitis in the area of the pustules, which may occur near the eye. Secondary bacterial infection is often suspected because of the intense inflammatory reaction due to the virus. Vaccinia infections of the eye usually have a history of vaccination of the patient or a contact about a week before. Herpes simplex virus infections of the eye are usually associated with some evidence of gingivostomatitis.

Possible Etiologies. The reported series of cases of orbital cellulitis have not had enough positive blood cultures to give reliable information about the frequency of various bacterial causes. Nose or eye culture results are not conclusive. Presumably, the three bacterial agents which are the most frequent causes of otitis media are also the most frequent causes of orbital cellulitis secondary to sinusitis. *H. influenzae*, pneumococci, and beta streptococci and *S. aureus* are the most common bacteria recovered from a blood culture when the patient has ethmoid sinusitis as the source of the infection and has not had previous antibiotic therapy.

When the cellulitis is secondary to a wound, nearby pustule or abscess, *S. aureus* is a frequent cause. Gram-negative enteric bacteria may also cause orbital cellulitis secondary to contaminated wounds.

Laboratory Approach. Pus should be Gram-stained and cultured, whether found in a wound near the eye, exuding from the conjunctivae, or present as a nasal or posterior pharyngeal discharge. The blood culture is positive in some cases and is therefore a useful procedure.

Treatment. Because of the severity of complications and the need for intravenous antibiotics, hospitalization is usually indicated. Intravenous ampicillin is usually the antibiotic of choice if the source is sinusitis because the usual pathogens are susceptible to ampicillin. If the patient is seriously ill or has proptosis, intravenous oxacillin and chloramphenicol may be indicated since there is less time available to observe the clinical response of 18 hours of ampicillin therapy. Oxacillin or some other penicillinase-resistant penicillin should also be used if the child is less than 3 months old, if Gram stain of pus from a wound indicates staphylococci, or if the infection is secondary to a wound and no satisfactory material is available from Gram stain. Oxacillin should also be considered if there is no improvement after 12 to 18 hours of intravenous ampicillin. Gentamicin and oxacillin should be used initially if there has been a grossly contaminated penetrating wound. Chloramphenicol may be indicated in severe illness if ampicillin-resistant *H. influenzae* has been observed in the community.

If sinusitis is present, nasal vasoconstrictor sprays (.25% phenyl-ephrine) may be of value to shrink nasal mucosa and allow drainage through the meatus.

Pus may be present behind or adjacent to the globe or in the ethmoid sinus. Operative drainage by an ophthalmologist may be necessary if there is no response to adequate antibiotic therapy, particularly if visual acuity is decreased.

Complications. Since the availability of antibiotics, complications are rarely seen. Compression or stretching of the optic nerve can produce loss of vision. Exposure keratitis can occur if the proptotic eye is not protected. Cavernous sinus thrombosis with bilateral proptosis and ophthalmoplegia is an extremely rare complication of ethmoiditis. In the past, it usually was secondary to staphylococcal furuncles near the nose. The eye involvement is typically bilateral and the retinal veins appear engorged. Meningitis, septicemia, and death are extremely rare in this antibiotic era.

Cervical Adenitis or Adenopathy

Cervical adenitis is defined as enlarged, tender lymph nodes in the neck. The anterior cervical (tonsillar) nodes under the angle of the jaw are most frequently involved. Adenitis rarely occurs in the posterior cervical nodes (behind the sternocleidomastoid muscle).

Cervical adenopathy is distinguished from adenitis by the absence of tenderness or erythma over the node. Although many patients without evidence of local inflammation have an infection, noninfectious causes are more likely. It often occurs in the posterior cervical area.

Infectious Etiologies. There is overlap between the causes of cervical adenitis and adenopathy, since the findings of tenderness or erythema may be made milder by previous antibiotic therapy, or by the partial immunity of the patient. Thus Group A streptococci, one of the most frequent causes of cervical adenitis, can also be a cause of cervical adenopathy.

Group A streptococci was the most frequent cause of cervical adenitis in a recent series of children who had not received antibiotics; this was determined by culture of the organism from needle aspiration, incision and drainage from the fluctuant nodes, or by evidence from antistreptolysin O titers. Sometimes beta-hemolytic streptococci are not recovered from the throat, even when recovered on needle aspiration of the node. Other recent studies have ranked beta-hemolytic streptococci second to *Staph. aureus* in frequency, regardless of prior antibiotic therapy.

Pneumococci, anaerobic peptostreptococci, or gram-negative rods rarely produce cervical adenitis, especially in young infants. Dental infections may be a predisposing factor for some unusual organisms, particularly anaerobes.

Infectious mononucleosis is a possible cause of cervical adenitis or adenopathy, especially in older children and adolescents. Anterior nodes associated with pharyngitis may be tender, but the enlarged posterior nodes are usually not tender. Splenomegaly is often present.

Atypical mycobacteria, previously called unclassified or anonymous mycobacteria, occasionally cause chronic cervical adenitis. Skin tests, using representative atypical mycobacterial antigens, can be compared with the reaction of a standard tuberculin test. In atypical mycobacterial diseases, the induration produced by an atypical antigen is larger than that produced by the standard tuberculin test. Culture of an atypical mycobacterium from the node is conclusive, but in one recent series only about one-third of children with the diagnosis based on skin tests had a positive culture. The mycobacterium can often be recognized as an atypical species on the basis of a yellow or orange color after only a few weeks, before growth is sufficient to allow metabolic differentiation from *Mycobacterium tuberculosis*. Some patients can be observed without therapy since the adenopathy often resolves spontaneously. If the node drains and forms a sinus tract, excision and therapy with rifampin is indicated.

Tuberculosis is now a rare cause of cervical adenitis in the United States. Usually an excised cervical node reported as showing acid-fast bacilli and typical histologic findings of tuberculosis can be assumed safely to be an atypical mycobacterial infection, while awaiting the results of the culture.

Cat-scratch fever may produce enlarged nodes in the head or neck. Cat scratches are found in the majority of patients. Fever over 101°F (38.3°C) occurs for about a week in about 25 per cent of patients. A rash, conjunctivitis, or parotid enlargement may be noted. The enlarged regional lymph node is noted about 2 weeks after the scratch but may occur as late as 7 weeks or as early as 3 days after the scratch. Suppuration and liquefaction of the node occurs in 10 to 25 per cent of the cases.

Toxoplasmosis is an occasional cause of cervical adenopathy in the United States.

Diagnostic Approach. White blood count and differential may reveal a leukocytosis that implies a bacterial adenitis. Atypical lymphocytes suggest infectious mononucleosis, but rarely toxoplasmosis. A slide serologic test for infectious mononucleosis should be done. Serologic evaluation for histoplasmosis, coccidiomycosis, or toxoplasmosis may be indicated.

A tuberculin test is usually indicated in the case of a patient with cervical adenitis which does not respond to initial penicillin therapy and persists longer than 2 weeks. Equivocal reactions may be the result of cross reactions from atypical mycobacterial infection, and skin testing with atypical mycobacterial antigens should then be done if antigens are available.

Chest radiograph is characteristically abnormal in tuberculous cervical adenitis but is usually normal in atypical mycobacterial adenitis. It may reveal mediastinal adenopathy if cervical adenopathy is caused by a neoplasm.

Needle aspiration or incision and drainage with Gram-stain and culture of the pus are often conclusive. Anaerobic culture of the pus may be useful. Smear and culture of the pus for acid-fast organisms should also be done in selected cases. Biopsy or excision of the node, with histologic examination, may reveal the granulomatous lesion of mycobacteria or a fungus, the sulfur granules of actinomycosis, or the eosinophilic histiocytes of toxoplasmosis. A skin test with cat-scratch antigen may be helpful if the antigen is available.

Treatment. Local warmth may be of value for symptomatic relief in mild cases. Penicillin is indicated initially for most patients with cervical adenitis because of the probability of beta-hemolytic streptococcal infection. Usually the nodes decrease gradually during penicillin therapy. If there is no improvement in 2 or 3 days, needle aspiration of the node should be considered, and antibiotic therapy should be changed to treat a penicillin-resistant staphylococcus. If there is still no decrease in the size in another 3 days, incision and drainage of the node will probably be necessary, and antibiotics may be stopped. When the mass becomes fluctuant, the abscess should be incised widely and the septae broken up, usually under general anesthesia.

Antituberculous chemotherapy and surgical excision are indicated if *M. tuberculosis* is found. Excision is sufficient for atypical mycobacterial adenitis, but rifampin is useful if there is a chronic draining sinus.

Complications. Torticollis (wryneck) may occur as a complication of cervical adenitis or peritonsillar infection. Occasionally it is mistakenly believed to be associated with dislocation of the cervical vertebrae.

Parotitis

Parotitis can be defined as enlargement of the parotid gland, accompanied by fever. Sometimes the parotid gland may appear to be enlarged, when in reality the tonsillar lymph nodes are enlarged. The clinician should try to distinguish cervical adenitis from parotitis by looking carefully at the anatomic location of the swelling. When the parotid gland is enlarged, the location of the swelling occurs both above and below the angle of the jaw, although dependent edema may result in slightly more swelling below. In contrast, when cervical nodes are enlarged, the center of the swelling is located below the jaw. Minimal parotid swelling can best be detected by seeing enlargement of the parotid area, rather than by palpation.

Several other findings are helpful in recognizing parotitis. Parotid enlargement may occur rapidly if the major ducts are obstructed. Parotitis is usually somewhat painful because of stretching of the capsule, and is made worse by foods which stimulate production of saliva. A bacterial infection, such as a cervical abscess, is tender to palpation, whereas parotitis is usually not tender, unless it is a suppurative parotitis.

Mumps Versus Parotitis. The word "mumps" originally referred to the swelling seen in epidemic parotitis. Mumps virus infection is the usual cause of parotitis, but parotitis is occasionally caused by other viruses. In addition, mumps virus often produces infection without parotitis. Therefore the word "mumps" should not be used as if parotitis and mumps virus infection were identical. The best diagnostic phrasing is "parotitis, probably due to mumps virus infection." Outbreaks of parotitis, or cases of parotitis that can be related to exposure to another person with parotitis, are almost always caused by mumps virus.

Possible Causes. Mumps virus infection is the usual cause of parotitis. Classical mumps virus infection is painful parotitis, with enlargement of the parotid glands and fever. Edema of the openings of Stensen's ducts in the mouth can often be seen. The other salivary glands may also be enlarged. Edema of the neck or presternal area can occur in severe cases. Headache and vomiting may be very severe. (See Table 32-5.)

Parainfluenza virus is probably the second most common cause of acute parotitis. Very rare causes of parotitis include lymphocytic choriomeningitis virus and coxsackie viruses. Presumably other agents can cause

Table 32–5. Acute Parotitis or Cervical Adenitis

Problem pattern	Most probable etiologies
Parotitis: Parotid enlargement (mostly above angle of jaw), usually with fever.	Mumps virus, if known exposure Parainfluenza virus Coxsackie virus Rarely lymphocytic choriomeningitis virus, bacterial parotitis
Cervical adenitis: fever or erythema and anterior cervical lymph node enlargement (below angle of jaw; in front of sternocleidomastoid muscle)	Group A streptococcus *Staph. aureus* Possibly anaerobic bacteria from mouth Infectious mononucleosis Rarely atypical mycobacteria, cat scratch fever, toxoplasmosis

parotitis, since infection with the previously mentioned viruses were excluded by laboratory results in a study of children developing parotitis months or years after being immunized with live mumps virus vaccine.

Staph. aureus is the usual cause of bacterial parotitis, and rarely occurs in the newborn period. Purulent material can often be expressed from the ducts. Postoperative suppurative parotitis is rare in children.

Persistent or Recurrent Parotid Enlargement. There is no laboratory confirmation of the widespread belief of the public that mumps virus infection can produce parotitis more than once. However, parotitis with isolation of mumps virus in spite of past live mumps virus vaccine has been documented. A second episode of parotitis might result from a virus other than mumps, but several other possibilities should always be considered. These include parotid duct narrowing (sialectasis), presumably secondary to past inflammation; drug hypersensitivity, such as to iodides; and swelling of the mandibular joint because of rheumatoid arthritis.

Complications of Mumps Virus Infection. The frequency of various complications of mumps has seldom been studied adequately in a prospective fashion. Some case reports of serious complications may in reality have been coincidental, since mumps parotitis was a frequent disease before vaccine was available.

Orchitis is a complication that occurs in about 10 to 20 per cent of adult males with mumps parotitis, during outbreaks. Oophoritis appears to occur less frequently than orchitis; atrophy of the ovary apparently does not occur, presumably because the ovary is not surrounded by an inelastic tunica albuginea, as is the testis. Deafness is exceedingly rare. It apparently does occur, but there are no adequate data on the frequency of this complication.

Aseptic meningitis syndrome is very common, but significant permanent neurologic sequelae are extremely rare. The patient may have severe headache and transient delirium, but brain involvement (encephalitis) is rare, if defined as a severe and persistent disturbance of consciousness with a CSF lymphocytosis. Death due to mumps virus infection is sometimes reported on death certificates and can occur as a complication of encephalitis; but death due to mumps rarely has been documented by virus isolation, with exclusion of other causes. Pancreatitis is probably less frequent than is commonly believed. The elevated serum amylase comes from the parotid gland rather than from the pancreas.

Very rare complications can include diseases which may have been coincidental. A causal relationship remains unproved for illnesses commonly listed as rare complications. Prospective studies of mumps infections in pregnancy have not indicated any adverse effect except an increased risk of abortion, although endocardial fibroelastosis in infancy appears to have a statistical association with a positive skin test for mumps. Other "rare complications" include arthritis, thyroiditis, myocarditis, facial paralysis, transient psychosis, thrombocytopenic purpura, and transverse myelitis. Diabetes mellitus in children has been suggested as a possible late sequella of mumps virus infection, but this has not been proved.

Laboratory Studies. Mumps virus is isolated relatively easily in laboratories equipped for virus isolation. The virus produces a typical cytopathic effect on rhesus monkey kidney cells, and hemadsorption occurs when guinea pig erythrocytes are added to the infected cell cultures.

Paired sera should be obtained if serological studies for mumps virus antibody are desired. The complement fixation is usually done.

Serum amylase is elevated in patients with parotitis due to any cause. It may be useful as a laboratory guide to distinguish parotitis from cervical adenitis or other masses in the neck. However, amylase elevation is not specific for mumps parotitis. Amylase elevation persists a few days in some patients after the parotid swelling disappears, so that elevated amylase may indicate recent parotid gland disease. The elevation probably does not indicate pancreatitis, since it is proportional to the severity of parotitis rather than to the severity of the abdominal pain.

Treatment. There is no specific treatment for mumps parotitis. Bed rest is of no proven value to prevent orchitis, which can occur in postpubertal males. In one controlled study of orchitis, steroids were of no value in relief of pain, swelling or tenderness, and apparently did not influence testicular atrophy on evaluation 6 months after infection. Aspirin or codeine and support of the scrotum usually provide some relief.

Prevention. The commercially available mumps skin-testing antigen appears to be relatively unreliable as a guide to immunity. Postpubertal males who have not had clinical parotitis should be given the attenuated mumps virus vaccine (see Chapter 4 on immunization). The commercially available hyperimmune serum has not been proved to be of value in preventing mumps after exposure.

MIDDLE RESPIRATORY SYNDROMES

The phrase "middle respiratory infections" is not used often by physicians, but the concept is very useful. Infections of the middle and lower respiratory airways are as common and as important a cause of hospitalization and death in children as pneumonia syndromes. A patient's acute middle respiratory infections can be classified as laryngitis, bronchitis, bronchiolitis, and influenza-like illness. The distinction between bronchiolitis, asthmatic bronchitis, and acute bronchial asthma is also described below. Subglottic laryngitis, described below, should be distinguished from supraglottic laryngitis, a life-threatening infection described on page 529.

Subglottic Laryngitis (Croup)

This is a syndrome with several possible causes, although it is usually viral. Croup is characterized by inspiratory stridor and a typical brassy cough, but the epiglottis is normal, whether visualized directly or outlined by lateral roentgenogram of the soft tissues of the neck. High fever, marked leukocytosis, a very ill appearance, or drooling suggest epiglottitis rather than subglottic laryngitis. Subglottic laryngitis is about 100 to 1000 times more common than epiglottitis. Epiglottitis requires an artificial airway in at least 50 per cent of cases, whereas ordinary croup is rarely severe enough to require an airway, although it may be necessary in prolonged illnesses or in infants who become fatigued.

Croup is often referred to as "viral croup" because the usual cause is a virus, especially a parainfluenza virus. A foreign body or diphtheria is a rare cause of the croup syndrome. "Spasmodic croup" refers to an illness which tends to be recurrent in some children and is associated with laryngospasm, possibly precipitated by cold, allergens, aspiration of secretions, or a viral illness.

Mist and humidified oxygen are probably helpful in moderate to severe illnesses. Racemic epinephrine by aerosol is often used, but has not been proved to be of value in a controlled study. Antibiotics are probably not indicated, and they have not been adequately studied in a controlled study. However, antibiotics are often used if the patient has marked fever or leukocytosis. Observation of the patient for hypoxemia, as manifested by restlessness and anxiety, is important, as intubation or a tracheotomy may be needed if the patient becomes worse in spite of mist and oxygen.

Acute Bronchitis and Influenza-like Illness

These two syndromes are discussed together because of their similarity. Both illnesses are manifested by cough, without clinical evidence of pulmonary involvement. It is useful to regard coarse inspiratory rhonchi which clear with coughing as essential for the diagnosis of bronchitis, but fever is usually moderate or absent (Table 32–6). In an influenza-like illness, headache, sore trachea, and moderate to high fever are usually present, but fatigue or myalgia is essential for the diagnosis if fever is absent. Neither tachypnea nor inspiratory rales is found in either if these diseases are uncomplicated. Vomiting or diarrhea is usually absent, although lay persons often mistakenly refer to acute gastroenteritis as "the flu."

Bronchitis. A virus infection is the usual cause of bronchitis in children. Measles should be suspected in an unimmunized child with acute febrile bronchitis if conjunctivitis is prominent, since this is the typical clinical appearance of measles for a few days before the rash occurs. Whooping cough occasionally is manifested as an acute bronchitis, with episodes of a stacatto cough, but the typical inspiratory whoop may not

Table 32–6. Comparison of Influenza-like Illness and Acute Bronchitis

Symptom	Influenza-like illness	Acute Bronchitis
Cough	Prominent	Prominent
Muscle aches, fatigue	Prominent	Absent
Headache	Often present	Absent
Rhonchi which clear	Unusual	Typical
Usual fever pattern	Moderate to high	Moderate to absent
Rapid breathing	Absent	Absent

occur early in the illness or in young infants. Parainfluenza virus, *Mycoplasma pneumoniae*, respiratory syncytial virus, and foreign body are important possible causes of acute bronchitis.

Influenza-like Illness. In a civilian outbreak, influenza virus is the usual cause. In sporadic cases, adenovirus, parainfluenza virus, and *Mycoplasma pneumoniae* are common causes, although the myalgia and fatigue are much less prominent than with influenza virus infection.

Laboratory Approach. Respiratory virus infections are identified most conveniently by antibody studies of paired sera, which are easily transportable. Most respiratory viruses can also be cultured in a reference laboratory, but the specimen must be obtained early in the illness and transported promptly.

Treatment. Muscle aches and fever are usually treated with aspirin or acetaminophen. Rest should be encouraged for patients with fatigue. Antibiotics are unnecessary, unless pneumonia, a rare complication, occurs.

Bronchiolitis, Asthmatic Bronchitis and Asthma

These three syndromes closely resemble each other. However, it is clinically useful to distinguish them (Table 32–7). In each there is tachypnea and expiratory obstruction. In severe expiratory obstruction, the breath sounds are decreased. In mild to moderate obstruction, the breath sounds are low-pitched and coarse, and wheezes are usually present.

Bronchiolitis. This syndrome characteristically occurs in infants less than 2 years of age. After a few days of mild cough and rhinitis, the infant develops rapid respiration and is taken to a physician. The breath sounds may be decreased throughout or may be coarse, with coarse rales throughout. Chest radiographs shows little or no pneumonia, but the diaphragms are low ("air-trapping"). The cause is usually viral, particularly respiratory syncytial virus. Treatment consists of humidified oxygen, although it is rare for mechanical ventilation to be needed in extremely severe cases. Bronchodilators are typically of no value.

Asthmatic Bronchitis. This is the same syndrome that the British call "wheezy bronchitis." The child usually is about 1 to 4 years of age.

**Table 32–7. Differentiation between Bronchiolitis,
Asthmatic Bronchitis, and Asthma**

Feature	Bronchiolitis	Asthmatic Bronchitis	Bronchial Asthma
Usual age	Less than 2 yrs.	1–4 yrs.	4 yrs. and older
Recurrences	Rare	Sometimes	Repeated
Presumed location	Bronchioles	Small bronchi	All bronchi
Response to epinephrine	Little or none	Variable	Usual
Differential auscultatory features	Coarse breath sounds, wheezes, rhonchi and occasionally rales	Wheezes, rhonchi	Musical wheezes
Usual etiology	RS virus	Viral infections	Allergens: inhalants, food or infections

Asthmatic bronchitis resembles the bronchiolitis syndrome, except that the child often has a history of one or two previous similar episodes. This syndrome can be considered an early or mild form of acute bronchial asthma precipitated by infectious bronchitis; it may not necessarily progress to the more typical pattern of acute bronchial asthma. The etiology is usually viral, including rhinoviruses, which in an ordinary host produce only the common cold.

Acute Bronchial Asthma. This syndrome usually can be recognized after 2 years of age and is characterized by a history of repeated attacks of bronchospasm, relieved by epinephrine. In severe episodes unresponsive to epinephrine (status asthmaticus), hospitalization is indicated for humidified oxygen, corticosteroids, and intravenous high-dose theophylline (monitored by blood level, if possible).

COMMON EXANTHEMS

An exanthem is defined as a skin rash typically associated with fever. An enanthem is defined as lesions of the mouth, associated with a skin rash. Exanthems are best classified by reference to the classical disease they most nearly resemble (e.g., measles, rubella, and chickenpox, Table 32–8.

Table 32–8. Possible Etiologies of Rash Syndromes

Problem pattern	*Most probable etiologies*
Measles-like rashes	Measles virus, if susceptible Drug reactions
Rubella-like rashes	Rubella virus, if susceptible Ampicillin rash Adenovirus Echovirus or coxsackieviruses
Roseola-like rashes	Unknown etiology, presumably an unidentified virus Coxsackieviruses and echoviruses
Maculopapular exanthem (not like rashes above)	Echoviruses or coxsackievirus Unidentified causes
Rose spots	Typhoid fever Shigellosis Echo- or coxsackie viruses

Scarlet fever-like rashes	Group A streptococci
	Staph. aureus
	Drug reactions
	Erythema infectiosum involving
	  cheeks
	Rarely mucocutaneous lymph
	  node syndrome (Kawasaki
	  disease)

Vesicular or pustular rashes	Chickenpox
	Gonococcal or other
	  bacteremia
	Zoster
	Herpes simplex
	Hand-foot-mouth syndrome
	  (coxsackievirus)
	Stevens-Johnson syndrome

Petechial or purpuric rashes	Meningococcemia Rocky Mountain spotted fever Endocarditis, if petechial Anaphylactoid purpura Rarely, atypical measles Thrombocytopenia Adenoviruses Group A streptococci
Multiforme-urticarial rashes	Urticaria ("hives") Erythema multiforme *Mycoplasma pneumoniae*

Uses of the Word Rubella. This classification is illustrated best by the concept of a rubella-like rash. It is useful to distinguish the clinical diagnosis of a rubella-like rash from a laboratory-documented rubella virus infection. Rubella-like rash is a legitimate description of a rash and can be used as a problem-oriented syndrome diagnosis. Rubella-like illness is a descriptive diagnosis that implies that other typical features are present, such as lymphadenopathy or arthralgias. Rubella virus infection is a laboratory-confirmed etiologic diagnosis. "Rubella" without further modification is a term that should be avoided, since it is not clear whether the word is being used as a problem-oriented descriptive diagnosis meaning a rubella-like rash, or a laboratory-confirmed etiologic diagnosis.

Classification, Definitions, and Possible Causes. The following classification of rashes is based on the typical or classical clinical patterns. A patient's rash can be classified first by reference to the pattern it most nearly resembles. The possible etiologies for each syndrome are listed in Table 32–8, in order of probability.

Maculopapular Rashes

Measles-like Illness. Classical measles-like illness has severe cough, severe conjunctivitis, high fever, Koplik's spots, and a generalized confluent maculopapular rash which lasts 7 days. The cause is measles virus infection in at least 95 per cent of cases. In milder forms, modified by transplacental antibodies or gamma globulin, some of the typical features are absent.

Rubella-like Illness. Classical rubella-like illness has no remarkable fever. There is a generalized non-confluent rash, generalized lymphadenopathy (especially in postauricular or occipital areas) and occasionally splenomegaly or arthralgia. Rubella virus infection is the usual cause of this syndrome when it is observed in outbreaks. Other causes of rubella-like illnesses include adenovirus, echoviruses, and coxsackieviruses (Table 32–8). If there is a possibility of exposure to a pregnant woman, a suspected rubella virus infection should always be evaluated by the laboratory, usually by serologic tests.

Roseola-like Illness. Classical roseola-like illness occurs in an infant less than 2 years of age. The infant has 2 to 4 days of high fever, often as high as 104°F (40°C), without the child appearing seriously ill. Then the temperature abruptly returns to normal and it is noted that the child has a sparse, faint maculopapular rash. In most cases, attempts at virus isolation have been unsuccessful, so that the usual cause of the syndrome is probably an unidentified virus, although Coxsackie and echoviruses occasionally produce this syndrome.

Enterovirus-like Illness. This is a useful preliminary diagnosis to describe an illness with a maculopapular rash which does not resemble measles, rubella, or roseola. This diagnosis can be used to describe a variable relationship of the rash to the fever. Enterovirus infections often occur in small outbreaks, particularly in the summer or fall. This variable pattern can be caused by echoviruses, coxsackieviruses, adenoviruses, rubella virus, and measles virus infection modified by antibody.

Rose Spot-like Rash. Rose spots are sometimes seen in typhoid fever. These are rose red macules 1 to 4 mm. in diameter, usually only 6 to 12 in number, and seen predominantly on the trunk. High fever and febrile delerium are often present. Typhoid fever is a rare disease. A sparse macular rash is more likely to be caused by an enterovirus.

Erythematous Rashes

Scarlet Fever-like Rash. Classical scarlet fever-like illness has a generalized red macular rash which blanches and occurs in areas of the body not exposed to the sun. The rash may look and feel papular (like fine sand paper) and is sometimes sparse and sometimes confluent. Streptococcal pharyngitis or a streptococcal wound infection producing erythrogenic toxin is the usual cause. Mucocutaneous lymph node syndrome (Kawasaki disease) is a recently recognized syndrome of unknown cause which resembles scarlet fever. Allergy, sunburn, and even rubella virus infection may resemble scarlet fever.

The red cheeks of erythema infectiosum are sometimes mistaken for scarlet fever. Erythema infectiosum usually occurs in an asymptomatic child. The child is first noted to have red cheeks and later a lacey, gyrate rash. This disease often occurs in outbreaks, but the presumed virus that causes this disease has not been isolated.

Vesicular or Pustular Rashes

Chickenpox-like Illness. Chicknpox usually is associated with a known exposure. There is a generalized rash which evolves in stages from vesicle to pustule to scab. Initially, the rash appears as a few clear vesicles on a red base; there is mild fever and shallow ulcerations of mucous membranes. More than one stage of the lesions are present at any one time and these are often grouped. This illness is almost always caused by *Herpesvirus varicellae* (varicella-zoster virus), but occasionally *Herpesvirus hominis* produces an illness which may resemble mild chickenpox. Smallpox is not a likely differential diagnostic consideration in the United States in recent years.

Zoster-like Illness. The lesions are identical with those of chickenpox, but are located in one or two sensory nerve dermatomes. As with chickenpox-like illnesses, this is almost always caused by *Herpesvirus varicellae*, but it can rarely be produced by *Herpesvirus hominis*.

Septic-like Pustular Rashes. Septicemia due to some bacteria can produce isolated sparse lesions which evolve from papule to pustule, and later to hemorrhagic, purple to black bullae or ulcers. High fever and possibly shock may be present. Bacteremia due to *Staph. aureus*, *Pseudo. aeruginosa*, or *Neisseria gonorrheae* are the most likely etiologies.

Hand-foot-mouth syndrome is an illness typically caused by coxsackieviruses, usually occurring in the summer or fall. There is a papular, vesicular, or pustular rash predominantly found on the palms, soles, and buttocks. Shallow white ulcers may occur in the mouth, on the gums, or the buccal mucosa. Some of these features may be absent in any individual patient.

Petechial-Purpuric Rashes

Meningococcemia-like Illness. The rash may consist of petechiae (1 mm., non-blanching pink macules which evolve to darker red and then to purple), and purpuric spots (1 to 20 cm. non-blanching red macules which quickly become purple, like a bruise). High fever, toxicity, and hypotension often are present. If in doubt about the diagnosis, patients should be treated as if they have meningococcemia. Rocky Mountain spotted fever should be considered, especially in the middle Atlantic states. Thrombocytopenic purpura, anaphylactoid purpura, or infective endocarditis also should be considered.

Pruritic Rashes

Bite-like Rash. This preliminary diagnosis can be made when there are itchy papules, often with the tops scratched off by the patient. These can be due to mosquitoes, fleas, mites (scabies), molluscum contagiosum (a virus), spiders, or chiggers.

Multiforme-Urticarial Rashes. Urticaria, or hives, is characterized by itchy intradermal edema forming large irregular patterns of erythema. Often there is central clearing. Erythema multiforme is a dermatological diagnosis applied to a generalized irregular erythematous rash which often has a central clearing with a circular, target appearance; itching usually is not prominent. However, erythema multiforme and urticaria sometimes are difficult to distinguish.

Enteroviruses have been recovered concurrently with both of these rashes, but such isolations may be coincidental. *Mycoplasma pneumoniae* infections are occasionally associated with an urticarial or multiforme-like rash. Usually the cause of urticarial or multiforme-like rashes is not found, but is presumed to be an allergic reaction.

URINARY INFECTIONS

Diagnosis

A presumptive clinical diagnosis of urinary tract infection can be made on the basis of typical clinical manifestations and pyuria, but a laboratory-confirmed diagnosis depends on the demonstration of significant bacteriuria. These characteristics need further definition.

Clinical Manifestations. Fever implies infection. In adults with a urinary infection, high fever (> 103°F or > 39.5°C) usually indicates renal involvement. However, this is not the case with children, who may have high fever without renal involvement. Frequent or urgent urination implies bladder irritation. Burning on urination implies urethral irritation.

Cloudy urine may be caused by bacterial growth in the bladder urine but may also result from precipitated solutes.

Foul-smelling urine implies bacterial growth but occasionally the patient regards concentrated urine as foul smelling. Suprapubic pain or tenderness implies infection involving the bladder. Flank pain or tenderness implies infection involving the kidney.

In infants and young children, symptoms may be absent, mild, or perhaps not even traced to the urinary tract. Therefore, a careful urinalysis should be done in a child with unexplained fever. Asymptomatic infections are detected in about 2 per cent of school-age girls when screening cultures are done.

Pyuria. There is no widely agreed upon definition of pyuria, so that the upper limit of normal for leukocytes in the urine is defined by the laboratory or the physician doing the examination and depends on the method used. Usually, the number of leukocytes in the urine is more than the observer normally finds and can be clearly recognized as pyuria. Clumps or casts of white blood cells usually indicate pyuria. Pyuria can also be defined as more than five or 10 leukocytes per high power field in the centrifuged sediment. Pyuria cannot be excluded by the microscopic examination of uncentrifuged specimens unless a large volume is examined quantitatively in a hemocytometer.

Microscopic Bacteriuria. Microscopic examination for pyuria also is useful for immediate recognition of the presence of bacteria. Experienced observers can usually give a semi-quantitative estimate of the number of bacilli in the sediment, which usually correlates well with culture of the urine. The absence of bacteria in the centrifuged sediment does not exclude urinary infection, but rod-like bacteria can usually be seen in large quantities in the sediment if the culture is going to result in >100,000 bacteria/ml. A methylene blue-stain or Gram stain of a drop of uncentrifuged urine is an equally accurate test for microscopic bacteriuria; some physicians prefer this method.

Microscopic bacteriuria with a negative culture can have several possible explanations. Most frequently, the bacteria seen are contaminants which are not detected by the usual bacteriologic media (e.g., diphtheroids or vaginal lactobacilli). Artifacts and technical errors in collection and culture are much more likely explanations than failure to grow a fastidious pathogen, such as an anaerobe.

Significant Bacteriuria. Quantitative culture of the urine ("colony counts"), is a significant advance in the study of urinary infections. In a clean voided urine >100,000 bacteria/ml. usually indicates urinary infection. The difficulties with this figure of 100,000 do not lie with the accuracy of the counting, which is well within the capabilities of office bacteriology, but rather lie with the collection of the specimen. The value >100,000 bacteria/ml. should not be taken as significant by itself, since it depends on the method used to collect urine as well as a number of other variables.

Preliminary Classification

Using the three factors—clinical manifestations, pyuria, and bacteriuria—it is possible to classify any patient into one of the following eight logical possibilities (Table 32–9). The use of such a preliminary diagnostic category aids the clinician by giving guidance toward making a more specific diagnosis. The logical preliminary diagnoses can have a number of possible etiologies.

Typical Urinary Infection. If all three features of clinical findings, pyuria, and significant bacteriuria are present, the illness is a typical urinary infection.

Suspected Urinary Infection Without Pyuria or Bacteriuria. This should be the preliminary diagnosis when there are signs and symptoms suggesting a urinary tract infection but no pyuria or significant bacteriuria. There are several possible causes of this pattern. Urethritis due to a variety of causes (see p. 586) is a common cause. Recent or current chemotherapy that has suppressed cultural confirmation of the infection is one of the most frequent causes. Over-hydration with rapid urine flow and frequent voiding of urine before bacteria can reach high concentrations is another cause.

Fastidious or anaerobic organisms causing a bladder or kidney infection is a very uncommon cause of this pattern. However, *Hemophilus influenzae*, which will not grow on the plating media usually used for urine, should be considered a rare cause of this pattern. Suppression of bacterial growth by contamination of the urine with the disinfectant used to prepare the urethral area is also a very unlikely cause. Adenoviral cystitis is an uncommon cause of microscopic hematuria and pyuria without bacteriuria. Polycystic kidney, with intermittent obstruction of infected portions of the kidney, is a possible cause of variable urinalysis or culture results.

Presumptive Urinary Infection Without Bacteriuria. Urethritis is probably the most frequent cause of this pattern. Gonorrhea and non-gonococcal urethritis are discussed on page 586. Medications such as atropine-like drugs are an occasional cause of frequent urination. Unilateral pyelonephritis with complete ureteral obstruction is an unusual cause of this pattern.

Probable Urinary Infection Without Pyuria. This pattern is uncommon, but may occur several days after the onset of an infection when pyuria has decreased. The urinalysis and urine culture should be repeated to clarify the situation if antibiotics have not been administered.

Asymptomatic Bacteriuria and Pyuria. This pattern can be the manifestation of a urinary infection that has signs and symptoms suppressed by recent or current chemotherapy. It may also be due to poor technique in collecting a voided urine when there is no true urinary infection, especially if there is a delay in inoculation of the specimen. This is es-

Table 32–9. Logical Combinations of Three Major Variable Observations in Urinary Infections.

Diagnostic classification	Clinical findings suggesting infection	Pyuria	Bacteriuria
Typical urinary infection	+	+	+
Suspected urinary infection without bacteriuria	+	0	0
Presumptive urinary infection without bacteriuria	+	+	0
Probably urinary infection without pyuria	+	0	+
Asymptomatic bacteriuria and pyuria	0	+	+
Asymptomatic bacteriuria without pyuria	0	0	+
Asymptomatic pyuria	0	+	0
No bacterial urinary infection	0	0	0

(From Moffet, H.L.: Urinalysis and urine cultures in children. Urol. Clin. North Am. *1*:387–396, 1974)

pecially likely if there is vaginitis or in an uncircumcised male with unretracted foreskin.

Asymptomatic Bacteriuria Without Pyuria. This pattern can occur several days or weeks after the onset of the infection, after the initial clinical manifestations and pyuria have disappeared. It can rarely occur after the suppression of symptoms and pyuria by inadequate chemotherapy. This pattern also can be caused by poor collection of a voided urine as described above.

Asymptomatic Pyuria. This type of pyuria has many possible causes, several infectious. A bacterial urinary infection suppressed by chemotherapy may produce this pattern. Urethritis can be gonococcal, nonspecific, or chemical, as discussed below. Renal tuberculosis should also be considered.

Poor urine collection is a possible cause. Pyuria without infection often occurs after urethral instrumentation or bladder surgery. Noninfectious subacute or chronic renal disease can be associated with pyuria, but proteinuria, casts, or hematuria are often present. Fever in a patient with chronic renal disease may stimulate pyuria. Pyuria is also observed during convalescence from acute glomerulonephritis or toxic nephritis, but some hematuria is usually present. Extreme dehydration can also produce pyuria.

No Bacterial Urinary Infection. All three variables are negative in most normal children, provided there has been no recent chemotherapy.

Management

Chemotherapy. Sulfisoxazole or ampicillin is used most often to treat a first infection (see Table 33–1), but nitrofurantoin is equally effective.

Two weeks of therapy is usually adequate. A follow-up culture obtained about 1 week after stopping medication is essential to be sure there is no relapse. If a follow-up culture is positive, antimicrobial susceptibility tests should be obtained to guide selection of the drug used in the second course of therapy.

Urologic Evaluation. An intravenous pyelogram is probably advisable after the first infection for males and females. It certainly is advisable in infants. More complete urologic investigation with a cystourethrogram and cystoscopy is advisable after the first infection in boys.

Other Therapy and Follow-up. Children with a recent urinary infection should have several follow-up urine examinations and cultures for one year, even if no abnormalities have been noted. Culture can be done easily using a quantitative loop in the physician's office. As an alternative, the parent can test the child's first voided urine in the morning with a dip stick type of chemical test.

Children with recurrent urinary infections and no anatomic abnormalities seem to be helped by prophylactic therapy with low dose nitrofurantoin (Table 33–1) and extra oral fluids.

GENITAL INFECTIONS

Genital Ulcers

This general category includes ulceration of the skin or mucosa on or near the external genitalia. A syphilitic chancre is a shallow ulcer about 1 to 2 cm. in diameter, with hard, elevated edges. The chancre is painless if located on the genitalia but may be painful if it is extragenital. It is overlooked easily if it is on the cervix or in the rectum. The incubation period between exposure and appearance of the chancre is 10 to 90 days (usually about 3 weeks).

Chancroid or soft chancre is a chancre-like ulcer caused by *Hemophilus ducreyi.* This disease is about as common as syphilis. The lesion begins as a papule or vesicle that later ruptures and leaves a shallow, painful ulcer. Most patients have two or more soft chancres. Later there are large ulcers in the genital area with beefy red granulation tissue. The incubation period is 3 to 5 days.

Herpesvirus hominis infection in the genital area (herpes progenitalis) can result in small painful ulcerations. In children, genital herpes is not always spread by sexual contact.

Granuloma inguinale is a rare disease due to a gram-negative bacillus. The lesion begins as a non-painful nodule that erodes to leave a beefy red exuberant granulation tissue. The incubation period is 1 to 12 weeks, usually about 7 weeks.

Other possible causes of genital ulcers include moniliasis, psoriasis, scabies, molluscum contagiosum, erythema multiforme, and simple friction ulceration.

Laboratory Approach. The Venereal Disease Research Laboratory (VDRL) test may not be positive when the syphilitic chancre first appears, but usually becomes positive within a few weeks. The VDRL should be obtained as soon as the chancre is seen and repeated in about 3 weeks. Antisyphilitic therapy should be given as soon as the ulcer is seen by the physician, without waiting for the VDRL results.

All positive VDRL results should be confirmed in a reference laboratory by specific tests such as the fluorescent treponemal antibody absorption test (FTA-ABS), since biologic false-positive VDRL's are common in adolescents. False-positive FTA-ABS tests can also occur, so that this test should not be used for screening purposes.

Dark field examination of material from a chancre-like ulcer may reveal the spirochetes of syphilis, but dark field facilities with experienced observers are usually not available except where the disease is frequently seen. Gram stain of the smear of a chancre-like ulcer may reveal rows and chains of gram-negative rods, characteristic of *Hemophilus ducreyi*. Special stains of a smear from crushed tissue preparations are necessary to demonstrate the oval Donovan bodies found in granuloma inguinale.

Treatment. Genital ulcers are best treated with an antisyphilitic regimen until follow-up serologic tests determine syphilis has been excluded. Syphilitic chancre in an adolescent or adult is conventionally treated by 2.4 million units of benzathine penicillin, given intramuscularly in two sites. Tetracycline 500 mg. 4 times daily for 15 days is an alternative therapy for adults allergic to penicillin. Fever, malaise, and intensification of skin lesions (Jarisch-Herxheimer reaction) occur in many patients within 12 hours of the onset of therapy.

Chancroid responds to sulfonamides. Granuloma inguinale is treated effectively by tetracycline or erythromycin, but not by ampicillin. Treatment of herpes simplex lesions of external genitalia is currently controversial with no controlled studies showing benefit from any kind of therapy.

Inguinal Adenopathy

Enlargement of inguinal or femoral lymph nodes can be due to many causes unrelated to genital diseases and in children is usually a result of infections of the leg. However, tender or suppurative nodes in a postpubertal person should raise the question of a genital infection. Lymphogranuloma venereum (LGV), caused by *Chlamydia lymphogranulomatosis*, is rare. The first manifestation of disease is a tender inguinal node (bubo). Typically, the primary lesion, a small papule or erosion which occurs 1 or 2 weeks after exposure, is not noticed or reported. Then the bubo appears 2 to 4 weeks after exposure. The bubo may proceed to suppuration.

Syphilis and chancroid also may produce inguinal adenopathy, and should always be considered because the primary ulceration may have been overlooked.

Laboratory Approach. The diagnosis of lymphogranuloma venereum can be confirmed by a skin test (Frei test), but determination of serum antibodies is more reliable. Syphilis should be excluded by a VDRL in sexually active persons with inguinal adenitis and should be repeated at monthly intervals for 3 months.

Treatment. Lymphogranuloma venereum can be effectively treated by a 21-day course of tetracycline or sulfonamides. Aspiration of fluctuant nodes is also helpful.

Urethritis

Urethritis is defined by redness of the urethra or pain in the urethra on voiding. Urethritis can be classified as purulent or non-purulent, depending on the appearance of the discharge. Urethritis can also be classified as gonococcal or non-gonococcal, according to the results of culture of the discharge. This is similar to the classification of pharyngitis as streptococcal or non-streptococcal.

Purulent urethritis occurs most frequently in the male and is usually caused by the gonococcus. Symptoms of gonorrhea in the male begin about 3 to 5 days after exposure. Urination is painful, and there is a yellow discharge. Fever is usually absent. Urethritis is more likely to be gonococcal if there is a spontaneous discharge. Because the symptoms are acute, the male seeks medical care within a few days of the onset. The Gram stain of the discharge is usually unequivocally positive for Gram-negative diplococci, if the culture is going to be positive for the gonococcus.

In females, findings of urethritis are usually absent, and the gonococcal infection is more likely to cause cervicitis or salpingitis. Gonorrhea is one of the possible causes of painful urination with negative urine culture for the usual urinary tract pathogens (see page 582). Gonorrhea in females is often asymptomatic, but can spread to the endometrium and fallopian tubes. Dissemination with fever and arthritis may be the first sign of disease.

Bacteria other than the gonococcus are occasionally recovered from a purulent urethral discharge. Enteric bacteria, *Staph. aureus,* or streptococci are occasionally recovered, but the etiologic significance is not easily proved. It is rare for purulent urethritis to be caused by an *Acinetobacter* species (formerly called *Mima polymorpha,* so named because of its ability to mimic the gonococcus by Gram stain). Occasionally, non-purulent urethritis can be caused by the same bacteria which usually produce a purulent urethritis.

Non-purulent urethritis may have a number of causes including gonorrhea, but usually a bacterial cause is not found. Non-gonococcal non-purulent urethritis is common in sexually active adolescents. Urethritis may also be caused by physical irritation. Some strains of mycoplasma, called T-strains for the tiny colonies, have been regarded as a possible cause of non-gonococcal urethritis. However, recent studies indicate little or no role for mycoplasmas and a major role for chlamydiae.

Chlamydia species, probably *C. trachomatis*, seem to be the usual cause of non-purulent urethritis. This disease has an incubation period of about 10 days and responds to tetracycline.

Trichomonas vaginalis is a protozoan which can cause urethritis in the male or female.

Vaginitis

This syndrome can be defined by redness and exudate of the vaginal mucosa. Non-infectious causes predominate in prepubertal girls and include poor perineal hygiene, foreign bodies, and chemical irritants. Gonorrheal vaginitis can occur in prepubertal girls and should always be considered. The squamous epithelium of the postpubertal female is relatively resistant to infection by the gonococcus, so that vaginitis is rarely gonococcal in mature females.

The most likely infectious causes in postpubertal females include *Candida albicans* (moniliasis), *Trichomonas vaginalis*, and *Corynebacterium vaginale (Hemophilus vaginalis)*. Bacteria other than the gonococci appear to account for nearly half of all cases of vaginitis in adult women. A purulent, copious gray discharge with a characteristic offensive odor is suggestive of *Coryne. vaginale*, as has been demonstrated by inoculation of volunteers.

Candidiasis appears to account for the majority of cases of infectious vaginitis in children. Itching is prominent and the discharge is curdy. In prepubertal girls, beta-hemolytic streptococcus is also a possible cause. Shigella infection is a rare cause of vaginitis in prepubertal girls.

Laboratory Approach. A fresh wet preparation and Gram stain should be examined. Recent douching or menstruation can interfere with these studies. In one study, the wet mount preparation was inadequate, compared to culture, for candida or trichomonas. "Clue" cells, which are rounded epithelial cells with intracellular granules, suggest *Coryne. vaginale*. Culture should be done to exclude gonococcus in all cases. Special techniques are necessary for candida, trichomonas, or *Coryne. vaginale*, so that the laboratory should be informed when one of these organisms is suspected on the basis of clinical or microscopic evidence. Culture should be done if the wet preparation is negative.

Treatment. *Trichomonas* vaginitis is treated with metronidazole. *Coryne-bacterium vaginale* vaginitis appears to respond to ampicillin, but it has not been studied in a controlled fashion. Triple sulfa cream applied locally is also effective. *Candida albicans* vaginitis can be treated with nystatin or miconazole cream.

Orchitis

The acute onset of swelling and pain in one or both testicles in a postpubertal boy suggests acute orchitis, but the clinician should consider non-infectious etiologies including trauma and torsion.

Epididymitis is a clinical diagnosis based on palpation that localizes the swelling and tenderness to the epididymis and not to the testicle. Urinary tract anomalies may be the underlying reason for acute epididymitis in prepubertal boys, and a urological investigation should be carried out to look for such anomalies. Anaphylactoid purpura is another possible cause of epididymitis.

Mumps virus infection is an important and relatively frequent cause of orchitis and a rare cause of isolated epididymitis. Typically, the patient has parotitis and has had a known exposure to another individual with parotitis. Before mumps vaccine was available, mumps was the most common cause of orchitis.

The prognosis for fertility after mumps orchitis is probably very good. In one study of 105 cases of testicular causes of infertility with bilateral testicular biopsy, only two patients had a histologic diagnosis of atrophy due to past mumps virus infection, and in these cases a history of mumps orchitis was needed to support the histologic diagnosis.

In a controlled study, cortisone did not have any favorable effect on mumps orchitis in terms of acute symptoms or testicular size 5 months later.

Coxsackie B virus has been recovered from a testicular biopsy of a patient with orchitis, confirming the etiologic relationship implied by the increased frequency of orchitis in patients with pleurodynia.

Infectious mononucleosis is rarely complicated by orchitis. Other infections which are rare causes of acute orchitis include the viruses of chickenpox, dengue, and lymphocytic choriomeningitis.

BIBLIOGRAPHY

General

Krugman, S., Ward, R., and Katz, S. L.: Infectious Diseases of Children. St. Louis, C. V. Mosby, 1977.

An excellent source of information about common childhood diseases.

Moffet, H. L.: Pediatric Infectious Diseases: A Problem-Oriented Approach. Philadelphia, J. B. Lippincott, 1975.

A detailed discussion of infectious syndromes in children

Upper Respiratory Infections

Barton, L. L., and Feigin, R. D.: Childhood cervical lymphadenitis: A reappraisal. J. Pediatr., 84:846–852, 1974.

Cases proved by needle puncture.

Brunell, P. A., Brickman, A., Steinberg, S., and Allen, E.: Parotitis in children who had previously received mumps vaccine. Pediatrics, *50*:441–444, 1972.

Viral studies of this syndrome.

Moffet, H. L., Cramblett, H. G., and Smith, A.: Group A streptococcal infections in a children's home. II. Clinical and epidemiologic patterns of illness. Pediatrics, *33*:11–17, 1964.

Clinical details about streptococcal pharyngitis.

Moffet, H. L., Siegel, A. C., and Doyle, H. K.: Nonstreptococcal pharyngitis. J. Pediatr., *73*:51–60, 1968.

Viral and serologic studies of non-streptococcal pharyngitis.

Parrott, R. H., Wolf, S. I., Nudelman, J., Naiden, E., Huebner, R. J., *et al.*: Clinical and laboratory differentiation between herpangina and infectious (herpetic) gingivostomatitis. Pediatrics, *14*:122–129, 1954.

Clinical distinctions between herpes simplex and herpangina.

Polson, A. M.: Gingival and peridontal problems in children. Pediatrics, *54*:190–195, 1974.

Stomatitis is not necrotizing ulcerative gingivitis (trench mouth).

Taranta, A., and Moody, M. D.: Diagnosis of streptococcal pharyngitis. Pediatr. Clin. North Am., *18*:125–143, 1971.

Laboratory studies for suspected streptococcal pharyngitis.

Townsend, E. H., Jr., and Radebaugh, J. F.: Prevention of complications of respiratory illnesses in pediatric practice. A double-blind study. N. Engl. J. Med., *266*:683–689, 1962.

Lack of value of antibiotics in minor respiratory illnesses.

Otitis, Sinusitis

Bernstein, L.: Pediatric sinus problems. Otolaryngol. Clin. North Am., *4*:127–142, 1971.

A good review of sinusitis.

Bluestone, C. D., and Shurin, P. A.: Middle ear disease in children. Pathogenesis, diagnosis, and management. Pediatr. Clin. North Am., *21*:379–400, 1974.

An excellent review of otitis media.

33

Principles of Antimicrobial Therapy

Hugh L. Moffet, M.D.

Recommendations about antimicrobial therapy are based on past studies of the usual susceptibilities of the various microorganisms, the pharmacology of the antimicrobial agents, and clinical studies of the treatment of human infections. Many review articles and textbooks deal with these principles in detail and in depth. The purpose of this chapter is to provide a simple introduction to these principles and to indicate some special differences in the pediatric age group.

WHETHER TO USE ANTIBIOTICS

The severity of the illness is an important factor in deciding whether to use an antibiotic. A child with a small skin abscess usually does not need to be treated with an antibiotic in addition to incision and drainage; but a large skin abscess, poorly localized, with surrounding erythema usually should be treated with an antibiotic.

Young age or underlying host disease often influence the clinician to use an antibiotic as an exception to the general rule. For example, a small skin abscess in a newborn infant should be treated with an antibiotic because of the newborn's poorer resistance.

The patient's cooperation is another important factor. In some situations in which the patient is unlikely or unable to return for medication or to fill a prescription, antibiotic therapy may be used if a delay would ordinarily be made for culture or re-examination. For example, intramuscular benzathine penicillin may be appropriate in an emergency room for a child with exudative pharyngitis before results of the throat culture for beta-hemolytic streptococci are known, if follow-up contact is unlikely.

CHOICE OF ANTIBIOTIC

Clinical evaluation of the severity of the illness is very important in the choice of an antibiotic. The most potent drug should be used in a serious illness in spite of some risk of toxicity, but the antibiotic of least toxicity or no antibiotic at all should be used for minor illness.

The Gram stain is a very simple bacteriologic technique which can be done immediately, and can be an extremely useful guide to the selection of antibiotics. Pus should always be Gram stained as a preliminary guide to the likely organism. If no material is available for Gram stain, the initial choice of an antibiotic should be based on the clinical diagnosis, which implies a probable infecting organism. Table 32-1 lists recommended choices of antibiotics for selected clinical situations, classified by the anatomic areas involved.

After the bacteriology laboratory results have been reported, many drugs may appear to be effective on the basis of *in vitro* susceptibility tests. The antibiotic selected should be based both on the susceptibility

Table 33-1. Recommended Antibiotic Therapy of Selected Pediatric Infections

Clinical diagnosis	Antibiotic	Dose
Streptococcal pharyngitis	Benzathine penicillin, I.M.	0.3 to 1.2 million units depending on weight
	or	
	Penicillin V, oral	20–50 mg./kg./day, 10 days
	or	
	Erythromycin, oral	30–50 mg./kg./day, 10 days
Otitis media	Ampicillin, oral	50–100 mg./kg./day
First urinary infection	Sulfisoxazole, oral	150 mg./kg./day
Prophylaxis of urinary infections	Nitrofurantoin, oral	2–4 mg./kg./day
H. influenzae meningitis	Chloramphenicol, I.V.	100 mg./kg./day
Meningococcal or pneumococcal meningitis	Penicillin, I.V.	100,000 to 250,000 units/kg./day
Staphylococcal pneumonia	Oxacillin, I.V.	100–200 mg./kg./day
Staphylococcal abscess or wound infection	Dicloxacillin, oral	25–50 mg./kg./day

test results and on clinical experience with the particular organism. The *Medical Letter on Drugs and Therapeutics* publishes guidelines for the choice of antibiotics, revises them frequently, and gives authoritative and accurate comments on new information about antibiotic therapy. Guidelines for selection of antibiotics in children, with dosages and toxicities, appear periodically in review articles in pediatric journals, and should be consulted for the most current information.

Convenience and cost are other factors involved in the choice of antibiotics if all other factors are equal.

PHARMACOLOGIC PRINCIPLES

Absorption of antibiotics in children is similar to that in adults. However, excretion and inactivation of antibiotics in newborn infants deserves some special consideration. In the first week of life, conjugation and excretion by the immature liver is limited, so that chloramphenicol blood levels may increase to toxic levels and produce vascular collapse and death (gray syndrome). Because of this possibility, chloramphenicol is not used in the newborn period, except in special situations where it is clearly a superior drug and when blood levels can be monitored.

The renal excretion of many drugs is decreased in the first week of life, so that recommended dosages are decreased, especially in the case of aminoglycosides such as gentamicin. In low birth weight infants, renal and hepatic function are even more decreased than in term infants, so that even lower dosages, based on past pharmacologic studies, are recommended. The current *Physician's Desk Reference*, or the package circular, can also be consulted for appropriate antibiotic doses for newborn infants and for children with renal or hepatic disease.

In children, intramuscular injections are often limited by the muscle size of young infants or patients with muscle atrophy. In some diseases, intramuscular injections might interfere with observation of the function of the leg (e.g., paralysis or osteomyelitis involving a leg). Skin diseases, particularly burns, limit muscles available for injection. Inaccurately placed injection into the gluteal area can cause sciatic nerve palsy, particularly in young children. Excessive injections into the anterior thigh can cause quadriceps-femoris contractures in infants. Use of 1½-inch needles in the lateral thigh of infants can cause thrombosis of the femoral artery. If the lateral thigh is used in small infants, a 1-inch needle should be used and inserted obliquely into the muscle mass. If anatomic landmarks and proper direction of the needle perpendicular to the surface are utilized, the gluteal area can be used in children over 2 years of age who have developed their gluteal muscles by walking.

TOXICITY AND SIDE EFFECTS

An antibiotic should usually be discontinued at the first clinical or laboratory sign of a known associated toxic effect. Toxic effects that are especially important in children are shown in Table 33-2.

SPECIFIC ANTIBIOTICS

Some general comments can be made about specific antibiotics with respect to their use in children.

Penicillin

Oral and intramuscular penicillin preparations are quite useful in pediatrics, particularly when pneumococcal or Group A streptococcal infections are suspected. Penicillin allergy is uncommon in children, probably because it may take a number of exposures to become sensitized. Papular or erythematous rashes really caused by scarlet fever or by com-

Table 33-2. Most Common Adverse Effects of Antibiotics in Infants or Children

Antibiotic	Most common adverse effects
Ampicillin	Diarrhea, maculopapular rash
Methicillin	Hematuria
Oxacillin	Transaminase elevation
Erythromycin estolate	Allergic hepatitis
Sulfonamides	Hyperbilirubinemia, in newborns
Gentamicin	Vestibular damage
Tetracycline	Teeth staining, a cosmetic problem in children less than 8 years old
Chloramphenicol	Aplastic anemia (very rare); reversible bone marrow depression (dose-related); gray syndrome in newborns
Clindamycin	Enterocolitis (rare in children)
Nitrofurantoin	Nausea, vomiting
Trimethoprim	Bone marrow depression

mon minor virus illnesses may be mistaken for an allergy to the penicillin being given, so that penicillin allergy may be over-diagnosed. However, an urticarial rash (hives) occurring during penicillin administration is probably due to a penicillin allergy. The history of some kind of poorly described rash or reaction to penicillin should not be disregarded, as there is a small risk of a serious adverse reaction in this situation. Skin testing for penicillin allergy can be done, but erythromycin is often used as a substitute for penicillin when this history is given.

In the first week of life intramuscular aqueous (crystalline) penicillin is used instead of procaine penicillin to decrease local reaction at the injection site. Because of the decreased renal excretion, the aqueous penicillin injection can be given every 12 hours.

Ampicillin

This antibiotic is widely used for children less than 6 years of age because of its effectiveness against *H. influenzae*. The first ampicillin-resistant strains of *H. influenzae* were observed in the United States in 1974, and have been noted with increasing frequency. For this reason, chloramphenicol is becoming used more frequently as an alternative to ampicillin for life-threatening infections, but not for minor infections.

A maculopapular rash occurs frequently with ampicillin therapy. It does not appear to represent an allergy to the drug, which can be continued or readministered without adverse effects.

Amoxicillin is a derivative of ampicillin which is better absorbed and can be given three times a day instead of the usual four times a day. The total cost of a comparable course of ampicillin is about the same. Amoxicillin is less effective than ampicillin for the treatment of shigellosis.

Penicillinase-Resistant Penicillins

Methicillin was used for several years for parenteral therapy of staphylococcal infections before nafcillin or oxacillin became available. All three of these drugs appear to be comparable in clinical efficacy. Some authorities believe methicillin is associated with a greater frequency of hematuria, but accurate prospective studies comparing the adverse effects of these three drugs have not yet been done.

Cloxacillin, dicloxacillin, and nafcillin are comparable in efficacy when used orally. The local cost of comparable courses of therapy is the best guide to selection.

Carbenicillin

The usual use of this drug is in combination with gentamicin for the treatment of serious *Pseudomonas aeruginosa* infections in compromised hosts. It should be reserved for this kind of situation, and should not be used when ampicillin or penicillin would be equally effective.

Cephalosporins

These drugs have little importance in pediatric infections and are overused. No cephalosporin has yet been shown to be more effective than ampicillin in clinical trials if the bacterial agent is susceptible to both drugs. The cephalosporins are ineffective in the treatment of *H. influenzae* or meningococcal meningitis, probably because of poor penetration into spinal fluid. Penicillin allergy is rare in children, so this indication for a cephalosporin rarely applies in pediatric practice.

Erythromycin

This drug is fairly useful for minor infections due to staphylococci, Group A streptococci, or *H. influenzae* in a child allergic to penicillin. The estolate preparation is associated with rare and reversible allergic hepatitis, and has not been shown in clinical trials to be more effective than other oral preparations.

Clindamycin

This drug is a form of lincomycin that has superceded lincomycin in general use. It can be used (instead of chloramphenicol) for therapy of suspected infection with bacteroides, as in appendiceal abscesses. It is associated with severe colitis in adults, but this adverse effect appears to be rare in children.

Tetracycline

This drug should not be used in children less than 8 years of age because of the adverse effect of dark staining of the teeth. There is no advantage to using it instead of less toxic antibiotics.

Chloramphenicol

The use of this drug in pediatrics is generally limited to life-threatening infections caused by *H. influenzae*. Occasionally it may be used for bacteroides infections, although clindamycin is usually as effective. In hospitalized patients whose blood counts can be followed easily, the drug can be stopped as soon as hematologic toxicity is noted. When bone marrow depression occurs, it is almost always reversible. Aplastic anemia is a rare complication, and has usually occurred in out-patients receiving the drug orally, without regular blood counts. In addition, some cases of aplastic anemia attributed to chloramphenicol have probably been idiopathic aplastic anemia occurring in children coincidentally receiving chloramphenicol.

This antibiotic is rarely used in the newborn period, because of concern for the adverse effect called *gray syndrome*. This illness is characterized by lethargy, a pale or gray color due to shock, and sometimes death. It is especially a risk when high doses of chloramphenicol are used in the first week of life, when the newborn's immature liver is less able to conjugate and detoxify chloramphenicol. However, because of caution about the gray syndrome, the drug is rarely used in newborn infants, even in the very low doses now recommended for the rare situations when chloramphenicol is the best drug for older infants. If chloramphenicol is ever used in patients with liver disease or in the newborn period, serum concentrations of the drug should be monitored.

Gentamicin and Other Aminoglycosides

Gentamicin has had extensive pharmacologic and clinical studies in newborn infants and other children, so that the dosage, clinical efficacy, and toxicity are well defined. Gentamicin is more effective than kanamycin against more enteric bacteria and *Pseudomonas aeruginosa*. Newer aminoglycosides are still being investigated in children, but are unlikely to replace gentamicin unless a clear advantage of greater efficacy or less toxicity is demonstrated. Amikacin and tobramycin are other aminoglycosides which are becoming more frequently used for gentamicin-resistant bacteria.

Sulfonamides

These drugs attach to bilirubin-binding sites on albumin, resulting in increased bilirubin levels in the newborn, and so are contraindicated in the first week of life. Sulfisoxazole, or a comparable sulfonamide, is frequently used for uncomplicated urinary infections or as part of the treatment of otitis media in children allergic to penicillin. It appears to be useful in preventing recurrent ear infections in young children. It can be used daily to prevent streptococcal pharyngitis in children allergic to penicillin with past rheumatic fever, but is not effective in preventing rheumatic fever if used to treat streptococcal pharyngitis after the symptoms have begun.

Trimethoprim

This drug is synergistic with a sulfonamide and was available in 1977 only as a fixed combination with sulfamethoxazole. In 1977, it was approved in the United States for children under 12 years of age. It is used most for urinary infections, but has additional uses being investigated for typhoid fever and for pneumonia caused by *Pneumocystis carinii*, which is very rare except in hosts with immunologic problems such as leukemia.

Nitrofurantoin

This urinary antiseptic is most useful as a daily oral drug taken to prevent recurrent urinary tract infections in girls with this problem. Nausea or vomiting are the most frequent side effects.

Isoniazid

This antituberculous drug is used most frequently to prevent the development of tuberculous disease in otherwise normal children who are found to have a positive tuberculin test or who have been exposed to an adult family member with active tuberculosis. Adverse effects of hepatitis or neuropathy are occasionally seen in the adult but are rare in children. Supplemental pyridoxine to prevent neuritis is not necessary for children.

BIBLIOGRAPHY

Grossman, E. R., Walcheck, A., and Freedman, H.: Tetracycline and permanent teeth: The relation between dose and tooth color. Pediatrics, *47*:567–570, 1971.

A description of teeth staining by tetracycline.

Kagan, B. M.: Antimicrobial Therapy. Philadelphia, W. B. Saunders, 1974.

An excellent general reference.

Klein, J. O.: Current usage of antimicrobial combinations in pediatrics. Pediatr. Clin. North Am., *21*:443–456, 1974.

Discusses combinations of antibiotics.

Levine, B. B.: Skin rashes with penicillin therapy: Current management. N. Engl. J. Med., *286*:42–43, 1972.

Discusses ampicillin rashes.

McCracken, G. H., Jr., and Eichenwald, H. F.: Antimicrobial therapy: Therapeutic recommendations and a review of newer drugs. J. Pediatr., *85*:297–312, 451–456, 1974.

A recent review article.

Moffet, H. L.: Pediatric Infectious Diseases: A Problem-Oriented Approach. Philadelphia, J. B. Lippincott, 1975.

Chapter 21 is a more detailed discussion of principles and individual antibiotics.

Nelson, J. D.: Pocketbook of Pediatric Antimicrobial Therapy. Philadelphia, J. B. Lippincott, 1975.

A very useful list of recommended dosages.

Sutherland, J. M.: Fatal cardiovascular collapse of infants receiving large amounts of chloramphenicol. Am. J. Dis. Child., *97*:761–767, 1959.

A description and discussion of the gray syndrome.

34

Poisoning

Frank A. Oski, M.D.

Accidents, drownings, and poisonings are the leading causes of death in children between the ages of 1 and 16 years. Almost 1000 deaths per year occur from poisoning in children under 5 years of age; most of these are preventable.

In many instances of poisoning, parental negligence is largely responsible. In close to three-quarters of all poisonings in childhood, there is some evidence of disruption in the household. These include one-parent homes, mother-father strife, a recent move to a new home, an illness in some member of the household, or the presence of visitors in the home that have altered normal routines. In every instance of poisoning, a careful social history should be obtained. Help should be provided for the family in dealing with the basic family problem that may have been directly or indirectly responsible for the child's ingestion.

Poisoning, either acute or chronic, should always be suspected when there has been a change in a child's state of consciousness or pattern of behavior.

Parental counseling is the best way to prevent poisoning in the home. When parents have children 6 to 9 months of age, they must be warned to poison proof their homes. Soon the creeping infant or toddler can gain access to many dangerous items. Simple instructions should include:

1. Keep all drugs, pesticides and potentially poisonous household chemicals out of the reach of children and away from all foods.

2. Do not store poisons or inflammable materials in food containers or bottles.

3. Lock up all dangerous substances.

4. Never tell children that their medicine is "candy" in an attempt to induce them to take it. They may remember this at some future time and innocently eat it.

The principles of management of poisonings include:

1. Identification of the drug or chemical as quickly as possible
2. Evacuation of the poison from the stomach, except where contraindicated
3. Administration of a specific, or nonspecific, antidote if available
4. Symptomatic and supportive therapy, as necessary.

IDENTIFICATION OF THE DRUG OR CHEMICAL

Usually the ingested material can be identified by a careful history. Information regarding the specific ingredients in a commercial preparation should be available from a product label, a manufacturer, or a poison information center.

Always attempt to determine as rapidly as possible what and how much was taken. Assume that the largest estimated amount was consumed when planning therapy. All vomitus, urine, and containers should be saved to assist in identification of the poison when its identity cannot be established.

Clues to the nature of the poison can be obtained from the physical examination. Burns on the lip, mouth, or tongue, difficulty in swallowing or excessive salivation suggest that a corrosive substance has been ingested. A gasoline odor on the breath or clothing should suggest that a petroleum distillate has been swallowed.

Combinations of signs and symptoms that suggest specific types of poisons are listed in Table 34-1. In Table 34-2 emergency symptoms and signs are described.

REMOVAL OF THE POISON

Emesis should be induced following poisoning except when the material ingested is a corrosive, a petroleum distillate, or when the patient is comatose, convulsing, or is already vomiting bloody material.

Emesis is induced by the administration of 5 ml. of syrup of ipecac followed by the administration of 6 to 8 oz. of water. If no vomiting occurs within 15 minutes, the ipecac may be safely repeated in patients over 5 years of age.

If emesis has not occurred, gastric lavage should be performed. In comatose patients, lavage should not be attempted unless proper protection has been provided for the airway with an endotracheal tube to prevent aspiration. The patient should be placed on his left side, with his head hanging over the table during lavage. The contents of the stomach should be aspirated before lavage is instituted.

Table 34-1. Symptom Complexes Suggestive of Specific Poisons

Symptoms and signs	Possible poison
Agitation, hallucinations, dilated pupils, bright red color to the skin, dry skin, and fever	Atropine-like agents, LSD
Marked activity, tremors, headache, diarrhea, dry mouth with foul odor, sweating, tachycardia, arrhythmia, dilated pupils	Amphetamines
Slow respirations, pinpoint pupils, euphoria, or coma	Opiates
Salivation, lacrimation, urination, defecation, meiosis, and pulmonary congestion	Organic phosphates or poison mushrooms
Sleepiness, slurred speech, nystagmus, ataxia	Barbiturates or tranquilizers
Hyperpnea, fever, and vomiting	Salicylates
Oculogyric crisis, ataxia, and unusual posturing of head and neck	Phenothiazines

**Table 34-2. Emergency Symptoms and Signs
That may be Encountered in Poisoning**

Ataxia
  Alcohol
  Barbiturates
  Bromides
  Carbon monoxide
  Diphenylhydantoin
  Hallucinogens
  Heavy metals
  Organic solvents
  Tranquilizers

Convulsions and muscle twitching
  Alcohol
  Amphetamines
  Antihistamines
  Boric acid
  Camphor
  Chlorinated hydrocarbon insecticides (DDT)
  Cyanide
  Lead
  Organic phosphate insecticides
  Plants (lily-of-the-valley, azalea, iris, water hemlock)

  Salicylates
  Strychnine
  Withdrawal from barbiturates, benzodiazepines (Valium, Librium), meprobamate

Coma and drowsiness
  Alcohol (ethyl)
  Antihistamines
  Barbiturates and other hypnotics
  Carbon monoxide
  Narcotic depressants (opiates)
  Salicylates
  Tranquilizers

Paralysis
  Botulism
  Heavy metals
  Plants (coniine in poison hemlock)
  Triorthocresyl phosphate

Table 34-2. Emergency Symptoms and Signs
That may be Encountered in Poisoning (Continued)

Pupils

Pinpoint
Mushrooms
(muscarine
type
Narcotic
depressants
(opiates)
Organic phosphate
insecticides

Dilated
Amphetamines

Antihistamines
Atropine

Barbiturates (coma)
Cocaine
Ephedrine
LSD
Methanol
Withdrawal (narcotic
depressants)

*Nystagmus on
lateral gaze*
Barbiturates
Minor tranquilizers
(meprobamate,
benzodiazepine)

Pulse rate

Slow
Digitalis
Lily-of-the-valley
Narcotic
depressants

Rapid
Alcohol
Amphetamines
Atropine

Ephedrine

Respiratory alterations

Rapid
Amphetamines
Barbiturates (early)
Carbon monoxide
Methanol
Petroleum
distillates
Salicylates

Slow or Depressed
Alcohol
Barbiturates (late)
Narcotic depressants
(opiates)
Tranquilizers

*Wheezing &
pulmonary
edema*
Mushrooms
(muscarine
type)
Narcotic
depressants
(opiates)
Organic phosphate
insecticides
Petroleum
distillates

Paralysis

Organic phosphate
insecticides

Botulism

Mouth

Salivation
Arsenic
Corrosive
Mercury
Mushrooms
Organic phosphate
insecticides
Thallium

Dryness
Atropine
Amphetamines
Antihistamines
Narcotic depressants

Breath odor
Acetone; acetone, alcohol (methyl,
isopropyl), phenol, salicylates
Alcohol: alcohol (ethyl)
Bitter almonds: cyanide
Coal gas: carbon monoxide
Garlic: arsenic, phosphorus, organic
phosphate insecticides, thallium
Oil of wintergreen: methyl salicylate
Petroleum: petroleum distillates
Violets: turpentine

Skin color
*Jaundice
(hepatic or
hemolytic)*
Aniline
Arsenic
Carbon tetra-
chloride
Castor bean
Fava bean
Mushroom
Naphthalene
Yellow phos-
phorus

Cyanosis
Aniline
dyes
Carbon
monoxide
Cyanide
Nitrites
Strychnine

Red Flush
Alcohol
Antihistamines
Atropine
Boric acid
Carbon
monoxide
Nitrites

Violent emesis often with hematemesis
Aminophylline
Bacterial food poisoning
Boric acid
Corrosives
Fluoride
Heavy metals
Phenol
Salicylates

Abdominal colic
Black widow spider bite
Heavy metals
Narcotic depressant withdrawal

Gastric lavage becomes mandatory if ipecac does not induce vomiting. Ipecac left in the stomach is an irritant, and when absorbed, it is a cardiac toxin capable of producing conduction disturbances and myocarditis.

USE OF ANTIDOTES

Many drugs are absorbed by activated charcoal. It should never be given before or with ipecac because charcoal will absorb the ipecac and render it ineffective. The administration of 2 tablespoons of activated charcoal in 8 oz. of water should follow emesis or lavage when dealing with drugs for which charcoal is a useful antidote (see list, below). Specific antidotes are described in Table 34-3.

SUPPORTIVE THERAPY

The goal of supportive therapy is to maintain the patient in a satisfactory condition until normal renal and hepatic function rids the body of

Table 34-3. Poisons and their Specific Antidotes

Poison	Antidote
Arsenic, bismuth, chromium, cobalt, copper, iron, lead, magnesium, radium, selenium, and uranium	BAL
Lead, mercury, copper, nickel, zinc, cobalt, beryllium, and manganese	EDTA
Cyanide	Sodium nitrite
Narcotics	Naloxone (Narcan)
Warfarin, dicumerol	Vitamin K_1
Ferrous sulfate	Deferoxamine
Methanol, ethylene glycol	Ethanol
Insecticides that are cholinesterase inhibitors	Atropine
Amphetamines	Chloropromazine
Phenothiazines	Diphenhydramine
Carbon monoxide	Oxygen
Nitrite-induced methemoglobinemia	Methylene blue

the offending agent. Such therapy may include respiratory support, treatment of shock, correction of fluid losses, correction of anemia or coagulation disturbances, treatment of seizures, and treatment of renal or hepatic failure. Attention to detail is required in such circumstances in order to save the patient's life and reduce morbidity.

Drugs Absorbed by Activated Charcoal

Amphetamines	Morphine
Antipyrine	Muscarine
Aspirin	Nicotine
Atropine	Opium
Barbiturates	Parathion
Camphor	Penicillin
Cantharides	Phenol
Chlorpheniramine	Phenolphthalein
Cocaine	Primaquine
Colchicine	Propoxyphene
Digitalis	Quinine
Diphenylhydantoin	Salicylates
Glutethimide	Sulfonamides
Iodine	Strychnine
Ipecac	

BIBLIOGRAPHY

Arena, J.: Poisoning—treatment and prevention. JAMA, *232*:1272, 1975.

A review of the common causes of poisoning in children with suggestions for prevention.

Kaye, S.: Bedside toxicology. Pediatr. Clin. North Am., *17*:519, 1970.

Helpful clues to the establishment of prompt diagnosis in the poisoned patient.

Mofenson, H. C., and Greensher, J.: The unknown poison. Pediatrics, *54*:336, 1974.

This article provides the reader with clues to the interpretation of physical findings which may point to the poison ingested by the patient.

35

The Newborn

Margaret L. Williams, M.D.

Understanding normality and, therefore, abnormality in a newborn infant rests on a view of him or her as an individual within a circumscribed age frame—already a product of several months' growth and development but still far from the maturity that will allow survival without considerable manipulation of the environment. Evaluation of physical findings, recognition of aberrations from the norm and maneuvers in providing physical care all must be based on a knowledge of the normal progression of fetal to neonatal adaptation. This process, encompassing enormously rapid change, nevertheless produces an individual in whom every system has certain predictable immaturity; these "normal" peculiarities have significant impact on the infant's state of well being. It is against this background that neonatal care must be considered.

INTRAUTERINE RISK

Over the past decade it has become apparent that assessment of risk during pregnancy can identify before delivery as many as 50 per cent of infants who will have difficulty in the newborn period. An additional 30 per cent of such infants are identifiable by a second assessment of risk during labor. These statistics stress the importance of obstetrical information in understanding the newborn's condition. Although formal risk assessment encompasses the evaluation of a large number of factors, the following broad categories of prenatal risk should be investigated for each birth:

Pre-existing Maternal Disease. While any serious illness in the mother confers risk on the fetus, the presence of diabetes, chronic hypertension, renal or significant cardiac disease are most often associated with unfavorable outcome of the fetus. In addition, history of familial illness, not necessarily expressed in the mother, may be of great importance.

Difficulty in Previous Pregnancies. Rh sensitization, a previous fetal or neonatal death, low birth weight infant, or an infant with a major anomaly or with neurologic damage, statistically increase risk for the present infant.

Maternal Habitus and Life Style. Maternal age less than 17 years and greater than 35 years, shortness of stature, deficient diet, heavy smoking and poor socio-economic status may compromise fetal well being.

Morbidity in Present Pregnancy. Increased risk to the fetus is present with multiple pregnancies, evidence of poor fetal growth, third trimester bleeding, toxemia, hydramnios, Rh sensitization and premature rupture of the membranes.

Intrapartum Risk. Significant jeopardy to the infant is associated with prolapse of the cord, placenta previa and abruptio, premature labor, premature rupture of the membranes and eclampsia.

In addition to this historical information, a number of laboratory tests are now available which assess fetal well being. The results of these tests should be known to the pediatrician. The most widely used include maternal urinary estrogens as a measure of fetal-placental integrity, the amniotic fluid lecithin/sphingomyelin ratio as evidence of fetal lung maturity, and sonography to estimate fetal size. Intrauterine diagnosis of many inheritable genetic and metabolic disorders is also possible now. It is apparent that a thorough recognition of fetal compromise is essential information in caring for the newborn.

THE NORMAL NEWBORN

In the majority of births, the baby makes his way down the birth canal with no more serious difficulty than minor compression of the head, enters a world of air and light, is separated from his intrauterine supply of oxygen and nutrients, takes a first breath, alters his circulation to increase pulmonary blood flow from 10 to 50 per cent of the total cardiac output and is ready for extrauterine life within minutes of birth. This transitional individual is covered with vernix (a white cheesy material) and appears dusky but rapidly turns pink or red. First breaths are irregular but interspersed with lusty crying and the expulsion of much fluid from the upper airway. Tachycardia is present. In 15 to 30 minutes a calmer regular respiration is established, the heart rate drops and the infant falls asleep.

A complete examination should be conducted soon after birth. Alteration of usual adult examination techniques to avoid crying facilitates the procedure and serves to highlight findings unique to the infant. The following order is useful. This examination is generally geared to the full-term newborn infant who has no immediate indication of illness. Other specific physical signs will be discussed in a following section on the problem infant.

Inspection of the Total Undressed Infant

This examination should include assessment of the following:

Activity and Muscular Tone. The normal full term infant lies with all limbs flexed and has much spontaneous vigorous movement.

Color. The skin is normally pink with occasional duskiness of lips, perioral area or nails. Abnormalities to be noted include pallor, central (body) cyanosis and jaundice, best evaluated by inspecting skin blanched by fingertip pressure.

Skin Lesions. Pale wheals or papules with red bases, the so-called erythema toxicum are insignificant, but pustular, morbilliform or petechial rashes are of importance.

Umbilical Cord. One vein and two arteries should be identified. A single umbilical artery correlates with the presence of other congenital anomalies, often renal. A halo of erythema on the abdominal skin around the cord or a red line extending cephalad from the umbilicus is indicative of omphalitis.

Examination of the Chest

Contour. The normal infant chest is relatively flat: that is, the width is greater than the depth. An increased anterior-posterior diameter is generally indicative of air-trapping. Anterior bulging may be bilateral, unilateral (cardiac enlargement, diaphragmatic hernia), associated with a high diaphragm (diaphragmatic paralysis) or with a low diaphragm (overexpansion). Retraction or the pulling in of soft tissues suprasternally, subcostally or intercostally denotes respiratory obstruction. Depression of the sternum may be a primary anatomic abnormality or may be secondary to the retraction. Other indications of compromised respiratory function to be checked at this time include flaring of the alae nasae and audible expiratory grunting.

Respiratory Rate. Normal rate in a quiet infant should not exceed 60 breaths per minute. Irregularity of rate may occur. Some infants will show periodic breathing and the duration of the apnea should be noted along with observation of related bradycardia and/or color change.

Lungs. Percussion is generally of little value, although hyperresonance may be present with a massive pneumothorax. Evaluation of air entry by auscultation is easier in an infant than an adult and can generally be correlated with adequacy of ventilation. Directly after birth there are many adventitial sounds in the chest but persistence of rales, rhonchi or wheezes at 3 to 4 hours of age are suggestive of disease.

Heart. The point of maximum impulse of the heart is much closer to the sternum in an infant than an adult, due to the anterior position of the predominant right ventricle. Percussion of heart size is unrewarding but careful auscultation for murmurs along the left sternal border, in the pulmonic area and at the apex is important. Thrills are rarely felt. Cardiac rate of the quiet infant lies between 110 and 160, but is extremely variable with agitation. Brachial and femoral pulses are palpable, the absence of the latter suggesting coarctation of the aorta.

Abdominal Examination

Contour. Distention is an important symptom in infants, denoting possible intestinal obstruction, infection or food intolerance. A scaphoid abdomen may indicate displacement of abdominal organs as in diaphragmatic hernia.

Organ Size. The liver edge is generally right at the costal margin. Liver enlargement should be evaluated in terms of the position of the diaphragm. The spleen is rarely felt but a palpable tip is not abnormal. Both kidneys are usually palpable as 3.5–5.0 cm.-long masses and are best felt by bimanual palpation. The presence of a palpable bladder should be noted and the anal opening observed.

Head and Neck

Contour of Head. Mean head circumference in a normal full term infant is 35 cm. with a range of 33.5–37.0 cm. Percentile distribution of circumference is available for each gestational age. Although there is great variation in the size of the fontanelles and width of the sutures in newborns, excessively large fontanelles may indicate poor bone development as in intrauterine malnutrition, hypothyroidism, or osteogenesis imperfecta. Bulging of the fontanelle or sutures suggests increased intracranial pressure.

The compression of vaginal delivery can cause marked molding of the skull. Freely movable cranial bones can override one another at the suture lines causing considerable distortion of the head contour. In a full term infant, overriding of bones at the sutures should disappear within the first few days but in small prematures, particularly those with poor growth, it may be palpable for weeks.

With signs of trauma, careful palpation of the skull should be carried out to detect possible fractures. These may appear as depressions or crepitation may be palpated. Occasionally a "ping-pong" sensation is detected, usually near the suture lines. This also may represent a fracture or merely poor calcification. Thickened edematous tissue over the head—so-called caput succedaneum—may result from presentation of scalp through the cervix in advance of the bony skull. More localized fluctuant swelling overlying a single cranial bone represents subperiosteal bleeding or cephalhematoma.

Face. Facial palsies due to seventh nerve damage are quite common and fortunately are generally transient. They usually occur from peripheral compression of the nerve *in utero* or by forceps, and involve both the lower face and forehead. Facial palsies may originate in the central nervous system and then involve only the lower face. Easily confused with nerve weakness is hypoplasia of the depressor muscle of the mouth.

Eyes. Periorbital edema is often present at the first examination, the result of silver nitrate prophylaxis administered in the delivery room. Subconjunctival hemorrhages may be present, particularly with long labor or vertex delivery. Of more ominous significance is hyphema, or the presence of blood in the anterior chamber, which may be visible as a fluid level when the child is erect. Despite the difficulty in examining the eyes during the first day of life it is important to inspect the pupil for cataracts and the cornea for clouding of congenital glaucoma and to identify the pupillary-iris boundaries. Minimally, the red reflex from the eye grounds should be observed, although a more meticulous examination of the retina is best postponed.

Extraocular movements may not be well coordinated in the first days of life and varying degrees of strabismus are often present. Identification of true sixth nerve paralysis is important and can be gauged by the ability of the eye to travel laterally as the head is moved in the opposite direction (doll's eye maneuver).

Ears, Nose, Throat. Routine examination of the ears can be limited to inspection of the pinna for abnormalities and the determination that external ear canals are present. If distortion of the nose or the face is apparent, careful palpation for fractures is important. Examination of the mouth includes inspection of the gums on which cysts, varying from small mucosal tags to hard bony masses, or teeth may be present. The hard palate should be palpated as well as inspected for clefts. These may occur with or without clefting of the lip and may involve only the posterior palate. The presence of high arching of the palate with or without a cleft can be a clue to other developmental abnormalities. With the use of a tongue blade, the oropharynx can be seen easily and potentially obstructive cysts are occasionally detected.

Neck. Marked shortening of the neck due to missing cervical vertebrae is generally obvious. Redundancy of the skin of the neck has pertinence in defining certain syndromes (Turner's). Several types of cysts (thyroglossal, branchial cleft) present as neck masses both in the midline and laterally. The thyroid itself may be enlarged.

Examination of Extremities and Trunk

Clavicles. Crepitation is usually the only direct physical sign of clavicular fracture in the first day's examination but rapid callous formation permits palpation of a mass by the third day. A hint that a fracture may be present is determined by unilateral restriction of arm extension in the Moro reflex.

Upper Extremity Function. Similar restriction or absence of extension in a Moro reflex or mere inequality in the random movements of the arms may signal peripheral nerve damage resulting from brachial plexus injury. The most frequent form is Erb's palsy in which the affected arm hangs limply with internal rotation at the shoulder and pronation of the lower segment. Various modifications of this injury can be seen depending on the cervical nerve roots affected; an effort should be made to analyze the actual areas and degree of deficit.

Hands and Feet. Extra digits can occur as small pediculated appendages, usually without bone, or as perfectly formed sixth fingers or toes. Webbing, particularly of the toes, is a frequent anomaly. With abnormality of hand structure it is important to evaluate the position and function of the thumb in terms of its ability to oppose the fingers. On the hands, the presence of a simian (single transverse) crease is important to note because of its association with chromosomal abnormalities.

Hips. Congenital dysplasia is suspected when abduction at the hips is limited or produces a pronounced click as the head of the femur moves out of the acetabulum. Many minor clicks without a sense of displacement occur with the same maneuver and are not significant. These generally disappear by one week of age while the click of congenital dysplasia continues and requires evaluation by an orthopaedist.

Examination of the Genitalia

In the male, the presence of both testes in the scrotum or canals should be ascertained. On examination of the penis, the position of the urethral meatus should be checked if possible, although this is sometimes difficult in a non-circumcised child. With any visible abnormality of the foreskin it is imperative to determine the position of the urethral orifice by observation of the child voiding. Circumcision should be delayed if any abnormality is present.

In the female, the presence of a vaginal opening should be assured. Mucosal tags frequently present from the orifice and are generally insignificant; in contrast, bulging of the imperforate hymen with accumulated blood or mucus needs correction.

Immediate attention should be given to any ambiguity of the genitalia. Microphallus, clitoral enlargement, bifid scrotum or partial fusion of the labia should trigger rapid determination of the infant's sex and evaluation of potential management.

Neurological Evaluation

Complete evaluation of motor and sensory function of a newborn demands exceedingly subtle testing and correlates erratically with later neurological or cognitive development. Indication of generally intact neuromuscular function can be obtained through the following observations:

Tone. Best judged by extending flexed extremities and observing recoil.

Strength. Observed as equal spontaneous movements of extremities and resistance to manipulation, ability to raise head when pulled to sitting, ability to extend head to level of body when suspended in prone position, ability to place feet firmly on flat surface and "step" ahead.

Mass Reflex. The best known is Moro's reflex which involves extension and then flexion of the arms when an infant is startled. It is most easily elicited by the examiner dropping the baby's head into his other hand. The extent of the Moro is very dependent on maturity of the infant.

Reflex Coordination. Evaluated by observation of grasping, rooting, withdrawing of an extremity from pin prick.

Vision. With enough patience on the examiner's part, momentary focusing or even following by the eyes can be observed in almost every quiet, awake full-term infant.

Hearing. This is present in the newborn but very hard to demonstrate with surety.

GENERAL CARE OF THE NEONATE

In the Delivery Room

Throughout the United States and much of the rest of the world a standardized scoring system is used to evaluate an infant's condition in the immediate postpartum period. The Apgar score, which is most frequently recorded at 1 and 5 minutes of age, assigns values of 0 to 2 for each of five physical findings: pulse, respiration, color, tone and reflex irritability (Table 35-1). The sum of these scores is used as an index of well being; thus scores 8 to 10 reflect a healthy infant, 4 to 7 an infant who has suspicious signs of difficulty, and 0 to 3, an infant who needs immediate resuscitation. The 1-minute Apgar score indicates the degree of asphyxia present while the 5-minute score correlates more closely with mortality and morbidity in the newborn period and to some extent with long-range outcome.

Table 35-1. The Apgar Score

	0	1	2
Heart rate	Absent	Less than 100/min.	Greater than 100/min.
Respiratory effort	Absent	Slow; irregular	Strong cry
Muscle tone	Limp	Some flexion of extremities	Good flexion, active motion
Reflex irritability (when feet stimulated)	No response	Some motion	Cry
Color	Blue, pale	Body pink, extremities blue	Completely pink

The immediate needs of the usual healthy infant in the first minutes of life include gentle removal of oral and nasal secretions by bulb suction, towel drying to reduce heat loss through evaporation and the provision of a source of warmth. Prophylaxis against gonorrheal ophthalmia is administered by the instillation of a 1 per cent solution of silver nitrate into the eyes, followed 1 minute later by a water flush (the need for flushing is disputed). In most maternity services, 1.0 mg. of vitamin K is routinely administered intramuscularly to relieve the physiologic deficiency of vitamin K-dependent coagulation factors. Appropriate identification procedures, preferably fingerprinting, plus recording of data on a bracelet attached to the baby, must be completed before the child leaves the delivery room.

The baby with a low Apgar score needs medical support which may amount only to brief suctioning by catheter and provision of an enriched oxygen environment, or may include full scale resuscitative efforts. In the latter instance successive steps include the establishment of a clear airway, a short trial of positive pressure ventilation with 100 per cent oxygen by bag and mask, intubation of the trachea to ensure more adequate ventilation and, if necessary, cardiac massage. A glucose infusion is started and, if the infant is profoundly hypoxic or has circulatory failure, sodium bicarbonate is administered while positive pressure ventilation is continued. Throughout the procedure, careful attention is paid to keeping the child warm.

In the Nursery

On admission to the nursery, a full term infant is weighed and temperature, pulse, and respirations recorded. He is warmly wrapped and placed in a crib. If the rectal or axillary temperature is less than 36.0C (96.8°F), the baby should be placed on a radiant warmer or in an incubator and the temperature checked every 30 minutes until it reaches 36.5C (97.7°F).

Many mothers choose to nurse their babies in the Delivery Room and this should be allowed if the child is vigorous and can be kept warm. In the nursery feedings can be instituted at any time but the frequent persistence of excessive upper airway mucus in the first few hours make a 4-hour delay expedient as a routine. Depression or respiratory difficulty are cause to delay feedings further, but some type of fluid administration should be started by 12 hours.

Sterile water is offered first and if this is taken without difficulty, milk feeding can be initiated. The current overwhelming evidence that human milk is the most appropriate feeding for an infant imposes a responsibility on the physician to actively recommend breast feeding to mothers. It is obvious that this attitude should be modified if there is a physical or emotional reason for the mother to reject nursing, but there is little justification now for statements that formula is "just as good and easier."

If formula is to be used, any of several proprietary products containing 20 calories per ounce and 1.5–1.7 per cent protein will be adequate. Iron-fortified formulas should be used after the first week of life. All of the commercial formulas provide sufficient vitamins when they are fed in quantities that meet the infant's caloric requirements. Infants fed human milk may require a vitamin D supplement.

During the physician's daily visits to the infant in the nursery, the following data should be reviewed: temperature, weight, intake, voiding and stooling. The presence of hypothermia, duskiness, lethargy, poor feeding, vomiting, distention, or jaundice should be noted and appropriate investigation instituted. Observations of the mother-infant relationship and discussion with both parents of their fears and expectations can be extremely valuable to both the family and the physician. With the current trend toward early discharge it is particularly important to make an early appraisal of any potential problem, physical or emotional, and assure safeguards against increasing difficulty after discharge.

THE HIGH-RISK INFANT

The spectrum of neonatal disease is as wide as that of older individuals but many newborn problems either relate to antenatal adversity or reflect the immature physiological status of the patient. Of necessity the following descriptions of neonatal abnormality are brief but deal with the six most common areas in which problems arise. An attempt is made to focus on the observations needed for physicians to recognize and identify illness and to initiate appropriate management.

Low Birth Weight

Infants weighing less than 2,500 g. at birth are generally designated as "low birth weight" but in no way represent an homogeneous group. Any given birth weight may primarily reflect prematurity, or may represent a low rate of growth *in utero*. The terms "appropriate for gestational age" (AGA) and "small for gestational age" (SGA) are used to state this difference. Since intrauterine growth retardation can occur at any time during pregnancy, both premature and full term babies can be SGA. Prematurity is usually defined as gestational age of less than 37 weeks, while intrauterine growth retardation is variously defined as weight less than the 10th percentile or less than two standard deviations from the mean for gestational age. *In utero* development, both anatomic and physiologic, occurs in a reasonably predictable sequence; thus an analysis of characteristics of a newborn infant can be used to calculate gestational age (c.f. Dubowitz assessment) if date of delivery cannot be estimated by other means. Statistical charts such as the Lubchenco intrauterine growth curves (Fig. 35-1) are available; these charts relate gestational age to weight, length and head circumference on a percentile basis, thus allowing identification of the given infant as AGA, SGA or even LGA (large for gestational age).

The division of low birth weight infants into AGA or SGA categories is useful because of the marked differences in their neonatal problems. The true premature infant suffers most often as a result of immature respiratory function, poor weight gain, infections, apnea, jaundice, necrotizing enterocolitis and intracranial hemorrhage. The infant with intrauterine deprivation, on the other hand, rarely has evidence of the respiratory distress syndrome but frequently has birth asphyxia, hypoglycemia, seizures and a high incidence of congenital anomalies.

Respiratory Abnormality

The highest mortality in the first month of life is associated with the respiratory distress syndrome (RDS) or hyaline membrane disease in premature infants. The pathogenesis of this condition is instability of the terminal airways and alveoli resulting from deficiency of the phospholipid lining substance, surfactant, which ordinarily functions to reduce surface tension. The tendency of these immature lungs to collapse is associated in this disease with a failure of the pulmonary arterial circulation to dilate normally, leading to both extra- and intrapulmonary shunting of blood from the right to the left side of the circulation without becoming oxygenated. The result of these two processes is to produce a lung with both ventilation and perfusion variably decreased.

The infant with RDS generally has a gestational age of less than 37 weeks and often has a history of perinatal difficulty, frequently of fetal distress. Apgar scores are often, but not always, low. Respiratory distress may develop directly after birth or more slowly over the course of 6 to 8 hours. Flaring of the alae nasae, expiratory grunting, retraction, tachypnea and/or cyanosis are seen. The typical radiological appearance of the chest is one of homogeneous reticulogranular density with air bronchograms. Blood gases show a mixed metabolic and respiratory acidosis and a low PaO_2. Current therapy involves the use of increased oxygen concentrations, constant distending pressure (CPAP), and when necessary, ventilation by respirators. The course may vary from 72 hours to weeks during which time complicating factors include frequent pneumothoraces, intracranial hemorrhage, persistent patency of the ductus arteriosus and chronic lung disease secondary to high oxygen and positive pressure ventilation.

As opposed to the premature, the asphyxiated full-term or postmature infant may suffer meconium aspiration as the result of intrauterine gasping of meconium-contaminated amniotic fluid. The problem can be minimized by rapid removal of meconium from the naso-pharynx directly after birth. Infants who have aspirated meconium have over-inflated

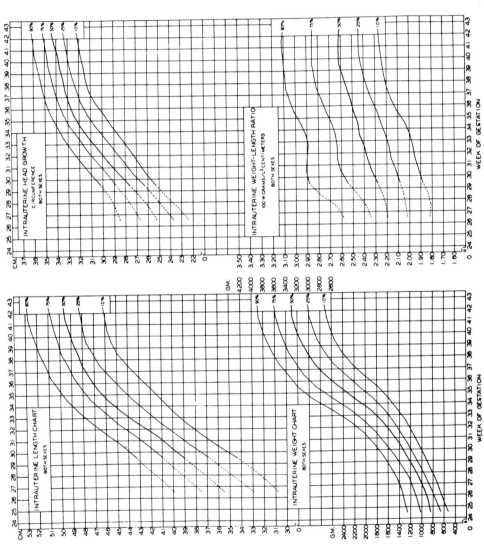

Fig. 35-1. Colorado intrauterine growth charts. (From Lubchenco, L. O., Hans-
man, C., and Boyd, E.: Pediatrics, 37:403, 1966.)

chests and irregular breathing with many auscultatory adventitial sounds. Chest radiographs show non-homogeneous coarse density and blood gases demonstrate marked hypoxia with accompanying acidosis. The course is variable, some chests clearing in 48 hours and others taking several days. The most frequent complication is pneumothorax.

Other respiratory diseases occurring in a newborn population include a group of moderately benign conditions, two of which are transient tachypnea of the newborn and the so-called type II respiratory distress syndrome. Each of these mimics RDS in symptoms and blood gas abnormalities but the radiograph appearance differs and the diseases are mild and limited in duration. Of much more serious nature are the congenital pneumonias; presently, the most frequent is that caused by group B beta hemolytic streptococcus. The radiographic appearance and symptoms are easily mistaken for RDS and the mortality rate is approximately 50 per cent. Finally, major confusion can exist in the differential diagnosis of respiratory and cardiac disease.

Congenital Heart Disease

The major presenting symptom of severe congenital cardiac anomalies is cyanosis which may appear at birth or at variable periods from hours to weeks thereafter. There may or may not be associated respiratory distress; in the former instance differentiation from pulmonary disease is most difficult. The failure of improvement in a low PaO_2 with the administration of supplemental oxygen is probably the most suggestive sign that the problem is cardiac in origin.

The customary signs of cardiac failure in a newborn are tachypnea, hepatic enlargement and increasing heart size. Peripheral edema is less common and most ominous. In terms of frequency, cardiac failure is most often seen in premature infants who have persistence of the ductus arteriosus. Infants with ventricular septal defects rarely have difficulty in the immediate newborn period, although they may have audible murmurs. Of the serious anomalies, translocation of the great vessels and hypoplastic left heart are most common.

Preliminary investigation of cardiac status includes auscultation of murmurs, detection of signs of cardiac failure, evaluation of the heart size and pulmonary vasculature by chest radiograph and analysis of the ECG.

Infection

The poor immunologic defenses of the newborn, particularly the premature infant, lead to a high incidence of infection in this age group. The responsible bacterial pathogens vary from decade to decade with the current offenders being primarily group B beta hemolytic streptococcus and *E. coli.* Coagulase-positive *Staphylococcus aureus* still poses a threat as a nosocomial agent but to a diminished degree as compared to previous decades. *Listeria monocytogenes*, enterococci and *Pseudomonas aeruginosa* infections also occur frequently in newborns.

The usual route of infection is by ascending vaginal organisms invading the uterine cavity following premature rupture of the membranes. With ruptured membranes, the incidence of infection increases rapidly beyond 24 hours; infection also appears to correlate with the stress of labor. Any infant who is not delivered within a 24-hour period post rupture should be considered suspect of infection and should be investigated by blood culture, white blood cell count and differential.

The usual infection of the neonate is septicemia without a localized site, although meningitis and pneumonia occur frequently. Sepsis presents with non-specific symptoms: lethargy, poor feeding, hypothermia, distention or vomiting. Such alterations in behavior should be investigated with cultures of blood, spinal fluid and urine, and the differential blood smear should be observed for leukopenia or the presence of band forms. Initiation of antibiotic therapy is indicated after cultures are obtained where suspicion of infection exists.

A group of non-bacterial agents including *Toxoplasma gondii*, cytomegalovirus, syphilis and rubella (STORCH) cause serious intrauterine infections which may be responsible for congenital malformations. Hepatosplenomegaly, cerebrospinal fluid pleocytosis and thrombocytopenia are the common presenting features.

Jaundice

Hyperbilirubinemia occurs frequently in the first days of life and unfortunately stems from multiple etiologies. Its danger lies in its potential to cause central nervous damage or kernicterus, but the level of serum bilirubin that is damaging varies with the maturity of the infant, the day of life, the partition between indirect and direct bilirubin and other factors such as oxygenation, pH and circulating substances interfering with albumin-bilirubin binding.

Investigation of the cause of jaundice is directed by the circumstances under which it appears. Thus, on the first day of life the possibility of a hemolytic process due to isoimmune sensitization is high, while jaundice which does not appear until the third day probably represents the physiologic inability of the immature liver to cope with the normal increased breakdown of cells. Serum bilirubin levels above 12 mg./dl. cannot be considered normal in a full-term infant and an etiological factor should be sought. Premature infants develop higher levels of physiologic jaundice but the cause of jaundice still merits careful investigation. Table 35-2 presents a standard scheme of investigation of hyperbilirubinemia based on the day of life the jaundice presents.

Current management of hyperbilirubinemia consists of phototherapy and exchange transfusion at bilirubin levels where the central nervous system is endangered.

Table 35-2. Schema for Diagnosis of Neonatal Jaundice

Jaundice appearing on first day of life

Known Rh sensitization

Cord blood: type, Rh, direct Coombs test, hemoglobin and bilirubin
Infant blood: CBC with smear, hemoglobin, and bilirubin at 2–4 hours

Unexpected jaundice

Type, Rh, direct and indirect Coombs, bilirubin, CBC with smear, reticulocyte count
If history or clinical evidence of infection: cultures of blood, urine, CSF
If suggestive evidence of intrauterine (STORCH) infection: IgM, VDRL, viral titers, platelets

Jaundice appearing on second day

Studies as in section above (unexpected jaundice)
RBC enzymes (G6PD, pyruvate kinase)
Physical examination for hematomas, concealed hemorrhage or signs of infection
Review of hydration, intake, weight, urine-specific gravity

Jaundice appearing in third day with indirect bilirubin greater than 12 mg./dl. in a full-term infant

Study as in section above (unexpected jaundice): Include IgM even without evidence of STORCH infection
Check for concealed hemorrhage
Check hydration

Persistent jaundice after third day

Carboxyhemoglobin to define hemolysis
Urinalysis and urine culture
Appropriate studies to rule out galactosemia, hypothyroidism, aminoaciduria
IgM, viral titers
Consider stopping breast feeding temporarily to note response of bilirubin level

Persistent jaundice with increased direct bilirubin

CBC and blood culture
Liver function studies
α-1-antitrypsin
STORCH serologies, VDRL
Vitamin E absorption test

Metabolic Disorders

The most common metabolic abnormality in the newborn is hypoglycemia. Blood sugar at birth is approximately 70 per cent of maternal glucose concentration but the level falls over the first 2 to 3 hours with stabilization in the full-term infant at concentrations of 45–60 mg./dl. With feedings, levels increase to 55–70 mg./dl. where they remain for the first week. Blood sugar concentrations of less than 30 mg./dl. can be considered hypoglycemia. Low birth weight infants have larger decreases in blood glucose than term infants and often have concentrations as low as 20 mg./dl. at 2 to 4 hours.

Symptoms of hypoglycemia in the neonate include limpness, high-pitched cry, apnea, cyanosis, twitching and occasionally convulsions or coma. However, there is poor relationship between symptomatology and blood sugar level and it is not unusual to find entirely asymptomatic infants with glucose levels less than 20 mg./dl. For this reason it has become common nursery practice to make Dextrostix measurements of blood glucose at frequent intervals in all infants at risk of hypoglycemia. These high-risk groups include infants of diabetic mothers, infants with intrauterine growth retardation and those who have suffered birth asphyxia, respiratory distress, infection, cold stress or other serious disease. In the case of the infant of a diabetic mother, the hypoglycemia results from hyperinsulinism generated in response to the mother's hyperglycemia, while in small-for-date infants the hypoglycemia is probably related to decreased liver glycogen stores or defective gluconeogenesis. The mechanism of the other secondary hypoglycemias is unsure.

There is little doubt that uncorrected symptomatic hypoglycemia can have permanent sequelae but confusion exists as to the danger of unsymptomatic hypoglycemia. It would appear prudent to attempt correction of any blood sugar less than 25 mg./dl. by intravenous infusion of glucose or the use of glucagon. As a routine, infants at risk of hypoglycemia should be fed early.

A second metabolic problem that occurs with some frequency is hypocalcemia. This can be defined as serum calcium less than 7.5 mg./dl. and is seen most often in premature infants, infants of diabetic mothers and infants with birth asphyxia. Symptoms are quire variable and include rapid, shallow respirations, apnea, duskiness or pallor followed by increasing agitation, tachycardia and finally, flaccidity. The carpopedal spasm, Chvostek's sign and stridor of classic tetany are generally absent. Treatment by intravenous infusion of calcium gluconate is effective.

Congenital Anomalies

Major congenital defects occur in approximately 2 per cent of all live births and can involve every organ system of the body. Many are life-threatening, some interfere with growth or development and others are cosmetically disastrous. The first category constitutes the bulk of neonatal surgical emergencies including problems of the airway (choanal atresia, laryngeal webs), the lungs (diaphragmatic hernia), the gastrointestinal tract (tracheoesophageal fistula, intestinal atresia) and the genitourinary tract (urethral obstruction, hydronephrosis). Early recognition of the problem is in most cases essential to adequate correction.

Investigation of etiology of anomalies is a later but important facet of their management. A search for the presence of teratogenic factors in pregnancy should be made. Particular care must be taken to detect any indication of inheritable abnormality; in these cases, genetic counselling should be made available. The physician who cares for a newborn infant with anomalies is responsible for starting the long-term planning process necessary for successful future development.

CONCLUSION

Over the past 20 years, reduction on the order of 30 per cent has taken place in neonatal mortality with the greatest decrease in the category of the small premature infant. Progress continues with attention now being focused both on intensive care of catastrophic illness and the subtler issues of optimal nutrition, growth, stimulation, and maternal-infant relationships. The new area of infant care during transport has arisen as a result of regionalization of perinatal facilities for the high-risk infant and mother.

The final results of neonatal care are hard to quantitate since outcome is measurable over a lifetime. Recent studies of development of low birth weight infants are generally optimistic with a decreasing number of major handicaps reported. However, the incidence of behavioral aberrations in this group continues to be high. Further improvement will rest not only on increased understanding of fetal and neonatal physiology but also on expansion of the availability of perinatal care.

BIBLIOGRAPHY

Avery, M. E., and Fletcher, B. D.: The Lung and its Disorders in the Newborn Infant. Philadelphia, W. B. Saunders, 1974.

> Contains good chapters on normal lung development and neonatal respiratory function as well as comprehensive discussion of all types of pulmonary abnormality in the newborn period.

Cook, L. N.: Intrauterine and extrauterine recognition and management of deviant fetal growth. Pediat. Clin. North Am., *24*: 431-454, 1977.

> A good description of fetal growth retardation and the SGA baby.

Dubowitz, L., Dubowitz, V., and Goldberg, C.: Clinical assessment of gestational ages in the newborn infant. *J. Pediatr.*, 77:1, 1970.

> Presents a scoring system for physical findings which allows estimation of gestational age.

Effer, S. B.: Biochemical and biophysical indices of fetal risk. Clin. Perinatol., *1*: 161-172, 1974.

> Reviews laboratory data used to delineate risk in a fetus.

Klaus, M. H., and Fanaroff, A. A.: Care of the High-Risk Neonate. Philadelphia, W. B. Saunders, 1973.

A thoroughly readable text covering common illnesses of the newborn period. Has a particularly good section on congenital heart disease.

Standards and Recommendations for Hospital Care of Newborn Infants. Evanston, Ill., American Academy of Pediatrics, 1977.

Recently published guidelines for delivery of newborn care.

Index

Numbers in *italics* indicate a figure; "t" after a number indicates a table.